NURSING CONCEPTS FOR HEALTH PROMOTION
Third Edition

Ruth Beckmann Murray, R.N., M.S.N., Ed.D.
Professor of Psychiatric Nursing, Assistant Dean
School of Nursing
St. Louis University
St. Louis, Missouri

Judith Proctor Zentner, R.N., M.A., C.F.N.P.
Director of Health Services
Corson Furniture Industries
Valdese, North Carolina

PRENTICE-HALL, INC., Englewood Cliffs, N.J. 07632

Library of Congress Cataloging in Publication Data

Murray, Ruth.
Nursing concepts for health promotion.

Bibliography: p.
Includes index.
1. Nursing. 2. Nurse and patient. 3. Health education. I. Zentner, Judith. II. Title. [DNLM: 1. Health Promotion–nurses' instruction. 2. Nursing. WY 100 M983n]
RT41.M9 1985 610.73 84-18210
ISBN 0-13-627332-7
ISBN 0-13-627308-4 (pbk.)

This book is dedicated to:

Our students—for their inspiration
Our families—for their patience

Editorial/production supervision: Karen J. Clemments
Interior design: Maria McKinnon and Margaret McNeily
Cover design: Lundgren Graphics, Ltd.
Manufacturing buyer: John Hall

Printed in the United States of America

10 9 8 7 6 5 4 3 2 1

ISBN 0-13-627332-7 01
ISBN 0-13-627308-4 {PBK.} 01

PRENTICE-HALL International, Inc. *London*
PRENTICE-HALL of Australia Pty. Limited, *Sydney*
Editora PRENTICE-HALL do Brasil, Ltda., *Rio de Janeiro*
PRENTICE-HALL Canada Inc., *Toronto*
PRENTICE-HALL Hispanoamericana, S.A., *Mexico*
PRENTICE-HALL of India Private Limited, *New Delhi*
PRENTICE-HALL of Japan, Inc., *Tokyo*
PRENTICE-HALL of Southeast Asia Pte. Ltd., *Singapore*
WHITEHALL BOOKS Limited, *Wellington, New Zealand*

Contents

To the Reader

We believe the nurse must consider the total health of the person and family. The physical, mental, emotional, sociocultural, and spiritual-moral needs are interrelated. Increasingly your emphasis must be on comprehensive health promotion rather than on patchwork remedies. This text, and the companion one, *Nursing Assessment and Health Promotion through the Life Span*, third edition, integrate material essential for such a nursing practice in any setting.

Often nurses study some of the topics presented in isolated courses with little or no application to the care of the client, the family, and the community. Therefore, an integral part of this book is the nursing application of such material, interwoven when appropriate, and emphasized in special sections at other times.

Your role in nursing is changing from that of working primarily for the physician or agency to that of being an advocate for the patient, client, or family. Today's physicians are often so specialized that the client feels fragmented and unable to understand how a specific disease process—the avoidance, modification, or elimination of it—will affect life and wellness. The person is afraid to ask, thinking that the physician is too busy and too engrossed in medical terminology. Most of us have been taught to seek the physician's help for illness and treatment rather than to maintain wellness. Thus *your* response to the client and to a family is crucial, whether they are well or ill. You are the one caring person who can interpret health care services, serve as a liaison between the physician, other health team members, and the client, and prevent fragmentation of health services.

The above paragraphs have been our opening statements to the reader beginning with our first edition in 1975. We think the statements are still appropriate in 1985; however, we are pleased that we see movement in the direction that we hoped these books would take nursing and health care in general.

Comprehensive health promotion is no longer a dream of only a few people. The wellness movement and self-care concepts have allowed some of our material not only to be included in nursing curricula but also to become part of lay reading and practice.

Also, we have seen the continued emergence of nursing as a profession that can stand on its own with its own body of knowledge and practice capabilities.

Finally, the patient/consumer/client is no longer always afraid to ask questions of the medical profession.

Before reading any chapter, you should orient yourself by studying the organization chart shown here, which illustrates the many facets that must be considered in nursing for health promotion. Next, read the Introduction. You can then gain a further orientation by (1) reading the table of contents, (2) looking at the objectives listed at the beginning of each chapter, (3) glancing at chapter headings, and (4) noting the terms in boldface which are followed by their definitions in italics.

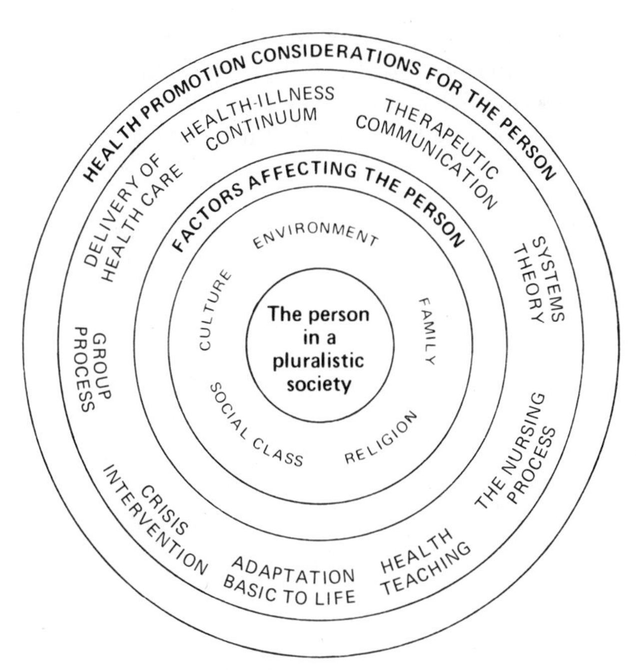

Organizational Chart

Consult the companion text, *Nursing Assessment and Health Promotion through the Life Span*, third edition, for a guide to physical and developmental assessment of each life era and for a study of death.

We invite you to be an active participant as you read. Our ideas are presented with conviction and directness, but we want you to integrate and modify our ideas into your specific circumstances. Each of you will have to adapt this information to your setting—be it independent practice, health maintenance organization, hospital, clinic, or home.

ACKNOWLEDGMENTS FOR THE THIRD EDITION

The authors appreciate the ideas received from students and colleagues that have been incorporated into the third edition.

We are again grateful to Sally Lehnert and Barbara Groneck for assistance in preparing the manuscript, to Frances Bruner for assistance with indexing, and to our families for their continued support and assistance.

Our thanks to the staff at Prentice-Hall, Inc., particularly David Gordon, College Editor; Dudley Kay, former College Editor; and Karen J. Clemments, Production Editor, who gave valuable guidance during the preparation of the third edition.

Finally, the following persons are acknowledged for reviewing the third edition manuscript: Louise Czupryna, University of Southern Maine; Jeanne Duffy, Salem State College; Allison Flower, D'Youville College; R. Hachel, George Mason University; and Gloria Weber, Doctor's Hospital of Opelousas.

RUTH BECKMANN MURRAY
JUDITH PROCTOR ZENTNER

General Introduction

This text on nursing in a pluralistic society is divided into two units. Unit I (Chapters 1-8) establishes a framework for health promotion in a complex society. As society becomes more complicated, nursing increasingly requires a framework—a set of concepts and tools—that can be used in any setting with a variety of people. Chapters 1-8 present topics whose sequential arrangement does not necessarily indicate that one subject must follow another. Rather, these topics are just important components of nursing knowledge, gathered from various sources and placed together into one unit for convenient reference.

Chapter 1 introduces the reader to the concept of health and its many meanings. Basic definitions of and variables influencing health and illness are examined. Systems Theory is introduced as a framework relating all of the concepts presented in this book.

Chapter 2 discusses the American health care system. You will get an overview of the system in which you work and suggestions on how to promote primary and comprehensive care, now and in the future.

Chapter 3 explores the meaning of therapeutic communication. Since you will observe and talk with persons and their families before, during, and after giving care, how you affect these people through your communication pattern will establish a basis for the nursing process, the topic of Chapter 4. Here the five steps of the nursing process, assessment, nursing diagnosis, planning, intervention, and evaluation, are described as a systematic method of providing health service to a person or group of persons, and the nurse-client relationship is explored as the basic unit of interaction in this process. The changing role of the nurse is also examined.

To help you learn and teach more effectively as a nurse, health teaching principles are discussed in Chapter 5. Attention is given to the creative process, the difference between child and adult learning, and methods that you may employ in teaching others to maintain or regain health.

Chapter 6 presents group process as a way of working with people who need health care. You are in a key position to do group counseling and teaching to promote health in any health care setting.

Chapters 7 and 8 provide two theories, along with suggestions for their practical application. The first, *Adaptation Theory*, considers how each aspect of the person or group must continually be adjusted to maintain wellness. The second, *Crisis Theory*, gives direction for helping the person, family, group, or community during crises, since many of the people you work with will be in some phase of crisis.

Unit II (Chapters 9-12) discusses factors influencing health development and use of the nursing process. In the past, the person's health status has usually been considered apart from the many factors that help define him/her—factors, moreover, that are an integral part of health (or lack of it). The American health care system rips the person out of his/her environment, often disregarding sociocultural, religious, or spiritual background and practices, and family life. Then we wonder why the client seems overwhelmed or disoriented in the health care setting.

Unit II takes a cosmopolitan view. Environmental pollution is considered as a world problem. Types of cultures and religions, in addition to those common in the United States, are examined. The individual's family life is discussed. You need to understand the physical climate from which he/she comes and the working and living conditions. Knowledge of the person's background will help you better plan the environment in which to work with him/her and the family. You need to know whether the culture emphasizes trust or mistrust in the medical profession. You need to understand the basis for and importance of religious rituals. You can better plan for care if you know the sociocultural values. You can also work more effectively with the whole family if you know whether it is an extended or a nuclear family. A knowledge of all these various background factors will enable you to treat each individual and his/her significant others or family with the special understanding that they deserve.

INTRODUCTION TO THE THIRD EDITION

The third edition of *Nursing Concepts for Health Promotion* has undergone several changes. Chapter 1, Basic Considerations in Health and Illness, has been expanded; Chapter 2, The System for Delivery of Health

Care, is expanded. General Systems Theory is introduced in Chapter 1 and is the focus of Chapter 2. Adaptation Framework is described in Chapter 7 and is spoken to throughout the text. Both sections of Chapter 7, on Biological Rhythms and Immobility, have been expanded and afford specific examples of adaptation. Crisis Theory as a framework is described in Chapter 8 and has application to Unit II. All other content is updated, including references, which have extensive additions.

The content of this book continues to furnish a basis for application of knowledge about the developing person, found in the companion text, *Nursing Assessment and Health Promotion Through the Life Span*, third edition.

The following list will serve as a quick guide to note the majority of changes and additions:

Chapter 1: Basic Considerations in Health and Illness

Definitions of health and illness expanded.
Factors that influence health and illness expanded.
General measures, practices, and choices that promote health expanded.
Wellness programs described.
Health education expanded.

Chapter 2: Delivery of Health Care

Content organized around major questions of:
What is health care? Who delivers health care? Where is health care delivered? How is health care paid for and evaluated?
Alternate health care system defined.
Levels of care expanded.
Health maintenance organizations.
Unmet consumer needs and consumer involvement.
Ethics/patients' rights.
Current legislation.
Health care in other countries expanded.
Present realities and future trends in health care.

Chapter 3: Therapeutic Communication

Nonverbal communication expanded.
Use of space in nonverbal communication.
Eye behavior in nonverbal communication.
Touch, including cultural aspects.
Listening process expanded.
Interviewing expanded.
Communication guidelines for hearing-impaired person.
Communication guidelines for visually impaired person.

Chapter 4: The Nursing Process

Five steps of nursing process: assessment, nursing diagnosis, planning, intervention, evaluation.
Historical background of nursing.

Characteristics of a profession.
Nursing definitions expanded.
Community assessment tool.
Nursing diagnosis process and examples expanded.
Care plans and discharge planning expanded.
Evaluation process and accountability expanded.
Nurse–client relationship expanded.
Maintenance phase of nurse–client relationship.
Guidelines for a helping relationship.
Characteristics of nontherapeutic relationship.
Models of nursing.
Nurse as primary practitioner.
Research in nursing expanded.

Chapter 5: Health Teaching

Health behaviors for teaching expanded.
Table of self-help books including title, author(s), publisher, and synopsis of content for each.

Chapter 6: Group Work in Nursing

Remains a basic introduction to group process and dynamics, applied to nursing.

Chapter 7: Adaptation Theory

Physiological, emotional, and cognitive responses to stress in Alarm and Resistance Stages of General Adaptation Syndrome expanded.
New examples of physiological adaptation.
Physiological mechanisms of defense expanded.
Manifestations of four levels of anxiety.
Suggestions for adaptation to stressors expanded.
Stress management—physical and mental techniques.
Section I:
Physiological and mental circadian rhythms in wellness and illness expanded.
Section II:
Mobility, immobility, and body mechanics expanded.
Relationship of physical and psychological mobility to adaptation.

Chapter 8: Crisis Intervention

Influences on crisis adaptation and resolution expanded.
Family, group, and community reactions to crisis.
Ineffective crisis resolution expanded.
Psychosomatic (mind-body) effects of stress/crisis.
Suicidal behavior in response to crisis expanded.
Care of hospitalized client after suicide attempt.
Aiding survivors after intentional death of loved one.
Physical assault/rape as a crisis.
Emergency care and psychological care of rape victim.
Family reaction to chronic illness and disability.
Nurses' reaction to loss, disability, and intentional death.

Chapter 9: Environment

Sources and effects of environmental pollution expanded.
Indoor air pollution.
Occupational hazards and effects expanded.
Taking occupational history guidelines.

Chapter 10: Sociocultural Influences

Values of mainstream America and subcultural groups expanded.
References listing information for 17 subcultures.
Social class information expanded.
Cultural influences on health expanded.
Cultural guidelines for nursing expanded.

Chapter 11: Religious Influences

Similarities and differences in major world religions expanded.
Nursing measures for spiritual care expanded.
Research on nursing practices in spiritual care.

Chapter 12: The Family

Tasks of family expanded.
Family adaptation patterns expanded.
Signs of destructive family relationships.
Family as social system expanded.
Extended family relationships.
Blended, restructured, or step-parent families expanded.
Current trends in family life expanded.
Nursing responsibilities in fourth trimester expanded.
Nursing responsibilities with parent education.
Nursing responsibilities with poor maternal-child relationship.

CONTRIBUTORS

Mildred Heyes Boland, R.N., M.S.N.

Assistant Professor, Retired, College of Nursing
University of Arizona, Tucson, Arizona

Joyce Patricia Dees Brockhaus, R.N., Ph.D.

Clinical Specialist in Child Psychiatry, In-Patient Child Psychiatry Program,
St. Louis Children's Hospital, and
Clinical Faculty, Child Psychiatry
Washington University School of Medicine, St. Louis, Missouri

Robert Herold Brockhaus, Ph.D.

Professor, School of Business and Administration
St. Louis University, St. Louis, Missouri

Ellen K. Duvall, R.N., M.S. in Nursing, M.A.Ed.

Clinical Specialist in Oncology Nursing
Incarnate Word Hospital, St. Louis, Missouri

Mary Ellen Grohar, R.N., Ph.D.

Assistant Professor of Medical-Surgical Nursing, School of Nursing
St. Louis University, St. Louis, Missouri

M. Marilyn Huelskoetter, R.N., M.S.N.

Associate Professor of Psychiatric Nursing, School of Nursing
St. Louis University, St. Louis, Missouri

Beverly Leonard, R.N., M.S.N.

Staff Nurse, Intensive Care Unit
Breckenridge Hospital, Austin, Texas

Virginia Luetje, R.N., M.S.N.

Adjunct Associate Professor of Psychiatric Nursing, School of Nursing
St. Louis University, St. Louis, Missouri

K. Michele McConville, R.N., M.S.N.

Staff Nurse, Psychiatric Intensive Care
Mesa Vista Hospital, San Diego, California

Norma Nolan Pinnell, R.N., M.S.N.

Instructor of Medical-Surgical Nursing, School of Nursing
Southern Illinois University, Edwardsville, Illinois

Eleanor Sullivan, R.N., Ph.D.

Assistant Dean, Assistant Professor, School of Nursing
University of Missouri–St. Louis, St. Louis, Missouri

UNIT I A FRAMEWORK FOR HEALTH PROMOTION IN A PLURALISTIC SOCIETY

1

Basic Considerations in Health and Illness

Study of this chapter will enable you to

1. Define *health* and *illness* and explain the meaning of the health–illness continuum.
2. Define *system* and identify characteristics of a system.
3. Describe the person and health care business as systems and the implications for nursing.
4. Identify needs that influence behavior and that must be met to maintain health.
5. Describe the external environmental and internal variables that affect behavior and health.
6. Examine measures that promote health of the individual and family unit.
7. Discuss nursing measures that are conducive to health promotion–wellness, considering factors that influence preventive health behavior.

"Al, are you ill?"

"No. Why?"

"Your face looks a little puffy."

Al, who thought he was well, suddenly decides he hasn't had his usual energy for several weeks. He thinks he'll make an appointment to see the doctor.

"I wish I knew what you meant by being sick. Sometimes I feel so bad I could curl up and die, but I have to go on because the kids have to be taken care of. Besides, we don't have money for the doctor. Some people can go to bed most anytime with anything, but most of us can't take time to be sick—even when we need to be."

These expressions immediately portray the difficulty in defining health and illness. Each person's definition is affected by cultural concepts, economic level, the value system of self and others, ethnic background, customs, and past experiences.

Baumann intensifies the subjectivity by identifying three ways in which a person defines himself as ill: (1) feeling "bad", (2) having distressing symptoms, such as pain, and (3) being unable to carry on daily activities. Thus both illness and health are what the person says they are. Person A may have the same symptoms as person B; but while A says "I'm well," B says "I'm ill" (1).

The well person usually has some small degree of illness—physical or mental. And the person who is physically very ill, even near death, may still have some health potential. Similarly, the emotionally ill person will manifest some health or appropriate behaviors.

Although *health* and *illness* are subjective and relative terms, Jourard believes that such qualities as hope, purpose, and direction in life can produce and maintain wellness, even in the face of stress. Similarly, demoralization through daily struggle for existence can help produce illness (60).

As a nurse, your concern, knowledge, and skill are directed to the health needs of persons from many different kinds of backgrounds and in various settings. It is essential, therefore, to understand the physical, mental, emotional, spiritual, and social aspects of wellness and illness; the factors influencing health and illness; and the basic regulatory mechanisms in the human body that normally maintain a state of health. The use of this information will assist you in helping others to maintain as well as regain health.

DEFINITIONS OF HEALTH AND ILLNESS

Working definitions of *health* and *illness*, although generalized, can give perspective. Traditionally they have been defined as opposites. An example is the definition given by the United Nations World Health Organization: *Health* is a "state of complete physical, mental, and social well-being and not merely the absence of disease" (3, 29). The only option in the absence of complete physical, mental, and social well-being, according to such a definition, is illness. No allowance is made for degrees of illness and wellness.

R. Dubois views *health* as adaptation, a function of adjustment. He believes a utopian state of health can never be reached because a person is never so perfectly adapted to the environment that life does not involve struggle, failure, and suffering (28).

H. S. Hayman defines *health* as a state of feeling sound in body, mind, and spirit, with a sense of reserve power. This perception of health is based on normal functioning of the body's physiological processes, understanding the principles of healthful living, and an attitude that regards health not as an end of survival and self-fulfillment in itself but as a means to a creative social adjustment and a richer, fuller life as measured in constructive service to humans (45).

H. Blum defines *health* as the person's capacity to function to the greatest capacity; to maintain a balance appropriate to age and social needs; to be reasonably free of gross dissatisfaction, discomfort, disease, or disability; and to behave in ways that promote survival as well as self-fulfillment or enjoyment (13).

F. and E. Rathbone formulate *health* as a wholeness of function, movement toward ongoing self-development, relating effective, creative use of potential, realistic interpretation of experiences, and coordination of attitudinal, physiological, and behavioral adaptations (82, 104).

Dunn defines *health* and *illness* on a graduated scale or continuum. Each person has neither absolute health nor illness but is in a relative and ever changing state of being, ranging from peak to "high-level" wellness to extreme poor health with death imminent (30).

High-level wellness refers *to the person's ability to* (1) *function in one or more domains at or above the expected norm, and* (2) *use inner potential continually in order to meet the demands of everyday life.* This definition involves a holistic approach that considers developmental levels, past experience, present situation, disabilities, and environment (30).

Health–wellness and *disease–illness* are now thought of as complex, dynamic processes on a continuum that includes physical, psychological (emotional, cognitive, and developmental), spiritual, and social components and adaptive behavioral responses to internal and external stimuli. Health depends on genetic, environmental, sociocultural, and spiritual influences that either help or hinder an individual in actively fulfilling the basic needs and reaching the highest health potential (103). The emotionally healthy person generally shows behavior congruent with events within or around him/her (8, 127). Key concepts in health–wellness include homeostasis, adaptation, dynamic nature of health–illness continuum, influence of internal and external environment, state of harmony with nature and people, comfort, safety, social relationships, and prevention of disease, disability, and social decay.

Men and women are socialized to define health and illness differently. Statistics show that women in the United States report more illnesses and disabilities, visit the physician more, and are hospitalized more often, including for emotional illnesses. The National Women's Health Network of Washington, D.C., states that about one-third of the hysterectomies done annually are unnecessary. Some people believe this is an example of male domination of women in the health care system. Recently, the media has publicized the numbers of unnecessary surgeries being done in the United States. Physicians are also more likely to prescribe drugs for women than for men, especially the mood-changing drugs (51). Often the physician does not take a complete history or learn of underlying problems that can be corrected other than through use of medication. Yet women have longer life expectancies than men and there is no difference between men and women in the incidence of psychosis (53). Perhaps the seeking of more health care by women reflects: (1) a different perception of illness or disability, (2) different cultural norms about health care behavior for men and women, (3) sex-role conflicts for women, which result in more illness, and (4) differences in diagnostic and treatment services for men and women. All these factors may be operating. The longer life expectancy of women may be the result of early diagnosis and treatment of disease, of inherent sex-linked resistance to disease, or of different exposure or response to noxious physical and social stressors (16, 53, 82).

A person's age influences the definition of health. Children define health as feeling good and being able to participate in desired activities. Children's ideas about health progress from a specific, concrete concern for health practices to future-oriented interests in optimal development and societal problems. Six-year-olds view health as completely different from illness and as a series of specific health practices, such as eating nutritional foods, getting exercise, and keeping clean. Nine-year-olds are less concerned with specific health practices and more concerned with total body states, such as feeling good or being "in shape." To them, health means being physically fit to do the activities of daily living; it is impossible to be partly healthy and partly unhealthy. Twelve-year-olds view health as long-term feeling good, not being sick, participating in desired activities, and as including mental as well as physical components. Some children include a fit environment as part of health. In contrast, adults typically define health as a state enabling them to perform at least minimal daily activities and including physical, mental, spiritual, and social components (85). The adult's perception, as well as life situation, influences the definition of health.

As used in this book, **health** *is a state of well-being in which the* *person is able to use purposeful, adaptive responses and processes, physically, mentally, emotionally, spiritually, and socially, in response to internal and external stimuli (stressors) in order to maintain relative stability and comfort and to strive for personal objectives and cultural goals.*

Emotional and social health *means that the feelings, emotions, interests, motivations, attitudes, and values of the person continue to mature and change over a lifetime, as the person engages in transactions with other people and the broader environment, manifests both flexibility and stability in adaptive abilities, accomplishes the developmental tasks appropriate to the life era and age, and fulfills social roles with a maximum of effectiveness and happiness* (81).

The definition of "disease" has progressed through several stages. Primitive people saw disease as an independent force that dominates and eventually overtakes the victim. Next, the medical-physiological view interpreted the human being as an active being with the ability to resist disease attack. The ecological definition looks at the environmental influence on health, whereas the equilibrium view emphasizes ineffective attempts to maintain homeostasis or adaptation. Finally, the social approach defines illness in terms of whether the person is performing expected cultural norms and social functions (127).

Illness is more than signs and symptoms. It is a process and an experience. **Illness** *is the failure of the person's adaptive powers to maintain physical and emotional balance and to use the usual health-promoting resources in the face of internal or external stressors. It is an experience that exists when there is disturbance or failure in the biopsychosocial development or adaptation of the person, with observable or felt changes, discomforts, or impaired ability to carry out minimal physical, psychological, or social behavioral expectations appropriate to customary roles and status* (82, 127). The person who has a disease may not consider the self ill; the person who considers the self ill may not have a disease or pathological state. The person does not consider the self ill or is not cognizant of disease unless the condition is considered significantly deviant from family, community, or ethic standards, regional customs, class values, or occupational attitudes (6, 81).

H. S. Sullivan defines **mental** *or* **emotional illness** *as inappropriate interpersonal behavior or behavior that is inadequate for the social context.* Sullivan believes that each person has some small degree of illness —physical or emotional—even when feeling and looking well. The illness may be minor aches, temper flares, inappropriate forgetfulness, or overuse of certain defense mechanisms such as rationalization or forgetfulness. Similarly, the emotionally ill person, including the psychotic patient, manifests some degree of health—some appropriate thinking and behavior—some of the time.

GENERAL SYSTEMS THEORY: UNDERSTANDING HUMANS, HEALTH, AND THE HEALTH CARE SYSTEM

Nothing can be studied as a lone entity: the macroenvironment, sociocultural components; politico-legal, religious, educational, and other social institutions; the person, family, groups, or community; or the health care delivery organization. All are interrelated. A theory to help you gain a comprehensive point of view and a holistic or interdisciplinary view of the person is *General Systems Theory*. According to this theory, there is probably nothing that is determined by a single cause or explained by a single factor.

A **system** *is an assemblage of interdependent parts, persons, or objects that are united by some form or order into a recognizable unit and that are in equilibrium* (11, 17, 67, 120).

People satisfy their needs within social systems. The **social system** *consists of groups of people joined cooperatively to achieve certain common goals of the individual or group, using an organized set of practices to regulate behavior* (9). The person occupies various positions and has defined roles in the social system. The person and his/her health are shaped by the system; in turn, people create and change social systems.

Characteristics of a System

The following elements or components are common to all systems (4, 11, 67, 120, 121). A given entity is not a system unless these characteristics are present.

1. **Parts** *are the system's components and they are interdependent units.* None can operate without the other. Change in one part affects the entire unit. The person as a whole system, for example, is made up of physical, emotional, mental, spiritual, and social aspects. Physically, he/she is made up of the body systems—neurological, cardiovascular, and so on. The health agency is one part of the health care system, and it, in turn, is made up of parts: the physical plant, employees, clients, departments that give services.
2. **Attributes** *are characteristics of the parts*, such as temperament or health of the person or the roles, education, or age of hospital employees.
3. **Information** *or* **communication**, *the sending of messages and getting feedback or the exchange of energy*, varies with the system but is essential to achieve goals.

4. **Boundary** *is a barrier or area of demarcation that limits or keeps a system distinct from its environment* and within which information is exchanged. The skin of the person, home of the family, or walls of the health agency are boundaries. Yet the boundary is not always rigid. Relatives outside the home are part of the family. The boundary may be an imaginary line, such as the feeling that comes from belonging to a certain racial or ethnic group.
5. **Organization** *is the formal or informal arrangement of parts to form a whole entity so that the organism or institution has a working order that results in established hierarchy, rules, or customs.* The person is organized into a physical structure, basic needs, cognitive stages, and achievement of developmental tasks. Hierarchy in the family or health agency provides organization that is based on power (ability to control others) and responsibility. Nursing care may be organized into primary or team nursing, as described in Chapters 2 and 4, which is a way of differentiating services. The specialization of medical practice is also a way of organizing care. Organization in an institution is also maintained by norms, roles, and customs that each member must learn.
6. **Goals** *are the purposes of or reasons for the system to exist.*
7. **Environment** *refers to the social and physical world outside the system, boundaries, or the community in which the system exists.* A constant exchange of energy and information must exist with the surrounding specified environment if the system is to be open, useful, and creative. If this information or energy exchange does not occur, the system becomes closed and ineffective.

A Person as a Social System

Every person is an open social system consisting physically of a hierarchy of such components as cells, organs, and organ systems; emotionally of levels of needs and feelings; and socially of a relative rank in a hierarchy of prestige, such as boss, worker, adult, or child. While internal stimuli are at work, such as those governed by the nervous and endocrine systems, outer stimuli also affect the person—for example, the feelings of others or the external environment. The boundaries or environment—such as one's skin, the limits set by others, one's status, home, and community—influence the person's needs and goal achievement. To remain healthy, the person must have feedback: the condition of the skin tells about temperature; an emotional reaction signifies a job well done or a failure; a pain signifies malfunction or injury.

A person is an open system, receiving stimuli from the outer world and, in turn, influencing that world through personal behavior.

Other social systems are the family; church; economic; politico-legal, and educational institutions; and health care agencies.

Linkage *occurs when two systems exchange energy across their boundaries* (4). Industry, the church, or the health agency, for example, draws energy from its linkage to the family. In return, industry is willing to contribute to family welfare funds, United Fund, mental health campaigns, or ecological improvements. The church maintains its role as prime defender of family stability. The health agency sets standards of health care.

Health Care as a System

Although much care to maintain health and overcome illness is given by a nurturing person in the home, formal health care can be thought of as a system having various subsystems—for instance, hospitals, neighborhood health centers, clinics, home health agencies.

The goal of any health care agency is to provide health, medical and nursing care by providing a variety of services related to health for a specifically defined population. How this goal is achieved depends on how the agency is organized.

In a highly organized system, such as a hospital, what one department does is crucial to another department. Action in a neighborhood health center may have little effect on any other health agency. Hierarchy is obvious and rigid in some agencies. For example, in some hospitals a staff nurse cannot take certain actions without obtaining permission from the head nurse. In other agencies the nurses are peers.

Social controls exist in each health agency and these controls create either coercion or cooperation. A nurse, for instance, may enlist the cooperation of a patient in establishing an oral drug routine or may quickly inject a medication when the patient refuses the oral medicine—a form of coercion.

Because each agency serves a specifically defined population, the subject of boundary becomes significant. Sometimes the environment is distinct: The neighborhood center services the northwest section of the city. Or the environment may be diffuse: Patients may come for hundreds of miles to a hospital for open-heart surgery. The hospital or home health agency may also relate with other health care subsystems in the environment, such as a nursing home, mental health association, Alcoholics Anonymous, or the Red Cross. Maintaining communication with and obtaining feedback from the community served are essential in serving the people's needs—the goal of the system.

Health care agencies may be categorized as being either (1) authoritarian or democratic or (2) *Gemeinschaft or Gesellschaft*. In the *authori-*

tarian system one person is in charge; other people follow. Ideas originate with the person at the top, flow down, and go unquestioned. People who are lower in rank have no power and little room for creativity. In the *democratic system* members are peers and all members are involved in decision making. Members arrive at solutions by discussion and consensus. Anyone may originate an idea and that person receives either negative or positive feedback about his or her ideas and behavior. All relationships in an agency are affected by the dominant pattern.

Table 1-1 contrasts the *Gemeinschaft* and *Gesellschaft* systems (116).

A health care agency may be one or the other, but typically it combines characteristics of these two ends of the continuum. Some nurses like to work in the informal but nonchanging *Gemeinschaft* atmosphere; they like feeling a part of a big, happy family. Other nurses are frustrated in the *Gemeinschaft* system; they enjoy the formal, efficient atmosphere of the *Gesellschaft* agency. They feel that they should concentrate on nursing as a job; they are not especially interested in the personal problems or joys of other workers.

An understanding of your own basic preference and a careful study of the philosophy and characteristics of the agency you plan to work for are useful in selecting a satisfying work position. Much of the mobility in nursing may be the result of a *Gemeinschaft* personality being employed by a *Gesellschaft* agency so that the person's emotional and social needs cannot be met. Economic rewards are always important, but some people also have strong needs for peer approval,

TABLE 1-1 Characteristics of Gemeinschaft and Gesellschaft Systems

GEMEINSCHAFT	GESELLSCHAFT
1. Person-centered. Value of person is based on who and what he/she is.	1. Task-centered. Person is valued for what he/she can do.
2. Relationships based on tradition and sentimentality.	2. Relationships based on roles and superficiality. Little interaction between members.
3. Low degree of organization or hierarchy. Norms and customs are unwritten. Group values determine person's behavior.	3. High degree of organization and hierarchy. Policies precise and detailed but changed by fiat.
4. Emotional aspects of person's life and the behavioral results are accepted. Much sharing occurs. Efficiency may decrease because of moods.	4. Emphasis on efficiency regardless of emotional status of person.
5. Variety of jobs done by one person; each helps the other with tasks as indicated.	5. Specialized task done by each person. If person can't function efficiently, he/she is replaced by another.

individual recognition for a job well done, or an affectionate relationship with the person in charge.

The health care system is further described in Chapter 2.

Application of Systems Theory for Nursing

Appreciating the complexity and interrelationships of the people, social institutions, and organizations giving health care will enable you to understand your role in giving health care. As a nurse, you will have a twofold purpose: to adjust at times to the system as it exists and at other times to work with people to produce necessary changes. The public increasingly expects you to do the latter to meet their needs.

Systems Theory takes the major responsibility for change from you as an individual person and recognizes the importance of the total situation in creating and maintaining problems that hinder change and are beyond the power of the individual to correct. Each aspect of life is so interrelated and people are so interdependent that you are unlikely to make much change in a situation unless you work with others and consider many factors.

Fundamental changes come from within the individual or system. They cannot be imposed from without, although an outsider can be an influence. The push for maintaining the status quo and the push for change exist simultaneously. If you strive for better conditions in a health agency, you may find that they can only be achieved by pressures for policy and administrative change on a high level *(Gesellschaft)*. Through your educational preparation, understanding of communication patterns, and experiences as a nurse, you will be in a position to promote changes in the health care system.

As a member of various health, education, welfare, and regulatory agencies in the community, you may function in the health care system in the following ways:

1. As an advocate for the person or family needing health services.
2. As a concerned, active community member.
3. As an expert in health affairs.
4. As a consumer of health services.

If you understand and are comfortable with Systems Theory, you can work more effectively for furtherance of health. You can also better understand the relationships that exist within the person you care for, in the agency where you work, and in the total health care field. The hospitalized patient may appear as a complex of unrelated parts while various specialists are examining the patient's/client's lungs, heart, head, or kidneys. You can help other health professionals perceive the patient as a whole. Disease affects the whole person, not just a single part. Community surveys, assessments, and demographic studies are tools that will help you use the nursing process in the social system of the community and specific health agency.

Intervention on the systems level includes talking with the nursing supervisor, clinical specialists, or dietitian about cold food at mealtimes or getting a wheelchair so that a patient can get out of the confining four walls of the room. You may be instrumental in creating a patient council that has at least some effect on improving the environment of a unit. Outside the institution you can participate in starting organizations for older or disabled persons that help to meet their individual needs and have an impact on the political life of their community or you may be instrumental in establishing a holistic health program for employees in the workplace or for athletes on a sports team.

Although you will not always strive for big institutional upheavals, avoid accepting the present situation as an unalterable fact. Frequently when working at the same place for some time, you adapt to distressing situations so that you do not even notice them, even though they cause considerable discomfort or suffering for the patient. Periodically survey your work environment as if you were a stranger to it. You might keep a diary of your reactions to the work setting when you are first employed and then refer to it periodically to determine changes you wish to initiate. In this way, you can better work as your patient's/client's advocate and as an advocate for nursing.

You may not always be able to make constructive changes in the system. Some changes take longer than others, but you should keep trying. Often an idea must be proposed several times before it gains acceptance by others.

Systems Framework helps you to remember that each patient/client is a system, interrelates with other systems, and is a part of a family, various groups and organizations, a job, and a community. In turn, the patient/client is affected by the various systems in which he/she participates. Therefore while you directly care for one system, you are indirectly caring for other systems as well.

Keep Systems Theory in mind as you read the rest of this book. The systems surrounding the person affect behavior and ultimately health. Nursing is a system because it consists of elements in interaction (46)—the patient/client, family, nurse—communicating or exchanging formation, engaging in the teaching-learning process or group work. A system must be adaptive to survive. Chapters 7 and 8 describe adaptation as a concept and crisis intervention as one way to help a troubled person or family system. Unit II looks at a variety of systems: the macroenvironment, the cultural, social, and religious groups, the family, and the relationship of these entities to health, illness, and the nursing process.

VARIABLES THAT AFFECT BEHAVIOR AND HEALTH

Basic Needs

Behavior *is the observable response to environmental stimuli, including verbal reports about emotional state, perceptions, and thoughts.* The primary purpose of behavior is to meet the needs of the person or the group (5).

Human needs are those aspects of the individual that must be satisfied for life to continue and that can be divided into three broad categories: physiological, libidinal (sensual and affectional), and ego developmental. *Physiological needs* are cyclic, perpetual, and imperative for survival. They include the need for oxygen, water, food, elimination, sleep, temperature control or shelter, safety, or movement (90).

Libidinal needs refer to sensual-sexual and affectional-emotional needs. *Sensual-sexual* needs are not uniformly rhythmic in humans, although hormonal rhythms of the menstrual cycle are correlated with affective and behavioral changes in some women. The basis of sensual-sexual needs is organic, but these needs take on psychologic meanings. *Affectional-emotional* needs are constant and are at the core of normal psychic dependence. The person must be given love, security, approval, respect, support, care, and protection for emotional and physical development (90).

Ego developmental needs refer to the need for cognitive, perceptual, and memory development (training and education). The person must have opportunity for and help with mastery of age-adequate behaviors, including motor coordination; emotional autonomy, independence, and self-identity; social skills; communication skills (speech, reading, writing, nonverbal); adaptive mechanisms; moral development; control of drives; problem solving; work skills; and the opportunity for development of creative and self-actualization behavior (90).

Libidinal and ego developmental needs emerge together; they influence each other and are equally significant for psychic and physical well-being. Ego development proceeds from mastery of simple to complex tasks (90).

Humans are very adaptable in meeting their needs, but adaptive potentials are not unlimited. In prehistoric evolution humans met many stresses, but their genetic constitutions were able to adapt over time. Now humans face threats created by modern technology that have no precedent in their evolutionary past. The rate of biologic evolution is too slow to keep up with the effects of technological and social changes (28). Thus certain needs may not be met as well; other needs may be created. Unmet needs affect health status.

In countries where the population continues to increase rapidly, there is a strain on all social and human resources, including economic and educational development, and many people will have unmet needs. In such countries, health promotion is an ideal; preventing starvation and providing shelter are already consuming the resources of many nations. When physiological needs are not met, the other needs described previously cannot be met. It is a challenge to international nursing to foster the meeting of basic needs, disease prevention, and health in the people of all nations (43).

External Environmental Variables

The external environment includes all stimuli, objects, and people impinging on the person.

The *physical environment* contains a wide variety of potential stimuli: gravity, light and sound waves, and meteorological stimuli, such as temperature variation, wind velocity, atmospheric pressure, humidity, solar radiation, air pollutants, ozone, oxygen, carbon dioxide and carbon monoxide levels, electromagnetic fields, day–night and seasonal periodicity, and infectious microorganisms (5). The physical environment, such as housing and sanitation facilities, affects health. Air, food, water, and other pollutants are directly or indirectly the cause of one-half of all cancers. Cigarette smoke is a form of indoor pollution for nonsmokers. Maternal smoking increases the risk of respiratory infection and asthma in the child. Nonsmokers who are chronically exposed to cigarette smoke in the workplace have pulmonary function similar to that of light smokers and poorer than nonsmokers in a smoke-free environment. Lung cancer is increased in nonsmoking wives of heavy smokers (37). Nonsmoking subjects seated adjacent to smoking environments were exposed to similar levels of carbon monoxide and showed similar physiological reactions as the smoker (88). Migrants moving from one environment to another develop the cancer pattern of the new geographic area (49). Mortality rates from cancer, as well as other disease, differ according to geographic region (91).

Meteorological stimuli are mediated primarily by the thermoregulatory centers of the hypothalamus and the autonomic nervous system. Seasonal variations affect every physiological system. In winter, calcium, magnesium, and phosphate blood levels are lowered; thyroid and adrenocorticord activities are elevated; hemoglobin levels are increased; and gastric acid secretion is high. These changes are gradual and reflect the thermostatic properties of the hypothalamus in conserving heat and energy during cold winter months (117).

Daily variations in *thermal stimuli* simultaneously affect the person. Responses to an approaching cold front include diuresis without increased fluid intake, increased thyrotropin production, elevated leukocyte and thrombocyte levels, elevated hemoglobin, lowered erythrocyte sedimentation rate, and increased fibrinolysis. The opposite changes occur during a heat wave (117). Any extreme fluctuation in environmental conditions results in a temporary disruption of internal environment and requires more energy to restore physiological adaptation.

Sociocultural attributes of climate and weather are reflected in the person's lifestyle, the kind of clothing worn, the food eaten, or the activities engaged in.

Psychological attributes of climate and weather relate to personal preference and symbolic interpretation. Some people have optimal performance in cold weather; others in warm weather. Some people associate fog and rain with depression; to others such weather symbolizes security (38, 117).

Although weather and climatic conditions affect the person in a given geographical setting, the *immediate physical environment* also provides multiple sensory stimuli. Room design and color, combinations of light and sound, and the arrangement of objects and persons in the room all form a *gestalt*, a whole pattern that may be perceived as either pleasant or unpleasant. One is sensitive to the physical and chemical stimuli in the environment that are of sufficient intensity and interest; some stimuli will not be perceived (5).

The *psychological environment* surrounding someone is difficult to ascertain because it has a specific meaning to that person; the person's perception of the environment is a major determinant of behavior. The reactions of others contribute to the development of self-concept and self-esteem, foster support to and involvement with the person, stimulate maturity, and convey limits on behavior (5).

To remain emotionally healthy, it is necessary to be with people who are healthy and in a group climate that contributes to developing one's optimal potential. Emotional health implies the capacity to love, learn, live fully, and share with others in the adventure of life. The emotionally ill person comes from an environment in which there is excessive tension, a barrier to emotional communication, an isolation between people, and in which emotional and social needs are not met. The emotional illness of one person in the family or group spills over so that all members are unhealthy to some degree (82).

Married and unmarried persons differ in their health status. Married men and women have lower morbidity rates for physical illness, use health services less frequently, and live longer than unmarried people. Although married women have a higher incidence of emotional illness than married men, single women have less incidence of emotional illness than single men. Married, employed women exhibit fewer physical and psychiatric symptoms than married, nonemployed women. Single men are at a greater risk for both physical and emotional illness. Sex-role expectations and lifestyle, as well as resultant emotional states, may be factors behind these statistics (53, 82).

Today, more women, married and unmarried, are employed than ever before. Many working women also bear the major responsibility of child care. Women are exposed to the same physical and emotional hazards of the work environment as men, plus the pressures created by multiple roles and conflicting expectations. The long-term health consequences of these complex changes are generally unknown; however, the National Institute of Health reports increased incidence of stress-related illnesses as a result of these changes (53).

The *sociocultural environment* includes the historical era, family, and other people and groups; social institutions, such as government, schools, and church; all sorts of social events; and shared values and moral, ethical, and religious beliefs. All groups have developed rules and regulations that assist an individual in the specific historical time in the process of becoming a useful and valued member of the group and that serve to constrain certain behaviors. Society helps an individual decide on the rules applicable in a particular situation, but it also grants the privilege of ignoring the rule if he/she so chooses. Punishment will be established for deviancy by the group if the rule is essential for the group's survival. Rules, values, and beliefs are fairly stable and resistant to change, thus giving the person variety with a basis for predicting outcome. Change occurs so rapidly in our society that old values and relationships no longer have the same importance or meaning. Social instability produces conflict and alienation between groups, creates lack of direction for members, and contributes to illness (5, 50).

The family contributes not only to genetic predisposition but also to the actual etiology of specific diseases through lack of hygiene measures, nutritional imbalance, transmission of social values, the socialization process of the child, and the family pattern of daily living and behavior (82). The family may also contribute to long-term health problems in its members through physical or emotional abuse or through sexual assault or incest.

Population density affects social behavior in animal studies and parallels human behavior in crowded conditions. Studies on small mammals show that uncontrolled population growth causes specific behaviors as population density increases: aggression, confusion as the number of social roles in the animal colony decreases, social withdrawal and avoidance of other animals, and loss of interest in tending young (18).

Socioeconomic class, occupation, and social roles influence behavior at various times of the day, preventive health measures practiced, and susceptibility to disease (24). Socioeconomic level influences health care accessibility. More affluent urban people can afford housing, food, and regular medical examinations that can promote health. Yet more affluent people may also be in executive positions or occupations or social roles that are highly stressful or that encourage overeating or social use of drugs or alcohol, thus predisposing the person to chemical dependency (112). The poorer rural person may not have an annual physical examination but may eat a diet composed primarily of simple carbohydrates, fish, and homegrown fruits and vegetables, which will contribute to health. Social roles are significant to health because they place various demands on the person and call for shifts and flexibility in attitude and behavior, which may be demanding to the point of illness. The occupational role is important. Whether the person is a farmer, nurse, coal miner, physician, executive, or clerk predisposes to different stressors and illnesses. The worker in an industrial plant may be exposed to carcinogenic materials. The miner living in poverty develops respiratory disease; he may realize his work is making him sick, but he is financially unable to change jobs or geographic locations. The middle-class person may work in a clean office, have conveniences to assist with housework, and see the dentist twice yearly for a checkup. The higher the socioeconomic class and occupational position, the greater is the variety of behavioral choices available to specific goals. When availability of resources becomes restricted because of economic or geographical reasons, lifestyle and behavior are restricted (5).

Internal Variables

Genetic inheritance influences the physical characteristics, innate temperament, the activity level, and intellectual potential of the person. Physical characteristics include sex and such features as skin and eye color, hair color and degree of curl, facial structure, and height. The physical characteristics influence the response of others as well as the person's response to the environment. The positive reinforcement and the interaction from the environment that a child or adult with desirable physical characteristics receives affect that person's self-concept development and relationship to others (5).

Intelligence, *the ability to deal with complex, abstract material*, is influenced by inheritance, environment, and sociocultural influences. The test score reflecting intelligence is influenced by many factors: motivation at the time of testing, what the test means to the person, level of anxiety, cultural and social class background of the person, physical environment of the testing situation, and the race and other characteristics of the tester (5).

Circadian and psychobiological rhythms are part of the internal processes of the person, are interdependent with the time–space aspects of the environment, and help to organize behavior (5). **Biological rhythms** *are self-sustaining repeating patterns* or inner clocks. They help explain why some people are mentally sharp at 6:00 A.M. while others work to full capacity at 10:00 P.M. Biological rhythms may be **exogenous,** *dependent on the rhythm of external environmental events, such as sunlight; or* **endogenous,** *arising within the organism and uninfluenced by the environment* (25). Biological rhythms are classified according to the length or occurrence of the rhythmic pattern (oscillation) as diurnal, circadian, ultradian, and infradian (25, 124). The terms *diurnal* and *circadian* were used in the past to mean a rhythm occurring once a day. The term *diurnal rhythm*, however, is ambiguous when applied to diurnal animals; so **diurnal** *rhythm is used to describe fluctuations in body processes confined to the working day, whereas* **circadian** *rhythm describes fluctuations occurring every 20 to 28 hours.* The terms **ultradian** and **infradian,** coined by Franz Halberg, *refer to rhythmic processes occurring less frequently than every 24 hours* and *on a weekly or monthly basis, respectively* (25). Biological rhythms are discussed further in Chapter 7.

Gender of the person affects disease susceptibility: certain genetic and acquired diseases are more common in one sex than in the other. *Sexual identity*, determined embryologically and molded through the influences of sociocultural environment, affects patterns of behavioral responses developed by that person. Cross-cultural studies show that division of labor is made on the basis of sex, although not all cultures designate home and child care as female functions. The environment makes distinctions in the expected and valued behaviors for each sex as well as to indicate which sex is more valuable.

Age and developmental level influence illness susceptibility as well as behavior. Response patterns and capabilities are minimal for the first few years of life and near the end of life. The infant has few response patterns available because of two factors: lack of experience and a state of physiological and psychological immaturity. The aged person has limited responses because of declining sensory-perceptual monitoring of the environment and declining physical abilities. The periods of greatest availability of responses to environmental and social demands are in young and middle adulthood; the peak years vary with each person and with occupational groups. Athletes peak earlier than physicians, for example (5).

Race of the person is related to cultural and ethnic experiences, values, and attitudes, as well as responses of others to the person. Behavioral patterns may vary with the race, as does susceptibility to illness. Descendants of African and Mediterranean people, for instance, are more prone to sickle cell trait and sickle cell anemia (5).

Self-concept *is the person's perception of self physically, emotionally, and socially, based on the internalized reactions of others to self.* The self-concept, self-expectations, perceived abilities, values, attitudes, habits, and beliefs affect how that person will handle situations and relate to others. How the person behaves depends on whether he/she feels positively or negatively and on how the person feels others expect him/her to behave in a specific situation. Additionally, the person discloses different aspects of self in various situations, depending on personal needs, what is considered socially acceptable, how others react, and past experience with self-disclosure. Thus the hospitalized patient's behavior may be different from the usual pattern; the person may behave according to others' expectations instead of how he/she desires. These variables also affect health practices and treatment sought. The incidence of cancer has been linked to geographical or environmental factors, for example. In the United States, Seventh Day Adventists have half as much cancer as the national average and rural Mormons in Utah have 60 to 75 percent less, apparently because of their lifestyle, which is related to their religion (49, 68).

The feelings of the person may be related to internal neuroendocrine processes, but they are also related to events in the external environment, including stressful events. A sense of hopelessness, despair, or extreme fear may cause death as well as disease. Many human and animal studies confirm this fact and the death that results from a hex being placed on a member is documented in various societies. When the person becomes an outcast and has nothing to live for, physiological processes stop and death occurs (64).

Although responses to stressful situations vary, anxiety is a common one. **Anxiety,** *a state of mental discomfort or uneasiness related to a feeling of helplessness or threat to self-image,* occurs in everyone, well or ill. Often there is no objective cause. The ill or hospitalized person may experience anxiety because of environmental changes. The individual exhibits signs of anxiety about the unknown: the outcome of surgery, the stability of job and family income, and possible death. The anxious person may experience the physical and behavioral effects that are described in Chapter 7 and Table 7-1. Other responses to stress include grief, mourning, and denial. These concepts will be covered in later chapters. Should the felt mental, emotional, or even physical disequilibrium become severe, mental or physical illness may result. Therefore the health of persons is directly related to and affected by their reactions to both the internal and external environment.

The **mind-body relationship,** *the effect of emotional responses to stress on body function, and the emotional reactions to body conditions,* has been established through research and experience (127). Emotional factors are important in the precipitation or exacerbation of nearly every organic disease and may increase susceptibility to infections. Stress and emotional distress, including depression, may influence function of the immunologic system via the central nervous system and endocrine mediation, which is related to incidence of cancer, infections, and autoimmune diseases. Apparently adrenal cortical steroid hormones may be immunosuppressive. Recurring or chronic emotional stress has a cumulative physiologic effect and eventually may produce chronic dysfunction, such as hypertension or gastric ulcers (55). The dynamics involve repression of certain feelings, such as rage or guilt, fooling the mind into thinking the feelings have disappeared. But the body's physiological functions respond to the feelings or perception of the effect (stressor) (108, 109, 111). *When physical or organic symptoms or disease result from feeling states, the process is called* **psychosomatic.** The opposite process, *feeling states of of depression or worry in response to physical disease states, is called* **somatopsychic.**

Feelings are often related to the person's perception of the event. The Social Readjustment Rating Scale (Life Change Scale) was devised to assess perceptions of the amount of adjustment required by 43 life events involving personal, social, occupational, and family changes. Certain life events, especially undesirable ones, are perceived by most people as stressful or as crises because of the amount of change or extent of readjustment required. Because change is stressful, and stress is a causative factor in illness, a relationship exists between the amount of recent change, number of crises encountered, and onset of illness (50, 101). Stressful events may even speed up death (50).

The determinants of behavior, health, and illness are multiple. Using knowledge from a variety of disciplines is useful in gaining a comprehensive view of the person under your care.

ROLE OF THE NURSE: PROMOTION AND MAINTENANCE OF HEALTH

ersonal Health Promotion

Until recently most of the focus in health care was on disease and death. Now more emphasis is being placed on how to achieve, measure, or maintain health. The goal of health promotion is to raise the levels of wellness in individuals, families, and communities. Wellness and illness may exist simultaneously with each of us; you must relate to both aspects of the person (8). If each person is to reach the goal of optimum health, you must place more emphasis on the fulfillment of health for you and your client through health education, preventive measures, and continuity of care. Since health is a purposeful, adaptive, total body response to internal and external stimuli to maintain stability and comfort, **health promotion** *includes those factors that help the person to maintain this necessary stability, to foster ongoing development*, and has been defined by Pender as *developing the resources that maintain or enhance well-being* (93, 94).

The following are considered factors that promote personal health for you and others (6, 8, 10, 20, 23, 27, 39, 40, 41, 47, 48, 70, 71, 91, 92, 94, 95, 97, 113, 118):

1. Assessing present health status regularly through periodic health examinations, including dental checkups, and participating in mass screening programs in the community. For a schedule, see Appendix II of *Nursing Assessment and Health Promotion Through the Life Span* (83).
2. Learning preventive measures and warning signals of disease, such as those published by the American Cancer Society and The American Heart Association.
3. Learning safety measures to prevent injury and emergency treatment to avoid excessive or unnecessary tissue damage if an accident or illness occurs.

   For example, everyone should know how to do the Heimlich Maneuver, named for the physician who developed it. This technique is done if the person is an adult and the airway is blocked by food or an object. First, ask the person if he/she can speak. If not, stand behind the person, place your arms around the waist slightly above the belt line, and make a fist with your right hand. Place your fist, thumb side against the victim's abdomen. Allow the person's head, arms, and upper torso to hang forward on your arm. Grasp your right fist with the other hand and press rapidly and forcefully several times into the victim's abdomen, slightly above the navel and below the rib cage, with a quick upward thrust. This reverse bearing pushes up on the diaphragm, compresses the air in the lungs, and expels the object blocking the respiratory tract. Repeat several times if necessary. If the victim is sitting, stand behind the victim and perform the maneuver in the same way. (See Figure 1-1.)

   Other important measures are to use sunscreening lotions, and avoid excessive exposure to sun and heat (to avoid heat exhaustion or heat stroke) or cold weather (to avoid frostbite). Plenty of fluids and cool clothing are important in extreme summer temperatures. Wearing several layers of warm clothing, covering the head,

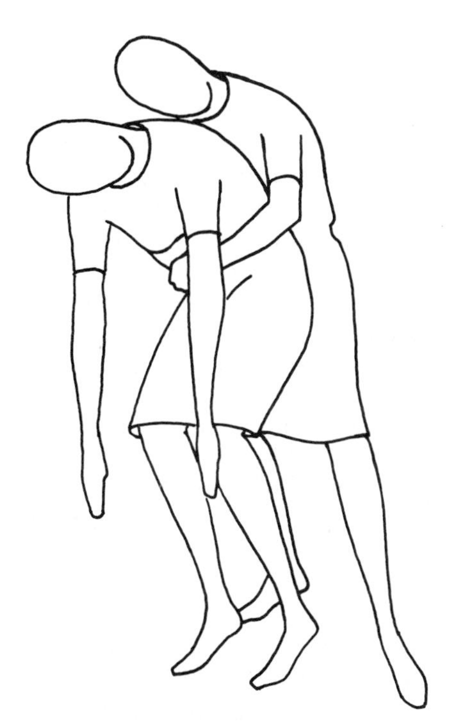

FIGURE 1-1 The Heimlich Maneuver

and avoiding the vasoconstricting effects of alcohol, nicotine, and fatigue are ways to prevent frostbite.

4. Securing anticipatory guidance for potential crises and for stresses related to developmental stage or lifestyle. See Chapters 3 and 8 for communication measures that promote anticipatory guidance.
5. Caring for the body functions, including those factors affecting the skin, mucous membranes, teeth, elimination, and sensory organs.
6. Avoiding products harmful to health—for instance, excess in caffeine, tobacco, any kind of drugs, alcohol, or food. Caffeine consumption has been linked to breast cancer and other diseases. Nicotine, excessive intake of most drugs, alcohol, and obesity are each linked to various diseases. Excessive or inappropriate use of prescribed or over-the-counter drugs frequently has serious consequences. A major problem involves overuse and inappropriate prescription of antibiotics, resulting in resistant strains of microorganisms and inadequate treatment of infections (107). The excessive and careless prescribing of mood-changing drugs may result in loss of behavioral control and even in physical and psychological addiction.

Taking a combination of many prescribed or unprescribed drugs may result in interactive effects that are toxic to the body. Alcohol is a major cause of many accidental injuries and deaths as well as of other diseases. Refer to Chapter 9 for discussion of other agents that are harmful to health.

7. Avoiding extreme stress, fatigue, or exhaustion, providing for adequate relaxation, rest, and sleep, and using relaxation techniques if necessary. Effectiveness of relaxation techniques has been demonstrated. These techniques are discussed in Chapter 8.
8. Maintaining essential nutrition and staying within 10 pounds of normal body weight. Nutritionists, in general, agree that the best diet is high in fiber, moderate in protein and fat, and low in sugar and salt. High-fiber foods include bran and other whole grains, raw fruits, and vegetables. These foods prevent constipation and apparently other gastrointestinal diseases, including cancer. Red meat should not be the main source of protein. Sources of saturated fats, such as red meat, butter, or whole milk, should be limited because they impair the body's ability to reverse cholesterol buildup. Processed foods should not be the mainstay of a diet. Coffee, tea, and cola intake should be limited, for excessive caffeine intake has been linked to feelings of increased stress. Cooking with herbs or using lemon juice, vinegar, or other condiments can decrease the need to use salt as a flavoring.
9. Using safety measures or devices, such as seat belts in cars, safety equipment in power machines, and sturdy ladders, to prevent injury.
10. Using principles of body mechanics can prevent injury. When you are moving or lifting objects, do the following to prevent muscle strain or musculoskeletal injury: (a) roll or slide the object rather than lift; (b) move objects on a flat or level surface if possible; (c) keep objects close to the center of gravity in the body; (d) use the largest and strongest muscles to apply force—for instance, thighs, legs, arms, and shoulders; (e) use leverage to apply force or move an object when possible rather than relying on body weight; and (f) reduce friction if possible when moving an object. Injury is also prevented by using the proper chair in the workplace. The back of the chair should be high enough to come about 2 inches above the lower tip of the shoulder blades and should tilt backward about 10 degrees. The back of the seat should be 3 degrees higher than the front edge. This will place you forward a bit so that you can lean back to maintain balance, thus putting your body in a good natural position. The depth of the seat should be such that the front edge comes to within 1 inch of the back of your knee, allowing your thighs to rest on it without putting pressure on your knees or

calves. Feet should rest on the floor. The person should also be advised not to cross knees which interferes with circulation. The aches and strains that develop in workers who sit or stand in poor posture daily can finally result in feeling ill and even in injury.

11. Preventing, when possible, and attending to any infection or injury that occurs. First aid measures can be obtained from the Red Cross or can be found in a medical-surgical nursing text.
12. Securing necessary immunization for the children and adults in the family, especially with outdoor exercise and athletic programs, wide travel, and resurgence of communicable diseases.
13. Maintaining a regular, moderate exercise program to enhance physical and emotional health. The exercise should involve large muscle groups in dynamic movement for about 20 minutes three or more days a week and should require 60 percent or more of a person's cardiorespiratory capacity. The exertion should be within limits appropriate to the physical status and needs of the person and should also be accompanied by a sense of excitement, flexibility, strength, and energy. At the end of exercise the person should feel replenished rather than bored, burned out, or excessively fatigued. Furthermore, the personal need to increase exercise to the point of competitive winning or achievement of maximal physical performance may contribute to eventual anatomical, physiological, and psychological breakdown (56).

    There is no evidence that running is better than other aerobic physical exercise, such as fast walking, swimming, bicycling, or dancing. The benefits of running are that it allows for psychomotor expression without the hazards of contact sports and is adaptable to a wide range of weather or geographical conditions, time schedules, personalities, and body types. Running can be social or asocial or organized or unorganized as an activity (56).

    Running, or any strenuous physical exercise, also has some hazards. It can become addicting because release of endorphins in the body causes the person to feel euphoric and oblivious to pain or injury while running and very anxious when the exercise is omitted or delayed. The person who engages in intense exercise may engage in other health promotion measures or may feel invulnerable to disease and death. That myth may prevent engaging in other health promotion measures (56). The long-term effects on joints and organs of regular, long-distance running is currently unknown; some orthopedic physicians report musculoskeletal damage resulting from the "pounding" effects. Some physicians also report that breast tissue is damaged if inadequately supported by a brassiere, and pelvic organs in women may suffer prolapse from excessive long-distance running. Other physicians disagree.

14. Taking time for play, leisure, or diversional activities and spiritual pursuits that are (a) rewarding emotionally, (b) done voluntarily rather than out of obligation, (c) outside of ordinary life routines, (d) absorbing in attention, (e) are not necessarily productive in earnings, and (f) have definite time and space boundaries (56). Lafferty lists a number of suggestions that will contribute to physical, intellectual, spiritual, emotional, and social health and to a healthy lifestyle (62).

    In addition to the measures already listed, Lafferty suggests the following measures (62):

1. Intellectual health is stimulated by (a) decreasing the amount of time spent in watching television, except for education or scientific programs, (b) developing a daily routine for study, reading, and adding a vocabulary word, and (c) attending special lectures and programs when available.
2. Spiritual health is promoted through (a) daily meditation, prayer, and devotional reading, (b) discussing spiritual or religious topics with another person, (c) identifying the weakest personal characteristic in order to work on overcoming it, and (d) reaffirming personal values and strong personal characteristics as a guide to life and behavior.
3. Emotional health is enhanced by (a) recognizing and constructively expressing positive and unhappy or angry feelings, (b) identifying personal strengths and limits and working to overcome limits, (c) dealing appropriately with feelings toward the opposite sex, and (d) seeking professional help with serious adjustment problems or crises.
4. Social health is promoted by (a) showing affection rather than directing criticism to friends and family, (b) working to overcome prejudices or fears of people of another race, the opposite sex, or persons in authority, (c) fulfilling responsibilities to others, and (d) communicating verbally and non-verbally in a way that is honest and clear.

Many forces are in play as a person decides for or against what has been defined as health promotion or illness prevention behavior. Internal (personality), external (environmental), and various knowledge and emotional forces, some unknown to the person, all contribute.

Sometimes health promotion behavior is motivated by other than health factors. White teeth and a slim body are regarded as sexually attractive, for example. A person may brush teeth and lose weight for this reason rather than to delay tooth decay and cardiovascular failure. On the other hand, a person may know that losing 100 pounds will increase the life span by 6 years and allow a better functioning cardiovascular system and yet be unable to forego the immediate reward system of high-calorie, empty carbohydrate desserts.

See Chapter 5 for the necessary steps in establishing value and attitude changes.

Preventive health behavior is related to subjective ideas about vulnerability and present health state, the value placed on health and early detection of illness, and the sense of internal versus external control (78). Pender defines **prevention** as *activities that protect from potential or actual health threats and their harmful consequences* (93, 94).

Family history is important; the greater the incidence of specific illness within the family and the closer the blood relationship of the affected persons to an individual, the more likely the person will feel vulnerable. Feeling weak or fatigued, having been ill within the year, or identifying self as part of a high-risk group also increases the sense of personal vulnerability. Anticipating a health problem can motivate the person to do something to prevent it (78, 93).

Four factors contribute to the perceived seriousness of any given health problem: (1) degree of threat, (2) overt visibility of illness or disability, (3) degree of interference with a person's lifestyle, family, or occupational roles, and (4) communicability of disease to others. The person's concern for the welfare of others may be greater than for personal health. Thus preventive measures are more likely to be followed for communicable disease than for those that affect only the individual (78, 93, 94).

The person chooses the preventive services that are perceived as being most effective in lowering the threat of illness. The higher the educational or socioeconomic levels, the more will people be aware of the entire range of preventive health alternatives available (93).

The person who feels powerless or unable to control the environment is not likely to try preventive health behavior. The person who feels able to control the self internally perceives self as less vulnerable to ill health and usually takes preventive health actions (93).

Four key factors influence the decision to seek preventive health services. First, the person may seek health care because of family encouragement. Second, patterns of using preventive services are learned in the family. The level of the mother's education correlates highly with preventive practices because the mother is often the decision maker in this area. Third, expectations of friends are powerful motivators to seek preventive health care, for parents especially want to fulfill the expectation of peers, neighbors, or friends about what "good parents should do." Fourth, information and respectful care from health professionals also increase the readiness to engage in preventive health behavior, especially if the health professional is seen as knowledgeable and caring. The small-group approach to giving information is more effective than teaching only one person. However, knowing what is healthful is no guarantee that the person will follow healthful patterns of living (93).

Situational determinants that influence the decision to practice preventive measures include cultural values on health and prevention, group norms and pressures, and information from mass media (93).

Yet various barriers impede a person's action even after the decision to take action: high costs, inconvenience, unpleasantness of treatment measures or facilities, pain, fear of findings from early detection measures, inability to decide which course of action would be best, psychological needs that are fulfilled by the illness, or prescribed changes in lifestyle that are perceived as undesirable (93, 94).

You should do everything possible within the agency to structure policies and the environment to meet the needs of those who present themselves for preventive health care. Unnecessary waiting lines; a cold, harsh manner; excessive noise, heat, or cold in the waiting area; architectural barriers that impede movement by persons with wheelchairs, walkers, or canes can be eliminated or minimized in order to avoid discouraging those who come or who might return for care. Some services could be taken to the clients' homes, places of employment, and schools. Additionally, churches, playgrounds, laundromats, and beauty shops could be viewed as centers to provide certain teaching or screening services periodically.

Increasing emphasis will be placed on preventive health behaviors because of the trend initiated by federal legislation and an active consumer.

The nurse-client relationship must be viewed differently than previously. The client becomes pivotal in all interactions whereas the nurse functions as an encourager, facilitator, teacher, counselor, or assistant who promotes adaptation and self-care by the client. Both parties must agree to the plan of care and responsibilities in the relationship (99).

Wellness Programs

Traditionally the main health concern for employees in the workplace was that of safety and accident prevention. A yearly physical examination was also included in many industries.

Today industries and some hospitals and other work settings are adding programs for their employees that generally include emphasis in four areas: stress reduction, exercise, smoking cessation, and nutritional and weight guidance, particularly for obesity and sodium and cholesterol reduction. Some industries have also established Employee Assistance Programs to help the chemically-dependent employee reduce alcohol or drug intake and remain a safe, dependable worker.

Facilities may vary from the Mercy Hospital in Des Moines, Iowa, which boasts nearly 24-hour availability of a fully equipped exercise room, gymnasium, handball court, and whirlpool baths, to a rough running track that has been measured out around a furniture factory in rural North Carolina. In Cape Breton, Nova Scotia, the Glace Bay General Hospital has decided to designate more money for keeping people well rather than focusing on existing illness (106). In some cities the employer uses existing exercise facilities in various clubs or organizations, such as the local chapter of the American Heart Association, for screening or teaching programs. In Hamilton, Ontario, a nurse using YMCA facilities oversees such a program (23).

The leaders in the preceding programs are convinced that such programs do more than enhance the corporate image. Helping their employees make changes that reduce their risks for heart disease and the lifestyle-related cancers not only cut their long-range health insurance costs but also promote the current well-being and productivity of their employees. Chen reviews some major health programs in industries, their rationale, useful resources, and the factors that contribute to program success (21). For more on this subject, see Chapter 5 and references by Allen, Chase, Cunningham, Hackler, Lange and Ardell, McCormack, Peipre, and Zohman (2, 20, 26, 39, 40, 63, 74, 75, 92, 128).

Health Education

Health education *is the learning process by which persons and groups learn to promote, maintain, or restore health.* Health education should be a constant part of people's lives. It is important for them to understand the impact that such factors as stress, smoking, exercise, excess weight, chronic disease, air pollution, recreation, and occupation have on health. Once a person has been exposed to a health education program, the desired outcome is a change in health behavior or attitude (57).

Health education must be adjusted to learning levels and directed to situations of immediate interest for the particular age group. For example, a 10-year-old boy is concerned with increasing his muscular prowess via proper food and exercise whereas the 16-year-old is concerned with the effects of smoking, drugs, and alcohol consumption. Adults are increasingly concerned about the effects of stress, pollutants, smoking, and drugs on long-term health.

As a health educator, you must learn about the health and health needs of each person by determining knowledge, values, attitudes, and practices related to personal health promotion, plans for health protection, and present mental and emotional health status. The individual who has a positive self-concept and who feels a sense of control over health and personal life is more likely to practice health education beliefs and preventive measures (42). All these points must be considered before the actual planning and during implementation of any health education program. Chapter 5 on health teaching discusses these points in detail.

You also play an important part in health education by promoting local and state control of infection and disease through mass screening or immunization and by supporting and promoting community projects for improved housing, adequate sanitation facilities, vermin control, slum clearance, and control of leaded paint and gasoline. You may also be involved in the use of mass media for health education. Turnbull found that television publicity about disease and disease prevention can increase use of health promotion measures, such as breast self-examination (118). Or you may help people explore less traditional forms of health promotion or healing, such as concepts used in Oriental or other folk medicine.

Teaching parents about child care, nutrition, normal patterns of development, how to manage given budgetary and other limitations, and realistic expectations for themselves and their children can promote adaptation to the ordinary stresses of family living and childrearing. Helping parents to feel "good" or positive about themselves and their children is basic to any teaching. By promoting the adaptive capacities of parents, you can help prevent child abuse. All these items are interrelated to enhance the health—physically, mentally, emotionally, and socially—of the person, family, and community.

In the past, health education was handled mainly by nurses. Today health educators, social workers, dietitians, and others are contributing to this process. Teaching about healthy lifestyles is one of our most effective techniques of fostering health promotion. More and more the consumer from all backgrounds expects a holistic or total approach to health care and prevention. The client increasingly expects a wellness orientation that includes body, mind, spirit, and cultural background considerations. The balance of lifestyle, environment, and relationships must be considered. Traditional and nontraditional methods of health care must be used. A holistic approach respects the right of the person to make choices about health care and to assume responsibility for those choices. Positive attitudes are promoted in a holistic health practice. The result of holistic health is an ever higher expression of potential and fulfillment.

The remainder of this book explores in greater depth the information that you can use to promote the well-being of yourself and others in a **pluralistic society**—*a society containing diverse groups of people distinctive in environmental setting, racial or ethnic origins, sociocultural patterns, and religion, who maintain independent lifestyles within the confines of a common civilization.* Information about developmental norms that will assist you in understanding people in a pluralistic society is also available (83).

REFERENCES

1. **Aiken, Linda,** *Health Policy and Nursing Practice.* New York: McGraw-Hill Book Company, 1981.
2. **Allen, Jim,** "New Insurance Policies Pay for Staying Healthy," *Hickory Daily Record,* August 27, 1980, Sec. B, p. 12.
3. **Anderson, Olin,** "Health Services Systems in the United States and Other Countries: Critical Comparisons," in *Patients, Physicians and Illness,* ed. E. Gartley Jaco. New York: The Free Press, 1972.
4. **Anderson, Ralph,** and **I. Carter,** *Human Behavior in the Social Environment.* Chicago: Aldine Publishing Company, 1974.
5. **Auger, Jeanine,** *Behavioral Systems and Nursing.* Englewood Cliffs, NJ: Prentice-Hall, Inc., 1976.
6. **Balog, Joseph,** "The Concepts of Health and Disease: A Relativistic Perspective," *Health Values: Achieving High Level Wellness,* 6, no. 5 (1982), 7–13.
7. **Baumann, Barbara,** "Diversities in Conceptions of Health and Physical Fitness," in *Social Interaction and Patient Care,* eds. James Skipper and Robert Leonard. Philadelphia: J. B. Lippincott Company, 1965, pp. 206–18.
8. **Beeson, Gerald,** "The Health-Illness Spectrum," *American Journal of Public Health,* 57, no. 11 (1967), 1901–4.
9. **Bell, Earl,** *Social Foundations of Human Behavior.* New York: Harper & Row, Publishers, 1961.
10. **Benson, Herbert,** "Your Innate Asset for Combatting Stress," *Nursing Digest,* 3, no. 3 (1975), 38–41.
11. **Berrien, F. Kenneth,** *General and Social Systems.* New Brunswick, NJ: Rutgers University Press, 1968.
12. **Blomquist, K. B.,** "Physical Fitness Programs in Industry: Applications of Social Learning Theory," *Occupational Health Nursing,* 29, no. 7 (1981), 30–31, 49.
13. **Blum, Henrik L.,** *Planning for Health: Genetics for the Eighties* (2nd ed.). New York: Human Sciences Press, 1981.
14. **Bower, Fay Louise,** *The Process of Planning Care: A Model for Practice.* St. Louis: The C. V. Mosby Company, 1977.
15. **Brailey, A. G., Jr.,** "The Promotion of Health Through Health Insurance," *New England Journal of Medicine,* 302, no. 1 (1980), 51–52.
16. **Briscoe, M.,** "Sex Differences in Perception of Illness and Expressed Life Satisfaction," *Psychological Medicine,* 8, no. 2 (1978), 339–45.
17. **Buckley, Walter,** *Sociology and Modern Systems Theory.* Englewood Cliffs, NJ: Prentice Hall, Inc., 1967.
18. **Calhoun, John,** reported by Daniel Rice. *Health Services World,* 8 (1973), 3.
19. "Cancer's Connection to World Geography—A Scientific Detective Story Begins Unfolding," *St. Louis Post-Dispatch,* June 9, 1976, Sec. D, p. 12.
20. **Chase, Marilyn,** "Ounce of Prevention Is Worth a Pound of Cure, Or So Say

Proponents of 'Wellness' Movement," *The Wall Street Journal*, September 15, 1981, p. 56.

21. **Chen, Moon S.**, "Wellness in the Workplace: A Review of Literature," *Health Values: Achieving High Level Wellness*, 6, no. 5 (1982), 14–17.
22. **Chin, Robert**, "The Utility of Systems Models and Developmental Models for Practitioners," in *Conceptual Models for Nursing Practice*, eds. Joan Riehl and Sister Callista Roy. New York: Appleton-Century-Crofts, 1974. pp. 46–63.
23. **Ciliska, Donna**, "Lifestyle Changes Are Our Business," *The Canadian Nurse*, 79, no. 4 (1983), 26–27.
24. **Clemen, Susan, Diane Eigsti,** and **Sandra McGuire,** *Comprehensive Family and Community Health Nursing*. New York: McGraw-Hill Book Company, 1981.
25. **Conroy, R. T. W. L.,** and **J. N. Mills,** *Human Circadian Rhythms*. London: J. & A. Churchill, 1970.
26. **Cunningham, Robert M., Jr.**, "Keeping Them Well Is Good Business Too," *Hospitals*, October 1, 1979, pp. 94–96.
27. **Delbanco, T. L.,** and **W. C. Taylor,** "The Periodic Health Examination," *Annals of Internal Medicine*, 92 (February 1980), 251–52.
28. **DuBois, Rene,** "Man Overadapting," *Psychology Today*, 4, no. 9 (1971), 50 ff.
29. _____, *Mirage of Health*. Garden City, NY: Doubleday & Company, Inc., 1959.
30. **Dunn, Halbert J.**, *High-Level Wellness*. Washington, D.C.: Mount Vernon Publishing Company, Inc. 1961.
31. **Elhart, Dorothy, Sharon Firsich, Shirley Gragg,** and **Olive M. Rees,** *Scientific Principles in Nursing*. St. Louis: The C. V. Mosby Company, 1978.
32. **Engel, George L.**, "A Unified Concept of Health and Disease," *Perspectives in Biology and Medicine*. Chicago: University of Chicago Press, Summer 1960.
33. **Erikson, Erik,** *Childhood and Society* (2nd ed.). New York: W. W. Norton & Co., Inc., 1963.
34. **French, Ruth,** *The Dynamics of Health Care* (2nd ed.). New York: McGraw-Hill Book Company, 1974.
35. **Fuerst, Elinor, LuVerne Wolfe,** and **Marlene Weitzel,** *Fundamentals of Nursing* (6th ed.). Philadelphia: J. B. Lippincott Company, 1979.
36. **Georgopoulous, B.,** and **F. Mann,** "The Hospital as an Organization," in *Patients, Physicians and Illness*, ed. E. Gartly Jaco. New York: The Free Press, 1972.
37. **Gortmaker, Steven, Deborah Walker, Francene Jacobs,** and **Holly Ruch-Ross,** "Parental Smoking and the Risk of Childhood Asthma," *American Journal of Public Health*, 72, no. 6 (1982) 574–78.
38. **Griffith, W.**, "Environmental Effects on Interpersonal Affective Behavior: Ambient Effective Temperature and Attraction," *Journal of Personality and Social Psychology*, July 1970, pp. 240–44.
39. **Hackler, Tim,** "Holistic Medicine: The Maintenance of 'Wellness'; An Assault On Dis-ease!," *Mainliner*, February 1981, pp. 92–96.
40. _____, "Prevention: The Most Powerful Medicine," *MCMS Bulletin*, July 1980, pp. 20–23.

41. _____, "New Studies Confirm Value of Exercise, Low-Cholesterol Diet," *Employee Health and Fitness*, February 1981, pp. 13-17.
42. **Hallal, Janice,** "The Relationship of Health Beliefs, Health Locus of Control, and Self-Concept to the Practice of Breast Self-Examination on Adult Women," *Nursing Research*, 31, no. 3 (1982), 137-41.
43. **Hamburg, David,** "Disease Prevention: The Challenge of the Future," *American Journal of Public Health*, 69, no. 10 (1979), 1026-33.
44. **Haro, Michael, Edward Hart, Guy Parcel,** and **Robert Werog,** *Explorations in Personal Health*. Boston: Houghton Mifflin Company, 1977.
45. **Hayman, H. S.,** "An Ecologic View of Health and Health Education," *Journal of School Health*, 35 (1965), 3.
46. **Hazzard, Mary,** "Symposium on a Systems Approach to Nursing," *Nursing Clinics of North America*, 6, no. 3 (1971), 383-462.
47. **Helsing, K.,** and **G. Comstock,** "What Kinds of People Do Not Use Seat Belts?" *American Journal of Public Health*, 67, no. 11 (1977), 1043-53.
48. **Mettler, B.,** "Wellness Promotion on a University Campus," *Family and Community Health*, 3, no. 1 (1980), 77-95.
49. **Higginson, John,** "A Hazardous Society? Individual Versus Community Responsibility in Cancer Prevention," *American Journal of Public Health*, 66, no. 4 (1976), 359-66.
50. **Holmes, T.,** and **R. Rahe,** "The Social Readjustment Scale," *Journal of Psychosomatic Research*, 11, no. 8 (1967), 213-17.
51. **Howell, Mary,** *National Women's Health Network Newsletter*, Fall 1982, pp. 1-4.
52. **Hoyman, Howard,** "Models of Human Nature and Their Impact on Health Education," *Nursing Digest*, 3, no. 5 (1975), 37-40.
53. **Ibrahim, Michel,** "The Changing Health State of Women," *American Journal of Public Health*, 70, no. 2 (1980), 120-21.
54. **Jahoda, Marie,** *Current Concepts of Positive Mental Health*. New York: Basic Books, Inc., 1956.
55. **James, Sherman,** and **Donald Kleinbaum,** "Socioecologic Stress and Hypertension Related Mortality Rates in North Carolina," *American Journal of Public Health*, 66, no. 4 (1976), 354-58.
56. **Jarrett, Paul,** "Some Mental Aspects of Physical Fitness," *Journal of Florida Medical Association*, 67, no. 4 (1980), 378-89.
57. **Jarvis, Linda,** *Community Health Nursing: Keeping the Public Healthy*. Philadelphia: F. A. Davis Company, 1981.
58. **Johnson, Miriam,** and **Harry Martin,** "A Sociologist's Analysis of the Nurse Role," *American Journal of Nursing*, 58, no. 3 (1958), 373-77.
59. **Jones, P.,** "An Adaptation Model for Nursing Practice," *American Journal of Nursing*, 78, no. 11 (1978), 1901-11.
60. **Jourard, Sidney,** *The Transparent Self*. New York: D. Van Nostrand Company, 1971.
61. **Kuller, L., J. Neaton, A. Caggiula,** and **L. Falvo-Gerard,** "Primary Prevention of Heart Attacks: The Multiple Risk Factor Intervention Trial," *American Journal of Epidemiology*, 112, no. 2 (1980), 185-99.
62. **Lafferty, Jerry,** "A Credo of Wellness," *Health Education*, September-October 1979, pp. 10-11.

63. **Lange, Mary E.,** and **Donald B. Ardell,** "Wellness Programs Attract New Markets for Hospitals," *Hospitals*, November 16, 1981, pp. 115–16.
64. **Langone, John,** "When Hopelessness Kills," *Discover*, October 1980, p. 116.
65. **Leahy, Kathleen, M. Marguerite Cobb,** and **Mary C. Jones,** *Community Health Nursing* (4th ed.). New York: McGraw-Hill Book Company, 1982.
66. **Leininger, Madeline,** *Nursing and Anthropology: Two Worlds to Blend*. New York: John Wiley & Sons, Inc., 1970.
67. **Loomis, C. P.,** *Social Systems*. Philadelphia: D. Van Nostrand Company, 1960.
68. **Lyon, J., et al.** "Cancer Incidence in Mormons and NonMormons in Utah, 1966–1970," *New England Journal of Medicine*, 204 (January 15, 1976), 129–33.
69. " 'Magic Walk': Hospital's Half-Mile Exercise Stretch," *Medical World News*, 21, no. 11 (1980), 47–48.
70. **Mallison, Mary,** "Updating the Cholesterol Controversy: Verdict—Diet Does Count," *American Journal of Nursing*, 78, no. 10 (1978), 1681.
71. **Malotte, C. Kevin, Jonathan Fielding,** and **Brian Danaher,** "Description and Evaluation of the Smoking Cessation Component of a Multiple Risk Factor Intervention Program," *American Journal of Public Health*, 71, no. 8 (1981), 844–47.
72. **Marshall, James, Saxon Graham,** and **Mya Swansen,** "Caffeine Consumption and Benign Breast Diseases: A Case-Control Comparison," *American Journal of Public Health*, 72, no. 6 (1982), 610–12.
73. **McClure, Diana,** "Wellness: A Holistic Concept," *Health Values: Achieving High Level Wellness*, 6, no. 5 (1982), 23–27.
74. **McCormack, Patricia,** "Diagnosis: Higher Medical Care; Rx: Stay in Shape," *News and Observer, Raleigh, N.C.*, January 6, 1981.
75. ——, "As Companies Jump on Fitness Bandwagon," *U.S. News & World Report*, January 28, 1980, pp. 36–39.
76. **Mechanic, David,** "Illness Behavior, Social Adaptation, and the Management of Illness: A Comparison of Educational and Medical Models," *Journal of Nervous and Mental Diseases*, 165 (1977), 79–87.
77. **Merton, Robert,** *Social Theory and Social Structure*. New York: The Free Press, 1968, Chapters 6 and 7.
78. **Mileo, Nancy,** "A Framework for Prevention: Changing Health—Damaging to Health—Generating Patterns," *American Journal of Public Health*, 66, no. 5 (1976), 435–39.
79. **Milsun, J. H.,** "Health, Risk Factor Reduction and Life-Style Change," *Family and Community Health*, 3, no. 1 (1980), 1–13.
80. **Morgenson, Donald,** "Death and Interpersonal Failure," *Canada's Mental Health*, 21, nos. 3 and 4 (1973), 10–12.
81. **Morris, N. M.,** "Pediatric Health Promotion Through Risk Reduction," *Family and Community Health*, 3, no. 1 (1980), 63–76.
82. **Murray, Ruth, M. Marilyn Huelskoetter,** and **Dorothy O'Driscoll,** *Psychiatric/Mental Health Nursing: Giving Emotional Care*. Englewood Cliffs, NJ: Prentice-Hall, Inc., 1983.
83. **Murray, Ruth,** and **Judith Zentner,** *Nursing Assessment and Health Promo-*

tion Through the Life Span (3rd ed.). Englewood Cliffs, NJ: Prentice-Hall, Inc., 1985.

84. **Nashold, Raymond,** and **Ellen Naor,** "Alcohol-Related Deaths in Wisconsin: The Impact of Alcohol on Mortality," *American Journal of Public Health*, 71, no. 11 (1981), 1237–41.
85. **Natapoff, Janet,** "Children's View of Health: A Developmental Study," *American Journal of Public Health*, 68, no. 10 (1978), 995–99.
86. **National Institute of Mental Health,** *Biological Rhythms in Psychiatry and Medicine.* Washington, D.C.: United States Department of Health, Education, and Welfare, 1970.
87. **Nowlis, H. H.,** "Coordination of Prevention Program for Children and Youth," *Public Health Reports*, 96, no. 1 (1981), 34–37.
88. **Olshansky, Stuart,** "Is Smoker/Nonsmoker Segregation Effective in Reducing Passive Inhalation Among Nonsmokers," *American Journal of Public Health*, 72, no. 7 (1982), 737–39.
89. **O'Neill, Mary,** "Patients with Hypertension: A Study of Manifest Needs with Self-Actualization," *Nursing Research*, 25, no 5 (1976), 349–51.
90. **Parens, Henri,** and **Leon Saul,** *Dependence in Man.* New York: International Universities Press, Inc., 1971, pp. 143–51.
91. "Patterns Found in Regional Cancer Study," *St. Louis Post-Dispatch*, January 9, 1977, Sec. C, p. 38.
92. **Peipre, Mall,** "The Canadian Employee Fitness and Lifestyle Project," *Athletic Purchasing and Facilities*, December 1980, pp. 10–21.
93. **Pender, Nola,** "A Conceptual Model for Preventive Health Behavior," *Nursing Outlook*, 23, no. 6 (1975), 383–90.
94. ______, *Health Promotion in Nursing Practice.* Norwalk, CT: Appleton-Century-Crofts, 1982.
95. "Pesticide Risk to Laborers Called Great," *The Nation's Health*, 9, no. 1 (1979), 4.
96. **Peters, Ruanne, H. Benson,** and **D. Porter,** "Daily Relaxation Breaks in a Working Population: I. Effects on Self-Reported Measure of Health Performance and Well-Being," *American Journal of Public Health*, 67, no. 10 (1977), 946–53.
97. ______, and **J. Peters,** "Daily Relaxation Response Breaks in a Working Population: II. Effects on Blood Pressure," *American Journal of Public Health*, 67, no. 10 (1977), 954–59.
98. **Ponte, Lowell,** "Biomagnetism: An Awesome Force in Our Lives," *Reader's Digest*, October 1982, pp. 157–60.
99. **Porter, Dawn,** and **Judith Shamian,** "Self-Care in Theory and Practice," *The Canadian Nurse*, 79, no. 8 (1983), 21–23.
100. **Quesada, Gustavo,** "Campaigning for Health Programs," *American Journal of Nursing*, 80, no. 5 (1980), 952–53.
101. **Rahe, R.,** and **R. Arthur,** "Life Change Patterns Surrounding Illness Perception," *Journal of Psychosomatic Research*, 11, no. 3 (1968), 341–45.
102. **Rinehart, Joan,** "Psychosocial Factors Related to Health Maintenance Behaviors of Pregnant Women," in *Readings for Nursing Research*, eds. Sydney Krampitz and Natalie Pavlivich. St. Louis: The C. V. Mosby Company, 1981.

103. **Romano, John,** "Basic Orientation and Education of the Medical Student," *Journal of the American Medical Association*, 143, no. 5 (1950), 411.
104. **Room, R.,** "The Case for a Problem Prevention Approach to Alcohol, Drug, and Mental Problems," *Public Health Reports*, 96, no. 1 (1981), 26-33.
105. **Schuster, Clara,** and **Shirley Ashburn,** *The Process of Human Development: A Holistic Approach*. Boston: Little, Brown & Company, 1980.
106. **Scott, Sandra,** "A Hospital-Based Health Promotion Program," *The Canadian Nurse*, 79, no. 8 (1983), 32-33.
107. **Seligman, Jean,** and **Charles Glass,** "Overdosing on Antibiotics," *Newsweek*, August 17, 1981, p. 77.
108. **Selye, Hans,** *The Stress of Life*. New York: McGraw-Hill Book Company, 1956.
109. **Shontz, F.,** "Somatopsychology: Concept and Content," *Rehabilitation Psychology*, 12 (1965), 20-27.
110. **Skipper, James,** and **Robert Leonard,** *Social Interaction and Patient Care*. Philadelphia: J. B. Lippincott Company, 1965, pp. 229-33.
111. **Solomon, G., A. Amkrant,** and **P. Kasper,** "Immunity, Emotions, and Stress," *Annals of Clinical Research*, 6 (1974), 313-22.
112. **Stammell, Marcia,** and **Jane Doe,** "The Plight of Executive Junkies," *P.D.-St. Louis Post-Dispatch*, December 19, 1982, pp. 14-16.
113. **Stewart, Elizabeth,** "To Lessen Pain: Relaxation and Rhythmic Breathing, *American Journal of Nursing*, 76, no. 6 (1976), 958-59.
114. **Suckman, Edward,** "Social Patterns of Illness and Medical Care," in *Patients, Physicians and Illness*, ed. E. Gartly Jaco. New York: The Free Press, 1972.
115. **Sullivan, Harry S.,** *Conceptions of Modern Psychiatry*. New York: W. W. Norton & Co., Inc., 1953.
116. **Toennies, Ferdinand,** *Community and Society. Gemeinschaft and Gesellschaft*, translated by C. P. Loomis. East Lansing: Michigan State University Press, 1956.
117. **Tromp, S. W.,** "Weather, Climate, and Man," in *Handbook of Physiology: Adaptation to the Environment*, eds. D. Dill, E. Adolph, and C. Wilber. Washington, D.C.: American Physiological Society, 1964, pp. 283-93.
118. **Turnbull, Eleanor,** "Effect of Basic Preventive Health Practices and Mass Media on the Practice of Breast Self-Examination," *Nursing Research*, 27, no. 2 (1978), 98-102.
119. **Turnbull, Sister Joyce,** "Shifting the Focus to Health," *American Journal of Nursing*, 76, no. 12 (1976), 1985-86.
120. **Van Gigch, John P.,** *Applied General Systems Theory*. New York: Harper & Row, Publishers, 1974.
121. **von Bertalanffy, Ludwig** *General Systems Theory*. New York: George Braziller, Inc., 1968.
122. "Weather, How It Affects Human Behavior and Moods," *St. Louis Globe-Democrat*, January 3-4, 1976, Sec. F, p. 1.
123. **Wesson, Albert,** "Hospital Ideology and Communication Between Personnel," in *Patients, Physicians and Illness*, ed. E. Gartly Jaco. New York: The Free Press, 1972.
124. **Weston, Lee,** *Body Rhythm: The Circadian Rhythms Within You*. New York: Harcourt Brace Jovanovich, 1979.

125. **Wilson, Robert,** "The Social Structures of a General Hospital," in *Social Interaction and Patient Care*, eds. J. Skipper and R. Leonard. Philadelphia: J. B. Lippincott Company, 1965, pp. 233–44.
126. "World Population to Double," *The Nation's Health*, 10, no. 6 (1980), 13.
127. **Wu, Ruth,** *Behavior and Illness*. Englewood Cliffs, NJ: Prentice-Hall, Inc., 1973.
128. **Zohman, Lenore R.,** *Beyond Diet . . . Exercise Your Way to Fitness and Heart Health*. CPC International, 1974.

2

The System for Delivery of Health Care

Study of this chapter will enable you to

1. Define, describe, and give examples of the types of health care available in the United States.
2. Relate General Systems Theory to the American health care system and analyze a health care agency by using Systems Framework.
3. Discuss major health care legislation and its impact on the health care system and professionals.
4. Explore the many kinds of health care workers and the effects of this variety on the quality of health care.
5. List the characteristics of a medical quack and discuss how you can help people avoid hazards of medical quackery.
6. Describe the various health care agencies or settings, their major characteristics, and the unique place each has in the total care of the person.
7. Discuss criteria that you could use to help a client, patient, or the family select a nursing home or other health care agency.
8. Compare various modes by which health care is financed.
9. Determine factors, including obstacles and various approaches, to consider in evaluating the effectiveness of health care given to the person or family.

10. Examine a health care issue or problem from an ethical perspective.
11. Explore the importance of consumer rights and involvement in formulating health care policy and in maintaining quality of care.
12. Discuss groups in your area whose health care needs are not adequately met and ways that could be implemented to improve their health care.
13. Analyze the differences between health care in the United States and other countries.
14. Discuss the nurse's role in various health care settings, including in primary care and in an expanded and extended role.
15. Collaborate, through appropriate referral, with personnel from various health care agencies to promote continuity of care.
16. Examine the implications of changes in the health care system and future trends in nursing practice.

INTRODUCTION

The American health care system and its various local agencies can be analyzed by using General Systems Theory discussed in Chapter 1. The main components of the general health care system in the United States are people, buildings, goals, norms, and values related to health and health care, and channels of communication, which are found in the subsystems of doctor's office, health center, home health agency, hospital, or nursing home. Each institution or agency giving health care can be analyzed and understood by using the Systems Theory.

The social environment greatly affects the local or national health care system. Federal legislation, various funding sources, and insurance companies, for example, influence which illnesses are considered serious enough to receive reimbursement. Local business and political leaders may have considerable influence on whether an agency is remodeled or built as new.

The people components of the health care system are **patients** or **clients**, *those seeking health care*; the **practitioners**, *those prescribing and giving health care*; and the many other workers who are directly or indirectly involved in health care. Sometimes these social components of the system are at variance. The patients/clients are interested in how they feel and in getting back to normal function. The practitioners are sometimes mainly interested in organic disease. And often the other workers are so organized by status levels that communication can take place only from the top of the hierarchy downward or within one category of work description. To illustrate, nurses, nurse aides, or medical secretaries usually talk with other nurses, nurse aides, or medical secretaries about problems and work conditions. Generally each group eats and socializes together during breaks and lunch periods. More will be discussed on this organizational problem later in the chapter.

Unit II is Factors Influencing Health Care in a Pluralistic Society. Levin and Idler called two of these factors, *religion and family—in addition to community and mutual aid groups*—the **Hidden Health Care System.** The authors say that although these areas are often overlooked because they are completely taken for granted, *by way of these institutions, lay people are the actual primary providers* (28).

Another term, **the alternate health care system,** has also emerged. Although *it includes some of the Western traditional health care givers, it represents an attitude and philosophy that can include such health care practitioners as optometrists and chiropractors, and often encompasses such adjunct healing forms as yoga and nutrition.*

The **health care system** may then be called *a complex part of a social system composed of individuals needing health care and a variety of individuals and/or groups who provide direct or peripheral service aimed at meeting these health care needs.*

The following discussion is organized around several basic questions: What is health care? Who delivers health care? Where is health care delivered? How is health care paid for? How is health care evaluated?

These questions are answered in relation to the traditional Western health care system. Patient's rights and ethics in relation to health care, the involvement of the consumer, the growing emphasis on self-care, people lost to the system, aspects of health care delivery in other countries, the nurse's role, present system realities, and future trends are also discussed.

WHAT IS HEALTH CARE?

Health care *is a service that people seek when they cannot manage their own health and related needs because of lack of knowledge, physical or emotional status, or lack of social support.*

Health care can be divided into community health and personal health service. **Community health services** *are directed toward maintaining health in groups of people.* Such services include water purification, sewage disposal, garbage collection, mosquito or rat control, or food or housing inspection. Communicable and other diseases or injuries would be rampant without legislation and activity to maintain a livable, safe, and clean environment. **Personal health services** *deal directly with the person/family in health promotion and maintenance or disease prevention* (46). Such services include assistance from the nurse, medical doctor, dentist, chiropractor, podiatrist, physical therapist, nutritionist, and others, as well as health education presented by official and voluntary health agencies.

Some services are both communal and personal in nature. For example, the person is immunized, but the community at large benefits, too. Community services have a preventive aim; personal services are often curative or restorative in nature because treatment is emphasized. One current concern of the health care system is that preventive care is often inadequate for the person/family. But with an emphasis on self-care, people are learning health care measures from professionals and then assuming varying levels of responsibility for their own health course.

Levels of Personal Health Care

Health care or treatment can be divided into various levels, such as acute and chronic care; primary, specialized, and inpatient care; or primary, secondary, and tertiary care (42, 46).

Acute or short-term care *refers to treatment given to the person whose illness has a rapid onset and is of brief duration.* Treatment may be managed in the doctor's office, emergency room, clinic, or hospital, depending on the seriousness of the illness and the availability of services.

Chronic or long-term care *refers to treatment given over time for an illness that may not be curable but that may improve somewhat, become regulated, or go into remission.* Such care may be managed in the doctor's office, clinic, patient's home, health clinic of an industry or school, a rehabilitation center, or a nursing home. At times the patient may be admitted to the hospital for diagnostic procedures or for better control over the illness. The Ontario Ministry of Health believes the hospital will be the leader and coordinator of long-term health services for the community, especially for the aging population (22). Because more people live longer and receive better initial and long-term medical care for chronic disease and severe injuries, defects, or health problems, care of the chronically ill is becoming a major health care problem. In the future you will be caring for more chronically ill people—helping them to maintain whatever level of health and function is possible and to prevent further illness.

Primary care or prevention *has been classified as ambulatory care, screening for and identifying potentially harmful factors or practices, preventing and treating acute diseases and disability, managing common chronic disorders, guiding and counseling persons/families, plus personal preventive measures* (46). **Primary care** also *refers to the place where the person enters the health care system, such as the doctor's or dentist's office, school, clinic, emergency room, drugstore, neighborhood health center, home, or hospital.* Assistance may initially come from the physician or nurse, pharmacist, social worker, nutritionist, physical therapist, occupational therapist, health planner, community worker, or home health aide.

The overwhelming majority of health complaints seen at the primary or ambulatory care level are uncomplicated and do not require specialists. Common problems include respiratory or gastrointestinal infections, skin lesions, minor emotional problems involving lifestyle disorders and problems of youth and old age, and chronic problems with bones, joints, and muscles. Yet today's medical doctors are being trained in an atmosphere of increased technology and specialization. The American Medical Association recognizes at least 63 medical specialties. One author blames this scientific technologic medicine for the near collapse of primary health care, which emphasizes compassion and the relationship between emotional factors and illness (7).

Greater emphasis is increasingly placed on primary care services in medical and nursing practices. Recently we have seen the rise of two specialists who give primary care to all age groups: the family nurse practitioner and the family practice physician. For further details, see references 5, 9, 11, 30, 33, 40, 45, 53, 59. A center that has successfully set up a primary care program is described in reference 9.

Specialized care *is given by a specially trained practitioner, usually to those people who need secondary care, who are too ill, or who have distinct problems that cannot be handled in a primary care setting.* A few medical specialties are urology, pediatric allergy, ophthalmology, neurosurgery, and aerospace medicine. Nursing is also increasingly specialized, usually following the specialization areas created by the medical profession. The clinical nurse specialist may focus care on clients with certain diagnoses, such as renal, cardiac, or psychiatric disorders, or she/he may be a specialist in caring for age groups, such as neonates, infants, adolescents, or the aged. These nurses may encounter a wide variety of medical, surgical, or psychiatric problems within any one age group.

Inpatient care *is provided in institutional beds, such as a hospital, extended care facility, or nursing home, and is normally supervised by a primary or specialized practitioner.* This situation is also called **sec-**

ondary care or prevention *because the person has an illness either acute or chronic, that needs early treatment so that disease duration is shortened or complications are prevented.* Initial prevention of the health problem is no longer possible if it was not accomplished in the primary care setting. **Tertiary care or prevention** *involves treating and reducing the sequelae or complications of an illness, fostering return to whatever productive capacity is possible, aiding readjustment to the condition, and maintaining whatever health remains.* It is also given in the inpatient setting and is often considered chronic care. Rehabilitative measures may be implemented and may or may not be successful.

Legislation

From 1960 to 1980 attention centered on comprehensive health planning, and the Congress passed a variety of health-related bills or granted money for various health care projects. Pressure for a national health insurance plan waxes and wanes from sectors in the federal government. The National Health Planning and Resources Development Act of 1974 (PL-93-641) has been called one of the most significant laws affecting national health. In this Act, health planning, done through regional health system agencies (HSA), superseded the traditional disease category approach and encompassed delivery of care in hospitals, clinics, and neighborhood centers. The law ensured balanced representation by both consumers and providers; some nurses gained positions on the governing boards. Essentially this Act was an attempt to provide equal access to quality health care at a reasonable cost (5). At present, however, HSA's no longer exist. Presently the federal government is more concerned about cost effectiveness of care than any other issue, and regulations and legislation are aimed at this goal.

Nurses can no longer avoid the political process. They are often heard to say that paying dues to the American Nurses Association yields nothing. Yet the message should be clear. It takes money to organize to be heard. It also takes personal involvement. Joining together to deal with certain issues at various political levels is a significant way to promote change. At one local nurses' association meeting various prospective political candidates were invited for a "meet your candidate forum." Not only were most candidates unaware of the key issues that nurses wanted them to consider in upcoming legislation, they also did not understand how many nurses were in the area, what their scope of professionalism was, or how low their salaries were compared to professionals of equal educational requirements and responsibility.

WHO DELIVERS HEALTH CARE?

Health care is one of the largest industries in the United States (32). This care has various origins, controls, and reimbursement systems. Care is provided in the public sector by various branches of the federal, state, and local governments and in the private sector by institutional (profit and nonprofit) and noninstitutional providers. Almost all of the latter are fee-for-service individuals or groups.

Professional nurses are the most numerous providers of care. In 1979 there were 1,375,208 registered nurses in the United States who held a license to practice. About 75 percent were employed in nursing (19). Health care is also given by many other professionals: physical therapists (P.T.), occupational therapists (O.T.), dietitians (R.D.), social workers (S.W.), medical doctors (M.D.), chiropractic physicians (D.C.), osteopathic physicians (D.O.), dentists (D.D.S.), orthodontists, optometrists (O.D.), ophthalmologists, and podiatrists (D.P.M.).

New categories of health workers are continuously evolving, to care for each age group, as well as do specific tasks. These categories include medical anthropologists, health educators, technologists in various departments, among them biomedical engineering technologists (BMET) and physician's assistants. The BMET provides servicing for the vast and growing amount of electronically operated medical equipment, used mainly in hospitals. The Physician's Assistant Program is modeled somewhat after the "feldsher" in Russia (49). The physician delegates certain jobs formerly done by the physician to the assistant.

Incompetence and Quackery within the Health Care System

Standards are set by professional organizations, among them the American Medical Association and the American Nurses Association. However, the "incompetent" or careless doctor has been ignored or "unseen" until recently. Published findings revealing unnecessary operations and fatal reactions from inappropriate antibiotics are making people more aware of their need to use certain standards for choosing and using a doctor (43). Additionally, self-styled health workers and "quacks" are also offering services. The self-styled health worker may emphasize certain herbs for healing or a special "hand-me-down" formula and does not rely on professionally set standards. A **quack**, *one who makes pretentious claims about the ability to treat others with little or no foundation*, may be found representing any health profession. The quack raises false hopes and causes loss of money and time—often money and time that could be better used for proven treatment.

Why do people go to quacks? Probably the main reason is *fear*: fear of mutilation from surgery, of pain, of dying. Some may go out of ignorance. Some may go to seek a miracle cure. Others may go because they lack patience with the traditional, approved treatment methods. Some have tried everything else—the quack is the "last resort."

You can help people avoid quacks by helping them set realistic health goals and by helping them recognize the following typical behaviors of the false practitioner:

1. Claims use of a special or secret formula, diet, or machine.
2. Promises an easy or quick cure.
3. Offers only testimonials as proof of healing power.
4. Claims one product or service is good for a variety of illness.
5. States that he/she is ridiculed or persecuted by traditional health professionals.
6. Promotes products through faithhealers, door-to-door health advisors, or sensational ads.
7. Refuses to accept proven methods of research.
8. Claims the treatment is better than any prescribed by a physician.

You should be aware of quackery in your community. For further reading on the subject, see reference 12. Examine the claims of the quack against standard treatment plans. Be willing to compare approaches with the client. Do not ridicule the person who has gone the nontraditional route. Above all, this person needs your listening ear and understanding guidance.

Remember that people think in terms of having symptoms and eradicating them. If the latter takes place to their satisfaction, they will place their trust in the health care worker who was responsible for their improvement, regardless of his or her credentials. What you call a *hoax* others may call *hope*.

WHERE IS HEALTH CARE DELIVERED?

Health care is delivered in a number of settings: physicians' offices, hospitals, including emergency rooms and outpatient departments, neighborhood health centers, local health department centers, industrial health centers, schools, and sometimes in people's homes.

Three recent trends for ambulatory care in the United States are group practice, neighborhood comprehensive health centers, and health maintenance organizations (HMOs).

Group Practice

Group practice means that *two or more doctors share the same facility*. This group may take on numerous variations, however. One group may simply share space, not patients. Another group may consist of the same kind of specialists who share patients. Yet another group may be made up of doctors from various specialties who share patients. Sometimes a group practice will include health professionals other than doctors—for example, nurse clinicians, physical therapists, or social workers.

A few groups who offer comprehensive services offer a **prepaid plan**. *Members pay a flat fee in advance in return for unlimited health care within a specified period.*

Neighborhood Health Centers

The **neighborhood health center** became popular in the 1960s and *was established to give comprehensive care to people of a certain geographic location*, often in a city. Usually the multidisciplinary approach is used with nurses, social workers, physicians, neighborhood health workers, and sometimes even lawyers serving the people. NHCs have been successful in some areas, but their major problem is financing. Originally sponsored by the Office of Economic Opportunity (OEO) and later by the Department of Health, Education, and Welfare (HEW), these centers must justify their existence for huge start-up costs as well as yearly operating budgets. In general, the people receiving care cannot afford to pay for it (29).

Health Maintenance Organizations

A **health maintenance organization (HMO)** *is a prepaid group practice*. Clients pay a fee that entitles them to all medical and necessary hospital services for a given period. The financial success of an HMO, at least initially, depends on preventing serious and long-term illness; thus health promotion is at the forefront.

One HMO of long standing (although not called an HMO until recently) is an option in the Kaiser-Permanente system. It started on the West Coast in the 1930s when Kaiser Industries needed to develop some mechanism of hospital and medical care for its employees at remote construction sites. By 1976 it operated in 6 states, had 2 million members, 3000 full-time physicians, 25 community hospitals, and 66 medical office facilities. Membership is voluntary (42).

One writer has said than an HMO is a socialist concept trying to function in a capitalist society (46). For further reading on HMOs, see references 33 and 46.

Hospitals

Basically the two kinds of hospitals are federal (such as Veterans' Administration) and nonfederal (including state and local governmental and private hospitals). Hospitals can be further classified in a number of ways: according to illness category (such as tuberculosis), age group served (pediatric or adult), profit or nonprofit, kind of ownership, short-term (patients staying under 30 days) or long-term (patients staying over 30 days), teaching or nonteaching.

As a subsystem of the health care system, the hospital is more than a building, nurses, doctors, and patients. The people components of this social system include those who are less visible but who have more power—the Board of Trustees. Although general norms and values that exist in the hospital are similar to those of the overall health system, each hospital has its own special atmosphere *(Gemeinschaft* or *Gesellschaft)*, its own special way of doing things. Norms and customs are influenced by the consumer of care (patients and families of an area) to some degree, as well as by administrative personnel and professional and nonprofessional workers.

Sometimes the stated norms and customs differ from those carried out. Channels of communication are maintained in the hierarchy of workers from the administrator, who is in ultimate control of the hospital but responsible to the Board of Trustees, down to the housekeeping or maintenance staff. The administrator has access to the most information and controls how much everyone else in the hierarchy is to have. Thus some workers get only brief statements telling them what to do; the reasons for what they must do are often omitted. Nurses have their own hierarchy within the overall bureaucracy. Often (in military fashion) the director of nurses is in command, followed by associate and assistant directors, supervisors, head nurses, and charge nurses; then come "the troops," the staff nurses. Certainly some nursing directors are democratic leaders who try to allow the nurses as much decision making as possible. It is to the director's advantage to see that the nurses perform as safely and competently as possible, for the power wielded by those high on the bureaucratic scale carries the price of being responsible for and accountable for those below.

Although the individual nurse works hard to give holistic and humane care, many factors interfere:

1. Lack of authority equal to responsibility.

2. Lack of opportunity to make decisions about policies that ultimately affect patient and nurse.
3. Lack of direct care by the nurse while she must coordinate and supervise care given by many other employees.
4. Lack of qualified staff.
5. Lack of supplies or equipment.

Because the chain of command goes down for each department, communication across departmental lines is sometimes minimal. And appropriate interdepartmental communication that reaches the patient is even more minimal. The stated goals of most hospitals include comprehensive care, recovery of the patient, and health teaching. But goals are often poorly implemented. One study indicated that hospitals were definitely not a source of health information to the patients interviewed (29). One anonymous author described her hospital stay as anything but holistic, personalized, and humane. The admitting clerk insisted that she had already been admitted. She received the wrong diet and incorrect medication. Staff behavior was nonprofessional. No wonder the writer bemoans the system in which her semiprivate room alone cost hundreds of dollars (1).

Increasingly nurses and other hospital employees are being reminded that the hospital is a business, especially as legislative, community, and consumer constraints become stronger. Every task is to be done with the dollar sign in mind. The current movement is designed to eliminate unnecessary waste—of supplies, employee hours, or equipment—but the ultimate effect of health care as a business on *quality* of patient care is unknown.

One trend that is becoming evident is the multihospital system or the move from single-entity hospitals to aggregate hospitals. This situation is seen in the investor-owned as well as in the not-for-profit institutions. Advantages are evident: ability to purchase in larger quantities for less cost; maintenance of a management pool; and sharing of equipment, library services, educational services, and billing procedures. The patient should benefit. Money used previously for duplication of services in free-standing hospitals can be used to hire additional staff who, because they have more time and in-service education, should provide better patient care (10).

One example of a multihealth care system is American Medical International. In 20 years AMI has gone from a two-hospital system to a 75-hospital system in ten countries. AMI also provides a broad range of specialized services to non-AMI hospitals, such as financial information, shared medical services, computer-aided hospital planning and design, and medical records consulting (4).

Although nurses and most hospital workers are paid by salary or hourly wage, the physician has a unique salary status, as well as a unique relationship to the hospital and staff. Usually the doctors are not employees of the hospital but are treating their patients in the hospital on a fee-for-service basis. Thus the hospital has little authority to discipline or manage the physician. Even if it did, it might prove ineffective because hospitals might not even exist as social institutions (at least as we know them) if there were no patients (which doctors provide).

Nursing Homes

The term **nursing home** refers to *a health facility that provides medium- or long-term care, generally to persons over age 65.* Nursing homes have become a major part of the health industry as a result of an increasingly aging population, the breakdown of the extended family, and governmental provision of funds through Medicare and Medicaid (discussed in a later section).

Since the Social Security Amendment of 1972, nursing homes are categorized as skilled nursing facilities or intermediate-care facilities. Although both facilities provide health care, the former provides the higher level of skilled care. (The skilled nursing facilities were formerly called extended care facilities (ECFs) under Medicare and skilled nursing homes under Medicaid). Certification for the skilled nursing facilities comes from the Secretary of HHS (42).

A skilled nursing facility is not intended to be a permanent home. Instead, it is to serve as a transition between hospital and home. The nursing home's goal is to provide continuous supervision by a physician, 24-hour nurse coverage, hospital affiliation, written patient care policies, and specified services in dietary, restorative, pharmaceutical, diagnostic, and social services (42). Unfortunately, few facilities meet this goal, even though they are licensed and receive government funds. Often the person never returns home, and quality care by prepared staff is lacking.

The intermediate-care facilities (ICFs) are also certified and meet federal standards, but most enforcement is by the individual state. These facilities have regular nursing service but not around the clock. Most ICFs have rehabilitation services, but greater emphasis is placed on personal care and social services (42).

Numerous reports have revealed blatant neglect of elderly persons in nursing homes. Standards were not enforced and profit was sometimes more important than care. Often the residents cannot bring effective attention to the situation. The roots of this problem lie in history. Nursing homes originated in the county poorhouses that housed the aging, homeless poor. Little attention was given to the needs of this group.

As they evolved, nursing homes were funded and operated by churches and fraternal and proprietary groups, in addition to the government. Generally those sponsored by church or fraternal groups produced the highest quality care (42).

Although the nursing home as a subsystem has its own unique characteristics, those discussed in relation to the hospital also apply to the nursing home, especially those that have large numbers of residents and are commercially run. In fact, many hospitals also have skilled nursing facilities under their management, and some will have "swing beds" that can be used as either SNF (skilled nursing facility) beds or acute beds, depending on the current need.

You may be in a position to assist a family and patient in selecting a nursing home. The following questions should be asked in order to make a careful selection.

1. What kind of home is it and what is its licensure status?
2. What are the total costs and what is included for the money?
3. Is the physical plant adequate and pleasant? How much space is allowed per person?
4. What kinds of care are offered (acute as well as chronic)?
5. What is the staff-resident ratio? What are the qulifications of the staff?
6. What services are provided by a physician, nurse practitioner, or nurse clinical specialist? Is a complete physical examination given periodically?
7. What therapies are available?
8. Are pharmacy services available?
9. Are meals nutritionally sound and is the food tasty?
10. Are visitors welcomed warmly?
11. Do residents appear well-cared for, content, and appropriately occupied (observe on successive days and at different hours)?
12. How is the residents' money handled? Who handles the money or financial affairs of the residents?
13. Do residents have an individual voice, representatives, or governing body to deal with administrative matters?

A check with the Better Business Bureau can further determine if any problems have been reported.

Home Health Care Agencies

Skilled health care is given to the person at home by visiting nurse associations, local health departments, or other private or hospital-affiliated home health care departments. Such care is given to avoid hospitalization of the ill person or to assist the person after discharge from the hospital or nursing home. Services are given by the nurse, home health aide, physical or occupational therapist, nutritionist, and social worker, and usually they are directed toward the dying, chronically ill, elderly, or the young mother and baby. Many people can use the services of a home health care agency, however, including the patient who is discharged from the hospital after extensive surgery or who is recovering from an injury prior to returning to work. Also, the family who is in need of mental health counseling may respond better to therapy given in the home than in the office.

Home care has advantages for the person who needs help but does not need acute, specialized hospital services or who has a home (rather than the nursing home) to return to for rehabilitation or long-term care. The person can remain in a familiar setting where personal preferences and routines can be maintained. Moreover, the cost of care is considerably less to the patient or family or taxpayer. Increasing emphasis is being placed on home health care services.

Miscellaneous Health-Related Services

Various health and social welfare agencies and services exist in the community to assist citizens of various age levels. Sponsorship may be by the federal or state government (official) or by certain voluntary groups within a local community or region. The network is very complex and fragmented in most cities, but few such resources exist in many rural areas. The services rendered may be either community or personal or both.

Hospice is a program that provides care for terminally ill patients and their families. The hospice may be a unit in a hospital or a community agency.

State and local health departments are responsible for health care planning and policies. At the local level, the health department provides direct services, such as maternal-child or venereal disease clinics; immunizations and chest x rays; blood lead level screening; testing of water supplies or air pollution levels; or rabies control. In some counties or cities the health department provides school or home nursing services.

Although all the following agencies or services are not directly included in the official health care system, they do contribute to the physical and emotional health of citizens and can be considered as part of the hidden health care system. Consider the state child abuse hot line, child welfare services, foster child care services, day care centers, or crisis hot lines that assist parents and children. Consider transportation, handyman, homemaker, or meals-on-wheels services that assist the elderly. The geriatric day-care center is a relatively new resource. It is a place where the elderly person who cannot remain at home alone goes during the day, receives a meal and certain kinds of health care, and can enter into social activities. While family members are at work and in school, the elderly person receives necessary supervision and does not feel isolated.

You can learn about the many health-related services in your community from the Community Service Directory published by the United Way, the telephone directory, or a local Information and Referral Service. Explore resources in your community so that you can make appropriate referrals.

HOW IS HEALTH CARE PAID FOR?

"The nation's health care business is very costly and generally noncompetitive. It is a business that needs profound reform." (government official)

"The reason for the present mess in hospital and health care costs is the government itself." (lay person)

"Americans are getting more and better health care in better facilities than citizens in any other country." (medical doctor)

"Americans should support sensible reforms in U.S. health care. But they should oppose any attempt to bureaucratize the health care industry and put it under the nation's worst managers in Washington." (hospital administrator)

Thus continues a war that has been raging for years. Should the United States have a national health plan under government control or should private fee-for-service care be upheld?

The following facts will not answer this question, but they will present some financial realities.

Federal Spending

In a single decade since the adoption of Medicare and Medicaid, hospital charges increased about 300 percent (33).

Created by Congress in 1965 through a series of amendments to the Social Security Act known as Title XVIII, **Medicare** *is a program paying hospital, physician, and certain other types of medical expenses for persons 65 and over.* The patient pays a certain percentage of every charge. When money became available, fees for services escalated, as did expectations about the services to be received and the use of available services. Formerly, the payment was made retroactively, which encouraged inflationary costs. With the signing of HR 1900 (P.L. 98-21), the Social Security Amendment of 1983, the prospective payment system became a reality. Based on 467 diagnosis-related groups (DRGs), hospitals and other treatment institutions will be paid a specified fee for care regardless of treatment. Private insurance companies are expected to follow this procedure (48).

Medicaid, known as Title XIX, is an amendment to the Social Security Act and is really *50 different programs, one for each state, which pay medical costs for the medically indigent.*

Because these programs are so complex, and especially because the Medicaid program varies in each state, you will need to guide your patients or clients who are eligible for either program to Social Security Administration representatives who can help them with proper procedure. Sometimes information is difficult to obtain because waiting lines are long or telephone lines are busy. In addition, the information is complicated. Nowhere is your helpful guidance and interpretation more needed than in this area.

Other direct government expenditures are for Veterans' Administration, United States Public Health Service, Armed Forces health service, mental hospitals and other state-operated facilities, municipal and county hospitals, and health department care services (52). *A program of compensation to an employee for injury or occupational disease suffered in connection with employment is called* **Worker's Compensation.** This reimbursement is paid under a government-supervised insurance system contributed to by employers.

Private Spending

Private spending for health falls into two categories: insurance benefits and out-of-pocket expenditures.

There are two kinds of insurance companies: not-for-profit companies and commercial companies that are in business for profit.

Blue Cross is an amalgam of approximately 70 not-for-profit insurance companies that provide mainly hospital insurance. *Blue Shield* is a group of not-for-profit companies that provide mainly for physicians' in-hospital services and some office visit coverage.

Commercial companies, such as Aetna, also write health insurance. Additionally, they offer major medical policies that cover catastrophic illness and hospital cash policies that pay a flat sum per each day of hospitalization.

Several independent plans, such as Kaiser-Permanente, can be employer–employee based or community based. They may involve group medical practice, private medical practice, or both. They may be limited to physician office care or they may include hospitalization benefits (46).

Health insurance is paid after a claim for services is made. Sometimes the company pays directly to the health care provider; sometimes it pays to the patient who, in turn, pays the provider. In some cases, the insurance policy covers all costs, but usually the patient has some initial or uncovered out-of-pocket expenses. Millions of the United States civilian population are *not covered* by some form of hospital insurance; the figure is difficult to calculate (42).

Overview of Spending

No matter how the spent money is categorized, we citizens of the United States are paying for our health care either through taxes or private insurance or both. If the insurance companies operate at a loss, they simply raise the premium—as does the government.

From 1969 to 1977 total health care expenditures in the United States increased from $60.6 to $162.6 billion. The latter figure represents 8.8 percent of the Gross National Product (GNP); of this amount, $721 per capita was for the treatment of illness and only $16 for prevention and health promotion. These costs represent only the direct health costs. If the indirect costs are figured (value of the individual in terms of losses in productivity or wages due to morbidity or mortality), 18 percent of the GNP in 1977 went into health care expenditures. Based on both direct and indirect costs, 22 to 25 percent of the GNP may be reached by 1985 and by the year 2000 we will be spending $416.4 billion on health care (39).

A general alarm has arisen throughout the country in the last few years, especially by business and industry leaders who are acting as brokers for their employees' health and insurance packages. One furniture company executive reported spending more on illness care than he did on a basic staple for his furniture business.

Many illness costs are directly related to lifestyle problems, such as smoking, alcohol and drug use, nutrition, and weight problems (which in themselves cost money), and would respond to the less costly health promotion-prevention activities.

HOW IS HEALTH CARE EVALUATED?

As early as the mid-1800s Florence Nightingale was drawing the world's attention to the lack of hospital facilities and high mortality statistics and advocating health outcomes as an indicator of quality of care (37).

In the medical field Dr. Ernest Codman was perhaps the first to talk about "end result analysis" (42). Only in recent years, with the federal government's increased involvement in the reimbursement of health care costs, has there been a persistent demand for assuring quality.

At "the heart" of the service professions of medicine and nursing there has always been the desire to give quality care. Without measurable standards, however, defining quality of care is impossible. One nurse may think that she has given quality care after giving a complete bed bath, changing the bed, feeding the patient, and giving a back rub. Another nurse may feel that she has given the same patient quality care after assisting the patient to bathe, arranging the food so that the patient can feed himself, and assisting him in a short walk. Variables are abundant and there is no agreement on what the patient needs in order to progress toward health; in fact, without agreement about what "health" is for this patient, the term "quality care" is nebulous.

Quality refers to the *degree of excellence inherent in a person, thing, or action* (26). Quality is measured by stating which actions are desired in giving care and then determining a way to measure whether the actions or outcomes were achieved.

Perhaps we should first consider the following obstacles to evaluating outcomes in health care accurately.

1. Society and the professions, such as medicine and nursing, have a "social contract." Society grants the profession authority over specific functions and permits considerable autonomy. In turn, society expects the profession to act responsibly, but society has not had criteria with which to evaluate the effectiveness of this assigned responsibility (41).
2. The highest quality of care might be given, but the outcome may be poor simply because medical science may not have the answers to the cause of the disease (such as multiple sclerosis) or because the patient's physical or mental state may not respond to the treatment given.
3. The outcome criteria may be irrelevant to the patient's problem—for example, when survival is the outcome criterion used, but disability rather than death is the usual result (such as in arthritis).
4. Many factors other than medical care influence outcome—for example, family size, health status prior to illness, or living conditions.
5. Some diseases have periods of remission and exacerbation. True "outcome" may only be measured over a period of many years—more years than are available in the study time.
6. Because legal action against health workers is a constant threat, health workers will hesitate before studying and publishing their poor results.

7. Colleagues in any professional group have difficulty evaluating each other (41).

Components of a Program

In trying to ensure quality, the evaluator can ask these questions: (1) What condition *should be* present? (In order to answer this question, the evaluator must have **criteria**, *predetermined desired outcomes of treatment and care*.) (2) What condition *was* present? (3) What were the gaps? (4) Did the action taken close the gaps between what *should be* and what *was* present? (26).

Kinds of Evaluation

There are three types of evaluation: structure, process, and outcome.

Structure is one approach to evaluation. This study may ask the following questions about an agency: Is the physical plant adequate and well maintained? Are there special diagnostic and treatment facilities? How many employees are there? How well is the staff educated? Essentially these questions answer something about the basics of facilities and personnel available, but they tell little about how they function and nothing about their ability to give high-quality care.

Process analysis is another approach to evaluation and answers the question: How is the system working? Process analysis may take (1) the statistical approach, (2) the record review approach, or (3) the practice-observation approach.

In the *statistical approach*, utilization rates are often studied—for example, the number of consultations, the length of hospital stay by diagnosis, or autopsy rates.

The *record review approach* is also called *peer review* or the nursing or medical audit and may be derived from the information gleaned in the statistical approach. Additionally, it may involve detailed review and analysis of the agency records by qualified staff or by an independent evaluating group. Sometimes chart review is done only by a committee of nurses or doctors; the trend is for a multidisciplinary team to do chart review or audit.

The *practice-observation approach* is probably the most accurate assessment of process. Instead of using records as in the other two approaches, the practitioner is directly observed by other qualified practitioners. If no mistakes are being made, perhaps little is gained by the procedure. But if mistakes or omissions are obvious, direct confrontation with the caregiver is an effective method of changing behavior or techniques (29).

Basic to any process of evaluation must be standards that define not only expected *outcomes* of care but also the expected performance or credentials of professional personnel, the specifications of the physical plant, and the regulation and administration of facilities and programs (26).

Even after evaluation the following questions still remain: Did the time spent, human resources used, and quality assurance activities chosen really improve the health status of the population served? Or have we reached the point of diminishing returns? Are we putting too much money into *medical care* instead of into *health*? Into structure and process instead of patient satisfaction?

Instead of continuing to feed the health care machine resources that do not add to positive health, we should direct our resources toward providing better nutrition, improved housing, educational and recreational opportunities, and a cleaner environment for children, teenagers, adults, and the elderly (50).

ETHICS AND PATIENTS' RIGHTS IN THE HEALTH CARE SYSTEM

A 1982 issue of *Ethics and Medics, Catholic Perspectives on Moral Issues of the Health and Life Sciences,* tackles such subjects as future technology and morality; technology judged by contribution to peace; Jehovah's Witnesses and blood: How far can their belief be respected?; and the imperative to alter: Is there an obligation to use genetic technology (18)?

Models for ethical decision making are abundant (8, 18, 35). These models rely on values clarification and a problem-solving approach. But often specific questions need to be asked when in a quandary.

1. What is going on in the care? Distinguish the scientific facts from the values and moral questions.
2. By what criteria should decisions be made? Professional codes provide one source. Nursing has an American Nurses Association Code (Code for Nurses) (14) and an International Code of Ethics (25). A religious perspective provides another source. Philosophical reasoning is a third source.
3. Who should decide? Patient, nurse, doctor, family, administration?
4. For whose benefit is the decision made? Do commitment and loyalty to the patient have priority?
5. How should professionals decide and act (34, 35)?

In 1973 the House of Delegates of the American Hospital Association approved a Patient's Bill of Rights (see Table 2-1) (55). Later the

TABLE 2-1 The Patient's Bill of Rights (86)

1. The patient has a right to considerate and respectful care . . . .
2. The patient has a right to obtain from his physician complete current information about his diagnosis . . . .
3. The patient has a right to receive from his physician information necessary to give informed consent to the start of any procedure and/or treatment . . . .
4. The patient has a right to refuse treatment to the extent permitted by law . . . .
5. The patient has a right to every consideration of his privacy concerning his own medical care program . . . .
6. The patient has a right to expect that all communications and records pertaining to his care should be treated as confidential . . . .
7. The patient has a right to expect that within its capacity a hospital must make reasonable responses to the request of a patient for services . . . .
8. The patient has a right to obtain information as to any relationship of his hospital to other health care and educational institutions insofar as his care is concerned . . . .
9. The patient has a right to be advised if the hospital proposes to engage in human experimentation affecting his care and the right to refuse to participate in such research projects . . . .
10. The patient has the right to expect reasonable continuity of care . . . .
11. The patient has the right to examine and receive an explanation of his bill regardless of the source of the payment . . . .
12. The patient has the right to know what hospital rules and regulations apply to his conduct as a patient.

*Reprinted with permission of the American Hospital Association, Copyright 1975.

National League of Nursing published a seven-statement document explaining what people can expect from modern nursing service. Some associations built on this foundation and published patient booklets, such as *Your Rights as a Patient*, which expanded the Bill of Rights and covered such subjects as patient representatives, scrutinizing bills, being a part of research, and confidentiality of medical records. While these lists are not legal documents, they give ethical guidelines for hospital policy and practice (61).

Although many patients did not hear about or think about their rights, a general feeling was building about consumer involvement, not only after the consumer became a patient, but also before the sick role was entered.

CONSUMER INVOLVEMENT

Lay people are becoming more aware of their need to participate in decisions about their health. Television, popular magazines, and newspapers are increasingly featuring such subjects as "How to Go About

Finding a Good Dentist," "How to Cut Hospital and Other Medical Costs," and "Legal Drugs Can Kill."

In 1976 a fourth-year medical student published his first issue of *Medical Self-Care*, now a quarterly publication. In his first editorial he said of his first year on the hospital wards, "About half the patients I saw that year had a preventable illness. Every time I saw a smoker with lung cancer or emphysema, a heavy drinker with liver disease, a fat, sedentary businessman with a heart attack, or a woman who'd only come to the doctor when her lung cancer was long past any chance of cure, I realized that medical care is not something to be left to doctors and other health care workers" (20).

Evaluation of inpatient and outpatient care needs to be increased, not only from a technological and disease control viewpoint, but also from the perspective of patient satisfaction and prevention of further complications.

Consumers should respond to the following questions.

1. Have you investigated the variety of health care services offered by your community, and do you feel comfortable in searching for any type of health care service that you think you need?
2. Do you have some planned criteria by which you select your primary care?
3. Do you visit your primary care practitioner on a regular basis in order to practice health promotion or do you contact the appropriate practitioner only when you have severe, persistent, or recurrent symptoms?
4. If you must be hospitalized and have a choice of institutions, have you selected one or two institutions by thoughtful planning? Have you developed a plan for possible emergency services?
5. Do you attend appropriate health care classes, such as first aid or cardiopulmonary resuscitation, when offered by a community health agency?
6. Do you question health practitioners about their methods, evaluation of your health status, and recommendations?
7. Do you budget for health care? Do you shop for the best quality? Price? Do you look for programs that might assist you in paying your medical bills?
8. Do you post important phone numbers, such as police, ambulance, emergency room, and primary care practitioner, by the home and work telephones?
9. Do you obtain necessary immunizations? Do you keep health records for yourself and your family?
10. Do you follow health promotion measures, e.g., exercise, weight control?

11. Do you report suspected health care frauds to the proper authorities?
12. Do you exercise your voting power in relation to health matters?

Consumers need a working knowledge of the health care system and how it functions. Also, with the rapid move into computerized and business, industrial, or government-controlled personal medical information, people need to be concerned about the confidentiality of their medical records and various personal or family information (54).

National Health Care is a subject about which most consumers do not have adequate information. The average person does not understand such programs in other countries (the USSR and England, for example) and they do not have any clearcut way of appraising how they would be affected if they changed from a private, fee-for-service or partially subsidized health program to a completely government-controlled health program. Additionally, the campaign for a government-sponsored program of health insurance spans about three-fourths of a century and has evolved considerably in its emphasis as American political life and economics of health care have changed. The most recent emphasis has been on a program that will emphasize cost containment.

Today the United States is the only major industrial nation without a national health insurance plan. Seventy countries throughout the world have public health insurance programs for medical care systems for the entire population. At this writing, however, there seems to be no strong political movement for a comprehensive national program (51).

UNMET NEEDS IN THE HEALTH CARE SYSTEM: PEOPLE LOST TO THE HEALTH CARE SYSTEM

In a health care system such as that in the United States some groups of people can easily "fall through the cracks." Such groups are the rural and urban poor, the aged, immigrants, and **migrant workers (migrants)**, *those who find work by moving with the seasonal harvesting of crops* (47).

Although the Migrant Health Act was passed in 1962 and has been a major source of funding since then, recent emphasis on cutbacks puts these people in great jeopardy. In a 1981 Report of a Select Panel for the Promotion of Child Health, migrants were described as living in marginal environmental and social circumstances that are, if anything, getting worse rather than better (47).

In 1981 migrants were thought to compose about 800,000 to 1.5

million of the population. Median income for a family of six, with the children working, was $3900 yearly. Living conditions are often worse than for inner-city dwellers. Without toilet facilities or drinking or washing facilities in the field, many women who will not use a hedgerow for a toilet hold their urine and consequently have a high rate of urinary tract infections. Food, usually sandwiches, is held with hands full of pesticide and then eaten. Lack of drinking water causes dehydration and susceptibility to a host of illnesses (47)*.

HEALTH CARE IN OTHER COUNTRIES VERSUS HEALTH CARE IN THE UNITED STATES

Because evaluation of health care in the United States is difficult, evaluating health care in other countries is even more difficult if not impossible. When representatives travel from country to country to study medical care and facilities, the host country naturally presents the best it has to offer.

Nevertheless, a few helpful comments can be made. The criticism of health care in the United States often centers around cost and ineffectiveness: although costs continue to rise, people are not necessarily gaining an equal measure of health.

One example might be that no controlled nutritional system exists in the United States. The individual has the final decision in a democracy about what to eat or to feed his/her children. While health authorities are advocating nutritional diets, many schools are still supplying their students with food machines that deliver "junk food" and giving high-fat and carbohydrate lunches.

By contrast, in Norway the government plans to guide its people's nutritional choices through standing policies, public education, and research. It will, for example, favor the purchase of skim milk over whole milk and of fish and poultry over meat. It will discourage the use of feed concentrate in cattle and dairy operations (44, 60). Recently, in Norway, a model for Health Service Management Program determined that the elderly and those with physical disabilities needed the most coordinated health service, yet the current focus seemed to be on acute care of the 18- to 85-year-olds. Through a determined effort, a match between the target populations and the tasks or services to be provided were met (62).

In the United States the individual has the final decision about how many children are wanted, although financial pressure has caused

*For information on migrant farm issues, write to Migrant Legal Action Program, Inc., Suite 600, 806 15th St. N.W., Washington, D.C., 20005 (47).

birthrates to drop. In China family planning has been carefully guided through education, group discussions (persuasion), and group approval because of a population that tops the billion mark. Appropriate behavior change is praised until the new attitude and way of life become habit (57). Additionally, financial incentives exist. Loss of income, free education, and free health care result if a couple has more than one child.

The People's Republic of China has an organized health care system that includes the number one hospital in Peking with the renowned reconstruction surgeon as well as the barefoot doctor and the smallest clinic in the rural area. A system of referral in terms of geography as well as intensity of illness is tightly controlled. The system is a composite of Eastern traditional medicine with its herbs and acupuncture and Western traditional medicine. Western medical techniques are used to make the diagnosis, but Eastern medicine may be used for the treatment (23). In the years since liberation the life span of the Chinese rose from 42 to 71 years for males and from 45 to 75 years for females. The Chinese are now encountering what the Western world is dealing with —diseases of longevity, especially cardiovascular disease. Attention is being given to nutrition, exercise, appropriate medication, and education (23). For more information on the health care system in the People's Republic of China, see references 15 and 21.

Great Britain presents an example of a National Health Service in a noncommunist country. The system initially enrolled over 90 percent of the population and covered all health costs. At present, people are paying for some dental work, eyeglasses, and prescriptions. The doctors reportedly do not like the system because they feel dictated to and dependent on the state. Patients seem generally satisfied with the British system even though waiting lines are long, both to see the doctor for an office visit and to have elective surgery. For those who are dissatisfied, private physicians and hospital beds are still available, although in a small percentage. Fees are still controlled, however, by the government.

Other differences in health orientation among countries exist. One study comparing hospitalized Americans with hospitalized Scots, for instance, found that Americans received almost twice as many drugs as their Scottish counterparts who had the same symptoms (27). Another study showed that Swedish hospitals do less extensive x rays and laboratory testing per patient than do United States hospitals (36).

Why these differences exist is difficult to say, but perhaps some of the reasons are that

1. The United States is a drug-oriented society.
2. Doctors in the United States are using "tools" (drugs or x rays) more than clinical insight and counseling.

3. The threat of lawsuit in the United States causes doctors to do more diagnostic work.
4. Patients in the United States may be more demanding than their counterparts in other countries.

People in the United States value their independence and ability to choose—whether it be a specific doctor, a certain food, or an over-the-counter drug. Americans prefer to make some wrong choices rather than have all choices made for them. Because of this basic philosophy, a national health insurance must be tailored to democratic ideals, not an easy task.

THE NURSE'S ROLE

Nurses are being taught to be more creative; yet they often work in a bureaucratic system that denies innovation. Nurses are being taught concepts to promote health, the emphasis of this book; yet they continue to function mainly in jobs that require care of episodic illness. Frequently the nurse is not permitted or encouraged to use her knowledge or creativity. In some agencies the role is limited to technical functions. In other agencies the nurse is assigned extra tasks delegated by the physician.

Professional nursing is changing for a number of reasons. Paramount is the consumer's demand for better care. Other factors are the increasing emphasis on primary care and the use of qualified practitioners, not just the physician, combined with an educational emphasis on skills that prepare the nurse to do more thorough assessment and to understand better the rationale for treatment and care. Nursing leaders are creating a new public image of the profession and are attempting to influence the legislative process from the local level to the national level.

Nurses in some hospitals are reorganizing their method of giving care into **primary nursing** *in which the nurse carries a designated caseload of patients.* Thus the nurse uses the educational preparation to give care directly to a group of patients. Together the nurse and patient make decisions regarding care. This method eliminates the need to have a nurse supervising other employees who give care and trying to determine from employees what has been done to the patient. Certainly, with primary nursing care, the nurse is in a much better position to be the patient's advocate. Primary nursing is discussed further in Chapter 4.

Home health agencies are asking their nurses to do complete health histories on and physical examinations of their patients. Although more time-consuming, this approach makes the nurse more fully aware of the patient's condition, an especially important factor when the nurse is in the home and solely responsible for noting changes in condition and for adapting care accordingly.

A new phase of nursing practice began in 1971 when Idaho revised its Nurse Practice Act to authorize registered nurses who had special preparation to diagnose and treat patients within certain specified limits (11). Other states have followed Idaho's lead, with each state responding somewhat differently in what is allowed. Almost all states that have revised Nurse Practice Acts are including nursing diagnosis as a function of the nurse.

The following nursing actions are judged appropriate by the U.S. Department of Health and Human Services.

1. Eliciting and recording a health history.
2. Making physical and psychosocial assessments; recognizing the range of normal and the manifestations of common abnormalities.
3. Assessing family relationships and home, school, and work environments.
4. Interpreting selected laboratory findings.
5. Making diagnoses in selected situations.
6. Choosing, initiating, and modifying selected therapies in selected situations.
7. Assessing community resources and needs for health care in the community.
8. Providing appropriate emergency treatment, such as in cardiac arrest, shock, or hemorrhage.
9. Providing appropriate information to the patient and the family about a diagnosis or plan of therapy.
10. Making prospective decisions about treatment in collaboration with a doctor, such as prescribing symptomatic treatment for coryza, pain, headaches, or nausea.
11. Initiating actions within a protocol developed by medical and nursing personnel, such as making adjustments in medication, ordering and interpreting certain laboratory tests, and prescribing certain rehabilitative and restorative measures.
12. Conducting nurse clinics for health screening and case finding for health problems in people of all ages.
13. Conducting nurse clinics for continuing care of selected patients.
14. Assessing community long-term care needs and participating in the development of resources to meet them.
15. Assuming continued responsibility for acquainting selected patients and families with implications of health status, treatment, and prognosis (59).

Some nurses are carrying out additional functions or former functions more independently within established institutions. In one study nurses with additional educational preparation in assessing, making nursing diagnoses, doing diagnostic procedures, teaching, and handling other treatments were employed for a one-year demonstration project. Results of the study showed that patients cared for by these nurses received significantly different care from patients cared for routinely by physicians. Both quality and quantity of care were greater.

Actually, some nurses have been expanding their role for years by making diagnostic decisions and giving a quantity of health services, especially in rural areas or industrial plants. Often the nurses did not recognize the scope of their services. Nurses have played an elaborate game that puts the physician at the head of the team—the only one capable of decision making (11). Women have been socialized to consider the man dominant (most nurses are female; most doctors are male) and smarter. The nurse who remained submissive in the bureaucratic system kept the system running smoothly but at the expense of patient care and her own self-actualization.

Nurses owe it to themselves to analyze what they can do and to stand up for their abilities. Keeping up with the nursing association, legislation, and social and technological trends is essential.

The nurse's educational level and degree of responsibility should be reflected in a salary that matches that received by people with an equal educational background and responsibility. Historically such is not the case, although salaries have improved in the last several years (17).

In January 1982 the average yearly salary for a full-time registered nurse in the United States was $19,381. A high level was realized by nurses in hospital administration at $27,865 and a low was realized by physician office staff nurses at $12,872 (17).

You can affect the health care system in another way. If you discover a patient or family problem, regardless of your position or care setting, you can take positive action. Perhaps no organizational source of health exists or a present source may be unable to meet the needs of the persons in question. What would you do? Your combination of creative ability and practical working knowledge can develop a program to meet the specific need. The following are proper steps to take should you find yourself in a position to make changes in organizational sources of help, and as a nurse in the primary care role you may indeed be in such a position.

Be very specific in identifying the problem. An epidemiological study may be needed. Note the number of people who are affected. If only a few isolated people are affected, redirect your plans to meet their needs within the existing care system. Once the problem is identified and found significant, write out the proposed solutions. Involve your supervisor throughout; perhaps that person can help you find unknown resources. Think about attaching the proposed program to one that already exists. If attachment is possible, costs can be cut drastically. Whatever your course—attachment or creation of a new program—inform your agency about your plans and ask for its support.

You are now ready to begin convincing others in the community that a new program is needed. Begin with the power structure of the community—the people known for "getting things done." Select people from various occupations and professions; get a cross section of the community. Visit each personally and ask for advice, suggestions, and support. Get permission to mention the names of those who react positively when discussing the proposed program with others.

Plan the first group meeting. Invite those people with whom you spoke, plus a variety of others from the community. Continue to look for support from valuable individuals or oganizations. Don't forget the consumer! At the meeting present your proposal verbally in addition to distributing a written outline. A temporary chairperson and interim steering committee need to be elected. The purpose of the committee is to review the proposed program in its entirety, determine cost details and ways of funding, investigate whether it is necessary to develop a new agency or if an existing one can be used, and, finally, prepare a written report of the findings.

The findings of the steering committee are presented at the second group meeting. A permanent board of directors should be elected. All involved people not on the board should be on the advisory council. The board is responsible for making policies, adopting bylaws, and writing a formal, detailed program proposal, including job descriptions of needed staff and facilities. The board must be prepared to state how the program will be financed. It should also solicit letters of commitment from organizations and agencies that will give free services. Program proposals may need to be written several times to meet particular funding requirements. Many meetings may be necessary to achieve your goal. (63).

Convincing people that a new program is needed may take determination and fortitude. While keeping your goal in mind, you will constantly integrate new ideas that may change your direction somewhat. Worthwhile programs are created through this difficult process, but time and effort are needed. Such action is an extension of the nursing process described in Chapter 4.

PRESENT REALITIES AND FUTURE TRENDS

In the decade ahead the people component of the health care system must come to terms with working in a helping institution in a capitalist society. Health care continues to be seen as a right at a time when both financial aid for health care and other resources are diminishing. Nurses should keep up to date in knowledge, attitudes, and performance as the philosophy of health care changes and as advances in technology and knowledge continue to have an impact on the profession of nursing and health care delivery. As a nurse in the future, you will be more likely to practice in a nonhospital setting; ambulatory or outpatient care and home care are increasingly emphasized in an effort to meet client needs better and to reduce health care costs. You will be more likely to care for people with chronic illness and the elderly. You may participate in research to find ways to prevent chronic diseases or disability, just as infectious and acute diseases or conditions are now preventable. You will be expected to work effectively with the client as someone who is responsible for self-care and with a variety of other health care professionals and paraprofessionals. Accountability for your practice is increasingly emphasized, which means that your practice will be evaluated by the consumer as well as other health care professionals.

Because of efforts of the nursing organization, the American Nurses Association, and nursing leaders, nurses will realize a new personal and professional self-worth and increased autonomy in the profession. Primary nursing will be a key way of delivering nursing service. Nurses will be increasingly successful and valued as clinical specialists, independent practitioners, client educators and educational administrators, consultants in nursing practice, education, and management, and lobbyists and politicians. More and more, nurses will be using knowledge about Systems Theory to work in the health care system and to improve the system.

REFERENCES

1. "A Consumer Speaks Out About Hospital Care," *American Journal of Nursing*, 76, no. 9 (1976), 1443–44.
2. **Ahmed, Mary,** "Taking Charge of Change in Hospital Nursing Practice," *American Journal of Nursing*, 81, no. 3 (1981), 540–43.
3. **Aiken, Linda,** "Nursing Priorities for the 1980s: Hospitals and Nursing Homes," *American Journal of Nursing*, 81, no. 2 (1981), 324–30.
4. *AMI Personnel Handbook*. Beverly Hills, CA: AMI Corporation, 1980.
5. **Andreoli, Kathleen G.,** "The Ambulatory Health Care System," *Nursing Digest*, 5, no. 1 (1977), 16–21.
6. *A New Opportunity for Health and Human Services Cost Optimization*. Morganton, NC: Institute for Health Management, n.d.
7. **Battistella, Roger,** "The Right to Adequate Health Care," *Nursing Digest*, 4, no. 1 (1976), 12–17.
8. **Bergman, R.,** "Ethical Concepts and Practice," *International Nursing Review*, 20, no. 5 (1973), 140–62.

9. **Bowar-Ferris,** "Loeb Center and Its Philosophy of Nursing," *American Journal of Nursing*, 75, no. 5 (1975), 810-15.
10. **Brown, Montague,** "Multihospital Systems in the '80s—The New Shape of the Health Care Industry," *Hospitals*, March 1, 1982, p. 71.
11. **Bullough, Bonnie,** "Influences on Role Expansion," *American Journal of Nursing*, 76, no. 9 (1976), 1476-81.
12. **Burkhalter, Pamela O.,** "Cancer Quackery," *American Journal of Nursing*, 77, no. 3 (1977), 451-53.
13. **Chaisson, G. Maureen,** "Correctional Health Care—Beyond the Barriers," *American Journal of Nursing*, 81, no. 4 (1981), 737-38.
14. "Code for Nurses with Interpretive Statements," Kansas City, MO: American Nurses Association, 1976.
15. **Donley, Rosemary,** and **Mary Jane Flaherty,** "Through a Looking Glass: Life and Health Patterns in New China," *Image*, 14, no. 3 (1982), 68-70.
16. *Enhancing Our Health Care System: WNCHSA Planning Highlights 1876-1982*. Morgantown, NC: Western North Carolina Health Systems Agency, n.d.
17. "Estimated Average Salaries of Registered Nurses by Employment Setting and Position (Full-Time)," *The American Nurse*, March 1982, p. 5.
18. *Ethics and Medics, A Catholic Perspective on Moral Issues in the Health and Life Sciences*, 7, no. 1 (1982).
19. *Fact Sheet on Registered Nurses*. Washington, D.C.: American Nurses Association, Government Relations Division, 1981.
20. **Ferguson, Tom,** Editor's Page in *Medical Self-Care*, vol. 1, no. 1 (1976).
21. **Henderson, Gail E.,** and **Myron S. Cohen,** "Health Care in the People's Republic of China: A View from Inside the System," *American Journal of Public Health*, 72, no. 11 (1982), 1238-43.
22. **Henderson, Jane,** "Issues in Rural Health Care Planning," *The Canadian Nurse*, 78, no. 1 (1982), 30-33.
23. **Hoskins, Olga,** Report on Trip to China, 1982. Lecture on Nov. 16, 1982, in Hickory, NC.
24. *Hospital Statistics* (1975 edition). Chicago: American Hospital Association, 1975.
25. "International Council of Nurses Code of Ethics," *American Journal of Nursing*, 68, no. 12 (1968), 2581-85.
26. **Laing, Mary,** and **Margaret Nisk,** "Eight Steps to Quality Assurance," *The Canadian Nurse*, 77, no. 10 (1981), 22-25.
27. **Lawson, D.,** and **J. Hershel,** "Drug Prescribing in Hospitals: An International Comparison," *American Journal of Public Health*, 66, no. 7 (1976), 644-48.
28. **Levin, Lowell S.,** and **Ellen L. Idler,** *The Hidden Health Care System: Mediating Structures and Medicine*. Cambridge, MA: Ballinger Publishing Company, 1981.
29. **Lutz, Carol,** "Communication Patterns of Hospitalized Patients," *Michigan Nurse*, January 1977, 8-10.
30. **Manley, Mary,** "Clinical Privileges for Nonhospital-Based Nurses," *American Journal of Nursing*, 81, no. 10 (1981), 1822-25.
31. **McLemore, Melinda,** "Nurses as Health Planners: Our New Legal Status," *Nursing Digest*, 5, no. 1 (1977), 59-60.

32. *Medical Care Chartbook* (7th ed.). Ann Arbor: University of Michigan Health Administration Press, 1980.
33. **Miller, Alfred E.**, and **Maria G. Miller**, *Options for Health and Health Care: The Coming of Post-Clinical Medicine*. New York: John Wiley & Sons, Inc., 1981.
34. **Mooney, Mary Margaret**, "The Ethical Component of Nursing Theory," *Image*, 12, no. 1 (1980), 7–9.
35. **Murphy, M. A.**, and **J. Murphy**, "Making Ethical Decisions Systematically," *Nursing '76*, 6, no. 5 (1976), 13–14.
36. **Neuhauser, Duncan**, and **Egen Jansson**, "Doctors and Hospitals in Sweden," *Scandinavian Review*, September 1975, p. 23.
37. **Palmer, Irene**, "Florence Nightingale: Reformer, Reactionary, Researcher," *Nursing Research*, 26, no. 2 (1977), 84–89.
38. **Pardee, Geraldine, D. Hoshaw, C. Huber**, and **B. Larson**, "Patient Care Evaluation Is Every Nurse's Job," *American Journal of Nursing*, 71, no. 10 (1971), 1958–60.
39. **Pender, Nola J.**, *Health Promotion in Nursing Practice*. Englewood Cliffs, NJ: Prentice-Hall, Inc., 1980.
40. **Pennell, Y.**, and **D. B. Hoover**, "Allied Health Manpower, 1950–1970," *Health Manpower Source Book*, Publication 263. Washington, D.C.: U.S. Public Health Service, 1970, Sec. 21, pp. 2, 3, 6, 66, 67.
41. **Phaneuf, Maria**, *The Nursing Audit: Profile for Excellence*. New York: Appleton-Century-Crofts, 1976.
42. **Raffel, Marshall W.**, *The U.S. Health Care System Origin and Functions*. New York: John Wiley & Sons, Inc., 1980.
43. **Remsberger, Boyce**, "The Problem of the Incompetent Physician," *St. Louis Post-Dispatch*, February 15, 1976, Sec. G, p. 3.
44. **Ringer, Kurt**, "The Norweigian Food and Nutritional Policy," *American Journal of Public Health*, 67, no. 6 (1977), 550–551.
45. "R. N. Opens Office for Insurance Health Assessment," *American Journal of Nursing*, 81, no. 10 (1981), 1891, 1910, 1912.
46. **Salloway, Jeffrey Coleman**, *Health Care Delivery Systems*. Boulder, CO: Westview Press, 1982.
47. **Satchell, Michael**, "Bent, But Not Broken," *Parade Magazine*, October 10, 1982, pp. 6–7.
48. **Shaffer, Franklin**, "DRG's: History and Overview," *Nursing and Health Care*, 4, no. 7 (1983), 386–96.
49. **Sidel, V. W.**, "Feldshers and 'Feldsherism': The Role and Training of the Feldsher in the U.S.S.R.," *New England Journal of Medicine*, 278 (1968), 981.
50. **Skipper, James**, "The Right to Adequate Health Care: Nursing Implications," *Nursing Digest*, 4, no. 1 (1976), 17–18.
51. **Starr, Paul**, "Public Health Then and Now: Transformation in Defeat: The Changing Objectives of National Health Insurance, 1915-1980," *American Journal of Public Health*, 72, no. 1. (1982), 77–88.
52. *Statistical Abstract of the United States*, 1975 (ed. 96). Washington, D.C.: Bureau of the Census, U.S. Department of Commerce, 1975.

53. **Stuart-Burchart, Sandra,** "Rural Nursing," *American Journal of Nursing,* 82, no. 4 (1982), 616–18.
54. **Templin, H. Elaine,** "The System and the Patient," *American Journal of Nursing,* 82, no. 1 (1982), 108.
55. The Patient's Bill of Rights. Chicago: American Hospital Association, 1973.
56. **Townsend, C.,** *Old Age: The Last Segregation* (Ralph Nader's Study Group Report on Nursing Homes). New York: Grossman, 1971.
57. **Wan, Virginia,** "Application of Social Science Theories to Family Planning Health Education in the People's Republic of China," *American Journal of Public Health,* 66, no. 5 (1976), 440–45.
58. **Weinstein, Edwin,** "Developing a Measure of the Quality of Nursing Care," *Journal of Nursing Administration,* 6, no. 6 (1976), 1–3.
59. **White, Susan,** "The Expanded Role for Nurses," *Nursing 77,* 7, no. 10 (1977), 90–93.
60. **Winikoff, Beverly,** "Nutrition and Food Policy: The Approaches of Norway and the United States," *American Journal of Public Health,* 67, no. 6 (1977), 552–57.
61. "Your Rights as a Patient." St. Louis: Lutheran Mission Association, 1975.

Interviews

62. **Jackson, Osa,** R.P.T., Ph.D., personal interview, May 15, 1983.
63. **Zentner, Reid,** personal directives on project establishment, May 1984.

3

Therapeutic Communication: Prerequisite for Effective Nursing

Study of this chapter will enable you to

1. Define *communication* and describe the elements in the communication process.
2. Identify the levels of communication and use this knowledge in nursing.
3. List and describe the tools used in communication.
4. Discuss ways to use language of size, time, space, and color, as well as words, effectively.
5. Observe various clients and situations and determine whether your observations meet the criteria and what factors influenced your observations and perceptions.
6. Describe the different types of nonverbal behavior and how each affects communication.
7. Analyze silent periods to determine the type of silence and its effect on communication.
8. Practice attentive listening and explore its impact on the other person.
9. State the definition and purposes of an interview.
10. Discuss interviewing methods and rationale for steps in the method.

11. Interview a person, well or ill, using the correct methods, and analyze the principles used and the effectiveness of the interview.
12. Describe methods of therapeutic communication and the rationale for each method.
13. Analyze the pattern of communication, using knowledge of rationale, after practice of therapeutic communication with a client.
14. Describe modifications in communication approach that will be effective with a child or adolescent.
15. Discuss ways to modify a communication approach to be effective with clients who have communication disorders.
16. Discuss barriers to and ineffective methods of communication, identify personal use of them, and analyze why they are ineffective.
17. Explore how use of effective communication methods is basic to nursing care and contributes to health and the functioning of systems.

> My Spanish friend looked puzzled when I said, "Let's keep in touch." I meant, "Let's talk to each other periodically."
>
> He heard the literal meaning. Often we don't communicate because we use words symbolically rather than literally, as further illustrated by the following statement:
>
> "I know you believe you understand what you think I said, but I am not sure you realize what you hear is not what I meant."—Anonymous

The ability to communicate should not be taken for granted; it is not a simple process but rather a complex system by which the world's work gets done.

Communication is the matrix for all thought and relationships between persons and is bound to the learning process. Early sensory experiences shape subsequent learning abilities in speech, cognition, symbol recognition, and in the capacity for maturing communication. Perception of the self, the world, and one's place in it results from communication. Verbal and nonverbal communication is learned in a cultural setting; if the person does not communicate in the way prescribed by the culture, many difficulties arise, for that person cannot conform to the expectations of society. Disordered thinking, feeling, and actions result, along with mental anguish, and perhaps even physical illness.

Communication is the heart of the nursing process, for it is one of the primary methods used to accomplish specific and general goals with many different kinds of people. It is used in assessing and understanding the patient and family as well as in nursing intervention. Communication helps people express thoughts and feelings, clarify problems, receive information, consider alternate ways of coping or adapting, and remain realistic through feedback from the environment. Essentially the client learns something about the self, how to identify health needs, and if and how he/she wishes to meet them.

DEFINITIONS

The word *communication* comes from the Latin verb *communicare*, "to make common, share, participate, or impart." **Communication** *establishes a sense of commonness with another and permits the sharing of information, signals, or messages in the form of ideas and feelings.* A series of messages exchanged between persons forms an interchange or communication (69). Communication is a continuous dynamic process by which one mind may affect another through written or oral language, gestures, facial expressions, music, painting, sculpture, drama, dance, or other signs.

Communication pattern *refers to the relatively consistent network of messages sent and received in short- or long-term exchanges, the habitual way of interacting with others.* Part of this pattern is the **social amenities pattern,** *the interaction that uses socially prescribed rules, ceremonies, or customs* according to the situation and usually results in superficial communications. The social pattern includes **small talk,** *social chitchat that encompasses mundane topics* and is used to kill time, to test the reactions of others, to avoid involvement, or to serve as a bridge to significant conversation. The **information pattern** differs in that it *involves a request for or giving of information or orders* but it is not likely to establish intimate understandings because there is little disclosure of self. Neither the social nor the informational pattern is adequate by itself in the nursing process. The communication pattern in the nurse-client-family relationship should be a **dialogue**, involving *purposeful, reciprocal, close expression between the participants* and focusing on the problems of the one seeking help rather than on those of the helper. Yet there should be an openness that contributes to the growth of all participants involved (80).

THE COMMUNICATION PROCESS

Every communication process includes a sender, a transmitting device, signals, a receiver, and feedback, as shown in Fig. 3-1. The sender attempts to convey a message, idea, or information through the appro-

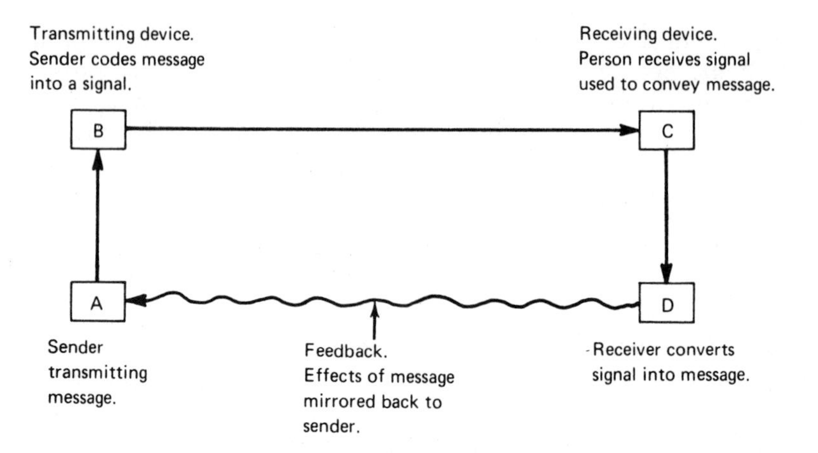

FIGURE 3-1 Elements in the Communication Process

priate use of symbols or signals directed to another specific person or group. That the message is sent does not guarantee that it will be received at all, let alone by the person for whom it is intended.

Many factors influence how the message is sent and whether, how, and by whom it will be received: the needs and condition of both the sender and the receiver, emotionally, physically, and intellectually; the occasion or setting; and the sender's knowledge about and relationship with the receiver. Other factors include the content of the message or the vocabulary to be decoded; the mood or attitude present in the situation; and the communication experience already in operation.

The receiver, in turn, perceives, interprets, and responds to the message. Through some process, feedback goes to the sender, confirming that the message has been received. The receiver at that point becomes the sender of a message. If the original message does not result in a response or feedback, there is no official interchange.

Communication involves feedback and each message sent, including feedback, affects the next message sent and its feedback. The process is circular; communication from A affects B and B, in turn, affects A.

Communication and related behavior can be studied only in context. Studying only the information, the command, the question—the words—is not enough. Behavior and the way of communicating are not static; they vary with the specific situation. In certain situations, seemingly inappropriate responses may be highly appropriate behavior. The apparently senseless talk of an emotionally ill person, for instance, may be the only feasible reaction in an absurd or untenable family communication context—the only way of achieving family equilibrium.

Or a child's aggressive behavior may be the only way of maintaining initiative and self when the mother communicates overprotection or "smothering" nonverbally. Communication is influenced by the family and social systems in which the person lives.

In the strictest sense, all behavior in the presence of others is communication and all communication affects behavior (84). How you gesture, posture, dress, move, speak, behave, or fail to carry out certain behaviors will provide an understandable signal for someone. To illustrate, two persons sitting side by side on a plane may neither speak nor look at one another. Yet there is a communiation process present, for the behavior of each conveys to the other a wish not to engage in an interchange of words, for whatever reason. Contrast this situation with two persons sitting side by side who do not speak but occasionally look at one another and smile. Then a few words are exchanged. The initial nonverbal expressions encourage the eventual verbal exchange. Thus anything perceptibly present or absent can serve as a signal of communication that need only be decoded to be meaningful.

Levels of Communication

Communication occurs on several levels because of the perceptions of each person involved in the communication, and each level becomes increasingly abstract (84), as demonstrated in Fig. 3-2. When two persons are communicating, the following levels may occur.

1. This is how I perceive me.
2. This is how I perceive you.
3. This is how I perceive you seeing and hearing me.
4. This is how I think you see me seeing you.

In a nurse-client dialogue, on level 1, you are thinking only of the self while talking to the other person. Self-awareness is important, but awareness must include more than that. Level 1 communication would not be very helpful to the person. On level 2, you are thinking of the self but also observing the client's behavior and hearing what is being said. This level of dialogue is more appropriate for communication of the other's needs. On level 3, you are aware of how the person might be perceiving you in addition to being aware of what both you and the person are saying, doing, and feeling. Thus you can better consider the effect of yourself on the other and his/her behavioral cues, and respond to them. In addition, you may ask for validation of personal perceptions—whether the client is actually perceiving you as you believe. For level 4 communication to occur, you must be very alert, feeling ener-

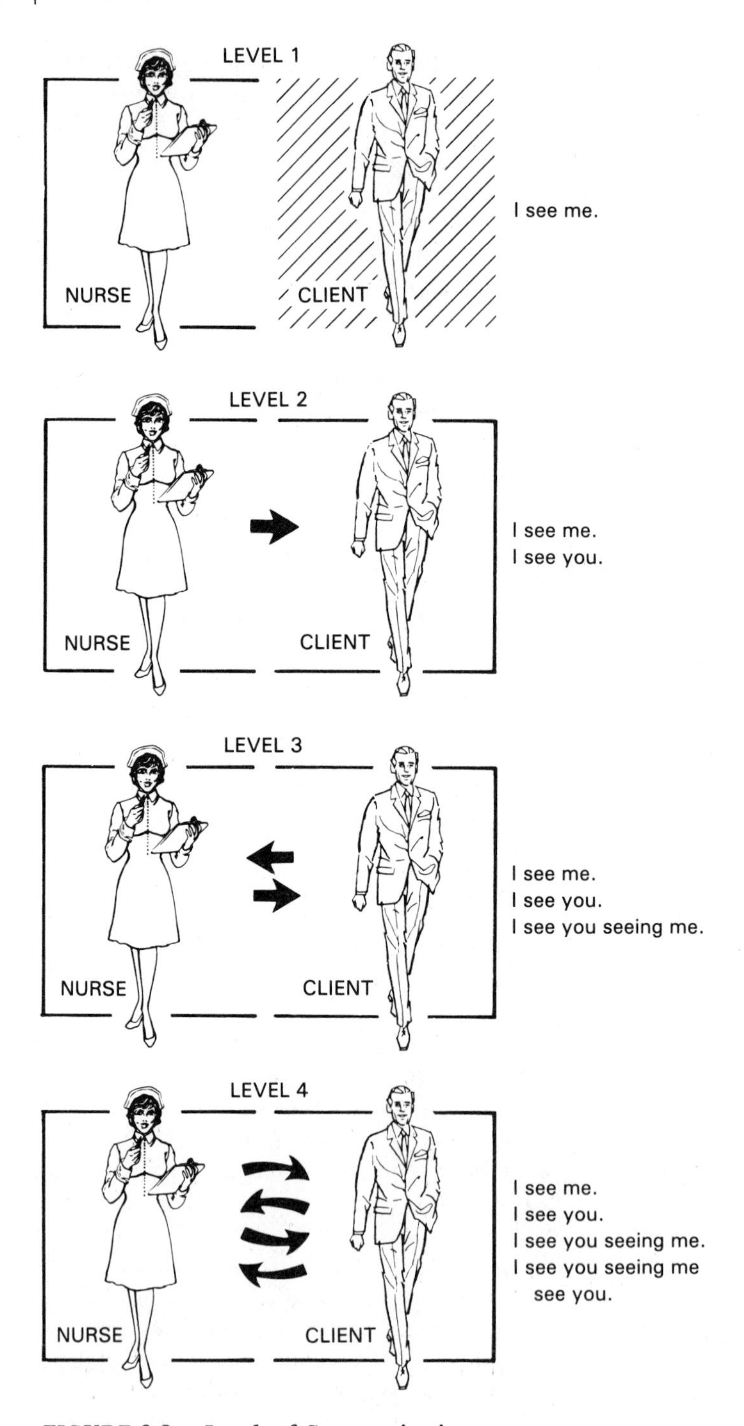

FIGURE 3-2 Levels of Communication

getic and attuned to the situation. Now, in addition to the foregoing levels, you consider how the person thinks you are perceiving him/her —your feelings and attitudes toward the person as *he/she* perceives them (84). Level 4 takes considerable empathy, but it will allow you to be most helpful in communicating with the client. These levels increase in complexity with increasing numbers of people. If you understand the levels of communication, you can anticipate the communication process, hear "hidden meanings," and recognize your impact on the process.

TOOLS OF COMMUNICATION

The tools of communication—language, observation and perception, nonverbal behavior, silence, and listening—are closely interrelated and are used simultaneously, although they are discussed separately in the following pages. Knowledge of these tools is essential before appropriately using the nursing process discussed in Chapter 4 and for your effective functioning in any system.

Language

Language is basic to communication. Without language, the higher order cognitive processes of thinking, reasoning, and generalizing could not be attained. Words are tools or symbols used to express ideas and feelings or to indicate objects; they are *not the same as the experience*, although words shape experience, communicate facts, convey interpretations, and influence relationships.

The functions of language can be classified as follows: expressive, arousal, and descriptive. A speech act is *expressive* if it informs us of a speaker's state of mind or emotions; it is also likely to serve the function of *arousal*, triggering an emotional response in the receiver of the message. The *descriptive* function serves to inform another person, to convey observations, memories, ideas, or inferences (84).

Visual images are more likely to serve the function of arousal than is language (24). Viewing a picture can arouse strong emotion, for much of the self can be projected into the image. Yet the visual image is unable to show the many contexts of description or tense of which verbal language is capable, for in listening, the personality of the speaker more easily strikes us.

The same words have different meaning for different people, and you must constantly be prepared to define the meaning of a word or phrase. Also, word meanings change over time in response to new inventions and to developments and changes in travel, mass media, and occupations. Thus language is a map of behavior and communication.

You select, consciously or unconsciously, the part of the world you wish to experience at any time. No two people are in exactly the same spot at exactly the same time; therefore all our experiences are, to some extent, different. Many problems in communication arise because we fail to remember that individual experiences are never identical. When two persons talk with one another, communication is established by determining mutual experience. If the experience being discussed is new to a person, he/she may have difficulty making sense of it. Much difficulty in introducing new ideas and much resistance to change arise from the fact that we must learn *what* to experience in the events we live through.

Words may be used both to express feelings and to avoid expressing them. When a man says he feels "fine," he may be functioning at optimum level—or he may be physically ill but wish to stop your further inquiry by responding with the word "fine." Words may also be used in deliberately obscure ways in order to convey hidden meanings, to test your interest in finding out such meanings, or the degree of your concern for the person, or to express hostility without fear of retaliation.

Nonlinguistic aspects of speech, such as silence, how much of the time and how fast the person talks, how soon the other person stops talking, interruptions, rate of speech errors, hesitations, such pauses as "ers" and ahs," and repetitions also give important signals. Many of these signals indicate anxiety or other feelings, as do loudness, high pitch, rapidity of speech, and breathiness. A depressed person talks slowly and at a low pitch and tolerates longer silences. An aggressive, dominating person talks loudly and rapidly, enunciates precisely, interrupts others more often, and may include ridicule, teasing, joking, or direct insult in speech (3).

In addition to the language of words, there is the language of size, time, space, and color.

The Language of Size, both physical and psychological, is related to the impact, influence, or potential for helping that one person has in regard to another. Large physical size conveys dominance, power, authority, and control. Large psychological size is perceived when someone is highly knowledgeable, extrovertive, aggressive, loud, rapid speaking, or moving; also, when someone is stern, distant, holds the body rigidly, places hands on hips, or keeps others at a distance by physical, verbal, or emotional maneuvers. The psychologically large person may be expected by others to solve problems, to see that all goes well, and to take care of them. Alternately, the psychologically large person may also be seen as someone to avoid, who stifles development and creativity, or who must have the final word. Regardless of the perception, size may interfere with communication (33). Examples of large psychological size include the business executive, teacher, doctor, or nurse as they relate with others in their environment (60).

The person who is large (psychologically and/or physically) will need to develop insight about and a feeling for others' perceptions and then develop methods to convey accessibility to and acceptance of others. Although changes in interpersonal communication take time and no one principle changes everything, using the principles of therapeutic communication described later in this chapter when interacting with others will be a positive move and help the person seem more empathic and approachable.

The Language of Time conveys feelings not expressed by words and may depend on the culture and one's concept of time. The nurse who frequently looks at her watch, who walks too fast for the patient to stay abreast, or who keeps a person waiting past the hour of an appointment may be conveying rejection, neglect, or lack of concern. Sitting at a patient's bedside conveys that you have time to listen.

The Language of Space—the distance between you and another—helps determine the nature of the communication. **Proxemics** *is the term for the study of human use and perception of social and personal space*. Physical distancing varies with the setting and the individual and is culturally learned. Placing a person near the center of a group is one way of saying that he/she is important. The amount of space given a person—the size of a desk or office, the size of the hospital room or ward cubicle—conveys differential importance or status to the person. The distance you maintain between the patient and yourself must be carefully determined, depending on the situation and the needs of the patient, for it may convey feelings to the patient that vary from concern to rejection (37, 74). You can also use physical space to foster communication and to bring people together. Place chairs in a circular arrangement to foster face-to-face contact, for example.

Territoriality *or* **personal space** *refers to an area with invisible boundaries surrounding the person's body*. According to studies by Hall, four distinct zones of interpersonal space exist, primarily in front of us. The intimate zone is reserved for someone who is highly attractive and ranges from 0 to 18 inches; the personal zone is from 18 inches to 4 feet; the social-consultative zone is from 4 to 12 feet; and the public zone from 12 feet and beyond. Different zones are appropriate for different interactions and relationships. The couple, the parent and child, or the nurse and patient, for instance, may interact in the intimate zone. The nurse and doctor may work together on a procedure with a patient in the personal zone but later remain in the social-consultative zone as they discuss the patient's progress. As you teach a class of expectant parents, you would tend to maintain the public zone. Attraction is also indicated by the zone. People who are attracted to each other at a business meeting stand farther apart than they would at a party. Everyone is expected to be closer at a party than at a meeting. Some details of the person's appearance are observable only in the intimate zone, although visual perception of the other may be slightly distorted. Persons talk softly or whisper; body heat and odors are transmitted. Touch is possible in the personal zone and visual perception and loudness of voice are normal. The social zone is used when impersonal business is conducted; sensory involvement is less intense. Distance of the public zone is outside the sphere of personal involvement. Others are perceived as somewhat smaller than life-size and verbal communication is formal (37, 38, 39, 60).

Knowledge of personal space or proxemics is useful in nursing. Research shows, for instance, that people need more space between them in a public area, such as a waiting room, than in an outdoor area. People tend to tolerate a stranger in their intimate or personal zones for about 10 minutes and then they are likely to move to a different location if at all possible. People use chairs or other objects or silence as barriers to protect their personal space. In one study chairs that were lined up in a nursing home corridor for residents and visitors were rearranged to promote corner-to-corner seating or face-to-face seating at a small table. After a 2-week period of adaptation interaction among the nursing home residents had doubled. The furniture rearrangement allowed for more eye contact and for more distance between individuals than had been possible in the row of chairs. (54). Minckley found that close proximity of beds (rows of beds 2 feet apart) in a recovery room, caused the patients to react with civil inattention to avoid one another's presence. Adjacent patients were not recognized; eyes remained closed; heads were under the covers or toward the wall (56). Patients apparently need more personal space in the morning than in the evening (54). The client's cultural background will influence use and need for personal space. Americans, Canadians, and British require the most personal space or territory; Latin Americans and Arabs need the least. People interpret another's spatial behavior according to their own cultural and personal patterns; friendly actions may be misconstrued as aggressive acts (54).

In health care, especially hospital admission, where the patient is deprived of most personal possessions, role, and social function, where close contact is necessary for many nursing interventions, and the person's body is hardly considered his/her own, it is essential to be mindful of the person's need for territory and privacy whenever possible in order to reduce feelings of threat and anxiety. Knock before entering the patient's room. Don't handle the patient's possessions without permission. Do not smoke in the patient's presence. Keep conversation focused on or with the patient rather than talking about an unrelated topic to another person in the presence of the patient. Raising the head of the bed to a height acceptable to the patient extends the sense of personal boundaries. Arrange furniture to decrease crowding when possible. Screen the patient adequately with drapes, curtains, solid dividers, closed doors, or other barriers when performing any procedure. Encourage the patient to place personal objects on the nightstand or chest table as a way to stake out his/her territory. Adapt your interventions to promote the person's sense of personal space and preserve personal identity.

The Language of Color elicits fairly specific responses. In American culture warm colors, such as yellow, red, and orange, stimulate creative, happy responses. Cool colors, such as blue, green, and gray, tend to encourage meditation and deliberation and have a dampening effect on equality of communication. Color in the environment can be better planned to be therapeutic and to enhance communication in nursing if you are aware of what is being conveyed to the client through the colors in the surroundings (7). You should also be aware of what the color of your uniform (or other dress) and hair means to the person. White clothing for example, may arouse fear in children with past illness experiences. Or the patient may perceive any redheaded nurse as quick-tempered or "sexy" until learning otherwise through observation.

Observation and Perception

The second tool of communication is observation and perception. **Observation** *is the act of noting and recording facts and events.* **Perception** *is the personal interpretation of observations.* Rarely do observations exist alone. Frequently the person attaches meaning to or makes judgments about observed events, based on one's knowledge, experience, and/or bias. The observer is part of the observed. What you communicate depends on the quality of your observations and your interpretation of them. Observations are made because of curiosity, a desire to understand others, a need for adequacy, security or self-preservation, or any combination of them. In nursing, each client's needs vary and constantly change. Because you are the one health team member who has continuous contact with the client and because the diagnosis, treatment, and prognosis frequently are determined by your observations, your keen perception will help guide the other team workers in their services.

Factors influencing observation and perception are similar to those influencing the communication process generally and include the following ones:

1. Physical, mental, emotional, social, and spiritual status, capabilities, limits, goals, and needs of the person.
2. Cultural, social, and philosophical background and values.
3. Number and functioning ability of the senses involved, length of time of contact with or exposure to the stimuli or event.
4. Past experiences associated with the present situation.
5. Meaning of the observed event to the self.
6. Interests, preoccupations, preconceptions, and motivational level.
7. Knowledge of or familiarity with the situation being observed.
8. Practice in purposeful observation; ability to focus on stimuli and maintain concentration.
9. Environmental conditions and distractions.
10. Availability of technical devices.
11. Presence, attitudes, and reactions of others—for if observations and perceptions are accurate but do not agree with group consensus, the person is likely to conform to the group.

One aspect of communication to remember in nursing is that when two sounds are presented simultaneously to both ears, any verbal signals, such as words, nonsense syllables, and separate speech sound, are more readily heard and identified by the right ear whereas music and environmental noises are better recognized by the left ear—*if* the person hears equally well with both ears (44). This information may be critical when you care for people who are depressed, medicated, or comatose.

Observations must fulfill certain criteria in nursing. They must be purposeful, planned, objective, accurate, complete and orderly. In *purposeful* observation, you decide what to observe, which are the general and which the specific factors, and why the observation is important. The *planned* observation considers timing, duration, interval between observations, and kind and location of observations. An observation is *objective* when it can be validated directly, indirectly, or through replication by others and is not based on personal bias. *Accuracy* involves use of knowledge, concentration, memory, and problem solving. A *complete* observation meets the purposes for which it is made. *Orderly* or systematic observation permits relating parts of data gathered, observing the commonplace and general data, and then focusing on minute details (63). Whenever you make an interpretation, it should be stated as such.

Perception of the same event varies from person to person and within the same person at different times, depending on personal feelings, preparation, and desires. In addition, the person often simplifies what is not understood, leaving out important facts or substituting others, even if distortion results. Recognize this factor in relation to yourself, the client, the family, and coworkers because perception of the event determines action.

Peplau describes four types of relationships between the observer and the observed in nursing.

1. The spectator relationship in which the person is not aware of being observed and the nurse is outside the focus of attention. This situation could occur when you observe the sleeping or critically ill patient.
2. The interviewer relationship in which the person is more or less aware of being studied and that you are taking notes of what he/she is saying in response to a situation or question. This situation could occur during the admission procedure or nursing rounds.
3. The collector relationship in which you use records or reports prepared by other health care workers to learn what has happened to the client. It occurs in the change-of-shift conference, team conference, or when reading the chart to assist in planning care.
4. The participant-observer relationship in which you engage in ordinary acts connected with nursing, such as morning care, and at the same time observe the relationship between the client and self. The person is aware of receiving care but not necessarily aware that his/her response to a situation and your attitudes about giving care are being observed and studied (63).

Action or Nonverbal Behavior

Movement or action is the third tool of communication—for example, finger pointing, head nodding, and other gestures; eye contact, a wink, gaze, eyebrow movement, smile, and other facial expressions; a touch or a slap on the back, general posture, body movement, and body sounds, such as belching, knuckle cracking, and laughing.

Nonverbal communication is powerful and honest and is culturally learned. Signals are often sent without the person's being aware of it. Research findings indicate that nonverbal behavior conveys 65 percent of the message (45). The skin flush, the tiny tremor around the eyes or corners of the mouth, and the brief hesitations in speech indicate stress or agitation in the person. Certain preening behavior has sexual overtones: stroking the hair, adjusting clothing, or changing position to accentuate maleness or femaleness (70). Our pupils dilate when we see an attractive person or object or are being presented with an attractive idea or positive line of reasoning, and they constrict whenever something unpleasant is encountered (42).

Several taboos related to nonverbal behavior exist in the United States. Touching, standing close to, or looking directly at a stranger, a person of the same sex, or someone we are not attracted to are all considered impolite and intrusive. As a relationship grows closer, the area open to touch increases, the amount of direct eye contact increases, and the distance between the two people decreases.

Eye Behavior

For most people, the eyes are an important part of nonverbal behavior and body image. The size, shape, and color of eyes often elicit a response from others as well as from self. Throughout history we have been preoccupied with the eye and its effects on human behavior, reflected by such phrases as

> She/He looks right through you.
> That was an icy stare.
> He's got shifty eyes.
> She's all eyes.
> Did you see the gleam in his eye?
> Now we're seeing eye to eye.
> He looked like the original Evil Eye.
> His eyes shot daggers across the room.
> She could kill with a glance.
> The eyes are the mirror of the soul.

Literature reveals numerous cases in which the eye is used as a symbol for either male or female sex organs.

Eye behavior begins at birth. An infant responds positively to its mother's eyes very early. Throughout childhood the person is subtly taught how to use the eyes during interactions, when to gaze and when not to gaze, and at whom and what to look.

Various eye movements and eye behaviors are associated with expression of feelings. Large pupil size may indicate, physiologically, either disease or use of drugs. Large pupil size may also indicate fear, anxiety, or arousal and feeling pleased with visual stimuli or the situation (42). Eyes opened wide with eyebrows raised are associated with wonder, naivete, frankness, fear, or terror. In anger, eyes fix in a hard, direct stare with the upper lid lowered and eyebrows drawn down (simultaneously, the lips are tightly compressed). A constant stare with immobile facial muscles indicates coldness. Eyes rolled upward may be associated with fatigue, a suggestion that another's behavior is inappropriate, or efforts at organizing thoughts. With feelings of disgust, eyes narrow (and the upper lip curls upward while the nose moves). During sadness the eyes look down, inner corners of the eyebrows raise (simultaneously, lips turn down and the lower lip may tremble). With embarrassment, modesty, or self-consciousness, the eyes look down and away —surprise is shown by raised eyebrows and direct gaze. Aggressive acts include threatening *gestures*, such as a direct look, a sharp movement of the head toward the other person, a frown, and handraising. Flight or defensive behaviors include closed eyes, bodily evasions, withdrawing chin into chest, and crouching (23, 24, 45).

Each society establishes eye-related norms. Eye contact in the United States is considered a sign of positive self-concept, a friendly mood, interest in the other person, persuasiveness, credibility, an obligation to engage in an interaction, monitoring of feedback, and attentiveness to events and communication with another. Decreasing, or brief avoidance of, eye gaze means lack of interest, insulation of self against threats, a wish to avoid interaction, impending leave taking, embarrassment, guilt, humility, deep thinking, talking rather than listening, or that the other person has a turn in the conversation if the person has been talking. Prolonged avoidance of eye contact is interpreted as a negative self-concept or feelings of worthlessness or inferiority, rudeness, or even a sign of mental illness. Yet our society also has norms about not looking too long at strangers in public places and not looking at various body parts under certain conditions. In interaction between Caucasians and people from other cultures, such as American Indians or Blacks, eye contact is avoided with the Caucasian until the other feels comfortable in the interpersonal situation.

In Latin America, southern Europe, Arab countries, and the Philippines, the use of eyes and eye contact during conversation is important. Eye contact is minimized in northern European countries. And it is taboo to various degrees in Far Eastern countries, such as Pakistan, India, or Vietnam. More than brief eye contact is generally avoided initially by the rural Appalachian, American Indian, or Black American.

Studies of blind children show that their spontaneous nonverbal expressions of feelings are the same as for sighted children. Remarkable similarities have been observed in the eye behavior of adults, infants, and children, blind persons, and nonhuman primates. These observations show the universality of nonverbal behavior, especially because blind children could not learn these behaviors from visual cues (23, 45).

Body Language

Through **body language,** *moving or positioning the body or some portion of it, a person conveys what he/she cannot or will not verbalize,* although this body language may be used simultaneously with verbal activity. Expression of self through movement is learned before speech so that under stress the person often reverts to preverbal communication. Thus an individual may overtly manifest the expression that he/she feels is expected in the existing situation—for example, the smile that is only a facade—rather than show what is really felt. Nevertheless, nonverbal behavior is more likely to express hidden meanings, although they must be interpreted with extreme care. Laughter is not always a sign of humor or happiness; it may be a device to cover anxiety, show ridicule, or seek attention.

Aggressive, controlling, manipulative acts include threatening gestures, such as a direct look, a sharp movement of the head toward the other person, a frown, and handraising. Flight behaviors include retreat, bodily evasions, closed eyes, withdrawing chin into chest, and crouching. These defensive behaviors often occur when a dominant person sits too close to a subordinate. Notice these behaviors, along with other signs of tension, such as rocking, leg swinging, or foot tapping, so that you do not push yourself onto the client (74).

Posture also indicates feeling. A slightly relaxed, leaning-forward position indicates closeness, interest in, or attraction to a person, object, or event. The male indicates attraction by the closed posture: arms in front of body with legs closed. The female indicates attraction with a more open posture: arms down at the side, and sitting with legs apart or not crossed at the knees (38).

Body language is often a reliable index of the real meaning of what is being said or communicated because the person is generally unable to exert as much conscious control over this aspect of behavior as over the words used. But knowledge of the person's sociocultural heritage is essential here, for various body parts are used differently in different cultures to enhance conversation. The use of the eyes is all important, for example, in India and Greece, but in Africa the torso is frequently moved. And in America head nodding is common. The amount of movement also varies culturally.

Normal distance for conversation is much closer in Latin countries than in the United States. You may feel uncomfortable when the South American client stands in the intimate zone while describing symptoms to you. Touching between same-sexed pairs, including male pairs, rather than between opposite-sexed pairs, is more common among Arabs or South Vietnamese than among Americans. It may be misinterpreted as homosexual behavior in the United States. Subtle cultural variations in the use of nonverbal signals often lead to serious misunderstandings and resentments. Misinterpretations of nonverbal signals can sometimes be avoided only by verbal validation of their meaning, but speaking of the nonverbal signal may often cause embarrassment because many of these signals are sent without much, or any, thought (23, 37, 39).

Other cultural differences are also seen. Gestures are used by Americans and the English to denote activity and by Italian or Jewish persons to emphasize words. The use of facial expression varies with the culture. Italian, Jewish, Black, and Spanish-speaking persons smile readily or use facial movements, along with gestures and words, to express feelings—happy, unhappy, or physical pain. Oriental, American Indian, English, Irish, and northern European persons show less facial expression and verbalize less, in response to feelings, particularly with strangers (60).

In Asia it is customary to conceal emotions and bad news with a smile. Even verbal techniques vary. Americans put commands in the form of queries or suggestions. The English talk with considerable understatement so that they will not be considered boastful. Arab speech contains much emphasis and exaggeration. The Japanese kiss to show deference to superiors, a signal that would be interpreted as an insult and be rejected by the superior in the United States (3, 23, 38). Sentence length and speech forms also vary with the social class of a country. The working class typically uses short, simple sentences and is more direct than the more educated class of people (3).

You must observe the nonverbal behavior of the whole person in order to interpret communication correctly, for an isolated gesture or expression may require a completely different interpretation in proper context. In addition, you must also validate your impressions with other health team members who have observed the person, as well as the person, for the same nonverbal behavior can be interpreted differently by different people. Also, look for inconsistencies between nonverbal and verbal behavior. A person's eyes may be cold, for example, even though he smiles and sounds friendly. And the meaning of words may be altered or even contradicted by the way the words are said.

Touch

Touch is an important nonverbal tool in communication, for touching another with some part of the body or an extension of it is an outside event that stimulates a response. Touch, like movement, begins in utero and precedes speech as a form of communication; thus the relationship between touch and communication begins in infancy and remains throughout life as a means of returning to direct experience. Without tactile stimulation that is gentle and nurturing, the child may not live or may have seriously impaired development. Touching stimulates an infant's chemistry for mental and physical growth (6, 32, 57, 85).

On reaching school age, the child is touched less and less even by the parents. Americans teach their children not to touch themselves unnecessarily and to keep their hands off grownups' objects and others' possessions, in general, thereby dampening the child's natural curiosity and desire to explore (57).

Americans tend to associate touch or physical contact with sexual connotations. Other cultures also consider touching taboo; the English and Germans carry untouchability even further than Americans. On the other hand, highly tactile cultures exist—the Spanish, Mexican, Italian, Greek, French, Jewish, Puerto Rican, and South American (18, 60).

Within our culture differences also exist among socioeconomic classes in the use of and response to touch as a form of nonverbal communication. People in upper and middle socioeconomic levels use touch less in communicating and are generally less responsive to this type of behavior as a positive reinforcement tool than people in the lower socioeconomic level (57, 60).

Touch is considered magical and healing in some cultures. In American culture, however, there is still a considerable taboo on casual touching, partly because of residual Victorian sexual prudery (19). Certain health care workers, however, are beginning to combine laying on of hands (touch) and prayer with other forms of scientific treatment (46).

Touch must be used judiciously and not forced on anyone. Yet a great deal of communication, closeness, empathy, mutual encouragement, trust, protection, reality contact, comforting, gentleness, and caring can be conveyed between two people in rapport when they touch. Touch may convey a connection, excitement, approval, happiness, competence, or frustration, anger, punishment, physical or psychological assault, and the invasion of personal territory and privacy (16, 20). Touch can help to reintegrate body image and differentiate self from another. The message conveyed through touch depends on the attitude of the people involved and the meaning of touch both to the person touching and to the person touched. In general, the need for intimacy and touch is so strong that the satisfaction of that need is a greater influence on behavior than is the fear of closeness or possible rejection.

When another human being reaches out to you, it is hoped that you will be there as a fellow, caring human being. Touch can communicate feelings between people who care about one another, when words would fail. The therapeutic use of touch is indispensable in the healing professions. Thus touch is an important tool in the nurse–patient relationship and in the healing art of communication. The back rub, the hand on the shoulder, the squeeze of a hand, each encourages closeness and communication between you and your patient or client.

Silence

Silence is the fourth tool of communication even though silence may also interfere with communication. Because one of your essential tasks is to encourage verbal description, you need to intervene effectively when encountering silence. There are different kinds of silence (55, 83).

The blank, empty, or blocked silence occurs when the client says that there is nothing to say and yet nonverbal behavior reflects anxiety. In this type of silence you initiate speech and somewhat structure the interchange. You might ask "What are you thinking?" or "What is going on with you now?" A comment can be made about the person's daily routine. You may even suggest that the person think of something to say as a way to break the impasse.

The stubborn, resistive silence occurs when a feeling of anger is present. The person trying to set up a power struggle to gain control over you, a ploy that can stimulate reciprocal anger unless you understand the basis for the anger. A response of impatience perpetuates the power struggle. Sit out the anger; be undemanding but interested. Ask, "I wonder what is going on with you?" or "What are you feeling?" When the person recognizes the anger and understands its possible cause, he/she is more likely to give up resistive silence (55).

Fearful silence occurs when a person's previous experiences in similar or identical situations were excessively intimidating. Perhaps other people or hallucinations were threatening when he/she talked. Stay with the person, recognize efforts to talk, show a kind, positive approach, and accept what is said in order to reduce fears.

A thoughtful silence, when the person is resolving difficulties or doing problem solving, is productive. Do not interrupt unless the silence is prolonged. Then suggest that the person share thoughts with you.

Do not cut off silence prematurely because of your own anxiety. Much can be learned from the silence by examining the data preceding the silence and observing the person during the silence.

Listening

Listening is the fifth tool of communication. We have two ears and one mouth, which should give us a clue! Everyone loves a listener, but few persons are skilled listeners.

Because listening gives no chance for self-assertion, instruction, or giving opinion, most people think listening is a passive act requiring no special talent. The evidence is to the contrary. You must learn to listen attentively and curb the desire to speak.

The act of listening consists of more than just hearing. Listening occurs only when the mind is purposefully attentive to what is being said or communicated. The mind is a selective organizer and responder to experience. On the average, we receive thousands of exteroceptive and proprioceptive impressions every second. Thus a drastic selective process is necessary to prevent the brain's higher centers from being overwhelmed by irrelevant data. Decisions concerning what is relevant and essential and what is irrelevant vary from person to person and are determined by processes and criteria outside the person's awareness. A person may say something that another does not hear because of the latter's selective response, a selective inattention. Selective hearing and listening are influenced considerably by past experience and associations as well as by the need to decrease anxiety over what is being said in the present situation.

Listening is a faster process than speaking. No matter how fast the speaker's mind is racing, it is not possible to articulate more than about 200 words per minute, but the listener can take in words as quickly as he/she can think. The endings of most sentences can be guessed before they are completed. In fact, a person may hear the end of the sentence inaccurately because of the false sense of security and selective inattention caused by this phenomenon. In the nursing situation you should listen attentively throughout the length of each sentence rather than guess or assume what will be said.

Listening manners are vital and may have a subtle but powerful impact on the other person. Elements of good listening described by many authors, include the following points (25, 26, 28, 49, 52, 60, 76, 87).

1. Show the person that you are listening by looking at him/her; avoid extraneous or distracting movements. Some clients need continuous eye contact as an indication of your attentiveness; others feel uncomfortable and may prefer that you occasionally shift your gaze.
2. Change facial expression in accordance with the topic and personal

reactions. A client benefits from nonverbal expressions of face and body that are congruent with your words and feelings.

3. Put aside personal filters—values, biases, ideas, attitudes, and experiences—to the extent possible to avoid missing what the other is saying. Personal filters contribute to moralistic judgments, making assumptions before the other has finished speaking, or formulating an answer or interpreting too soon.
4. Be patient—willing to wait until the person has spoken. Then formulate your response. Silence during the dialogue promotes thoughtfulness.
5. Use multidimensional listening. Try to understand not only the content but also the intent, feelings, inconsistencies, and nonverbal behavior. Attend to all aspects of the communication, not just the obvious words. Some people call this "listening with the third ear."
6. Use validation. Restate what you heard and ask "Did I hear and understand you correctly (21, 30, 31, 64, 78)?"

A message is not a spear of thought thrust into the listener's mind by a speaker or writer. Meaning is transferred only when the listener rearranges his/her mind in accordance with the speaker's voice or printed word signals. Your attitude while listening to another person is an important form of feedback. Realize that you may have no control if a client, because of illness or particular feelings, blocks your efforts at communication. But learn to adapt and to control your own behavior in order to listen attentively and to stimulate the communication of others.

INTERVIEWING AS PART OF THE COMMUNICATION PROCESS

All activities in nursing involve communication and verbal communication with patients often involves interviewing.

Definition and Factors Involved in Interviewing

An **interview** *is a transitory relationship between two persons in which one seeks information from another without gaining personal advantage and the other gives information without suffering disadvantage*. The interview is a conversation directed to a definite purpose other than satisfaction in the meeting itself. Interviewing in the nursing situation involves the following five factors.

1. The interview is usually conducted in connection with other nursing activities in which you do something for the client so that he/she can see and feel the immediate effect of nursing efforts; or you use interviewing to determine how best to give care or to evaluate the effectiveness of care given.
2. Either you or the client can initiate the interview.
3. The situation of the interview is flexible in regard to the setting, interruptions, and availability of time for client and nurse. The setting may be the waiting room, home, office, factory, or bedside. Interruptions may occur from other health team members, other clients, or visitors. Time limits may be beyond your control, because of intervening demands, so that you may have to return several times to the person to achieve the purpose of the interview.
4. The client is usually physically and emotionally confined or restricted and is relatively dependent on you and the climate created by you.
5. There is a continuum of people who represent "the nurse" over a 24-hour period. Each nurse, in the process of continuity of care, participates within the framework of the total plan of care. Thus each nurse may achieve a portion of the purposes of the interview —for example, teaching or gathering information—and the entire nursing team together works toward the total purpose.

Purposes of the Interview

In nursing the purposes achieved through an interview are as follows:

1. Establishing rapport to convey to the person a sense of worth and the fact that someone cares; developing or maintaining feelings of self-esteem; diminishing feelings of isolation.
2. Establishing and maintaining the nurse-client relationship.
3. Listening in order to provide release of tension or allow expression of feelings.
4. Obtaining information; identifying and clarifying needs.
5. Giving information or teaching.
6. Counseling to clarify a problem; encouraging self-understanding and constructive problem solving in the person.
7. Referring the person to other resources of help as necessary (10, 12, 26, 34).

Your Role as Interviewer

Your self—your personality—is the principal tool of the therapeutic interview or communication. Your character structure, values, and sensitivity to the feelings of others influence your attitude and helpfulness toward people.

As a beginner, you are more likely to have certain problems in interviewing and therapeutic communication than your more experienced colleagues. Often there is a strong fear that you will do something wrong or be criticized by others. Defense mechanisms used to control your anxiety reduce your sensitivity to the emotional responses of others. Fear of being inadequate can be projected onto the client. You may feel competitive toward professional peers and wish to perform better. You may feel guilty about "using" or "practicing on" the client. With experience, you will learn to overcome or cope with these feelings and become increasingly aware of relationships and subtleties. Refer again to Table 3-2 for clarification on levels communication.

At first you may bombard the patient with questions. Later you will learn when a person has completed the answer to your question or when encouragement is needed to go on. As competence grows with experience, you will be able to hear the content of words and simultaneously consider how the person feels, deduce what is being inferred or omitted, and gauge your emotional response. In addition, you will be able to intervene actively when necessary rather than sit and passively listen.

In order to gain this competence, take careful notes during or after each interview. And regular sessions should be held with a teacher or supervisor who can guide you and promote self-understanding.

Techniques of Interviewing

Prepare for the interview as much as possible through use of records, by applying general knowledge to the specific situation, and by being alert and observant. Know or define what information is needed to achieve the purpose of the interview. What you ask or say depends on the purpose of the interview. Avoid, however, the "self-fulfilling prophecy," setting up the interview situation in such a way that the person tells you (or *seems* to tell you) only what you have predetermined will or can be told you. If selective inattention causes you to see or hear only what you wish, much information will be missed or misinterpreted and you will not be fully helpful to the person.

The personality and attitude of the interviewer influence the interviewee's responses. The emotional climate and immediate conditions surrounding the interview also affect you and the other person. The following techniques will help promote productive interviews (34, 41, 64, 65).

1. Establish rapport. Create a warm, accepting climate and a feeling of security and confidentiality so that the person feels free to talk about whatever seems important.

2. Arrange comfortable positions for both yourself and the person so that full attention can be given to the interview.
3. Control the external environment as much as possible. Doing so is sometimes difficult or impossible, but try to minimize external distractions or noise, regulate ventilation and lighting, and arrange the setting to reduce physical distance.
4. Consider wearing casual clothing without excessive adornment instead of a uniform when working in the school, home, or occupational setting. Consider what expectations the interviewee may have of you. In some cases, the person will respond more readily to your casual dress; at other times your professional dress may be needed as part of the image to help that person talk confidentially.
5. Use a vocabulary on the level of awareness or understanding of the person. Avoid occupational jargon or words too abstract for the interviewee's level of understanding or health condition.
6. Avoid preconceived ideas, prejudices, or biases. Avoid imposing personal values on others.
7. Begin by stating the purpose of the interview. Either you or the interviewee may introduce the theme. You may start the session by expressing friendly interest in the everyday affairs of the person or by discussing events related to the person to establish rapport, but avoid continuing trivial conversation. Maintain the proposed structure.
8. Be precise in what you say so that the meaning is understood. Ask questions that are well-timed, open-ended, and pertinent to the situation. This pattern allows the person to stamp his/her own style, organization, and personality on the answers and on the interview. Getting unanticipated data can be as useful in an interview as in giving care. Meaningless questions get meaningless answers. Questions that bombard the person produce unreliable information. Open-ended sentences usually keep the person talking at his/her own pace. Carefully timing your messages, verbal and nonverbal, and allowing time for the interviewee to understand and respond are essential in nursing.
9. Avoid asking questions in ways that induce socially acceptable answers. The interviewee often responds to questions with what he/she thinks the interviewer wants to hear, either to be well thought of, to gain status, or to show that he/she knows what other people do and what is considered socially acceptable.
10. Be diplomatic when asking questions about home life or personal matters. What you consider common information may be considered very private by some. Matters about which it would be tactless to inquire directly can often be arrived at indirectly by peripheral questions. If a subject you suggest meets resistance,

change the topic; when the anxiety is reduced, you can return to the matter for further discussion. Remember, what the person does not say is as important as what is said.

11. Be an attentive listener. Show interest by occasionally nodding or responding with "I see" or "uh-huh." Remain silent and control your responses when another's comments evoke a personal meaning and thus trigger an emotional response in you. While the person is talking, find the nonverbal answers to the following: What does this experience mean for him/her? Why is he/she telling me this at this time? What is the meaning of the choice of words, the repetition of key words, the voice inflection, the hesitant or aggressive expression of words, the topic chosen? Listen for feelings, needs, and goals. Recognize the levels of meaning in communication previously discussed. Do not answer too fast or ask a question too soon. If necessary, learn if the words mean the same to you as to the interviewee. Explore each clue as you let the person tell his/her story.
12. Carefully observe nonverbal messages for signs of anxiety, frustration, anger, loneliness, or guilt. Look for feelings of pressure hidden by the person's attempts to be calm. Encourage the free expression of feelings, for feelings often bring facts with them.
13. Encourage spontaneity. Provide movement in the interview by picking up verbal leads, clues, bits of seemingly unrelated information, and nonverbal signals from the client. If the person asks you a personal question, redirect it, for it may be the topic that the interviewee unconsciously (or even consciously) wishes to speak about. Only occasionally will it be pertinent for you to answer personal questions. Brief self-disclosure may help the person feel more comfortable and may elicit additional information for the client's benefit.
14. Ask questions beginning with What, Where, Who, and When to gain factual information. Words connoting moral judgments should be avoided; they are not conducive to a feeling of neutrality, acceptance, or freedom of expression. The How question may be difficult for the person to answer, for it asks "In what manner . . . ?" or "For what reason . . . ?" and the individual may lack sufficient knowledge to answer. The Why question should also be avoided, for it asks for insights that the person should not be expected to give.
15. Indicate when the interview is terminated and terminate it graciously if the interviewee does not do so first. Make a transition in interviewing or use a natural stopping point if the problem has been resolved, if the information has been obtained or given, or if the person changes the topic. You may say "There is one more

question I'd like to ask . . . ," or "Just two more points I want to clarify . . . ," or "Before I leave, do you have any other questions, comments, or ideas to share?"

16. Keep data obtained in the interview confidential and share it only with the appropriate and necessary health team members, leaving out personal assumptions. If you are sharing an opinion or interpretation, state it as such rather than have it appear to be what the other person said or did. The person should be told what information will be shared and with whom.
17. Evaluate the interview. Were the purposes accomplished? Recognize that not everyone can successfully interview everyone. Others may see you differently from the way you see yourself, thus preventing you from being helpful or obtaining information. Evaluate yourself in each situation.

You must be sincere, knowledgeable about the purpose of the interview, and skillful in using tools of communication during the interview as well as in establishing and maintaining a climate conducive to successful data collection. The effective interview takes a great deal of energy and attention.

THERAPEUTIC COMMUNICATION

Analysis of your communication pattern will help you improve your methods. Realize that you cannot become skilled in therapeutic communication without supervised and thoughtful practice. As you talk with another, however, don't get so busy thinking about a list of methods that you forget to focus on the person. Your keen interest in the other person and use of your personal style are essential if you are to be truly effective.

To be effective while communicating with the patient or family, use simple, clear words geared to the person's intelligence and experience. Develop a well-modulated tone of voice, especially with the sick person, for auditory sensitivity is increased during illness. Several authors have described principles, attitudes, and methods essential in therapeutic communication that are useful with individual persons as well as with groups (11, 12, 21, 25, 31, 35, 41, 49, 50, 63, 64, 65, 80, 86).

Effective Methods

The following methods are basic for conducting purposeful, helpful communication with a person, well or ill, along with their rationale. Some elaborate on earlier suggestions for interviewing.

Use Thoughtful Silence to Encourage the Person to Talk. Silence gives you and the person time to organize thoughts. It directs the person to the task at hand but allows him/her to set the pace, aids consideration of alternative courses of action and delving into feelings, conserves energy during serious illness, and gives time for contemplation and relaxation. There is a time not to talk. Always focus on the person you are talking with, especially during silence.

Be Accepting. This is a difficult task at times. Realize that *all* behavior is motivated and purposeful. Indicate that you are following the person's trend of thought. Encourage the client to continue to talk while you remain nonjudgmental, although not necessarily in agreement.

Help the Person Strengthen Self-identification in Relation to Others. *Always use you, I,* and *we* in their proper context. Do not say "We can take a bath now" but rather "You can take a bath now."

Suggest Collaboration and a Cooperative Relationship. Offer to share and work together with the person; offer to do things *with* and not *for* or *to* him/her. Encourage participation in identifying and appraising problems and involvement as an active partner in treatment. Tell the person you are available to help. "I'll stay with you" or "I'm interested in your comfort" are examples of statements that can help to reassure that you will stay and care regardless of the person's behavior.

State Open-ended, Generalized Leading Questions to encourage the person to take the initiative in introducing topics and to think through problems. Examples include: "Is there something you'd like to talk about?" "Tell me about it." "Where would you like to begin?" "Go on." "And what else?" "Would you like to talk about yourself now?" "After that?" Avoid conventional pleasantries after initial greetings because they constrict the person's expression of feelings and ideas. It is important for the person to talk about his/her mental and emotional distress and turmoil and questions, for often he/she cannot cope with feelings until the feelings are stated.

State Related Questions. Do not let a subject drop until it is adequately explored. Peripheral or side questions help the person work through larger issues and engage in problem solving. Explore by delving further into the subject or idea without seeming to pry. Many clients deal superficially with a topic to test if you are truly interested. Avoid questions that call for a yes or no answer. Explorative questions call for answers that elaborate, thereby helping the person to increase understanding and do further problem solving or clarifying.

Place Events Described in Time Sequence. In order to clarify relationships associated with a given event, determine how it happened, place it in perspective, determine the extent to which one event led to another, and seek to identify recurrent patterns or difficulty or significant cause-and-effect relationships. Ask such questions as "What happened then?" or "What did you do after that?"

State Observations That You Perceive About the Person. Statements such as "You appear . . . ," "It seems to me that . . . ," "I notice that you are . . . ," and "It makes me uncomfortable when you . . ." encourage mutual understanding of behavior. Such observations offer a basis on which the person can respond without your having to probe, and they call attention to what is happening to help him/her notice or clarify personal behavior. Using this technique, you and the other person can compare observations and you can encourage a description of self-awareness. In addition, when you openly acknowledge that another's efforts at a task or behavior are appropriate to the situation, you reinforce the behavior and add to the person's self-esteem.

Encourage Description of Behavior or Observation through statements like "What did you feel?" "Tell me what you now feel," "What does the voice seem to be saying?" and "What is happening?" You can better understand the person when you observe and understand matters as they seem to the client. There is the need to act out impulses and feelings if the person feels free to state them.

Restate or Repeat the Main Idea Expressed to convey that it was communicated to you effectively, thereby encouraging the person to continue. Restate the idea until the person does clarify. Reformulating certain statements and using different words bring out related aspects of material that might otherwise have escaped the client's (or your) attention.

Reflect by Paraphrasing Feelings, Questions, Ideas, and Key Words to encourage further talking. Indicate that the person's point of view is important; acknowledge the right to personal opinions and decisions. Encourage the person to accept personal feelings and ideas. Show interest in hearing as much as the person wishes to tell you. Emphasize the word *you* while conversing, as in "*You* feel . . . ," in order to reflect what the person has said. (However, do not just mindlessly parrot his/her words.)

Verbalize the Implied or what the person has hinted at or suggested in order to make the discussion less obscure, to clarify the conversation, to show that you are listening and interested, and that you accept what is said. Questions can be used as a subtle form of suggestion. As an example, you might ask "Have you ever told your wife how you feel?" or "Have you ever asked your boss for a raise?" Regardless of the answer, you have indicated that such an act is conceivable, permissible, and perhaps even expected.

Attempt to Translate Feelings into Words. Sometimes what the person says seems meaningless when taken literally. Hidden meanings of verbal expressions, as well as their actual content, must be considered and can be explored by describing the implicit feelings.

Clarify when necessary through statements like "I don't understand what is troubling you" or "Could you explain that again?" The person is usually aware if he/she is not being understood and may withdraw or cease to communicate. It is not necessary to understand everything stated as long as you are honest about it and do not pretend to understand when you do not. Attempting to discover what the person is talking about can help him/her become clearer to self.

Reintroduce Reality by voicing doubt or by calmly presenting your own perceptions or the facts in the situation when the person is being unrealistic. Indicate an alternate line of thought for consideration; do not attempt to convince him/her of error by arguing. Such action only provokes resistance and a determination to maintain the idea. Encourage the person to recognize that others do not necessarily perceive events as he/she does or draw the same conclusions. Encourage reconsideration and reevaluation (even though it may not change his/her mind) through statements like "What gives you that impression?" "Isn't that unusual?" and "That's hard to believe." Expressing doubts may reinforce doubts the person already has but has discounted because no one else shared them before. A doubting tone of voice can be as effective as any specific statement.

Offer Information. Make facts available whenever the person needs or asks for them. Well-timed teaching builds trust, orients, and gives additional knowledge from which to make decisions or draw realistic conclusions. Inappropriate, excessive, or partial information or advice may cause alarm or needlessly suggest problems to the person. Give the person information about what can be expected and what he/she can do to help self. At times it may be appropriate for you to disclose briefly your own thoughts, feelings, or experiences; do not elaborate on yourself.

Seek Consensual Validation. Search for mutual understanding; words should mean the same thing to both of you. Therapeutic communication cannot take place if both you and the other person attach autistic (private) meanings to the words you both use. Always ask yourself if what you heard could have a meaning other than what you think. As a person defines self for the listener, he/she also clarifies what is meant. Avoid words and phrases that are easily misinterpreted or misunderstood and encourage the person to ask whenever there is doubt about what you mean.

Encourage Evaluation of the Situation by the Person. Help the client to appraise the quality of the experience, to consider people and events in relation to personal and others' values, and to evaluate the way in which people affect him/her personally as well as understand how he/she affects others. A simple query may help the person understand feelings in connection with what happened and refrain from uncritically adopting the opinions and values of others.

Encourage Formulation of a Plan of Action by asking the person to consider examples of behavior likely to be appropriate in future situations. The client can then plan how to handle future problems or how to carry out necessary self-care.

Summarize. Summarize important points of discussion and give particular emphasis to progress toward greater understanding. Summarizing encourages both you and the person to part company with the same ideas in mind, provides a sense of closure at the end of discussion, and promotes a grasp of the significance of what was said.

The quality of any response depends on the degree of mutual trust in the relationship. Techniques can be highly successful or they can misfire or be abused, depending on how they are used, your attitude at the time, and the other's interpretation. There must be a feeling of caring, of safety and security in your company, and a feeling that you want to help the person help himself. The more important or highly personal a feeling or idea is, the more difficult it is to say. This situation causes hesitancy in revealing thoughts, feelings, or intimate needs. By using therapeutic principles, such as those previously listed, you will help the person and his/her family identify you as someone to whom ideas and feelings can be safely and productively revealed.

Communicating with the Client Who Has Communication Difficulties

You will need to gather data from clients with sensory impairments. When you interview a person with hearing impairment, inability to speak the language, or visual impairment, the basic principles still apply, although the specific condition will necessitate some adaptations. The guidelines presented in Tables 3-1 and 3-2 will be helpful. For anyone with a communication disorder, develop rapport and a trust relationship slowly to overcome the reticence or suspicion that might be present. Introduce yourself and your purpose. Use appropriate nonverbal behavior to convey ideas. Use an intermediary, such as a family member or interpreter, if available and necessary, but *not* to the exclusion of talking with the client (60).

Table 3-1 summarizes guidelines for communicating with hearing-impaired persons (2, 8, 22, 60, 71).

Table 3-2 summarizes guidelines for communicating with visually-impaired persons (60, 89).

Barriers to Effective Communication

Various authors have written about communication patterns to be avoided by persons in the helping professions and the rationale for their avoidance (12, 25, 34, 40, 41, 43, 53, 64, 72, 73). The following approaches and techniques will interfere with helpful communication with the client and family whether you are conducting an interview or communicating in any other nursing situation. Continually study your personal pattern of communication, verbal and nonverbal, to ensure that you *avoid* these practices.

Using the Wrong Vocabulary—vocabulary that is abstract or intangible, full of jargon, slang, or implied status; talking too much; or using unnecessarily long sentences or words out of context can be interpreted by the person as your unwillingness to communicate. But words alone do not block. Perhaps even more crucial can be your attitudes and prejudices resulting from personal and cultural background and your failure to understand the receiver's background. Think about what the message will mean to the person, depending on age, sex, personality, socioeconomic status, cultural background, occupation, religion, and degree and nature of illness.

Conveying Your Feelings of Anxiety, Anger, Strangeness, Denial, Isolation, Lack of Control, or Lack of Physical Health negatively influences your initial and continued responses to another. Such feelings also interfere with your ability to listen and will certainly cause the other person to withdraw, for rapport cannot be established. The appearance of being too busy, of not having time to listen, of not giving sufficient time for an answer, or apparently not really wanting to hear are equally forceful in "cutting off" another. Establishing contact on a social rather than a therapeutic basis also limits communication to the superficial issues.

TABLE 3-1 Communication with the Hearing-Impaired Client

1. When you meet a person who seems inattentive or slow to understand you, consider that hearing, rather than manners or intellect, may be the reason. Some hard-of-hearing persons refuse to wear a hearing aid. Others wear aids so inconspicuous that you may not see them at first glance. Others cannot be helped by a hearing aid.
2. Be sure the person's hearing aid is in place, turned on, and in working order. Batteries need frequent replacement.
3. The hard-of-hearing person may depend to a considerable extent on reading your lips to understand what you are saying even if wearing a hearing aid. No hearing aid can completely restore hearing. Always speak in a good light, face the person and the light as you speak, and do not have objects in or covering your mouth (gum, cigarettes, hand).
4. When you are in a group that includes a hard-of-hearing person, try to carry on your conversation with others in such a way that he/she can watch your lips. Never take advantage of the disability by carrying on a private conversation in his/her presence in low tones that cannot be heard.
5. Speak distinctly but naturally. Shouting does not clarify speech sounds; mouthing or exaggerating your words or speaking too slowly makes you harder to understand. On the other hand, try not to speak too rapidly.
6. Avoid excessive environmental noise, which, when magnified by a hearing aid, is distracting and distressing and overrides normal conversational tones.
7. Do not start to speak to a hard-of-hearing person abruptly. Attract attention first by facing him/her and looking straight into the person's eyes. If necessary, touch the hand or shoulder lightly. Promote understanding by starting with a key word or phrase—for instance, "Let's plan our weekend now." "Speaking of teenagers . . . ". If he/she does not understand you, don't repeat the same words. Substitute synonyms: "It's time to make plans for Saturday."
8. If the person you are speaking to has one "good" ear, always stand or sit on that side when you address him/her. Do not be afraid to ask a person with an obvious hearing loss whether he/she has a good ear and, if so, which one it is. The person will be grateful that you care enough to find out.
9. Facial expressions and gestures are important clues to meaning. Remember that an affectionate or amused tone of voice may be lost on a hard-of-hearing person.
10. In conversation with a person who is especially hard of hearing or having difficulty understanding, occasionally jot down key words on paper. The person will be grateful for the courtesy.
11. Many hard-of-hearing persons, especially teenagers, who dislike being different, are unduly sensitive about their handicap and pretend to understand when they do not. When you detect this situation, tactfully repeat your meaning in different words until it gets across.
12. The speech of a person who has been hard of hearing for years may be difficult to understand, for natural pitch and inflection are the result of imitating the speech of others. To catch such a person's meaning more easily, watch the face while he/she talks.
13. If you do not understand the person, ask for a repeat rather than ignore the person.
14. Use common sense and tact in determining which of these suggestions apply to the particular hard-of-hearing person you meet. Some persons with only a slight loss might feel embarrassed by any special attention you pay them. Others, whose loss is greater, will be profoundly grateful for it.

TABLE 3-2 Communication with the Visually Impaired Client

1. Talk to the person in a normal tone of voice. Being visually impaired is no indication that he/she cannot hear well.
2. Accept the normal things that a blind person might do, such as consulting a watch for the correct time, dialing a telephone, or writing a name in longhand, without calling attention to them.
3. When you offer assistance, do so directly. Ask "May I be of help?" Speak in a normal, friendly tone.
4. Be explicit in giving verbal directions.
5. Advise the person when you are leaving so that he/she will not be embarrassed by talking when no one is listening.
6. There is no need to avoid the use of the word "see" when talking with a blind person.
7. In guiding the person, permit him/her to take your arm. Never grab the visually impaired person's arm, for he/she cannot anticipate your movements. Proceed at a normal pace. Hesitate slightly before stepping up or down.

   When assisting the person to a chair, simply place his/her hand on the back or arm of the chair. This is enough to give location.

9. Never leave the person without a way to secure help. Have a call signal available.
10. Never leave a blind person in an open area. Instead lead him/her to the side of a room, to a chair, or some landmark from which direction can be realized.
11. A half-open door, low stools, or loose cords or rugs are dangerous obstacles for the visually impaired person.
12. When serving food to a visually impaired person who is eating without a sighted companion, offer to read the menu. As you place each item on the table, call attention to it. Food locations on a plate should be described according to the face of the clock. If the person wants you to cut food, he/she will tell you.
13. Be sure to tell who else is present in the environment.
14. Encourage use of a magnifying glass if it is helpful.
15. Read mail to the person and assist him/her with business matters if necessary.
16. Describe the environment, people, and events surrounding the person to enrich his/her experience and understanding.

Failing to Realize That the Person's Reluctance to Make a Message Clear (resulting from the feeling that what needs to be expressed is socially unacceptable or inappropriate) can prevent therapeutic communication. The client may be afraid to ask questions for fear of getting an obscure answer or of being reprimanded for such questioning. This fearful silence can cause a sense of futility and a closure of communication. Lack of dialogue prohibits evaluating the effectiveness of any message and blocks further attempts at communication. Also avoid interpreting cooperation or passivity as understanding. Sometimes the person answers yes to please you but really does not understand you at all.

Making Inappropriate Use of Facts, Introducing Unrelated Information, Offering Premature Explanation or Counseling, Wrong Timing, Saying Something Important When the Person is Upset or not Feeling Well and thus Unable to Hear What Is Really Said—all these provoke anxiety and prohibit problem solving on the part of the person.

Making Glib Statements, Offering False Reassurance by saying, "Everything is OK," or unfairly indicating that there is no cause for anxiety—these are dishonest ways of evaluating the client's personal feelings and communicate a lack of understanding and empathy. You cannot foretell the future accurately; therefore you cannot honestly say that there is nothing to worry about. Such verbal behavior belittles the person who feels he/she has legitimate problems, and it discourages further expression of feelings and trust, although it may relieve your own anxieties.

Using Cliches, Stereotyped Responses, Trite Expressions, and Empty Verbalisms stated without thought, such as "It's always worse at night," "I know," "You'll be OK," or "Who is to say?" makes the person uncomfortable and prohibits you from maintaining objectivity. Such statements, unfortunately common, do not allow expression of feelings or show understanding. You cannot understand who a person really is if you respond automatically. Also, do not jump to conclusions based on initial impressions.

Being Too Strongly Opinionated in any aspect of your conversation with another presents a barrier, for you do not allow for a different response. Neither can you be totally neutral; recognition should be given for accomplishments. Approval or agreement and disapproval or disagreement, however, carry overtones of judgment about the person.

Expressing Unnecessary Approval, stating that something the person does or feels is particularly good, implies that the opposite is bad and limits freedom of the client to think, speak, or act in ways that may displease you. Excess praise arouses undue ambition, competition, and a sense of superiority, closing off possible learning experiences because the person may continue to speak and act only in ways that will bring approval. This approach does not allow the person to live up to his/her potential. Similarly, *excessive agreement,* indicating the person is right, can be equally inhibiting, for you leave little opportunity to modify a point of view later without admitting error. Do not take sides with the person, but use the time to help him/her gather data in order to draw personal opinions and conclusions.

Expressing Undue Disapproval, denouncing another's behavior or ideas, implies that you have the right to pass judgment on the person's thoughts and feelings and that he/she must please you. This moralistic attitude diverts your attention away from another's needs and directs attention to your own. *Excessive disagreement,* opposition to another's beliefs or values, implies that he/she is wrong and you are right and puts the other on the defensive. Disagreement usually results in resistance to change and shows lack of respect. Similarly, *rejection,* refusing to consider, or showing contempt for, the person's idea and behavior, closes off the topic from exploration and also rejects him/her as an individual. We have all experienced some degree of disapproval, disagreement, and rejection in the past; but such responses from others reinforce loneliness, hopelessness, and alienation and may even contribute to illness. This person may then avoid help rather than risk further disapproval, disagreement, or rejection.

Giving Advice, Stating Personal Experiences, Opinion, or Value Judgments, Giving Pep Talks, Telling Another What Should Be Done—such behavior emphasizes yourself, elevates your self-esteem, and relieves your anxiety, but it implies that you know what is best and that the person is incapable of self-direction. Such behavior inhibits spontaneity, prevents struggling with and thinking through problems, and may unnecessarily promote a state of prolonged dependency. Certainly talking about yourself is of no interest or relevance to the person or family in need of help. Remember that when asking for your advice, opinion, or judgment, a client has frequently already made a decision and is actually seeking a sounding board or validation for ideas. (Instead such queries should be met with questions like "What have you been told to do?" "What would you like to do?" "What do you plan to do?" Then you can facilitate the person's problem solving by using the effective methods of communication previously described.)

Probing, Persistent, Pointed, or "Yes-No" Questioning places the person on the defensive and makes him/her feel manipulated and valued only for what he/she can give. Often data obtained will not be accurate because the person will give answers he/she feels you want to hear or, to protect self, will give no answers.

Requiring Explanations, Demanding Proof, Challenging or Asking "Why . . .?"—when the person cannot provide a reason for thoughts, feelings, and behavior and for events—forces an invention of reasons, partial answers, expanding delusions, or rationalizing, for he/she feels "on the spot." Emotionally charged topics should be avoided. If the person knew the "whys," the reasons, he/she could handle the situation.

Belittling the Person's Feelings (equating intense and overwhelming feelings expressed with those felt by everyone or yourself) implies that his/her feelings are not valid, he/she is bad, or that the discomfort is mild, temporary, unimportant, or self-limiting. Such statements indicate a lack of understanding and offer no constructive assistance. When someone is concerned with personal misery, he/she is not concerned about or interested in the misery of others but does expect you to be concerned and interested in his/her feelings and problems. Don't say "Everyone feels that way."

Making Only Literal Responses or asking questions related only to practical matters cuts off exploration of feelings. Persons often cannot state feelings directly or in conventional phrasing but must use symbolism or statements with hidden meanings. If you respond to symbolism on its literal level, you may be showing a lack of understanding. For example, if the person says, "I'm a real doll," it may mean that he/she feels likable, less than human, or conspicuous. Similarly, a statement such as "It's a gray day" may have no reference to the weather.

Interpreting the Person's Behavior or Confronting Him or Her with analytical meanings of behavior may cause great anxiety, denial, or withdrawal and indicates your limited confidence in his/her capacity to cope with, work through, or understand personal problems. Self-understanding does not come directly from someone else but from assistance from another.

Interrupting or Abruptly Changing the Subject takes control of the conversation, often to escape from something anxiety provoking. The new topic may be of no interest or relevance to the client. Such verbal behavior is rude and shows a lack of empathy. The other's thoughts and spontaneity are interrupted, the flow of ideas is cut off or becomes confused, and you will get inadequate information or be unable to do effective counseling or teaching. The relevance of what is being said may not be immediately apparent, but you should remain hopeful for later understanding.

Defending or Protecting Someone or Something (nurses, doctors, hospital) from verbal attack by the client is unnecessary and implies that the person has no right to express impressions, opinions, or feelings. Stating that the criticism is unjust or unfounded does not change feelings because his/her feelings are valid to the self. Moreover, what he/she is saying may be true. Genuine acceptance, understanding, and competent care of the client make defense unnecessary.

IMPLICATIONS FOR HEALTH PROMOTION

·Applications to Nursing

The first communication problem that you must control is that of personal emotions in the nurse-client-family relationship. Because the main barrier to communication is emotions, you must develop skill in building bridges over these barriers. The basic bridge to effective communication is feeling. Everyone seeks *warmth, security, assurance*, and *appreciation*. When these qualities are present, tough problems can be taken in stride, especially when commitment is combined with skillful use of the methods described in this chapter.

Study yourself to discover those points at which you could be responsible for blocking communication through your own shortcomings. Know your likes and dislikes; recognize them for what they are; and keep them under control. In order to accept another person, you must first accept yourself. You must be aware of your own needs in order to help another meet personal needs.

Cultivate an understanding of the part played by body language in human interactions and be as aware of what you are saying with your body movements as you are of what others say with theirs. Feelings are frequently expressed by gestures, attitudes, gait and body posture, and facial expressions. Refer to the following references for more information on the science of body language (3, 9, 13, 17, 22, 23, 24, 27, 37, 38, 39, 48, 54, 56, 70, 74, 75, 81).

In order to make full use of therapeutic communication, the person must feel safe with you, respected by and trusting of you. Revealing one's innermost thoughts and feelings to someone one scarcely knows is difficult for any individual, even when help is needed and expected. Use of communication techniques in counseling makes no attempt to influence the speed or direction of the person's problem-solving efforts; be a facilitator instead of a doer or a teller.

The nurse is in a key position to apply an understanding of the communication process and to carry out therapeutic communication methods in nursing while conducting routine procedures, teaching, and counseling or giving support. Thus you can enable the person and family to achieve optimum wellness and prevent future health problems. In addition, through communication, you will learn of the effectiveness of care you have given.

Application to Daily Living

Although this chapter has centered around nurse-client-family interaction, the discussions of the communication process, of interviewing, and of techniques and blocks to communication apply equally well to associations with your colleagues and other health team members. In fact, application of all information in this chapter to your everyday relationships with family and friends will promote an increasingly appropriate, harmonious living pattern. The smoother the communication system, the smoother all other systems will function.

Appropriate, realistic, constructive communication between persons is a basic step toward mental, emotional, and, indirectly (but no less significantly), physical health. Communication patterns that block or resist the other person reduce feelings of autonomy and equality and increase feelings of being misunderstood. The resultant emotions—frustration, anger, depression, and the like—will eventually affect the relationship between the persons involved as well as the physiological functioning of the body.

As a nurse, you will find yourself refining your personal pattern of communication, practicing therapeutic communication with others, and teaching others patterns of communication that promote health individually, within the family, and within community social groups.

REFERENCES

1. **Allport, Floyd,** *Theories of Perception and the Concept of Structure.* New York: John Wiley & Sons, Inc., 1955.
2. **Altshuler, K.** "Towards a Psychology of Deafness," *Journal of Communication Disorders,* 2 (1978), 159–69.
3. **Argyle, Michael,** *The Psychology of Interpersonal Behavior.* Baltimore: Penguin Books, Inc., 1967.
4. **Asch, S. E.,** "Effects of Group Pressure on the Modification and Distortion of Judgments," in *Groups, Leadership, and Men,* ed. H. Geutzkow. Pittsburgh: Carnegie-Mellon University, 1951.
5. **Ball, Geraldine,** "Speaking Without Words," *American Journal of Nursing,* 60, no. 5 (1960), 692–93.
6. **Barnett, Kathryn,** "A Theoretical Construct of the Concepts of Touch as They Relate to Nursing," *Nursing Research,* 21, no. 2 (1972), 102–10.
7. **Bartholet, M.,** "Effects of Color on Dynamics of Patient Care," *Nursing Outlook,* 16, no. 10 (1968), 51–53.
8. **Bender, R. E.,** "Communicating with the Deaf, " *American Journal of Nursing,* 66, no. 4 (1966), 757–60.
9. **Benthall, Jonathan,** and **Ted Polhemus,** eds., *The Body as a Medium of Expression.* New York: E. P. Dutton & Co., Inc., 1975.
10. **Bermosk, Loretta,** "Interviewing: A Key to Therapeutic Communication in Nursing Practice," *Nursing Clinics of North America,* 1, no. 2 (1966), 205–14.
11. **Bigham, Gloria,** "To Communicate with Negro Patients," *American Journal of Nursing,* 64, no. 9 (1964), 113–15.
12. **Bird, Brian,** *Talking with Patients.* Philadelphia: J. B. Lippincott Company, 1965.

13. **Birdwhistell, Ray,** *Kinesics and Context.* Philadelphia: University of Pennsylvania Press, 1970.
14. **Burkhardt, M.,** "Response to Anxiety," *American Journal of Nursing*, 69, no. 10 (1969), 2153–54.
15. **Burton, Genevieve,** *Persona, Impersonal, and Interpersonal Relations* (3rd ed.). New York: Springer Publishing Company, 1970.
16. **Cashar, Leah** and **Barbara Dixson,** "The Therapeutic Use of Touch," *Journal of Psychiatric Nursing*, 5, no. 5 (1967), 442–51.
17. **Christoffers, Carol,** "Movigenic Intervention: An Expanded Dimension," *Journal of Psychiatric Nursing and Mental Health Services*, 6, no. 6 (1968), 349–60.
18. **Davis, Flora,** *Inside Intuition: What We Know about Nonverbal Communication.* New York: McGraw-Hill Book Company, 1973.
19. **DeThomaso, Marita,** "Touch Power and the Screen of Loneliness," *Perspectives in Psychiatric Care*, 9, no. 3 (1971), 112–17.
20. **Durr, Carol,** "Hands That Help—But How?" *Nursing Forum*, 10 (1971), 392–400.
21. **Dye, Mary C.,** "Clarifying Patients' Communication," *American Journal of Nursing*, 63, no. 8 (1963), 56–59.
22. **Egolf, Donald,** and **S. Chester,** "Speechless Messages," *Hearing and Speech Action*, 43, no. 4 (1975), 12–15.
23. **Eibl-Eibesfeldt, I.,** "Similarities and Differences Between Cultures in Expressive Movements," *Nonverbal Communication*, ed. R. A. Hinde. Cambridge: Cambridge University Press, 1972, pp. 297–312.
24. **Ekiman, Paul,** and **Wallace Friesen,** *Unmasking the Face.* Englewood Cliffs, NJ: Prentice-Hall, Inc., 1975.
25. **Eldred, S.,** "Improving Nurse-Patient Communication," *American Journal of Nursing*, 60, no. 11 (1960), 1600–02.
26. **Enelow, Allen,** and **Scott Swisher,** *Interviewing and Patient Care* (2nd ed.). New York: Oxford University Press, 1979.
27. **Faust, Julius,** *Body Language.* New York: M. Evans & Co., Inc., 1970.
28. **Freund, H.,** "Listening with Any Ear at All," *American Journal of Nursing*, 69, no. 8 (1969), 1650–53.
29. **Gibran, Kahlil,** *The Prophet.* New York: Alfred A. Knopf, Inc., 1953, p. 21.
30. **Goffman, Irving,** *Relations in Public Places.* New York: Basic Books, Inc., 1971.
31. **Goldin, P.,** and **B. Russell,** "Therapeutic Communication," *American Journal of Nursing*, 69, no. 9 (1969), 1928–30.
32. **Goodykoontz, Lynne,** "Touch: Attitudes and Practice," *Nursing Forum*, 18, no. 1 (1979), 4–17.
33. **Grasha, Anthony,** *Practical Application of Psychology.* Cambridge, MA: Winthrop Publishers, Inc., 1978.
34. **Greenhill, Maurice H.,** "Interviewing With a Purpose," *American Journal of Nursing*, 56, no. 10 (1956), 1259–62.
35. **Grieshaw, Susan,** "My, These Are Beautiful Flowers," *American Journal of Nursing*, 80, no. 10 (1980), 1782–83.
36. **Haggerty, Virginia,** "Listening: An Experiment in Nursing," *Nursing Forum*, 10, no. 4 (1971), 382–91.

37. **Hall, Edward,** *Hidden Dimension.* New York: Doubleday Publishers, 1966.
38. ———, "Proxemics," in *Nonverbal Communication,* ed. Shirley Weitz. New York: Oxford University Press, 1974, pp. 205–29.
39. ———, *The Silent Language.* New York: Doubleday Publishers, 1959.
40. **Hardiman, M.,** "Interviewing or Social Chit-Chat?" *American Journal of Nursing,* 11, no. 7 (1971), 1379–81.
41. **Hays, J., and K. Larson,** *Interacting with Patients.* New York: The Macmillan Company, 1963.
42. **Hess, E. H.,** "Attitude and Pupil Size," *Scientific American,* 212 (April 1965), 46–54.
43. **Hewitt, H., and B. Pesznecker,** "Blocks to Communicating with Patients," *American Journal of Nursing,* 64, no. 7 (1964), 101–103.
44. **Jakobson, Roman,** "Verbal Communication," *Scientific American,* 227, no. 3 (1972), 73–80.
45. **Knapp, Mark,** *Nonverbal Communication in Human Interaction* (2nd ed.). New York: Holt, Rinehart & Winston, 1978.
46. **Krieger, Dolores,** "Therapeutic Touch: The Imprimatur of Nursing," *American Journal of Nursing,* 75, no. 5 (1975), 784–87.
47. **Kron, Thora,** *Communication in Nursing.* Philadelphia: W. B. Saunders Company, 1967.
48. **LaMeri, Russell,** *Dance Composition: The Basic Elements.* Lee, MA.: Jacobs Pillow Dance Festival, Inc., 1965.
49. **Litwack, Lawrence, Janice Litwack,** and **Mary Ballow,** *Health Counseling.* New York: Appleton-Century-Crofts, 1980.
50. **MacKinnon, Roger,** and **Robert Michels,** *The Psychiatric Interview in Clinical Practice.* Philadelphia: W. B. Saunders Company, 1971, pp. 1–64.
51. **Manthey, M.,** "A Guide for Interviewing," *American Journal of Nursing,* 67, no. 10 (1967), 2088–90.
52. **Mattes, Norman,** "Are You Listening?," *American Journal of Nursing,* 58, no. 6 (1958), 827–28.
53. **Meadow, Lloyd,** and **Gertrude Gass,** "Problems of the Novice Interviewer," *American Journal of Nursing,* 63, no. 2 (1963), 97–99.
54. **Meisenhelder, Janice,** "Boundaries of Personal Space," *Image,* 14, no. 1 (1982), 16–19.
55. **Mickens, Patricia,** "The Influence of the Therapist on Resistive Silence," *Perspectives in Psychiatric Care,* 9, no. 4 (1971), 161–66.
56. **Minckley, Barbara,** "Space and Place in Patient Care," *American Journal of Nursing,* 68, no. 4 (1968), 510–16.
57. **Montagu, Ashley,** *Touching: The Human Significance of Skin.* New York: Columbia University Press, 1971.
58. **Muencke, M.,** "Overcoming the Language Barrier," *Nursing Outlook,* 18, no. 4 (1970), 53–54.
59. **Muller, Theresa,** "Dynamics of Communication in Nursing," *American Journal of Nursing,* 63, no. 1 (1963), 9–16.
60. **Murray, Ruth,** and **M. Marilyn Huelskoetter,** *Psychiatric/Mental Health Nursing: Giving Emotional Care.* Englewood Cliffs, NJ: Prentice-Hall, Inc., 1983.
61. **O'Sullivan, Ann,** "Privileged Communication," *American Journal of Nursing,* 80, no. 5 (1980), 947–50.

62. **Paynich, Mary,** "Cultural Barriers to Nurse Communication," *American Journal of Nursing,* 64, no. 2 (1964), 87-90.
63. **Peplau, Hildegarde,** *Interpersonal Relations in Nursing.* New York: G. P. Putnam's Sons, 1952.
64. ———, *Basic Principles of Patient Counseling* (2nd ed.). Philadelphia: Smith, Kline and French Laboratories, 1969.
65. ———, "Talking with Patients," *American Journal of Nursing,* 70, no. 7 (1970) 964-66.
66. **Pirandello, L.,** "Language and Thought," *Perspectives in Psychiatric Care,* 8, no. 5 (1970), 230 ff.
67. **Prange, A.,** and **H. Martin,** "Aids to Understanding Patients," *American Journal of Nursing,* 62, no. 7 (1962), 98-100.
68. **Rodger, B.,** "Therapeutic Communication and Posthypnotic Suggestion," *American Journal of Nursing,* 72, no. 4 (1972), 714-17.
69. **Ruesch, Jurgen,** and **Gregory Bateson,** *Communication.* New York: W. W. Norton & Company, Inc., 1951.
70. **Scheflen, Albert,** *Body Language and Social Order.* Englewood Cliffs, NJ: Prentice-Hall, Inc., 1972.
71. "Simple Courtesy and the Hard of Hearing," St. Louis Hearing and Speech Center, St. Louis, MO, 1977.
72. **Skipper, James,** "Communication and the Hospitalized Patient," in *Social Interaction and Patient Care,* eds. James Skipper and Robert Leonard. Philadelphia: J. B. Lippincott Company, 1965, pp. 61-82.
73. ———, **D. Tagliacozzo,** and **H. Mauksch,** "What Communication Means to Patients," *American Journal of Nursing,* 4, no. 4 (1964), 101-3.
74. **Sommer, Robert,** *Personal Space.* Englewood Cliffs, NJ: Prentice-Hall, Inc., 1969.
75. **Speigel, John,** and **Pavel Machotka,** *Messages of the Body.* New York: The Free Press, 1974.
76. **Suhrie, Eleanor Brady,** "The Importance of Listening," *Nursing Outlook,* 8, no. 12 (1960), 687.
77. **Taylor, M.,** "The Process Recording: Aid to Interviewing," *Canadian Nurse,* 64, no. 10 (1968), 49.
78. **Thomas, M., J. Baker,** and **N. Estes,** "Anger: A Tool for Developing Self-Awareness," *American Journal of Nursing,* 70, no. 12 (1970), 2586-90.
79. **Tobiason, Sarah,** "Touching Is for Everyone," *American Journal of Nursing,* 81, no. 4 (1981), 728-30.
80. **Travelbee, Joyce,** *Intervention in Psychiatric Nursing.* Philadelphia: F. A. Davis Company, 1969.
81. **Underwood, P.,** "Communication Through Role Playing," *American Journal of Nursing,* 71, no. 6 (1971), 1184-86.
82. **Veninga, Robert,** "Communications: A Patient's Eye View," *American Journal of Nursing,* 73, no. 2 (1973), 320-22.
83. **Ward, Anita,** "My Silent Patient," *Perspectives in Psychiatric Care,* 7, no. 2 (1969), 87-91.
84. **Watzlawich, P., J. Beavin,** and **D. Jackson,** *Pragmatics of Human Communication.* New York: W. W. Norton & Company, Inc., 1967.

85. **Weiss, S. J.,** "The Language of Touch," *Nursing Research*, 28, no. 2 (1979), 76–80.
86. **Wicks, Robert,** *Counseling Strategies and Intervention Techniques for the Human Services*. Philadelphia: J. B. Lippincott Company, 1979.
87. **Wilson, L.,** "Listening," in *Behavioral Concepts and Nursing Intervention*, coord. C. Carlson. Philadelphia: J. B. Lippincott Company, 1970, pp. 153–70.
88. **Wu, Ruth,** *Behavior and Illness*. Englewood Cliffs, NJ: Prentice-Hall, Inc., 1973.

Interview

89. **Leighninger, R. D.,** Director, St. Louis Society for the Blind, St. Louis, MO.

4

The Nursing Process: A Method to Promote Health

Study of this chapter will help you to

1. Discuss major historical events and their impact on nursing.
2. Define the *conceptual approach* and describe some concepts used in nursing practice.
3. Describe *holistic care* and the importance of this approach in nursing.
4. Compare the scientific method with the nursing process.
5. List criteria and discuss essential attributes for professional practice.
6. List the steps of the nursing process and define *assessment, nursing diagnosis, planning, intervention,* and *evaluation.*
7. Discuss the purpose of an assessment tool and construct an assessment tool appropriate for patients/clients in each life era with various health problems.
8. Formulate nursing diagnoses from nursing assessments.
9. Differentiate nursing diagnosis and nursing history and write a nursing history on a patient or client.
10. Describe purposes, possible formats, and uses of nursing care plans.
11. Write a nursing care plan for a patient/client, using guidelines given in this chapter.

12. Explain the importance of scientific rationale and a nursing model for intervention.
13. Relate the step of evaluation to accountability in the nursing process.
14. Use the process recording and analysis of care to evaluate your effectiveness in patient-client care.
15. Differentiate between a social and helpful nurse-client relationship.
16. Describe guidelines for a therapeutic nurse-client relationship.
17. List and describe the phases of the nurse-client relationship and the effect of the nurse's and client's feelings on each phase.
18. Discuss the changing role of the nurse.
19. Compare problem solving and research and explore the importance of each to nursing.

Most nursing in the past, and even today, was practiced on an empirical basis. Care patterns established by early nurses, such as Florence Nightingale and Clara Barton, were chiefly concerned with procedures and aimed at providing an environment of cleanliness, comfort, and safety. Nursing's responsibility was to foster solely a reparative process and functions toward this end have accompanied the growth of technology in nursing—a tradition that is almost holy (63). Today, however, this limited approach has proved inadequate. Thus a conceptual approach to care has emerged, an approach that is essential in order to care for a diverse population in a complex society.

The **conceptual approach** *is the uniting, combining, modifying, and using of many theories or ideas from various disciplines into a new form; it is a holistic, dynamic approach.* Thus for resources or inspiration you might draw on methods or approaches of medicine, religion, education, psychology, sociology, or business. Your approach will be refined as you constantly look for ideas from other fields that are applicable to nursing. Learning theories that have been successful in psychotherapy, for example, can be translated to nursing and adapted to client/patient teaching. The conceptual approach does not isolate procedures. Instead it fits these aspects of nursing into a health-promotion emphasis, and it uses whatever knowledge is applicable, such as basic human needs and levels of wellness, stress, and adaptation. Although the conceptual approach is concerned with repair, it is also concerned with prevention of breakdown; even though it is concerned with practical measures, it is also concerned that sound scientific principles underly these measures.

HISTORICAL BACKGROUND

Some discussion of historic events will promote a deeper understanding of the nursing process. Events prior to, during, and after World War II and events of the last two decades have significantly influenced nursing.

Prior to World War II

In the early Christian-Judaic era, the needs of the sick were met by individuals through unselfish caring and love of neighbor augmented by the extensive use of apprentices. During the last centuries of the medieval period, the world experienced vast social and political changes, accompanied by great turmoil and unrest, and the practice of nursing reflected these changes in national and social structures. Religious orders devoted solely to the care of the sick emerged, but it was actually not until Florence Nightingale's time (1820–1910) that nursing began its long climb toward professionalism through efforts to attain a sound pattern of education combined with practice (63).

Ms. Nightingale was an innovator, a feminist before the term became popular, and an independent spirit firmly believing in her goals for nursing care. Defying all traditions, she built the foundation on which nursing rests today. She emphasized a clean environment, good nutrition, and use of knowledge; she was concerned that the nurse receive adequate remuneration; and she ardently proclaimed the need for advanced preparation for those in administrative and teaching roles (63).

Yet from the turn of the century until World War II nursing made little progress. Education and practice saw little change in the status quo. In fact, complacency existed in all the professions because of the overall letdown during and following World War I and the Great Depression of the 1930s.

During World War II

The propelling force of World War II with its patriotic spirit and large numbers of casualties, together with the explosion of technology and innovative materials, produced steadily on-going changes in health care. The doctor–nurse–client relationship gave way to the health team and this concept has continued to expand.

Ancillary personnel evolved in the health professions. Military corpsmen and nurses aides became essential to the delivery of care. Clinical medicine moved ahead, marked by such advances as early ambulation, new techniques in burn treatment, the discovery of new drugs, especially the antibiotics, and a whole complex of sophisticated mechanical and electronic devices for prosthetic and life support. These changes directly affected the practice of nursing.

The Postwar Years

The two decades following the war brought more rapid change to nursing than any other era. Everyone—lay public and health professionals alike—looked on the health care system in a new light. The public began to question what constitutes good care; the economy changed; health insurance was becoming more popular; the population escalated and the composition and climate of urban areas altered radically.

Scientific inquiry and development literally exploded with new therapies, medical discoveries, and newly perfected techniques. It became important to strive to keep people well and the whole realm of preventive medical and nursing care was opened to exploration and revelation.

The educational scene witnessed fresh developments. The GI Bill of Rights provided funds for those who otherwise might never have considered preparing for a career, and nursing schools, along with all others, were flooded with applicants for degrees. Education began to influence the practice of nursing. The concept of *total patient care* was born. The emergence of the *health team* forced nursing to reevaluate its role in health care, for teamwork was now fundamental.

The foregoing innovations produced so much confusion that the profession requested an unbiased nonnurse, Esther Lucille Brown, to evaluate the status of nursing. Her report in 1948 marked a major turning point in the lives of nurses and in their practice of the profession. Ms. Brown underscored, as did Ms. Nightingale, the deep concern that nurses be adequately remunerated for *quality service*.

During the 1950s more thought was given to the use of the term "professional" as well as to the expansion of health programs and the interpersonal relationships between nurse, client, and allied health personnel. Discussion was rife as to whether nursing was a profession.

As we moved toward the 1960s, various approaches in terms of nursing functions were used to establish nursing as a profession. Crucial questions arose. How does the nurse affect the client? How significant are the nurse's decisions and judgments for the welfare of the client? How complex are nursing actions with regard to education and experience? Is there an effective check on nursing actions? On what are the nurse's decisions based? Does performance improve with experience? With education? How can the consumer judge the nurse's actions?

At the core of these questions is the code of ethics published by the American Nurses Association. The existence of this code meets one criterion for a profession and it is today the basis on which action by the nurse is founded and the standard against which nursing actions are judged.

Nursing continues as an emerging profession, based on the criteria that describe a profession. Genevieve and Roy Bixler have identified seven characteristics of a profession. A profession:

1. Uses a well-defined and well-organized body of knowledge as the basis for practice.
2. Enlarges its body of knowledge and improves techniques of education and service through the scientific method.
3. Educates its practitioners in institutions of higher education.
4. Applies a body of specialized knowledge in practice services that are vital to human and social welfare.
5. Functions autonomously in the formulation of professional policy and in the control of professional activity.
6. Attracts people with above-average intellectual and personal qualities, who exalt service above personal gain, and who consider their profession as a lifework.
7. Strives to compensate its practitioners by providing autonomy of action while being accountable to the client, opportunity for continuous professional growth, and economic security (4).

Many leaders in nursing have contributed to nursing becoming a profession. It is impossible to mention all of them. Several nurses who have contributed to the profession through their development of a nursing model are mentioned in the following section.

The Nursing Model

In all fields of practice, regardless of the discipline, certain concepts are used to define the practitioner's role with the client. In nursing, observations, diagnoses, and the plans for action are based on a **nursing model,** *a set of concepts that assist the practitioner to simplify and organize the data into a manageable plan of action.* In discussing the nursing process, it becomes clear that the nurse brings to that process a mental profile of the client, the goals of care, and the role of the nurse in the execution of the plan. Thus the nursing model has become increasingly useful in practice for defining the nurse's role, and in research as a guide for collection and interpretation of data.

Some models that exist in nursing are the Systems Developmental-Stress Model (77), the Nursing Process Systems Model (10), Adaptation

Models (38, 81), Hierarchy of Needs Model (47), and the Interaction Model (8). Other models have been described by Peplau (5, 67), Travelbee (92), Patterson and Zdered (66), Rogers (80), Orem (62), and Johnson (32, 37).

The Nursing Process Today

The complex nature of *nursing* is evident in the many approaches that are used to define it. Everyone has a different image of the term. To define it, one can use actions, functions, roles, consumer images, images held by peers, the individual nurse's philosophy, settings in which nursing is performed, the value placed on the client, or in respect for the client as seen from the employer–employee standpoint.

The variety of nurses within the profession today and the diversity of their educational backgrounds further compound the problem. The engulfing proliferation of information and knowledge and the tremendous surge of technology in the health fields have had an overwhelming impact on the thrust of societal changes. The public is more deeply concerned with health and illness and the rights of the individual to attain maximum well-being. The evergrowing need for preventive health care and health maintenance presents a new challenge to nursing.

The rest of this chapter discusses concepts basic to the nursing process, the systematic method of nursing practice, ways to evaluate effectiveness of the nursing process, the use of a helpful nurse–patient relationship as one of the unique functions of nursing, and the changing role of the nurse. As you study this chapter, keep in mind that, in addition to acquiring a mastery of skills and knowledge necessary for your clinical area, you will also need to possess a zeal for continuing your learning and a commitment to the good of people rather than to self-aggrandizement. Moreover, you should view nursing as an art, a systematic but compassionate way of applying knowledge and skill to achieve clearly defined goals.

BASIC CONCEPTS

The Holistic Approach to People and Their Needs

A person is a system striving to maintain optimal balance by means of discharging and conserving energy. Your goal is to assist the person in maintaining or restoring this balance, to help him/her remain adaptive;

thus you will need an understanding of the nature of the person and his/her needs.

A person is a part of all that is within and around him—whether it be a cell, organ system, family, or society. He/she is more than the sum of all the parts. This view, called **holistic or total**, will provide a foundation for considering all the areas that affect health.

A person's **behavior,** *observable characteristics and responses,* can help you recognize needs. Although the person usually seeks to meet physical and psychosocial needs simultaneously, preservation of physical integrity is basic. According to Maslow, the human must maintain an optimal level of oxygen-carbon dioxide exchange, fluid and food intake, rest and activity, elimination of waste products, temperature regulation, and participation in procreation in order to guarantee the species' survival. Next in order are needs for safety, belonging and love, self-esteem, and self-actualization (realizing the best of one's potential) (47). In nursing, you help the person meet the basic needs that he/she is unable to meet. Knowing priority of needs will help you set your priorities of care. For example, you would not expect a person to concentrate on job safety while suffering from excessive hunger.

A Systematic Approach to Nursing Practice

You will be systematic in your nursing practice through use of the scientific method, long a part of research in other disciplines. The scientific method must also be an intricate part of nursing if goals of health care are to be effectively met.

As you work with patients/clients, you may not always follow the steps of problem identification, formulation of hypothesis, sampling, data collection, statistical analysis, and retesting of the hypothesis in a sophisticated manner. You can, however, readily see the similarity between steps of the scientific method and the steps of the nursing process.

Identifying the problem and formulating the hypothesis may be compared to the assessment and nursing diagnosis stages of the nursing process. The third, or planning, stage is analogous to the step in the research process wherein the design of the study is prepared and criteria are selected for dealing with sample population. Intervention, the fourth stage of the nursing process, may be seen as similar to the action stage of a research project in which a procedure is carried out by the investigator to test its effect on the sample. The fifth and final step in the nursing process, evaluation, is comparable to the conclusions about the value of a research study leading to further investigation, thereby producing a circular effect.

DEFINITIONS OF NURSING AND THE NURSING PROCESS

Definitions

Many leaders in nursing have defined nursing. You may want to read various references at the end of this chapter to help you formulate your own definition.

The authors define **nursing** *as an art and science in which verbal, nonverbal, tangible, and intangible health-related activities are systematically performed by a specially educated, licensed, and compassionate person. The purpose of these activities is to promote, maintain, or restore biopsychosocial and spiritual health of the person, family, and group, as well as to comfort, protect, or stabilize the same during life or in the face of death, and to aid in their recovery. These activities, legally defined, involve use of self and may be performed independently or collaboratively with other health team members but always with the person, family, group, or community as the central focus and as actively as possible in the process.*

The five steps of the nursing process are **assessment** (*identifying needs*), **formulating the nursing diagnosis,** *stating the client's needs as related to impairment of function, structure, or adaptation;* **planning** (*setting priorities and developing the care plan*), **intervention** (*implementing the care plan*), *and* **evaluation** (*validating the effectiveness of the care*). In this sequence of operations that uses the scientific method, your knowledge, plus available resources, will combine with your personality, compassion, and commitment to produce an effective art and science of nurturing. Thus the nursing process is what you do as a nurse. Every decision for action is carried out within the context of one of the five steps, whether it be an instantaneous decision in an emergency or a long-range plan that grows out of a team conference. Only the time factor varies. The process can be as simple as deciding to sit with a lonely elderly client or as complicated as intensive-care nursing. After you engage in a knowledgeable, purposeful series of thoughts and actions, you then evaluate their effectiveness.

Assessment

The first step in the nursing process is **assessment,** *study of the whole person to establish a baseline of information and determine the person's potential and need for help.* Once established, this baseline is fluid and your assessment is a continuous process. As changes in the person yield new data, nursing problems and objectives may require restatement or may no longer be relevant for care.

Assessment is accomplished through observation, the use of knowledge and resources, and communication.

Observation includes recognizing objective signs in the patient, family, or community; watching their interactions with one another; determining the response of the person or family to you; and discerning the way in which the person arranges personal belongings and speaks of self. Observation and perception are closely related and are more fully described in Chapter 3.

Knowledge from previous experiences and courses of study must be used in assessment. Knowledge of normal physiology and anatomy and of growth and development provides a basis for understanding pathological states and enables you to predict patient/client responses and plan care accordingly. Sociology, psychology, philosophy and theology are also examples of areas of information you must use to enhance your conceptual approach to care. Both units of this book, as well as other texts, present theory and facts on which to base assessment. Essential to assessment is a sound knowledge of the developing person (56).

Other Resources include data gathered from the person's chart and health history. The literature pertinent to the person's condition must be explored, including information about the medical regimen, such as treatments and drugs, and their implications for nursing care must be considered. A word of caution is needed about the use of literature in assessment. Do not attempt to fit the patient/client completely into a textbook pattern. Everyone's adaptational response is unique and any information gathered is to be used only as a guideline.

Communication as part of assessment involves a goal-directed approach to the patient, the family or significant others, the physician as your colleague, and other members of the health team. Verbal and nonverbal exchanges take place between you and the patient, ideally leading to the meeting of the minds—a sharing of the same meanings as each sees the other's point of view. Clarification of meaning is necessary when any doubt exists so that needs can be met in a way acceptable to patient and family.

Methods of effective communication and interviewing and barriers to communication are discussed in Chapter 3 and must be used for thorough assessment.

Assessment occurs on two levels. **First-level assessment** *is done on initial contact with a person to determine the perceived health threat, the adaptive ability, and priority care measures.* **Second-level assessment** *continues while the person is in your care and adds depth and breadth of understanding about the physical, emotional, mental, spiritual, cultural, social, and family characteristics and needs.* This more comprehensive view of the person enables you to plan and give more individualized care (7, 77, 82).

A visiting nurse, for example, is ordered into a home by a physician. Along with the client's name, address, phone number, age, and race, the nurse has the diagnosis of chronic degenerative arthritis and chronic bladder infection. The nurse is to change a No. 20 Silastic indwelling urinary catheter every two weeks and when necessary.

On the first visit the nurse finds a person who is essentially bedfast and who is crying because "my catheter hurts so much. And my stomach is swollen. Oh, I think I'm going to die."

The nurse will obviously act at the *first level of assessment.* She/he discovers a distended abdomen. The old catheter is removed; its openings are clogged. The pooled urine flows out with the insertion of a new catheter. The person's pain is gone. She stops crying and seems relieved and comfortable as the nurse explains what happened and how to avoid this problem in the future.

The nurse can now proceed to the *second assessment level.* Actually, she/he has been gathering information for this broader assessment while driving through the community by noting the kind of neighborhood the person lives in. From the moment the nurse walked in the door she/he has been taking mental notes: general home arrangement, family relationships (the manner in which members talk to each other), religious affiliation (church membership certificate hanging on wall), leisure activities (macramé purse in the making), cognitive state (verbal communication between nurse and client), emotional state (crying and then smiling), obvious physical status (breathing pattern, appearance of skin, body movements and limitations), elimination pattern (urinary catheter and "honey, I'm constipated,"), safety factors (arrangement of bed, rugs, etc.), sensory status (hearing and visual acuity), and nutritional status (obesity, snacks within reach).

The nurse will need to elaborate on each of these areas in the written report. She/he will also have to elicit health history, financial status, and a more detailed physical assessment.

Assessment Tools

Each profession has its tools and nursing is no exception. Nursing tools are not the devices with which treatments are carried out but rather the methodology through which assessment of needs is compiled or the vehicle through which *planning*, the third step, is carried out. These tools include the nursing history and a special format for systematic assessment of the patient's/client's functional areas, leading to a clear identification of *nursing diagnosis.*

The **nursing history** *is distinct from a medical history in that it focuses on the meaning of illness and health care to the person and family as a basis for planning nursing care*, whereas the medical history is taken to determine or rule out pathology as a basis for medical care (43, 68). Instead of recommending a specific format or a list of steps to follow, the following discussion explains the kind of data that a nursing history provides and the ways in which you can make use of this tool.

The initial interview with a person/family on entrance into a health care agency—hospital, clinic, physician's office or, if approved, home visits—must be done by the professional nurse if personalized care is to be planned effectively. Systematically collecting data will help you make maximum use of your limited time with the person.

Whether you use a standard form or an unstructured interview will depend on agency policy, your own ability to collect data, the effectiveness of your communication, and the time available. Techniques for this initial gathering of data are the interview, direct observation, and inspection. Subjective as well as objective data are collected and recorded. Analytical thinking and the knowledge you bring from the contributing sciences permit you to make judgments and decisions for care (48).

To be of practical use, a *nursing history should reflect the client's perception of the illness, the need to seek care, and expectations regarding the care he/she hopes to receive. The history must provide clues to personal needs and ability to deal with health problems*. These areas can be covered in an interview guide that includes

1. The meaning of illness and agency care to the person and to the important family members with whom he/she lives; interests; and projected care plans after discharge.
2. The person's specific needs and the extent to which nursing intervention will be required to help satisfy basic needs: hygiene, rest, sleep, relief of pain, safety, nutrition, fluids, elimination, oxygen, and sexuality.
3. Additional data that can be labeled "other," such as allergies, adverse reactions to medications, language barriers, educational level (prerequisites for successful communication and health teaching), emotional reactions, social situation, and *anything* the person thinks would be helpful to you in caring for him/her.
4. Your impressions and a summary of the initial interview. If a questionnaire is used, this last area could be completed away from the client.

The entire form can be the first nursing entry on the patient's/client's record and serves as a complete admission note, either on the traditional nurses' notes or in the Problem-Oriented Medical Record (3, 94).

Systematic assessment of the functional areas, using a specific guide, is basic to ongoing understanding of the person and the development of a nursing plan. This assessment tool is distinct from the nursing history, which focuses on relatively unchanging information that identifies potentials, strengths, attitudes, efforts, and weaknesses present on admission. The assessment focuses on areas that change, depending on the person's position on the illness–wellness continuum.

All working guides developed by nursing leaders cover the primary areas of physiological and psychosocial needs. Several typologies are in use and variations are emerging. Well known to nursing are the 21 problems suggested by Abdellah (1), the functional-abilities tool devised by McCain (48), and Henderson's activities of daily living (34). Geitgey describes a guide that makes use of the acronym SELF-PACING to identify needs and to emphasize the client's right to be as self-directing as possible (28). The letters stand for the past and current status of *S*ocialization and special senses; *E*limination and exercise; *L*iquids and factors influencing fluid balance; *F*oods and dietary modification; *P*ain, personal hygiene, and posture; *A*eration; *C*irculation; *I*ntegument; *N*euromuscular control and coordination; and *G*eneral condition. A guide that emphasizes wellness when assessing the external body has been devised by Turnbull. The four major health indicators for each body area are intactness, symmetry, nourishment, and productivity (93). A comprehensive assessment tool for use in occupational nursing has been devised by Serafini (86).

Figure 4-1 uses Deininger's framework for factors to be considered in identifying the needs of a hospitalized patient with emphysema (19). This is another way of looking at the person's functional areas during first-level assessment when establishing a baseline for the planning of care. Figure 4-2 shows a tool that could be used for a more extensive second-level assessment of biopsychosocial status during the patient's hospitalization or during the client's or family's use of other health care services.

Another method of assessment uses the Weed problem-oriented record (POR), a series of progress notes in which each problem is listed and numbered by the physician, the nurse, and other members of the health team. Under each listing are four subheadings, the initials of which form the acronym SOAP. The S stands for subjective data, O for objective data, A for assessments and interpretations, and P for plan of treatment (94). The following variation of the problem-oriented record is helpful when charting conventional nurses' notes, for it assists you in writing notes that reflect the nursing care plan. Begin each note with

FIGURE 4-1 Example of a Patient Assessment

Patient: Mrs. H. Age 50. Medical Diagnosis: Emphysema. 1-14-85

1. *Oxygen Utilization and Circulation*
   A. Respirations rapid; long inspiratory phase, short expiratory phase. Rate 28 per minute.
   B. Chest somewhat barrel-shaped.
   C. Lungs hyperresonant to percussion. Vocal fremitus decreased. Breath sounds faint and harsh.
   D. Flushed appearance. Purses lips on expiration. Pauses after every few spoken words.
   E. Apical and radial pulses regular at 92. Blood pressure 148/90. No heart murmurs noted.
   F. Frequent non-productive dry cough. No wheezing.
   G. Heavy smoker.
   H. Some clubbing of fingers.
   I. Lower extremities cool to the touch. Popliteal pulses absent.
   L. pedal pulse absent.

2. *Nutrition and Elimination*
   A. General diet. Appetite poor.
   B. 1000 c.c. of 5% D/W with aminophylline 500 mg. infusing I.V. at 100 c.c. per hour.
   C. Thin. Height 165 cm. Weight 42 kg. Skin dry with poor turgor. Nails dry.
   D. Drinks coffee and tea. No alcohol.
   E. Bowel pattern: hard stool 2 or 3 times per week; usually takes laxative (Ex-Lax) or soapsuds enema 2 or 3 times per month.
   F. Voiding: no frequency, urgency or pain.

3. *Comfort, Safety and Hygiene*
   A. No chest pain.
   B. Teeth in poor condition, some discoloration, gums retracted, back molars missing on both sides, plaque present.
   C. Body, hair, and nails clean.
   D. Prefers sitting position in bed; unable to breathe comfortably when supine.
   E. Anxious appearance—restless—constantly folds Kleenex.

4. *Activity, Rest and Sleep*
   A. Bathroom privileges only.
   B. Tires easily; unable to take own bedbath or shower.
   C. Restlessness interferes with ability to nap.
   D. Sleeps poorly at night—4 to 5 hours at most on "good" nights.

FIGURE 4-1 (cont.)

5. *Regulatory and Sensory Mechanisms*
   A. Oriented X 3—to time, place, person.
   B. No impairment of hearing. Able to hear soft whisper from 10 feet distance when awake.
   C. Wears glasses for reading. Able to see clearly 20 feet from bed.
   D. Postmenopause; states no untoward symptoms at this time. Last Pap smear 6 months ago.
   E. Hgb 11.0, Hct 47%, urinalysis negative on admission.
   F. Tolerating I.V. aminophylline well at this time. No nausea.
   G. Electrolytes and blood profile within normal limits. Exception: K^+ 3.0.

the subjective symptoms expressed by the person; add your observations about the person's current situation, and conclude with the intervention or nursing action that you carried out. Staff and students alike have found it useful to visualize this method of charting as follows: "What does the patient express?" "What do I see, hear, touch, smell?" "What did I do about it?"

Assessment of specific patient/client needs or problems can also be done. The medication history described by Parker, for example, can help you obtain detailed information about medications taken, both prescription and nonprescription, potential drug interactions, and effects of medications on the person (65). Forms can also be devised to obtain a nutrition history (12) or spiritual history (see Chapter 11). Cohen gives suggestions on how to assess mental status (16). Joyce Snyder and Margo Wilson describe the following factors to be included in the psychological assessment:

1. Response to stress and coping and defense mechanisms
2. Interpersonal relationships
3. Motivation and lifestyle
4. Thought processes and verbal behavior
5. Nonverbal behavior
6. Awareness and handling of feelings
7. Support systems
8. Talents, strengths, and assets
9. Physical health
10. Nurse's impression of the interview and interaction (88)

Janis Reynolds and Jann Logsdon describe a tool for assessing mental status that includes information about identifying data; responses based

FIGURE 4-2 Example of Second-Level Assessment Guide

Identifying Data

Name: Sex: Age:

Race/Ethnicity: Date of admission:

Referral source, if any:

Social Status

Environment (neighborhood, geographic area):

Home arrangement or retirement care:

Occupation: Educational level:

Leisure activities:

Organizational memberships:

Lifestyle usually followed; effect of illness on lifestyle:

Special preferences in care related to lifestyle:

Financial status; insurance; special concerns:

Family Relationships

Marital status: Number of children:

Other important family members: Other significant people:

Role in family:

Patterns of sexual relations:

Effect of illness upon family life:

Religious Practices

Church affiliation: Clergyman:

Special rituals/preferences in care related to religion:

Cognitive Status

Level of consciousness: Orientation:

Ability to communicate verbally and nonverbally:

Memory recall: Attention span:

Ability to grasp ideas, to think logically:

Apparent insight into health problem:

Special values related to health:

Emotional Status

Feelings about present illness/hospitalization:

Feelings about past experiences with health care agencies/staff:

FIGURE 4-2 (cont.)

Stressful event(s) prior to this illness:

Perceptual abilities (vision, hearing, touch, etc.):

Special awareness of any body part or function:

Feelings about self:

Prefer being alone: With others:

Attitude toward life:

Goals or aspirations:

Sources of pleasure: Displeasure:

Situations causing upset feelings:

Ability to cope with stress:

General behavior:

Health History

Usual health status:

Usual activity level, hours of work:

Pattern of biological rhythms:

Usual eating habits; fluid intake:

Usual sleep habits:

Use of beverages, alcoholic beverages, tobacco, drugs (prescribed, nonprescribed, legal, illegal):

Present illness and its onset:

Past illness(es), hospitalization(s):

Usual health care practices:

Usual source of health care:

Special home care needs/discharge plans:

Family illness(es):

Physical Status

Height: Weight: Posture:

Position of comfort: Body movements:

Appearance of head: Face:

Eyes: Ears: Nose:
Mouth: Teeth: Throat:

Appearance of skin: Temperature:

Circulatory status: Blood pressure:

Muscular build, tone:

FIGURE 4-2 (cont.)

Condition of chest (size, shape, movements, cough):

Heartbeat: Pulses: Respirations:

Condition of abdomen (soft, distended, rigid, painful, other symptoms):

Appearance of back:

Appearance of extremities:
Arms and hands:
Legs and feet:
Fingers and toes:
Range of motion:

Elimination pattern:

Body excretions/secretions:

Reproductive status; appearance of external genitalia:

Presence of pain:

Other signs or symptoms:

on the nurse's judgment, such as appearance, motor movement, and level of consciousness; and responses based on the person's self-description about illness, family, living arrangements, and life patterns (76).

In assessing a community, consider the following items:

1. Geographical area or neighborhood, including distribution of residences, industry, commercial establishments, or service facilities, and ecological factors such as natural resources or presence of pollutants.
2. Sources of income, income stratification, and the amount of interaction between various income levels.
3. Educational facilities, educational levels, and occupations of the population.
4. Cultural and ethnic background of the community and its residents.
5. Number, age, sex, and family-size distribution of the population.
6. Health facilities, their accessibility, and care available.
7. Other facilities, such as churches, leisure and recreational facilities.
8. Service people in the community, such as health care workers, police, clergy, social-welfare workers, and their use by the population.
9. Designated and informal community leaders and their roles.
10. Means of communication in the community, such as face-to-face interchange, directives, and nonverbal messages, as well as the formal communication systems and presence of media.
11. The decision-making process and enforcement of decisions in the community, including informal and governmental.

12. Acceptance and integration of new residents into the community.
13. Level of trust in the community between residents, between leaders and residents, and between leaders and service providers.
14. Changes that have occurred in the last several years, as well as rapidity of change, cause of change, and acceptance of change by the community.
15. Degree of cohesion in the community.
16. Acceptance of members who do not conform to the cultural norm.
17. History of the community (55).

Nursing Diagnosis

The nursing diagnosis is formulated as a result of judgments made after the assessment (75). The word **diagnosis** means to *state a decision of opinion or make a judgment after careful examination and analysis of facts*, and it is not limited to medical conditions (27).

Nursing diagnosis is a *"statement of a potential or actual altered health status of a client which is derived from nursing assessment and which requires intervention from the domain of nursing." It includes a statement of the etiology or possible causes and manifestations of signs and symptoms* (23). Nursing diagnoses are distinct from pathological states identified as being responsive to the physician's treatment. The area in which nursing diagnoses are made involve potential or current disturbances in life patterns, body functions, emotional states, spiritual aspects, or developmental level, including those occurring secondary to disease. The nursing diagnostic category suggests the status of the person, primary elements of the care plan, treatment, and potential outcome (27, 30). This framework tends to describe the client rather than the nursing activity. Instead of using functional concepts, such as "provide adequate oxygenation," for instance, you should shift the emphasis by evaluating why the person needs suctioning or any other nursing activity. The answer is found in a description of the client's state: potential respiratory dysfunction (30) resulting from (*condition*) as noted by (*signs and symptoms*). This approach forces the nurse to use knowledge of anatomy and physiology. Nursing diagnosis may be indicative of the medical diagnosis and, conversely, the medical diagnosis may indicate the nursing diagnosis. Thus a nursing diagnosis of respiratory dysfunction might be related to the medical diagnosis of pulmonary embolus. Similarly, the medical diagnosis of fracture might suggest the nursing diagnosis of impaired mobility. But the medical diagnosis remains the same, even during rehabilitation. The nursing diagnosis changes as the person's condition or reaction to the condition changes.

Other examples of nursing diagnosis include ineffective breathing pattern, alteration in bowel elimination, alteration in cardiac output, impaired mobility, alteration in nutrition, ineffective family coping, impaired verbal communication, ineffective individual coping, deficit in diversional activity, fear, anticipatory grieving, dysfunctional grieving, potential for injury, disturbance in self-concept, impairment of skin integrity (actual or potential), sexual dysfunction, spiritual distress, social isolation. The list could go on; it is still being added to, based on research.

The nursing diagnoses emerge quite naturally from the assessment of the client. These statements may express needs or concerns in any or all five areas of human experience and awareness: the biological, physical-environmental, sociocultural, psychological, and spiritual-humanistic realms and are applicable to health promotion as well as acute or chronic illness.

There are times when a specific diagnosis may be stated by several members of the health team—for instance, physician, social worker, and nurse. The physician's diagnosis of "anxiety" in a patient who has undergone a colon resection for cancer may refer to the patient's fear of a recurrence. The social worker may make the same observation of anxiety and be referring to the patient's worry over the cost of required colostomy equipment. The nurse may diagnose anxiety and be referring to the patient's difficulty in caring for his colostomy. Each will subsequently intervene in a different manner. The physician may prescribe a tranquilizer, the social worker arrange for financial assistance, and the nurse intervene by teaching and giving support to the patient as he learns colostomy care (23).

Given a general idea as to the meaning of a nursing diagnosis, the next step is to understand how it can be used in a practical sense. It will be helpful to think of it in terms of a specific, common situation that frequently confronts the nurse: that of a patient admitted to the hospital with a medical diagnosis of diabetes. This patient has not been adhering to his prescribed diet, has neglected his food care, and has been careless about taking his oral hypoglycemics. After a comprehensive assessment, the nurse will have formed some judgments regarding the patient's needs. How can they be expressed in writing? The answer lies in the ability to relate the patient's needs to something that is amenable to nursing care. When stated in these terms, which reflect the definition of nursing diagnosis, it will be helpful to all who care for this patient.

The following examples of a nursing diagnosis might be used for the preceding patient:

1. Nonadherence to prescribed drug therapy *related to lack of understanding of the disease process*, manifested by ______________ .
   (behavior, signs, symptoms)

2. Nonadherence to prescribed diet therapy *related to lack of knowledge of diet restriction*, manifested by ________ (behavior, signs, symptoms).

In each statement the cause of the problem is within the ability of nursing to alleviate, either directly by patient teaching or by referral to another health discipline.

Other examples that may serve to clarify the use of a nursing diagnosis might be

1. Potential skin breakdown over coccyx related to impairment of circulation, manifested by ______.
2. Urinary frequency related to bladder infection, manifested by ______.
3. Dehydration related to elevated temperature, manifested by ______.
4. Withdrawal related to embarrassment over odor, manifested by ______.
5. Impaired mobility related to necessity for continuous traction, manifested by ______.
6. Anxiety related to concern about surgical outcome, manifested by ______.

The accepted use of the term "related to" is necessary for clarity. It is useful in that it ties the need or problem directly to the area most apt to be responsive to nursing actions; at the same time it allows for other factors that may impinge on the problem and so is less confining in its meaning than the phrase "due to" might be.

To help nurses formulate diagnoses, lists have been developed at four national conferences and are available from the North American Nursing Diagnosis Association, St. Louis University School of Nursing, 3525 Caroline Street, St. Louis, Missouri, 63104.

The nursing diagnosis sets the stage for the fourth step in the nursing process—planning the care.

Formulating Nursing Care Goals and a Plan of Care

On the basis of your systematic study of the patient, decide which functional area is in most need of your help. The problems of care must be determined before you can set priorities. Then you will be able to state **goals,** *a positive statement of what is to be accomplished or the objectives for the person's return to wellness—the priorities for today, this week, and for eventual discharge to his/her usual life with optimum health for the individual.* Thus you formulate a **nursing care plan,** *a* *record summarizing all information required to carry out appropriate nursing care for an individual, family, or group at a given time. The plan is built on the nursing assessment and diagnosis of health needs and indicates specific goals to be reached with the client through designated nursing actions* (29). The goals and plan are established with the patient/client and family.

Essential to planning care is setting priorities. Once the nursing diagnoses are made, they are ranked in order of priority for care. This step is often a stumbling block for the beginning nurse. Here Maslow's Hierarchy of Needs model may be helpful; priorities can be set according to the Hierarchy.

Consider Mr. Denton, age 62, who sustained a cerebral vascular accident and has been in the hospital 24 hours prior to your being assigned to care for him. He has a right hemiplegia and is on complete bedrest. What are the immediate priorities of care? You might select his bath or the monitoring of his intravenous fluids. These steps are important but not ends in themselves; instead they are ways of meeting the needs of those functional states that are in varying degrees of maladaption.

Assuming that you know Mr. Denton's age, occupation, social-cultural background, and general response through a nursing history, you can decide what you hope to accomplish. Immediate priorities may be to establish rapport and guide his understanding of the situation, preserve musculoskeletal function, prevent skin breakdown, assist the family in the crisis situation, and establish adequate elimination and nutrition. Long-range goals may include rehabilitation to optimum physical function, a return to work, or help with the acceptance of a disability.

The nursing diagnoses on which you base Mr. Denton's care might be

1. Anxiety related to unfamiliar surroundings and personnel.
2. Immobility related to right hemiplegia.
3. Family apprehension related to concerns for Mr. Denton's care and comfort.
4. Dehydration related to his inability to help himself to fluids.
5. Erratic bowel pattern related to immobility.
6. Weight loss related to inadequate food intake.
7. Lack of communication related to aphasic speech.

It is not difficult to see from this list how priorities can be set and a plan formulated for Mr. Denton's care.

The *purpose of the nursing care goals and an established plan* is to improve care and minimize wasted efforts. Care plans can be very effective. However, if the plan is not kept up to date, the wrong care may be given.

Consider the experience of a nurse who was admitted as a patient to the hospital with a diagnosis of acute enteritis. The next day the cause of her illness was found to be pyelonephritis. During the ensuing 12 days, certain new team leaders who talked with the patient on their "walking rounds" approached her in the context of the diagnosis of enteritis. She was questioned about her bowel pattern to the exclusion of any concern for urinary function. The team leader would consult her care plan and ask such things as, "Why are you still on I & O?" or "Don't you think this cranberry juice you asked for will irritate your bowel?" The patient explained her revised diagnosis, but apparently no one had ever changed it on the record. If she had been a lay person instead of a nurse, this situation could have been most confusing and even serious in terms of possible errors in intervention.

Remember, too, that a diagnosis may be initially incorrect through faulty writing, misspelling, or incorrect transcribing by the admitting clerk or unit ward clerk.

On the other hand, care plans make the difference between poor care and adequate care. Consider the patient who is almost totally deaf but who is used to nodding and saying "Fine" to any comment. She was being taught how to irrigate her new colostomy. Although she kept smiling and saying "Fine," she never seemed to learn how to manage the procedure. Finally, a worker perceived that she was deaf (a rather late perception). This information, along with explicit instructions on how to teach under these circumstances, was incorporated into the care plan. Within several days the woman was managing the procedure adequately.

Not only are care plans useful for people with physiological problems, but people with communication barriers, as in the preceding examples, or those with psychological problems are also in need of an ongoing, up-to-date plan that each health worker can follow. The format used for the written care plan will vary from agency to agency, but in any situation the plan must be simple to use and capable of being readily understood by all workers. A nursing care plan or card usually contains spaces for basic information: diagnosis, age, activity, type of bath, diet, directions regarding intake, output, and vital signs, and space to note communication barriers (such as visual or hearing impairment, aphasia, or speaks a foreign language). Diagnostic tests, treatments, and medications, as well as a space for special instructions in administering them, are also noted. For example, the size and number of dressings to be used, any special way equipment should be arranged, and difficulties to be anticipated and avoided can be noted in a space under "Special Instructions."

Table 4-1 illustrates some of the entries that might appear on a nursing care plan for an elderly man with diabetes and arteriosclerotic-heart disease. Notice that the nursing diagnoses are stated in the context of a dysfunction in an area to which nursing care can be addressed for the necessary help or support.

Teaching begins at the time of the patient's admission and should appear in your care plan from the beginning. It may appear as a part of intervention aimed at a current need, such as explaining the importance of elevating the legs or of using foam pads. Or it may be geared to discharge arrangements, as is the plan for teaching a diabetic. Whatever the need, include it in your plan in such a way as to ensure teaching that can be carried out easily and consistently by everyone. Writing instructions is not enough. Conference discussions and individual help to team members in interpreting the need for teaching are necessary if instruction is to be productive.

In writing your care plan, be sure to use precise action verbs, such as raise, turn, move, place, direct, or apply. Put the nursing action in the most descriptive verb form: what is to be done or how it is to be done. Use modifiers for precision: gently, slowly, firmly, and so on. The which, what, and where are important: which joint, what position, where is it located. The time and frequency elements need to be stated: when, how often, how long. For example, "turn q.2h" may need to be stated so as to consider individual patterns: sleep habits, right- or left-handedness, sleep position most favored, time at which visitors may be expected, or time at which the patient may desire to read or watch television (43).

Table 4-1 Example of Entries for Nursing Care Plan

NURSING DIAGNOSIS	NURSING ACTIONS
1. Shortness of breath, related to respiratory dysfunction.	1. Head of bed 45°. Check position frequently. Keep footboard in place.
2. Mouth dry, related to constant mouth breathing.	2. Oral care T.I.D. Keep lips lubricated with chapstick.
3. Generalized edema, related to cardiovascular insufficiency.	3. Monitor IV flow carefully—15 gtts/min. Keep legs elevated when sitting in chair. Discourage sitting on edge of bed.
4. Reddened areas on back and extremities, related to pressure of bed on edematous areas.	4. Change position q. 2 h. Skin care 2x each shift. Use protective boots on feet.
5. Inadequate self-management of diabetes related to lack of knowledge of disease processes.	5. Set up teaching program for diabetic management with dietician and nurse clinician.

Because one tends to think of care plans in terms of a hospital setting, the example in Table 4-2 has been offered. It is important to note that planning for health maintenance and health promotion for the more than 70 percent of persons with chronic illnesses who are not in hospitals is an urgent need in our society today. Table 4-2 shows a care plan used in a Wellness Clinic in a retirement community for a female client with hypertension.

A nursing care plan is the nurse's responsibility. If the attendant admits the patient, taking vital signs, weighing the person and writing the results, she/he can also write other information: "says he often feels faint" . . . "has an artificial left leg" . . . "likes to sleep with the window open" . . . "requires kosher food." These observations can then be sorted out and used by the professional nurse to formulate care goals with the patient and family and to begin the written nursing care plan in a more formal sense. Much of the potential success of written plans lies in the ability of the professional nurse to involve team members on all levels in the task of keeping the plan current. If ancillary personnel are never consulted about the plan or coached in its use, it will never become a viable part of the scheme of care.

Although each member of the nursing team (including all three shifts) is to be involved in the task of updating the plan and keeping it current, the nursing orders must be one person's (head nurse, team leader, or primary nurse) overall responsibility and authority. Nursing strategies cannot change daily or at random if consistent care to meet established goals is to be given. There may be several approaches to a given problem, each one good in itself; when combined, however, they are likely to be less effective than each would be if used alone.

Discharge planning is an integral part of the nursing goal and care plan in any setting. Discharge planning must begin the day of admission and involve the patient and family unit. Because the entire plan of hospital care is geared toward discharge, it is only logical to consider the nurse as being primarily responsible for plans for continuity of care at home or for referral to a hospital-based home care department, a home health care agency, or other agencies. Other health team members who may contribute to discharge plans are the physician, social worker, dietitian, and physical therapist. The degree to which these people collaborate with the nurse depends on the patient's specific needs and the conditions of life to which the patient will return.

When a patient enters the hospital for a colostomy, for example, the postoperative progress will be followed by the nurse each day, often in conjunction with an ostomy therapist. Together they will do patient teaching, note how well the patient adapts to his colostomy, and evaluate the learning of self-care. The nurse is responsible for investigating

Table 4-2 Example of Entries for Nursing Care Plan

NURSING DIAGNOSIS	NURSING ACTIONS
Need for patient teaching	
Lacks knowledge of hypertension.	Encourage questions and discussion. Supply literature and explain same.
25 lbs. overweight.	Discuss effects of obesity on hypertension. Explore eating habits and suggest modifications in keeping with lifestyle and preferences.
Leads a sedentary life at age 70.	Supply literature on simple exercises to promote weight loss and strengthen muscle tone. Encourage walking.
Lacks understanding of medications.	Review purpose of medications, explain their action in lay person's terms and importance of consistency in dosages. Teach an awareness of possible side effects.
Lacks knowledge of high-salt food products.	Provide lists of salt content of various foods. Assist in planning a compatible diet regimen low in salt. Suggest ways of enhancing flavor of foods without the use of salt.
Need for emotional support	
Lost husband 2 months ago after a long illness.	Allow opportunity to express feelings and assist her in moving through the steps of grieving. Recommend Widows' Support Group at Senior Center nearby.
Difficulty in adapting to lifestyle change due to bereavement and subsequent feeling of having "time on her hands."	Encourage to participate in activities in retirement village where she lives, thereby establishing a new routine with other people. Suggest various volunteer activities to help others.

the need for home care and any necessary agency referrals, involving the family in all of this planning. How well the family members are coping with the patient's condition; their abilities, strengths, and limits; and the physical setting in the home all need to be explored. Similarly, the diabetic, the patient who has a stroke, and all patients in need of continuity of care will need this kind of planning.

Nurses are the best qualified members of the health care delivery team for discharge planning because they are familiar with all aspects of their patient's/client's care, they are able to interpret medical as well as nursing information, and they are in a position to transmit this information to those who will render follow-up care.

Nursing Intervention

All actions that you carry out to promote the patient's/client's adaptation constitute **intervention,** the fourth step in the nursing process. You **intervene** (from the Latin meaning "come between") *when you modify, settle, or hinder some action* in order to prevent harm or further dysfunction.

"Ministering" to people, carrying out "comfort" measures, or "caring" for the sick are terms often equated by lay people with conserving the ill person's energy by waiting on him/her. But your interpretation of *care* and *comfort* should encompass the overall goal of professional nursing: to assist the person to function as effectively and efficiently as the limits of illness permit and to encourage him/her to react to the situation in a unique way. Care that is limited to energy-conserving measures on the person's behalf may be very detrimental to his/her progress. You need a comprehensive data base, including a nursing history and assessment that encompasses all functional areas, a list of nursing diagnoses, and a plan that is based on goals so that your nursing actions are pertinent for the individual. In addition, you must know the **scientific rationale,** *the reasons, either physiological or psychosocial, for performing any action.* For example, do you bathe the patient because of a rigid schedule or because of physiological and psychosocial principles involving (1) increased circulation and aeration, (2) care of the integument, (3) preservation of musculoskeletal function, and (4) opportunity for communication, further assessment, and health teaching?

Nursing actions may consist of either dependent or independent functions: those depending on the medical regimen as outlined by the physician or those derived from nursing judgments. Through nursing intervention, you execute all those ministrations that help meet needs that the individual is not able to meet. Intervention includes all comfort and hygiene measures; safe and efficient use of medical techniques and skills; planning and creating an environment conducive to wholeness, including protection from risk and injury; and health teaching, formal and informal. It also includes the offering of oneself for strength and courage in coping with problems through counseling, listening, and socializing; and using information for referrals wherever indicated, either for in-agency care or as discharge planning.

The concept of rehabilitation could be considered almost synonymous with intervention, for from the very beginning of your relationship with the client/family intervention must be geared to restoration of the person's potential for optimum functioning. It is unquestionably tied in with teaching and discharge planning, discussed under the section on nursing goals and plan of care.

The importance of the written care plan to organize nursing intervention cannot be overemphasized. It is a powerful instrument that can be used in a variety of ways. The data base is invaluable as the groundwork for later evaluation and judgment regarding patient progress.

Nursing intervention occurs in many settings: hospital, local health department, visiting nurse association, nursing home, school, industry, doctor's office, neighborhood health center, and ambulatory clinic. Nurses also carry out intervention from other bases, such as the Red Cross, insurance companies, children's camps, health maintenance organization, and even through a telephone service (54).

Because the nursing process is a problem-solving mode of action using the scientific method, your nursing actions are hypotheses to be tested in practice. When they are shown to be effective and can be validated, specific actions or ways in which needs are best met become a part of the ongoing individualized nursing care plan. The fifth step of the nursing process, evaluation, is used to determine the validity of nursing actions, to decide to what degree goals have been met, to redefine nursing diagnoses, and to lay the foundation for a further plan of care.

Evaluation

Evaluation, *determining immediate outcomes and predicting long-range results*, cannot be entirely separated from the first four steps in the nursing process. A circular effect implies constant reassessment of the patient/client situation, redefining of nursing diagnoses, stating nursing goals, and updating of the nursing care plan for action. Interventions will then be modified or expanded and reevaluation will occur. Criteria for evaluating the care as to its effectiveness will evolve from the goals inherent in the nursing diagnoses: for instance, if the nursing diagnosis was "erratic bowel pattern related to immobility," the gain or lack of a consistent bowel pattern will be evidence to support the success or failure of the nursing actions taken to accomplish the goal. Validation must include feedback from the recipients of care—patient or family—and from members of the health team who are objective observers. Subjective symptoms, such as pain, and results of intervention are best evaluated by the patient. Observable signs may be evaluated best by the health team.

The goal of your chosen action within the nursing process is always to minimize objectively the negative consequences to the greatest degree possible and to capitalize on those outcomes that are positive. In evaluating results of intervention, you will seek to duplicate the positive effects and to determine the cause of unexpected outcomes, whether positive or negative. In a negative outcome, attempt to control or help the person control the events responsible so that the outcome does not recur.

Recognizing that an act may have more than one consequence, you must evaluate who will be affected by the act, what results can be anticipated, and the value of the consequences to those involved. Being aware of this evaluation process will help you appreciate that even the simplest activity is a means of achieving the goals you have set for the patient in striving toward wellness. Emptying a bedpan then becomes not an isolated menial task but a part of your intervention for carrying out some priorities of care, such as provision of needed rest and maintenance of elimination and fluid balance.

Evaluation of care is directly related to what is termed **accountability**, *the state of being responsible for one's acts and being able to explain, define, or measure in some way the results of decision making.* Accountability involves evaluating the effectiveness of care on the basis of "how," "what," and "to whom" (78, 89). Just believing that your care makes a difference is not enough. You must have criteria that justify both the need for and the effectiveness of your nursing actions.

The "how" is measuring your effectiveness against a set of criteria—a predetermined outcome to be observed. Noting that an immobile patient who has been given daily prune juice is now able to have a normal stool at reasonable intervals without requiring enemas or cathartics is one example of observing a predetermined outcome. You can evaluate the care of an individual patient, care given within a nursing unit, or care delivered by an entire community health agency or clinic.

The "what" of accountability involves intervention measures and intangibles, such as attitudes and subtle nuances. The nursing measures you carry out are important, but equally important is the meaning of care to the person.

In order to decide "to whom" you are accountable, you must first clarify for yourself the nature and the purpose of your care. You will be accountable to the patient/client, family, group, doctor, nursing staff, agency administration, and community.

One way in which nurses can contribute to improvement of care is by developing within their own agency a quality control system that applies specifically to nursing. This system must be one in which desired nursing criteria are identified and it must incorporate a way in which nursing practice can be compared to the established criteria.

Process standards rather than structure standards must be used. (The difference between process and structure standards can be illustrated by examples: *Structure*—Are written care plans used? *Process*—Is the written care plan appropriate to the patient. Does it consider personal needs, disease-related needs, and therapy-related needs? *Outcome*—What is the outcome in terms of mortality, morbidity, and social functioning?)

The scope of the system may be determined by the objectives and specific needs of the agency. It may be limited to patient care or may include administrative functions; it may be used for a particular department exclusively; or it may apply to a specific group of patients—for example, those with respiratory diseases. Once it has been determined, a form can be prepared, one with a format that is simple, easy to use, and readily interpretable by all who use it. Because the design will influence the way in which the standards are worded, the evaluation form must be prepared first (89).

Basic to any quality control system, or as it is sometimes called, a nursing audit, is a plan for recording accurate and objective observations of patients in their clinical record or chart. Without written data relevant to patient progress, patient response to therapy, and completion of physician's orders, the nursing process would be incomplete. *The nurse's charting must reflect the nursing care plan.* Only by validation of nursing actions can the profession hope to demonstrate its commitment to quality care.

Whatever system of charting is used—narrative nurses' notes, a problem-oriented record in which progress is noted by using the SOAP format, or a goal-oriented record—it must be capable of being analyzed in terms of the quality of care given. Such analysis includes both technical aspects and the "art of care." The "art of care" includes rules, manner, and behavior of care providers, and their communication with clients (95). This responsibility rests on the nurse and requires accountability to the patient, profession, other members of the health team, the institution, and, not least, oneself.

An essential part of the nurse's accountability is a personal commitment to continuing education that is related directly to the practice of nursing. The current explosion of knowledge, advances in technology, and public demand for more effective health care make it essential that nurses continue their learning beyond their basic education.

Lately there has been a move toward mandatory continuing education for nurses with arguments pro and con. Whether mandatory continuing education for licensure as a registered nurse becomes widespread, the responsibility for improvement of practice through education will always rest with the individual nurse.

TOOLS FOR EVALUATING YOUR EFFECTIVENESS

The Process Recording

Communication is essential to the nursing process and thus is repeatedly emphasized throughout the book. One tool for analyzing your communication pattern with patients is the process recording.

The **process recording** *is a written account of the responses of client and nurse and the analysis of these responses*, providing for the reconstruction of a nursing incident in order to identify and examine the elements in it. It may be written during the time the conversation or interview is occurring or from recollection. You should obtain the person's consent if you plan to take notes during an interview.

The reconstruction of an interview or conversation is valuable for picking out clues to behavior and for determining inconsistencies in your response to the person. The process recording allows you to evaluate your responses in relation to communication principles and methods, improve communication, focus more accurately on the person's needs, and make predictions about nursing intervention. In addition, you provide the person a seldom available opportunity to express self to someone who listens in a nonjudgmental way. Thus you help him/her to sort out thoughts and feelings. The process recording is also a teaching tool. When you share with other team members what you have told the person and his/her reaction to the illness, they can use this information as a guide in further therapeutic communication.

The forms used for process recordings vary, but all should provide columns in which the responses or perceptions of the nurse are separated from the responses of the patient. A third column is used to analyze the responses of either the nurse, or the client, or both. Table 4-3 is an example.

Although initially you may feel self-conscious when writing, most clients agree to this system when you tell them it will help you give better care. You may use shorthand or write only the first words of each statement by you or the client to enable you to reconstruct the interview. The interview you analyze through a process recording may occur in a variety of settings and may last from 5 minutes to an hour, depending on your purpose and the person's needs and condition.

You will build on the foundation of interviewing and therapeutic communication studied in Chapter 3. The person must be able to sense your regard and interest in his/her ideas, hopes, and fears. Your nonjudgmental attitude is essential to help the person sort out ideas and reach the solution that seems most feasible.

As soon as possible after the interview, reconstruct it from your

TABLE 4-3 Process Recording

CLIENT'S VERBAL AND NONVERBAL COMMUNICATION	NURSE'S VERBAL AND NONVERBAL COMMUNICATION	ANALYSIS OF COMMUNICATION PATTERN, THOUGHTS, AND FEELINGS
	I knock and enter the room to do preoperative teaching. I sit down on a chair near the bed and look at her with a serious expression and say, "Mrs. Jones, have you been told you're going to surgery tomorrow?"	Wanted to make sure she knew about surgery before I began teaching and to check her level of readiness for teaching. Sat down to show her I had time and was interested in her.
"Yes, that's what they told me." Facial expression is serious as she looks at me. She clenches the sheet; restlessly moves legs. Chin quivers as she speaks.		
	I pause briefly to let her continue talking if she wishes.	Noted her movements and that her pupils are dilated in a well-lit room, indicating anxiety.
She looks down.	"What are you feeling about going to surgery?" I lean slightly forward and maintain eye contact.	Asking open-ended question to encourage her to talk about feelings. Must relieve anxiety before she will be able to hear or utilize my teaching.
"Oh, honey, I'm scared to death!" She shifts position toward me. "You know, they're cutting on me for my gall-bladder. The doctor told me it was nothing, but I know of a person who died after gall-bladder surgery."	I nod as she talks to show acceptance of her feelings and to encourage further talking. I maintain silence.	Noted the use of words "cutting on me"—surgery can mean mutilation and be a threat to body image. Need to talk about feelings to resolve them.
	"You're afraid you'll die?" Speak softly, with acceptance.	Reflect back main idea to encourage further talking.
"Yes, I just might not wake up. People *die* with surgery." Pauses.	Silence.	Let her continue talking about this if she needs to. Nothing I say right now would make a difference.
"I keep telling myself that it's unlikely that I'll die, that my doctor is right saying I won't die, that I am in good hands."		

TABLE 4-3 (cont.)

CLIENT'S VERBAL AND NONVERBAL COMMUNICATION	NURSE'S VERBAL AND NONVERBAL COMMUNICATION	ANALYSIS OF COMMUNICATION PATTERN, THOUGHTS, AND FEELINGS
	"Yes, facing surgery is frightening, although your ideas about not dying and being in good hands are true. It takes courage to go to surgery, but in this case it is for your ultimate comfort."	Restate feelings, recognize and validate feelings, but also try to reinforce ideas so she can feel less worried.
She smiles, clenched hands relaxed. "You do understand! I thought maybe I was abnormal."		Noted she is beginning to relax. Being accepted and listened to as she talked helped reduce anxiety.
	Look toward her with a slight smile. "Your feelings are not abnormal. Tell me more about how you're feeling."	Validate with her about her feelings; show acceptance. Use open-ended question to encourage further talking if she needs to.
Stretches in bed, smiles, "Oh, I feel better just being able to tell you and having you understand."		
	"Do you feel ready to discuss the preparation you'll be having for surgery?"	Question phrased to get "yes or no" response. Want to check readiness for teaching.

brief notes and make an analysis of the verbal and nonverbal dialogue. This expansion can help you gain insight into yourself and the client and provide data for planning care. If your approach to the person seems unproductive, a process recording in which incidents are reconstructed may help identify the problem. Clues can be analyzed for their meaning by writing out what preceded certain of your or the client's responses. You can better realize ways in which you could have intervened in a more direct or helpful manner, perhaps by rephrasing or refocusing your portion of the dialogue.

Written Analysis of Nursing Care

Another tool for evaluating your effectiveness in the nursing process and nurse–client relationship is a **written analysis** *of nursing care*. The written analysis provides a way of looking at your assessment of needs, your intervention as a result of planning, the scientific rationale on which your intervention was based, and of evaluating the care you gave.

Assessments and Nursing Diagnoses may be put down in a sequential order if you wish or they may be sorted out according to functional areas. Table 4-4 gives an example of analyzing care according to functional areas.

Intervention, Together with the Reason for Your Action, is placed in a second column and shows the results of your planning. A stumbling block in this portion of your analysis is often the confusion of medical intervention with that of nursing. If the patient has an intravenous pyelogram done in x ray, for example, that is medical intervention. If you explain the test to the patient, allay fears through communication and teaching, and prepare him/her for the test by administering prescribed medication or treatments, these are nursing interventions.

You should justify or give the rationale for action on the patient's behalf, validating your rationale with the literature. Therefore familiarity with the current nursing literature, as well as an ability to use the literature of related disciplines, the natural and behavioral sciences and humanities, will be a necessary part of your continued independent study as you practice nursing.

Evaluation is the step often overlooked or given minimal attention. Yet it is the basis for reassessment and improvement of care and should be included in your written analysis. You may not always write an analysis, but you should have the same information firmly in mind and be able to describe it to others. You may be able to incorporate some of the process recording in your evaluation. Your reassessment is then based on a more complete data base and can be done with a number of interrelated facts, some of which, if missing, would considerably change your approach to the improvement of the patient's care. You may see, for instance, that the outcome of the bath you have given is increased relaxation for the patient, including a restful nap before lunch, but fail to evaluate the feeling of dependence and loss of self-actualization expressed by the person verbally and nonverbally. Rehabilitation may then be seriously impaired through inadequate evaluation.

Ensuring quality of care throughout the health care system is discussed in Chapter 2.

THE NURSE-CLIENT RELATIONSHIP IN THE NURSING PROCESS

Differences Between a Social and a Helpful Relationship

Establishing a helpful relationship is one of the unique functions separating nursing from other health services.

The **nurse-client relationship** *is a helpful, purposeful interaction*

TABLE 4-4 Analysis of Care, Sample Form

Name Mrs. S. Age 56 Date 2-1

Diagnosis Arthritis – R. total hip replacement – 2nd postop day

Nurse Mr. J.

ASSESSMENT (NURSING DIAGNOSIS)	INTERVENTION AND RATIONALE	EVALUATION
8:30 A.M. Obese female—appears in pain—has Buck's traction on R. leg. Foot plate is resting against foot of bed. (Pain related to surgery and position)	Had aide help me move patient up in bed to release pressure on footplate which interferes with efficiency of traction. Checked chart to see when pain medication was given last. Most pain medication is given no oftener than q. 3-4 hours to avoid oversedation and respiratory embarrassment.	Should help alleviate some of her pain by allowing a more even pull from traction. Must remember after this to check on time of last medication before seeing patient.
No pain medication given since 2:00 A.M.	Gave injection of Demerol 100 mg. IM before beginning bath to promote relaxation, relief of pain, and more ease in moving.	Mrs. S. more relaxed after about 20 minutes.
Has perspired during night. Breath is somewhat fetid—mouth dry. (Impaired personal hygiene and discomfort related to perspiration and dry mouth)	Gave oral care (preserves integrity of gums, prevents dental caries, and heightens enjoyment of food). Gave complete bed bath to refresh, provide chance for observation, stimulate circulation and aeration, and cleanse skin. Removed traction for skin care and gave back care q. 2 h. to prevent pressure areas by stimulation of areas over bony prominences. Did ROM exercises with unaffected extremities to maintain joint mobility, muscle tone, enhance circulation, prevent thrombus formation. Bath and exercises aid maintenance and reintegration of body image.	Appeared more comforable after bath and is in proper body alignment.

TABLE 4-4 (cont.)

ASSESSMENT (NURSING DIAGNOSIS)	INTERVENTION AND RATIONALE	EVALUATION
Talked during bath about fear of crutch walking. (Anxiety related to immobility and anticipated crutch walking)	Encouraged Mrs. S. to verbalize concerns about walking. Talking promotes anxiety reduction and enables patient to begin problem solving. My listening showed respect for and interest in her as a person, gave attention, promoted trust in nurse-patient relationship.	Explanation of pool therapy and therapist's help in P.T. seemed to help her figure out for herself that she should walk OK. Mrs. S. came to conclusion after our conversation that she would wait to see progress before assuming she would have trouble walking.

over time between an authority in health care, the nurse, and a person or group with health care needs, with the nurse focusing on needs of the client while being empathic and using knowledge. Through this relationship the nursing process is put to use, and it must be differentiated from mere association. Social contact with another individual, verbal or nonverbal, may exert some influence on one of the participants and needs may be met. But inconsistency, nonpredictability, or partial fulfillment of expectations often results. Characteristics of social relationship are as follows:

1. The contact is primarily for pleasure and companionship.
2. Neither person is in a position of responsibility for helping the other.
3. No specific skill or knowledge is required.
4. The interaction is between peers, often of the same social status.
5. The people involved can, and often do, pursue an encounter for the satisfaction of personal or selfish interests.
6. There is no explicit formulation of goals.
7. There is no sense of accountability for the other person.
8. Evaluation of interactions does not concern personal effectiveness in the interaction (55).

A nurse-client relationship is established *when the person's or family's needs are met consistently and unconditionally.*

A working nurse-client relationship is, by definition, good, helpful, therapeutic. There is no such thing as a poor nurse-client relationship; there are only poor or unsatisfactory experiences that prevent establishing the relationship. Interactions moving toward a relationship occur whenever direct patient care, health teaching, listening, or counseling are done, or when the person's/family's activities are being directed or modified in some way.

The following interactions are *not* helpful to the patient because needs are met inconsistently or conditionally:

1. Automatic, in which there is no meaning to either person.
2. Impersonally helpful, in which a service is expertly given but no personal interest or empathy is displayed.
3. Involuntary, in which "carrying out orders" is done as a duty, often the result of the nurse's perception of work as just a job to be done.
4. Inconsistent (that which is conditional in nature)—assisting the patient only when the situation is interesting or when it fulfills the nurse's needs (92).

The nurse-client relationship is one in which the person's real complaint is uncovered. The focus is on the client's needs rather than on your own. The person is not a social buddy. There is a giving of self in an objective way to the person and family; yet you do not identify with (feel the same as), pity, or reject the one seeking help. Neither do you feel you are the only person who can help the client. You use the resources that a team can offer whenever doing so is beneficial to the person or family.

The Effect of Feelings on the Relationship

Only through mutual striving for self-awareness and appreciation of the other person's reactions can a nurse-client relationship grow to maturity. Knowing that each person has needs to be met gives meaning to this relationship. You must expect both positive and negative feelings in yourself and in the other, and you must realize that both can be expressed either overtly or covertly.

The client's positive feelings may be those relating to a sincere desire to cooperate in his/her own care and may include a polite manner toward others. The feelings may be a result of educational, religious, or cultural background, or a combination of these factors. In any event, you are in a position to capitalize on such positive feelings in order to establish rapport and a sense of trust as a foundation for the nurse-client relationship. Additionally, make every effort to learn the person's negative feelings. Insecurity; distrust of unfamiliar persons, routines, and treatments; or helplessness or hostility because of a lack of control over his/her own responses—all may be present.

Unfortunately, when either positive or negative overt feelings dominate a patient's behavior, the person may be labeled "good" or "bad" by the staff. The "good" patient is the one who never complains, who accepts illness no matter how distressing or painful, and who receives the care given without question. The characteristics of the "bad" patient are usually described by staff as demanding, complaining, and displeasing physically and conversationally. Such a person is seen as not helping himself/herself, unappreciative, and uncooperative. Nurses often become upset or judgmental with the intransigent patient as well. He/she does not understand the rules in the same way that you do and interferes with the established routine. Yet the interference may be an expression of the very self-determination necessary for rehabilitation (92). Often the behavior of the person from a different culture, social class, or ethnic group is misinterpreted. When the person's behavior does not match your expectations, do not label it. Instead try to understand why the behavior might be different.

The positive feelings that you may have toward the client are strongly bound to your commitment to nursing as a way of life. They cannot develop if you are merely doing a job because the negative feelings we all possess can overpower the positive and interfere with the nurse–client relationship. Negative feelings, which may at times be expressed in your reactions, will provoke inappropriate behavior. Talking out your negative feelings with the staff is better than unloading them on the client or family.

The Effect of Behavior on the Relationship

To develop an awareness of the feelings that you take with you to the client, examine your behavior to determine whether it is modified for some people in a helping way and for others in a manner that hinders your effectiveness. Modification of your behavior with, or approach to, different persons is a valuable tool. Surely you would behave differently toward the child than toward the aged person. But behaving differently because a person is rich or poor, Black or White, quiet or boisterous, grateful or ungrateful, in agreement or disagreement with your value system may prevent you from meeting that person's needs.

Remembering that all behavior has meaning will help you to sharpen and improve those qualities you possess that produce a positive response in others. When inappropriate reactions do occur, analyze them in terms of what preceded them and of what happened after the incident. Search for clues to establish the meaning of feelings. Using the process recording format, you might record the event by writing the conversation and the nonverbal responses of both you and client for closer analysis. Discussing the incident with objective persons may help, perhaps in team conference. Become familiar with your own coping mechanisms; seek to understand their relative value and the ways in which you use them in your approach to nursing care. Take sufficient care of your personal needs outside the nursing setting so that you can give your best professional care to the person or family or group.

Although the relationship with a client is a reciprocal experience, the responsibility for establishing it and for making appropriate changes in it rests with you, not with the client. The relationship is based on each person's perceiving the other as a unique individual without stereotyping. Help the person *not* to see you as the command officer or the "angel in white" and avoid seeing the patient as a "gallbladder" or a room number.

You may unconsciously exhibit a middle-class tea-and-cookie niceness combined with Puritan morality that insists on uncompromising obedience on the part of nursing student, nurse, patient, and family alike. You may represent a punitive social system, and the person may sense your moral indignation toward health problems that some regard as stemming from "indiscretions": alcoholism, drug addiction, unwed motherhood, obesity, venereal disease, or even diabetes uncontrolled because of dietary carelessness. Superimposed on this attitude may be the ethic of cleanliness in which you loom as a threat to the other, judging the person in terms of how clean he/she is, internally as well as externally.

Hospital administrations sometimes contribute to stereotyping by commending the nurse as "good" if she/he gets the beds and baths finished, the pills passed, the treatments done. Because these things are tangible, they do not require time for involvement with patients' reactions, behavior, or qualitative responses of nurse to patient or patient to nurse. Tasks must be done and are vital to nursing care, but overemphasis on tasks leaves little time for exploring the meaning of the person's health status and health goals.

Carrying out the person's planned regimen for health maintenance or restoration will be accomplished more easily because of the nurse-client relationship, for it will naturally foster the tangible as well as the intangible aspects of your care. Above all, keep expectations mutual and remember that the major characteristic of the nurse-client relationship is that *the nursing needs of the individual or family are met in an emotional climate of warmth, support, and mutual trust* (92).

Guidelines for the Nurse-Client Relationship

If you consider your behavior an influence on the person's or family's behavior, you will be in a better position to advise specific approaches for bringing about change. You will want to develop characteristics of a helping, humanistic relationship. These characteristics include being

1. *Respectful*—Feeling and communicating an attitude of seeing the client as a unique human being, filled with dignity, worth, and strengths, regardless of outward appearance or behavior; being willing to *work* at communicating with and understanding the client because he/she is in need of emotional care.
2. *Genuine*—Communicating spontaneously, yet tactfully, what is felt and thought, with proper timing and without disturbing the client, rather than using professional jargon, facade, or rigid counselor or nurse role behaviors.
3. *Attentive*—Conveying rapport and an active listening to verbal and nonverbal messages and an attitude of working with the person.
4. *Accepting*—Conveying that the person does not have to put on a facade and that the person will not shock you with his/her statements; enabling the client to change at his/her own pace; acknowledging personal and client's feelings aroused in the encounter; to "be for" the client in a nonsentimental, caring way.
5. *Positive*—Showing warmth, caring, respect, and agape (love); being able to reinforce the client for what he/she does well.
6. *Strong*—Maintaining separate identity from the client; withstanding the testing behavior of the client.
7. *Secure*—Permitting the client to remain separate and unique; respecting his/her needs and your own; feeling safe as the client moves emotionally close; feeling no need to exploit the other person.
8. *Knowledgeable*—Having an expertise based on study, experience, and supervision; being able to assist the client in formulating goals.
9. *Sensitive*—Being perceptive to feelings; avoiding threatening behavior, responding to cultural values, customs, norms as they affect behavior; using knowledge that is pertinent to the client's situation.
10. *Empathic*—Looking at the client's world from his/her point of view; being open to his/her values, feelings, beliefs, and verbal statements; stating your understanding of his/her verbal or nonverbal expressions of feelings and experiences.
11. *Nonjudgmental*—Refraining from evaluating the client moralistically or telling the client what to do.
12. *Congruent*—Being natural, relaxed, trustworthy, and dependable, and demonstrating consistency in behavior and between verbal and nonverbal messages.
13. *Unambiguous*—Avoiding contradictory messages; using purposeful communication.
14. *Creative*—Viewing the client as a person in the process of becom-

ing, not being bound by the past, and viewing yourself in the process of becoming or maturing as well (79).

Other features that correlate highly with being effective in a helping relationship are being open instead of closed in interaction with others, perceiving others as friendly and capable instead of unfriendly and incapable, and perceiving a relationship as freeing instead of controlling another (55).

Establishing and maintaining a relationship or counseling another does not involve putting on a facade of behavior to match a list of characteristics. Rather, both you and the client will change and continue to mature. As the helper, you are present as a total person, blending potentials, talents, and skills while assisting the client to come to grips with needs, conflicts, and self (55, 67).

Working with another in a helping relationship is challenging and rewarding. You will not always have all the characteristics just described; at times you will be handling personal stresses that will lower your energy and sense of involvement. You may become irritated and impatient while working with the client. Accept the fact that you are not perfect; remain as aware as possible of your needs and behavior and your effect on the other. Remember that the most important thing you can share with a client is your own uniqueness as a person. As you give of yourself to the client, you will in return be given to—rewarded with warmth and sharing from the client.

Phases of the Nurse-Client Relationship

Unless the encounter is brief, the feelings between you and the client and the family and the work jointly done evolve through a sequence of phases. The phases are not sharply demarcated and they vary in duration. They can be compared to human developmental stages because of the degree of dependency-independency and feelings of trust involved: the orientation phase is comparable to infancy, identification to childhood, the working phase to adolescence, and termination to adulthood (67).

The Initial or Orientation Phase of the relationship begins when you first meet the person or family. You might carry out intervention measures shortly thereafter, as you function in the role of technical expert, counselor, teacher, referral person, or substitute mother. Your main tasks during this phase, however, are to become oriented to the other's expectations, health needs, and goals through assessment while simultaneously orienting the person to your role and health care goals and his/her role in the health care system. You formulate a tentative care plan. Establishing rapport and showing acceptance are vital for assessing and orienting the other person. Be aware of how you are affecting the person and how he/she is affecting you. During this period the person clarifies the health status and its meaning through your exploration of the many factors affecting him/her. Essential to this phase is caring for the person or family in such a way that a sense of trust and confidence in you is established.

The Second Phase, Called the Identification Phase, marks the time when the person has become better acquainted with you, places trust in your decisions and actions, works closely with you, follows your suggestions, and at times imitates your behavior. He/she sees you as "his/her nurse." You continue the nursing process, actively guiding him/her but also providing opportunities for participation in self-care. You accept dependency without fostering it excessively.

The Third, the Working Phase, is the time when the client is becoming more independent, actively using all services and resources offered by the health team. He/she becomes more assertive and no longer relies so heavily on you. By now he/she is usually regaining physical and emotional health—optimal function—so that behavior begins to change as he/she becomes more involved in decision making about certain aspects of the situation. Although the person seems more independent and even self-centered, you can now work as equal partners in meeting health goals. The client is preparing for convalescence and discharge from your services.

Maintenance Phase

Often the nurse who works in an acute care setting does not really experience the rewards of a relationship with the patient. The short stay typical of hospitalization or even the few visits given by a home health nurse allow nothing more than establishing rapport, if that.

The maintenance phase in the relationship is only possible in the setting in which a client is followed by the same nurse over a period of time—for example, in a rehabilitation center, nursing home, senior residence, or psychiatric-mental health agency. Also, the nurse in independent practice or in an ambulatory care clinic may see the same clients over a period of years.

In this phase, termination does not occur for a long time. Often termination only comes with the death of the person. The active, working, therapeutic stage goes on until the person has reached his/her potential. In this situation, the client has reached a plateau where support and maintenance are essential for daily living. The client may live at home, following your directions for health promotion measures, and may call on you for assistance only when chronic illness becomes uncontrolled or when a new condition of pathology or aging arises. Or the client may be in an institution and need maximal or minimal assistance with daily physical care. What characterizes this phase is that you must actively pursue interventions in order to maintain emotional and social well-being. The reward will be the gratification of seeing a person reassert his/her will to live, to become creative in coping with problems or making "ends meet," and to remain independent.

The Last Phase, Termination, is marked by the person's becoming as fully independent as possible, leaving the health care system to return to the community. Together you plan the management of the health situation after discharge, especially if the client requires any special lifestyle modifications, such as in exercise, hygiene, or diet. This is a time of separation and both you and the person must work through feelings about separation–sometimes past as well as present situations. Mutual attachment develops between you and someone you take care of for a long time and either one or both of you may feel uncertain about the person's ability to manage without you. Together you need to talk about feelings about separation and your confidence in the ability to be independent and remain healthy. Avoid increasing dependency on you at this time to meet your needs. When the client leaves the health care system, each of you should feel no regret about the termination. On the other hand, if there is need for follow-up visits after discharge, your interest and concern in the person or family extend to this ongoing care.

Without the nurse–client relationship, the person's needs are not met and the nursing process is not in force. Mechanical tasks become an end in themselves and the person is not helped to prevent or adapt to his/her illness.

There may be people with whom you cannot form a helpful relationship. There may be situations in which it would be best for the client if someone else were to work with him/her. You need to be aware of your own feelings of discomfort with a client and you should be able to accept the fact that you cannot work with certain people. Often the reasons will be obscure; you may want to work through the reasons with an instructor or supervisor for your own personal growth. Reference 55 gives more information on barriers to an effective nurse–client relationship.

THE CHANGING ROLE OF THE NURSE

The Nursing Process and the Expanded Nursing Role

The future of nursing in the face of a complete revision and updating of the American health care delivery system depends on a compatible fusion of nursing process and redefined role. Nursing is asserting itself as a profession and claiming the right to function independently of the medical profession in giving primary care. This movement began with the idea of the extended role, which has gradually been reworked into the expanded role. However, in nursing, *extended* has come to mean taking on new functions, often technical. *Expanded* has come to mean gaining depth and breadth of knowledge in order to function in a new and broader role in many settings and to make independent judgments to meet the holistic needs of the person or family. The nurse thinks of self in a new way—as an advocate for the client, not as a handmaiden to the doctor.

The nursing practitioner in the nontraditional setting, the family nurse practitioner, the pediatric nurse practitioner, the school nurse, nurse-midwife, and nurse clinician in industry are some examples of the changed role of the nurse. The nurse handles some diagnostic and care functions that in the past were done only by the physician, functions that were often neglected because the physician was too busy. Primary care services, such as physical and psychosocial assessment, history taking, health screening and diagnosis, referral, teaching, and counseling and working with the person or family over time for continuity of care, are examples of how the nurse has expanded the role. Technical and physical care are not enough. The increasing need for reorganized or refocused health care is changing the nurse's role to provide more than traditional nursing care.

In North Carolina a member of the state personnel department asked for a delineation of what was different about the nurse who had expanded the nursing role via a formal nurse practitioner program and one who had not. The roles were defined as similar, but the practitioner was approved (by a joint subcommittee of physicians and nurses) to interpret signs and symptoms of abnormalities, make appropriate diagnoses (medical as well as nursing), and initiate a medical care regimen, including prescribing medication. A nonpractitioner, for instance, would be expected only to distinguish abnormal from normal whereas the practitioner would diagnose the abnormal symptoms. A nonpractitioner would only order appropriately prescribed laboratory procedures whereas the practitioner would order the necessary procedures and interpret the findings and relate them to other patient data (36).

The model of the nurse practitioner was formally created in 1965 to expand the scope of nursing without changing its essential nature. Originally seen as a highly skilled, academically prepared, community health nursing specialist, this person was considered rather avant-garde—even maverick. The role has worn well, however, and is now considered the norm for qualified professional nurses in whatever facilities they may practice. The nurse practitioner–clinician is indeed a nurse for all settings (26).

The trend toward specialization in medicine has created a shortage of primary physicians available to care for people with ordinary or chronic illnesses for a modest fee and to do basic diagnosis for referral to specialty care. In 1978, the potential and actual family practice physicians, including some internists and pediatricians, constituted less than one-half of the physicians in practice. This situation provided the strongest impetus for the role expansion of registered nurses into ambulatory primary care with persons of any age group, including those with chronic disease or disability.

Inside the hospital itself advancing medical technology has expanded the scope of nursing practice, especially in the critical care units (adult and neonatal) in which nurses operate complex equipment and are called on to make on-the-spot diagnostic judgments. Primary nursing is being implemented on other patient care units in many hospitals. Primary nursing is a "philosophy and a modality of humanistic health care delivery in which the client becomes a contributor to as well as a recipient of his/her plan of care. The client is assigned a professional nurse who cares for him/her utilizing the nursing process and scientific inquiry. The primary nurse has authority, autonomy, and is accountable to the client. This modality may be applied in a variety of settings" (20).

In community health settings and outpatient clinics many nurse practitioners were working in the expanded role early in the 1900s: doing case findings, giving treatment for minor illnesses, teaching, referring people to community agencies. The nurse did family-centered nursing by assisting the individual and family with problems—medical, social, or economic—that interfered with the family's ability to cope with daily activities. With additional preparation, the community health nurse did complete psychosocial and physical assessment in order to give total care to clients.

Social trends have contributed to role expansion for the nurse, the women's liberation movement being a strong factor. More autonomy for women has erased many self-doubts about their assuming more responsible roles. Conversely, as sex stereotyping has decreased, more men have been attracted to nursing. They are not tuned to playing the "doctor–nurse game" and serve as healthy examples of change for their classmates in today's schools.

The changing age distribution in the population has contributed to the development of the nurse practitioner. The number of persons in the postretirement years is increasing and this is the group that suffers most from chronic illness. Long-range support and health teaching are important to the management of their symptoms. Nurse practitioners with a background in both the behavioral and biological sciences are ideally qualified to manage chronic illnesses in the elderly.

There is a distinct interrelationship between the law and social change. States are revising their nurse practice acts to provide for role expansion, thereby removing a significant barrier to role change. At the same time, these changes in the laws are inspiring nurses to seek specialty training so that they may move into more satisfying positions for health care delivery (11).

Nurse practitioners are found anywhere where nurses practice. One sees them in a variety of settings. The United States Public Health Service has nurse practitioners who staff clinics on Indian reservations where patients are seen regularly for primary care. Nurse practitioners function independently, with a backup of one or more consulting physicians in the nearest town whom they can use for referrals. Many use standing orders similar to those developed by the Frontier Nursing Service in Kentucky for their own nurse practitioners. Nurse practitioners also carry caseloads in outpatient clinics at medical centers. They are also found in school and occupational health and in geriatric and long-term care settings. The physician has found that the nurse prepared in the skills of physical and psychosocial assessment is a greater addition to the staff than the receptionist-filing clerk-office nurse of the past. In some doctor's offices the nurse has her own caseload, making hospital and home visits to patients/families as indicated in order to provide continuity of care, teaching, and counseling. Nurses have set up private practices in several cities and in some rural areas.

One of the more interesting examples of the nurse practitioner role was implemented at the University of Arizona College of Medicine in the academic year 1976-1977. A highly structured, sequential, competency-based physical examination course taught by nurse practitioners was instituted to instruct preclinical medical students in the complete physical examination of the asymptomatic adult. One of the writers of this chapter participated in this experimental course as a nurse practitioner instructor, teaching with residents and physicians. At the end of this course, the study concluded that no differences in the performance of a complete physical examination by first-year medical students were observed among groups taught by nurse practitioners, residents, or medical faculty. Regardless of the instructor, once the students received explicit criteria, all were able to demonstrate a performance indicating mastery of the skills involved (90).

Additional information can be gained by reading *Nurse Practitioners: A Review of the Literature 1965–1979* (60), and by reading references Simmons (87), Sullivan (91), Natkins (57), Ramsey (73), and Marchione (46). The American Nurses Association has the Council of Primary Health Care Nurse Practitioners as an organizational arm. Practitioners can also be nationally certified by taking the appropriate American Nurses Association examination. (Recertification is required every 5 years for a family nurse practitioner.)

The *nursing process* must remain the essence of nursing care in the changed or expanded role. To ensure that it does, the following components must be incorporated into all nursing practice:

1. *Separation of clinical from nonclinical activities.* Activities for assisting in the prevention, reversal, or arresting of maladaptive states in clients are clinical and demand your attention. All other activities should be surrendered to those who do not have your professional education. Clinical activities demand the methods and theory of science.
2. *Constancy of assignments.* The same client–nurse–physician teams should be established for primary or hospital care. The same nurse can be assigned to the same persons or families for the entire duration of care and thus can be responsible for all their clinical needs. Each nurse then has more knowledge concerning specific patients. The quality of care becomes more visible to the person, who can then more readily cooperate in personal care planning. Accountability can be monitored, too, and a strong colleague relationship can be built among physician, nurse, client, and family.
3. *Decentralization of authority and shared power.* Decisions need to be made where the need is "on-the-spot" if the nursing process is to function in making each person accountable for his/her actions. Authority must accompany responsibility if accountability is to have meaning. Shared power means that whoever has competence may intervene. Nurses and physicians with similar competence must work toward sharing clinical activities. At times the nurse will be solely responsible for the client or family.
4. *Increased flexibility of time with clients.* Innovations in time scheduling will be yours to make as a member of the new generation of nurses. One professional goal is the allocation of nursing time based on the clinical demands of the unit rather than on the traditional three-shift system. Lengthening work days and shortening work weeks are a way to provide more flexible structuring of time (64).

The nursing process may be considered within the framework of the Standards of Practice established by the American Nurses Association. These standards embody the five steps of the nursing process.

1. Collection of data as a continuous process.
2. Nursing diagnosis derived from health status data.
3. A plan of care that includes goals derived from nursing diagnoses.
4. A plan that includes priorities and prescribed nursing approaches.
5. Nursing actions that provide for patient participation in health promotion, maintenance, and restoration.
6. Nursing actions that assist the patient to maximize health capabilities.
7. The patient's gain or lack of progress toward the goals as determined by the patient-family-nurse in conjunction with other members of the health team.
8. This gain or loss directs a reassessment, a reordering of priorities, new goal setting, and a revision of the plan of care (59).

If each nurse fully implemented these standards in the practice of nursing, the problems of holistic care would be at a minimum. It is not difficult to see the nursing process reflected in the standards, to see how an initial assessment leads to a better evaluation of outcomes, to see the relevance of initial psychosocial and physiological data for eventual posthospital planning, and to relate the nursing diagnoses to the nursing actions that will facilitate the transition from hospital to home. It is the individual nurse's responsibility to provide a sense of patient advocacy along with a high quality of nursing care, to be aware of resources within the health care facility and in the community, to establish and maintain a collegial relationship with the other health team members, and to be willing to accept accountability for the results of nursing actions for specific patients/clients, regardless of the system of care delivery—functional, team or primary—in whatever setting nursing may be practiced (49, 59).

Individual people are always responsible for change—people willing to suggest, to offer alternatives, and to volunteer assistance with new ideas. Use your professional education with its problem-solving approach to work with others in making the nursing process an exciting reality.

Problem Solving Versus Research in the Nursing Process

In nursing you will do problem solving and research; both use the scientific method discussed in this chapter. Although problem solving and research are frequently thought of as synonymous, a fundamental difference in purpose exists between them.

The purpose of problem solving is to solve an immediate problem in a specific setting. The solution is not necessarily new knowledge and cannot be generalized to a larger population. Consequently, the precision of study is not so exacting, and statistical analyses are seldom done.

The purpose of research is to reveal new knowledge. All elements of the scientific method are precisely followed. The results of a research study cannot be expected to produce information to solve a specific problem.

Knowledge obtained through research may contribute to the solution of an immediate problem and problem solving may reveal new knowledge applicable beyond the immediate situation. But the basic difference remains. Problem solving as a health teaching method is discussed in the next chapter.

Research in Nursing

Historically nursing research has been scarce, although Florence Nightingale reportedly valued astute observation and gathering of evidence and indicated their importance for nursing (63). Research has been considered the exclusive domain of academicians, nurse-scientists, doctoral candidates—or worse, researchers from other disciplines who have found nurses a rich source of data for study in the behavioral sciences. Study of the nursing profession by behavioral scientists has resulted in certain benefits. Many pertinent facts have emerged that have given insight to nurses concerning their responses to patients and to each other. However, nursing cannot justify its worth as a separate discipline unless clinical research is performed by its own practitioners.

Staff nurses are extremely valuable resources for ideas that nurse researchers can use. At the bedside or in a one-on-one patient-client relationship in any setting, nurses can observe and report those areas of nursing care that need to be studied. Nurses can start listing ideas or problems that require further investigation and these items can be brought to the attention of someone interested in developing the idea. Staff nurses are invaluable in the collection of data. They know the patient's individual characteristics, limitations, and availability and thus can facilitate the researcher's work.

Although the Ph.D. is usually considered the research degree, many Master's level programs prepare nurses to do beginning-level research. All nurses are taught the problem-solving process, which is the basis of all research. The nurse without a doctorate who wishes to do research would be wise to consult a qualified researcher for assistance in developing the methodology of the project.

Most research in nursing is not funded. Countless small projects are carried out by individual nurses or groups of nurses with little or no financial help. Many faculty members in universities are able to do research with small amounts of money through some plan of the institution that encourages pilot studies. Larger studies may be supported by private foundations, such as the American Nurses Foundation, which is one of the most important to nursing. The ANF is supported primarily by nurses; it welcomes contributions so that it can grow and help nurses develop research that will enhance practice for all nurses. Most large research grants come from the federal government and are difficult to obtain. To qualify, one must have completed one or more pilot studies and have published the results of the research. In rare instances, organizations or institutions will support nursing research by providing released time for the nurse so that proposals may be developed and data collected and analyzed (50).

Nursing research begins with a **discrepancy,** *a perceived difference between two states of affairs,* or an uncomfortable feeling about the status quo. A difference is felt between what is occurring now and things as they could, ought, should, or might be. A gap might exist between what is known and what needs to be known to take action. Or there might be a discrepancy between sets of facts (21).

In the final analysis, the curiosity of the individual nurse and the belief in the value of nursing practice will determine whether significant research is done in nursing. Each nurse must be responsible for noting if certain situations or sets of circumstances produce specific patient responses. Collecting such data over a period of time can obviously result in increased knowledge for nursing. More importantly, if carefully analyzed and reported, the data can result in improved care for patients, families, and communities.

REFERENCES

1. **Abdellah, Fay, et al.,** *Patient-Centered Approach to Nursing.* New York: The Macmillan Company, 1960.
2. **Anderson, Marcia,** "A Psychosocial Screening Tool for Ambulatory Care Clients: A Pilot Study of Validity," *Nursing Research,* 29, no. 6 (1980), 347–51.
3. **Atwood, Judith, P., Mitchell,** and **S. Yarnell,** "The POR: A System for Communication," *Nursing Clinics of North America,* 9, no. 2 (1974), 229–34.
4. **Bixler, Genevieve,** and **Roy Bixler,** "The Professional Status of Nursing," *American Journal of Nursing,* 59, no. 7 (1959), 1142–46.
5. **Blake, Mary,** "The Peplau Developmental Model for Nursing Practice," in *Conceptual Models for Nursing Practice* (2nd ed.), eds. Joan Riehl and Sister Callista Roy. New York: Appleton-Century-Crofts, 1980, pp. 53–59.
6. **Boland, Mildred Heyes,** "Independent Practice via Pontoon Boat," *American Journal of Nursing,* 76, no. 8 (1976), 94–95.
7. **Bower, Fay,** *The Process of Planning Nursing Care: A Theoretical Model.* St. Louis: The C. V. Mosby Company, 1972.

8. **Brodish, Mary,** "Nursing Practice Conceptualized: An Interaction Model," *Image,* 14, no. 1 (1982), 5-7.
9. **Brown, Esther Lucille,** *The Future of Nursing.* New York: Russell Sage Foundation, 1948.
10. **Brown, Sally Jo,** "The Nursing Process Systems Model," *Journal of Nursing Education,* 20, no. 6 (1981), 36-40.
11. **Bullough, Bonnie,** *The Law and the Expanding Nursing Role.* New York: Appleton-Century-Crofts, 1975.
12. **Butterworth, Charles,** and **George Blackburn,** "Hospital Malnutrition and How to Assess the Nutritional Status of a Patient," *Nutrition Today,* 10, no. 2 (1975), 8-18.
13. **Carlson, Judith H., Carol Craft,** and **Anne McGuire,** *Nursing Diagnosis.* Philadelphia: W. B. Saunders Company, 1982.
14. **Chance, Kathryn,** "The Quest for Quality: An Exploration of Attempts to Define and Measure Quality Nursing Care," *Image,* 12, no. 2 (1980), 41-45.
15. **Clemence, Sister Madeleine,** "Existentialism: A Philosophy of Commitment," *American Journal of Nursing,* 66, no. 3 (1966), 500-05.
16. **Cohen, Stephen,** "Mental Status Assessment: Programmed Instruction," *American Journal of Nursing,* 81, no. 9 (1981), 1493-1518.
17. **Coleman, Leatrice,** "Orem's Self-Care Concept in Nursing," in *Conceptual Models for Nursing Practice* (2nd ed.), eds. Joan Riehl and Sister Callista Roy. New York: Appleton-Century-Crofts, 1980, pp. 315-28.
18. "Congress Passes Peer Review Reforms," *The WNCMPRF Newsletter,* 6, no. 1 (1983), 1.
19. **Deininger, Johanna M.,** "The Nursing Process—How to Assess Your Patient's Needs," *The Journal of Practical Nursing,* 25, no. 10 (1975), 32-34.
20. **Dickerson, Thelma,** "Introduction," in *The Realities of Primary Nursing Care.* New York: National League for Nursing Publication No. 52-1716 (1978), p. 1.
21. **Diers, Donna,** "This I Believe . . . About Nursing Research," *Nursing Outlook,* 18, no. 11 (1970), 50-54.
22. **Diers, Donna,** and **David Evans,** "Excellence in Nursing," *Image,* 12, no. 2 (1980), 27-30.
23. **Edel, Margie,** "The Nature of Nursing Diagnosis," in *Nursing Diagnosis,* eds. Judith Carlson, Carol Craft, and Anne McGuire. Philadelphia: W. B. Saunders Company, 1982.
24. **Feldman, Harriet,** "A Science of Nursing—To Be or Not To Be?" *Image,* 13, no. 5 (1981), 63-66.
25. **Ford, Jo Ann Garafolo, et al.,** *Applied Decision Making for Nurses.* St. Louis: The C. V. Mosby Company, 1979.
26. **Ford, Loretta,** "A Nurse for All Settings: The Nurse Practitioner," *Nursing Outlook,* 27, no. 8 (1979), 516-21.
27. **Gebbie, Kristine,** and **Mary Lavin, eds.,** *Classification of Nursing Diagnosis.* St. Louis: The C. V. Mosby Company, 1975.
28. **Geitgey, Doris A.,** "Self-Pacing; A Guide to Nursing Care," *Nursing Outlook,* 17, no. 8 (1969), 48-49.
29. **George, Madelon, Kazuyoshi Ide,** and **Clara E. Vamberry,** "The Comprehensive Health Team: A Conceptual Model," *Journal of Nursing Administration,* 1, no. 2 (1971), 9-13.

30. **Gordon, Marjory,** "Nursing Diagnosis and the Diagnostic Process," *American Journal of Nursing,* 76, no. 8 (1976), 1298–1300.
31. **Gortner, Susan,** "Nursing Science in Transition," *Nursing Research,* 29, no. 3 (1980), 180–83.
32. **Grubbs, Judy,** "The Johnson Behavioral System Model for Nursing Practice," in *Conceptual Models for Nursing Practice* (2nd ed.), eds. Joan Riehl and Sister Callista Roy. New York: Appleton-Century-Crofts, 1980, pp. 217–54.
33. **Hale, S.,** and **J. Richardson,** "Terminating the Nurse-Patient Relationship," *American Journal of Nursing,* 63, no. 9 (1963), 116–19.
34. **Henderson, Virginia,** *Nature of Nursing.* New York: The Macmillan Company, 1966.
35. **Hull, Richard T.,** "Responsibility and Accountability, Analyzed," *Nursing Outlook,* 29, no. 12 (1981), 707–12.
36. **Islen, Lois,** and **Betty Eller,** *Difference between Expanded Role and Nurse Practitioner.* Raleigh, NC, n.d.
37. **Johnson, Dorothy,** "The Behavioral System Model for Nursing," in *Conceptual Models for Nursing Practice* (2nd ed.), eds. Joan Riehl and Sister Callista Roy. New York: Appleton-Century-Crofts, 1980, pp. 207–16.
38. **Jones, P.,** "An Adaptation Model for Nursing Practice," *American Journal of Nursing,* 78, no. 11 (1978), 1901–5.
39. **King, Imogene M.,** *A Theory for Nursing.* New York: John Wiley & Sons, Inc., 1981.
40. **Kramer, Marlene,** "The Consumer's Influence on Health Care," *Nursing Outlook,* 20, no. 9 (1972), 574–78.
41. **Leininger, Madeleine,** "Caring: A Central Focus of Nursing and Health Care Services," *Nursing and Health Care,* 1, no. 3 (1980), 135–43.
42. **Lewis, Lucille,** "This I Believe . . . About the Nursing Process: Key to Care," *Nursing Outlook,* 16, no. 5 (1968), 26–29.
43. **Little, Dolores E.,** and **Doris L. Carnevali,** *Nursing Care Planning* (2nd ed.). Philadelphia: J. B. Lippincott Company, 1976.
44. **Lunney, Margaret,** "Nursing Diagnosis: Refining the System," *American Journal of Nursing,* 82, no. 3 (1982), 456–59.
45. **Mallick, M. Joan,** "Patient Assessment Based on Data, Not Intuition," *Nursing Outlook,* 29, no. 10 (1981), 600–5.
46. **Marchione, Joanne,** and **T. Neal Garland,** "An Emerging Profession? The Case of the Nurse Practitioner," *Image,* 12, no. 2 (1980), 37–39.
47. **Maslow, A. H.,** *Motivation and Personality.* New York: Harper & Row, Publishers, 1954.
48. **McCain, R. Faye,** "Nursing by Assessment—Not Intuition," *American Journal of Nursing,* 65, no. 4 (1965), 82–84.
49. **McKeehan, Kathleen M.,** *Continuing Care: A Multidisciplinary Approach to Discharge Planning.* St. Louis: The C. V. Mosby Company, 1981.
50. **Miles, Margaret,** an interview on "Nursing Research," *Mid-America Nursing,* 3, no. 3 (1982), 18–19.
51. **Miller, Judith,** and **Diane Hellenbrand,** "An Eclectic Approach to Practice," *American Journal of Nursing,* 81, no. 7 (1981), 1339–43.
52. **Mooney, Judith,** "Attachment-Separation in a Nurse-Patient Relationship," *Nursing Forum,* 15, no. 3 (1976), 259–64.

53. **Mooney, Mary,** "The Ethical Component of Nursing Theory," *Image*, 12, no. 1 (1980), 7-9.
54. **Murphy, Donna,** and **Eleanor Dineen,** "Nursing by Telephone," *American Journal of Nursing*, 75, no. 7 (1975), 1137-39.
55. **Murray, Ruth,** and **M. Marilyn Huelskoetter,** *Psychiatric/Mental Health Nursing: Giving Emotional Care*. Englewood Cliffs, NJ: Prentice-Hall, Inc., 1983.
56. **Murray, Ruth,** and **Judith Zentner,** *Nursing Assessment and Health Promotion through the Life Span* (3rd ed.). Englewood Cliffs, NJ: Prentice-Hall, Inc., 1985.
57. **Natkins, Lawrence,** and **Edward Wagner,** "Nurse Practitioner and Physician Adherence to Standing Orders Criteria for Consultation and Referral," *American Journal of Public Health*, 72, no. 1 (1982), 22-29.
58. **Neuman, Betty,** "The Betty Neuman Health Care Systems Model: A Total Person Approach to Patient Problems," in *Conceptual Models for Nursing Practice* (2nd ed.), eds. Joan Riehl and Sister Callista Roy. New York: Appleton-Century-Crofts, 1980, pp. 119-34.
59. **Nichols, M. E.,** and **Virginia G. Wessels,** *Nursing Standards and Nursing Process*. Wakefield, MA: Contemporary Publishing, Inc., 1977.
60. *Nurse Practitioner: A Review of the Literature 1965-1979*. Kansas City, MO: American Nurses Association, 1980.
61. **O'Brien, Margaret, Margery Manley,** and **Margaret Heagarty,** "Expanding the Public Health Nurses Role in Child Care," *Nursing Outlook*, 23, no. 6 (1975), 369-73.
62. **Orem, Dorothea,** *Nursing: Concepts of Practice*. New York: McGraw-Hill Book Company, 1971.
63. **Palmer, Irene Sabelberg,** "Florence Nightingale: Reformer, Reactionary, Researcher," *Nursing Research*, 25, no. 2 (1977), 84-89.
64. **Parker, Susan,** "A Conceptual Model for Outcome Assessment," *Nurse Practitioner*, 8, no. 1 (1983), 41-45.
65. **Parker, Wm.,** "Medication Histories," *American Journal of Nursing*, 76, no. 12 (1976), 1969-71.
66. **Patterson, Josephine,** and **Loretta Zderad,** *Humanistic Nursing*, New York: John Wiley & Sons, Inc., 1976.
67. **Peplau, Hildegard,** *Interpersonal Relations in Nursing*. New York: G. P. Putnam's Sons, 1952.
68. **Perry, Anne,** "Analysis of the Components of the Nursing Process," in *Nursing Diagnosis*, eds. Judith Carlson, Carol Craft, and Anne McGuire. Philadelphia: W. B. Saunders Company, 1982, pp. 41-54.
69. **Phaneuf, Maria C.,** *The Nursing Audit: Profile for Excellence*. New York: Appleton-Century-Crofts, 1976.
70. **Pluckhan, Margaret L.,** *Human Communication: the Matrix of Nursing*. New York: McGraw-Hill Book Company, 1978.
71. **Pohl, Margaret L.,** *The Teaching Function of the Nurse Practitioner*. Dubuque, Iowa: William C. Brown Co., 1978.
72. **Porter, Anne, P. Moschel, B., Liederman,** and **M. Pope,** "Patient Needs on Admission," *American Journal of Nursing*, 77, no. 1 (1977), 112-13.
73. **Ramsey, Janice, John McKenzie,** and **David Fish,** "Physicians and Nurse Practitioners: Do They Provide Equivalent Health Care?" *American Journal of Public Health*, 72, no. 1 (1982), 55-57.

74. **Ratliff, Bascom W.,** "The Emerging Specialty of Discharge Planner," in *Leaving the Hospital: Discharge Planning for Total Patient Care*, ed. Bascom W. Ratliff. Springfield, IL: Charles C Thomas, Publisher, 1981, pp. 23–25.
75. **Resler, Marion,** "Formulation of a Nursing Diagnosis," in *Nursing Diagnosis*, eds. Judith Carlson, Carol Craft, and Anne McGuire. Philadelphia: W. B. Saunders Company, 1982, pp. 55–76.
76. **Reynolds, Janis,** and **Jann Logsdon,** "Assessing Your Patient's Mental Status," *Nursing '79*, 9, no. 8 (1979), 26–33.
77. **Riehl, Joan,** and **Sister Callista Roy, eds.,** *Conceptual Models for Nursing Practice* (2nd ed.). New York: Appleton-Century-Crofts, 1980.
78. **Rinaldi, Leena,** "What to Do after the Audit Is Done," *American Journal of Nursing*, 77, no. 2 (1977), 268–69.
79. **Rogers, Carl,** *Client-Centered Therapy*. Boston: Houghton Mifflin Company, 1951.
80. **Rogers, Martha,** *The Theoretical Basis for Nursing*. Philadelphia: F. A. Davis Company, 1970.
81. **Roy, Sister Callista,** *Introduction to Nursing: an Adaptation Model*. Englewood Cliffs, NJ: Prentice-Hall, Inc., 1976.
82. **Saxton, Dolores,** and **Patricia Hyland,** *Planning and Implementing Nursing Intervention*. St. Louis: The C. V. Mosby Company, 1975.
83. **Schaefer, Jeannette,** "The Interrelatedness of Decision Making and the Nursing Process, *American Journal of Nursing*, 74, no. 10 (1974), 1852–55.
84. **Schlotfeldt, Rozella M.,** "Nursing in the Future," *Nursing Outlook*, 29, no. 5 (1981), 292–301.
85. **Schroeder, Mary,** "Symbolic Interactionism: A Conceptual Framework Useful for Nurses Working with Obese Persons," *Image*, 13, no. 5 (1981), 78–81.
86. **Serafini, Patricia,** "Nursing Assessment in Industry," *American Journal of Public Health*, 66, no. 8 (1976), 755–60.
87. **Simmons, Ruth S.,** and **Janet Rosenthal,** "The Women's Movement and the Nurse Practitioner's Sense of Role," *Nursing Outlook*, 29, no. 6 (1981), 371–75.
88. **Snyder, Joyce,** and **Margo Wilson,** "Elements of a Psychological Assessment," *American Journal of Nursing*, 77, no. 2 (1977), 235–39.
89. **Stevens, Barbara J.,** "Analysis of Trends in Nursing Care Measurement," in *Nursing Standards and Nursing Process*, eds. M. E. Nichols and Virginia G. Wessels. Wakefield, MA.: Contemporary Publishing, Inc., 1977, pp. 77–84.
90. **Stillman, Paula M., et al.,** "A Comparison of Physicians and Nurse Practitioners as Instructors in a Physical Diagnosis Course," *Journal of Medical Education*, 54, no. 9 (1979), 733–34.
91. **Sullivan, Judith,** "Research on Nurse Practitioners: Process Behind the Outcome," *American Journal of Public Health*, 72, no. 1 (1982), 8–9.
92. **Travelbee, Joyce,** *Interpersonal Aspects of Nursing*. Philadelphia: F. A. Davis Company, 1967.
93. **Turnbull, Sister Joyce,** "Shifting the Focus to Health," *American Journal of Nursing*, 76, no. 12 (1976), 1985–87.
94. **Weed, Lyle L.,** *Medical Records, Medical Education, and Patient Care: The Problem-Oriented Record as a Basic Tool*. Cleveland: The Press of Case Western Reserve University, 1969.
95. **White, Nicole,** *Ambulatory Medical Care Quality Assurance*. La Jolla, CA.: La Jolla Health Science Publications, 1977, p. 10.

5

Health Teaching: A Basic Nursing Intervention

Study of this chapter will enable you to

1. Discuss why teaching is a major nursing responsibility in all settings.
2. Differentiate the traditional and simple definitions of *teaching, learning,* and *education* from the nontraditional and complex.
3. Define *health education* and *self-care.*
4. Describe changing educational trends with an emphasis on the future.
5. Identify the varied opportunities for teaching health promotion.
6. List the fundamentals of teaching.
7. Explore and apply the many facets of creativity in teaching–learning.
8. Discuss and translate into practical examples various teaching–learning theories, including how they are affected by language, culture, and other factors.
9. Compare methods of teaching with various ages, including individual and group approaches, and predict when each might be appropriate.
10. Discuss how teaching may differ from institution to home setting.

11. Select self-care books and periodicals as resources to promote health behavior.
12. Sharpen your ability to identify significant teaching-learning opportunities through analysis of case studies.
13. Teach patients, families, and coworkers in the nursing setting when appropriate.

On entering nursing you may not have understood that to nurse is to teach. Teaching provides a major way to help another adapt. This chapter does not attempt to review the many teaching-learning theories. Instead it presents various theories and methods that seem applicable to nursing and that you can begin to use.

The authors have not attempted to emulate educational jargon, but they, too, are imprisoned in words. You must take the words and phrases and apply them to people, yourself included, making the ideas alive and active. Only then will you experience the teaching-learning process.

DEFINITIONS

Learning *is the process of acquiring wisdom, knowledge, or skill; an overt change in behavior may be observed.* **Teaching** *is the process of sharing knowledge and insight, or facilitating another to learn knowledge, insight, and skills* (19). These definitions are deceptively simple. Popular magazines, textbooks, and library shelves are full of theories and explanations about how these processes take place. Yet no one can say learning *will always* take place under certain conditions or teaching *will never* take place under certain conditions. In spite of myriads of information, people with their unique minds and personalities are always modifying the existing theories.

In actuality, teaching and learning cannot be separated, for while a person is teaching, learning is also taking place, or at least should be. Perhaps the substandard use of *learn*, as in the sentence "I'm going to learn you something" has more accuracy than people have thought. Both terms connote a lifelong process, an internalization (learning) of thoughts, attitudes, facts, and a consequent externalization (teaching) of those thoughts, attitudes, and facts. Teaching and learning can be conscious and formal, as in the announced situation "Today we are going to learn about the digestive system." Or they can be unconscious and informal, as when a mother frowns and says with a certain tonal emphasis "What is *that* smell?" The listening and watching child combines a certain smell with a negative mental attitude.

One word that connotes a chilly, stiff learning process is *pedagogy*. Originally the word meant teaching children, but today it refers generally to teaching. Unfortunately, most knowledge about learning has come from studies of children and animals and most knowledge about teaching has come from teaching children who are in compulsory attendance. Thus adults are often taught as though they were children. To combat this erring process, Knowles has coined a new word, **andragogy**: *helping adults learn* (29). Consequently, he turns from traditional pedagogical methods. His and others' ideas will be more thoroughly considered later in this chapter, for they are useful in patient teaching.

The word *education* has traditionally meant a process that transmits the culture. But the word originally came from a Latin word meaning "to draw out." Although we are more familiar with education as a cramming full of facts and information, the other side of the definition is to draw out the mysterious hidden qualities within a person. The amount of education a person has gained and retained has long been measured by IQ (intelligent quotient) tests. But many qualities cannot be measured this way. The IQ test cannot measure how much creative imagination a person has, how much ambition, perseverance, or willingness to cooperate (50). And these qualities are significant, although previously not often considered or given priority. Thus a balanced definition of **education** is the *continuing process of using immeasurable inner resources to gain external information.*

Health education *specifically transmits information, motivates the inner resource of the person, and helps people adopt and maintain healthful practices and lifestyles.* It is also concerned with the environment, professional training, and research to maintain and evaluate the process. Traditionally health education focuses on what the professional thinks is good for the patient/client.

Self-care, increasingly popular in recent years, *focuses on what the learner perceives as needs and goals to maintain or enhance health and well-being.* It is generally undertaken prior to illness rather than in response to disease.

EDUCATION: HISTORICAL PERSPECTIVE

Toffler says that the educational system is dying—a startling thought. He traces the stages of education in America (70). In stage 1 history was important. People looked to the past for knowledge, guidance, and strength. Teaching came primarily through family, religious institutions, and apprenticeships. The teacher and learner were spread throughout the community.

Industrialism and the mechanical age ushered in stage 2. New skills were required and the educational system took on a factory appearance. Assembly-line students were taught by specifically trained teachers in a central location. One writer relives such an educational experience (his elementary school). He feels his old fear of the factorylike structure with its castle facade. Perhaps his experience is extreme, but he doesn't associate school with learning, only with the necessity to get ahead, to compete with classmates, to make a good impression on the grim teachers who gathered the little robots (students) into the human factory to shovel food (knowledge) into the body (27). Adults educated in such a manner have difficulty with more open, democratic approaches (70).

Toffler insists that in our present stage 3, the new technological era, in which more sophisticated machines perform more frequently, in which communication systems connect most world points, and in which environments are ever changing, we need a superindustrial education. He calls for teachers and learners who can adapt to change, who plan for future change, and who understand the impetus toward the future. No longer can a person use the skills of the parents for the rest of his life. In fact, it may not even be possible to use what was recently taught in school. Teaching and learning must again take place in various settings within the community, but with much greater speed and flexibility than in stage 1. Education must be a lifelong process, not a phase of experience finished in 21 years (70).

Skills are then needed in four areas: learning, relating, choosing, and problem solving. People must learn how to learn. With such rapidly changing information, they must know the process of discarding obsolete data in order to take on new. They must learn to relate under new conditions. Mobility has caused less stable friendships. People now cope with more loneliness and less reliance on groups of people. With so many choices available for the person, some goals and priorities must be set. Along with data, people must acquire behavioral skills or "life know-how." The self-care movement is a part of this know-how.

Teachers, including yourself as nurse-teacher, must adapt to the present age, reexamine teaching methods and goals for effectiveness, and provide people with information about how to learn, what the future may hold for them, and how to adjust to these conditions. Teaching can no longer present all facts. The future must be considered.

THE NURSE AS TEACHER-LEARNER

As a staff nurse or unemployed nurse, you may be more of a teacher than someone actually called a "teacher." A history instructor may teach high school students from 9:00 A.M. to 3:00 P.M. 5 days a week.

But you can spend nearly every waking moment in teaching health promotion. You teach through example: through health precautions and personal hygiene as well as by words.

If you have a family, either children of your own or brothers, sisters, and parents, you constantly do health teaching. You may lock the medicine and caustic material in a cabinet, explaining the dire results of taking too much internally. You may notice early diabetic symptoms in your father and direct him to an internist for tests. You may quickly take the proper first-aid action when your sister fractures a bone. You will additionally be a teacher to your neighbors and friends.

Teaching those near you takes on unprecedented magnitude when you analyze the barrage of so-called health information directed at us daily through communication-advertising media: natural or organic foods are superior to processed foods; certain vitamins and minerals will provide pep and sexual vigor; certain exercises will promote breast development. Or again, certain procedures will grow hair on a bald male head or remove hair from a female face; a particular cream will slow down the aging process; a certain diet will cause drastic weight reduction; certain medications will wake you up, put you to sleep, or remove all your aches in moments.

Obviously Americans are concerned with staying slim and appropriately masculine or feminine, with looking young and retaining their vigor. They have a fear about their own and their loved ones' health. You can supply sound information on the essentials of good nutrition, exercise, and rest while pointing out that people must accept periods of strain, fatigue, lesser energy, and the aging process. You won't always teach with words alone. Your standards of cleanliness—for example, how frequently you wash your hands—will be imitated by your children and observed by your patients.

You will teach no matter what professional position you hold. The staff nurse can teach while giving a bath. The nurse in the doctor's office or clinic can do spot teaching while preparing a patient for examination. The public health or visiting nurse can teach while working with specific situations in the home. The industrial nurse can teach while taking down worker information. Of course, the nurse is also a teacher while instructing students, but teaching is more basic than a professional job. Also, your teaching is not limited to the task at hand. One industrial health nurse in a 2-week period encountered 40 problems offered by the employees that were unrelated to their treatments. Most problems concerned health needs of family members (73).

In trying to help each individual reach the maximum health potential, you must consider the total person. The particular culture, social class, religion, environment, definition of health and illness, developmental stage, whether the person is in a crisis, and what kind of communication he/she responds to will affect understanding and your consequent teaching. Thus this entire text and *Nursing Assessment and Health Promotion through the Life Span* together provide a foundation from which you may glean teaching and learning concepts (43) in order to practice **holistic health care,** *care that encompasses the whole person.*

You might ask yourself: What does the person want to learn? How can he/she best be taught? Can I help the person project a positive image of what he/she will be in the future? For example, can I help the person who is a diabetic think of self as slim, healthy, and enjoying the proper foods rather than as a deprived person who will moan and reminise about delicious sugary desserts? Can I help the person understand that he/she must continue to learn about the disease and possible new treatments as medical research probes now-unknown possibilities? Can I improve my skills, and the person's skills, in the four crucial areas of learning, relating, choosing, and problem solving?

FUNDAMENTALS OF TEACHING

Although no set rules can be laid down as absolute standards for effective teaching, the following suggestions are recommended.

1. Be trustworthy and consistent.
2. Have self-esteem and enthusiasm. Generate a sense that what you are teaching will benefit the learner.
3. Don't discuss your personal problems with a client.
4. Think through your teaching image. What do patients learn from your cleanliness (or lack of it), dress, posture, tone of voice, gestures, yawns, and facial expressions?
5. Determine what the client *wants* and *needs* to learn before you begin your instruction.
6. Know your teaching area. Organize and present your material so that patients feel you know what you are doing.
7. Utilize available teaching methods, resources, various emotional climates, and referral systems when appropriate. Encourage practice of skills and use repetition if it is needed.
8. Respect the client as more important than a procedure, a potential disease process, or a research project.
9. Involve the client actively in the learning process in order to enhance learning.
10. If you ask the client to do something, explain why. Be sure that what you ask is realistic.

11. Distinguish between lack of intelligence and misunderstanding caused by cultural, ethnic, or religious differences, and do not equate intelligence level with educational level.
12. Strive for learning from inner motivation through recognition of need, not from outward pressure.
13. Practice sensing the moment of learning. A sense of appropriate timing is essential in teaching, based on assessment of the learner's interest, knowledge, motivation, and values.
14. If you write instructions, write legibly.
15. Plan for interruption.
16. Don't overwhelm with technicalities or excessive, complex facts.
17. Reinforce progress. Give positive feedback when appropriate.
18. Accept errors in the learning process without harsh judgment but with correct information.
19. Don't allow your racial bias to control your attitude about another's ability to learn.
20. Don't reinforce destructive thinking. When a client says "My mother died of this disease," don't reply "It's a real killer. My two aunts died from it, too."
21. Record your teaching experience and share these notes with other staff members (or teachers from other disciplines) who may instruct the patient.
22. Be realistic about teaching and learning. Accept good days and bad days. Sometimes you will be elated, sometimes depressed, about results.

CREATIVITY

Assume that your best teaching device is you. You may be open to new knowledge and you may agree with the fundamentals of teaching but not always know how to implement them. Thus you will benefit from the following investigation of creativity and its application to teaching and learning.

What is *creativity*? The word has been used freely. It has been defined as a process, a product, a personality, and an environmental condition. **Creativity** *is the ability to sense gaps or problems with known information, forming ideas or hypotheses about what should be done, testing and modifying those ideas, communicating those ideas, and taking appropriate action in a unique way* (72). From this process you will obtain ideas or carry out activities that are new, unique, and useful to you even though they may not be new, unique, or useful to other people.

An appropriate question might be "How do you sense gaps and

problems?" Without this essential tension in thinking, the rest of the process will not follow. One answer is to improve your observation. People can look at a slowly changing object for years and not notice the change, as the exterminator proves who points to a foundation beam largely devoured by termites. The astonished homeowner says "I've gone by here every day for a year but didn't notice the change." Or less dramatic, can you describe in detail from memory the tree outside your kitchen window?

These are two examples (or at least one, if you can describe that tree in detail) of lack of sight perception. Other senses that need sharpening are sound, touch, sensation of movement, taste, and smell. Recreate in your mind the following sensations: the voice of your mother or father when you were little and being reprimanded, the feel of the hair on your pet dog, the sensation of your body as you hiked the last 100 feet of the mountain last summer, the taste of lemon juice, the smell of cooking broccoli. Practicing this kind of observation exercise of your sensory memory will improve your teaching because you will have a broader sensitivity base from which to sense gaps and problems.

Observing emotional reactions is also significant as you work with patients. Can you recreate the emotion of despair you felt when, after working hard and counting on a certain achievement, you failed the test, were disqualified in the race, or didn't get the job or school position you wished? How did you feel when you lost the love and understanding of someone you were counting on? You really can't walk a mile in the patient's shoes, but your helpful understanding of his/her emotions, through understanding your own, can increase the value of your teaching.

Lowenfeld lists this quality of sensitivity in observation among his criteria for creativity, along with fluency of ideas, flexibility, originality, and the ability to redefine or rearrange, analyze, synthesize, and coherently organize problems (33). You might display fluency of ideas as you think of the various ways you could apply a bandage, form recipes, or adjust meals in a particular situation. You might show flexibility as you quickly incorporate changing circumstances into a situation. For instance, a procedure doesn't work because a previously unknown factor has been introduced. Instead of saying "It won't work," you take the factor into account and get desirable results.

Originality is variously defined. Some say there are no new ideas and hence no true originality. Others say that every time you associate or combine two or more ideas that you already have and come up with a new perspective, you have been original.

The rest of Lowenfeld's criteria work into a systematic process. You redefine a disease process with new research results or you rearrange a procedure with the new knowledge that the patient is left-handed instead of right-handed. You analyze, or take apart, the significant factors involved in an unwed mother's situation. You synthesize, or put the parts back together, when you help a senior citizen create a new way of life. You exhibit coherence or organization when you arrange all the aspects of any teaching plan to form a unified working unit (33).

Creativity, then, conjures up visions of curiosity, imagination, discovery, innovation, and invention. It is a number of abilities rather than a single characteristic. The creative person often has a high degree of psychologic health, is persistent, self-assertive, energetic, dominant, individualistic, and playful. The creative person can see many relationships among elements, relationships that baffle the conformer, the person who does only what is expected and does not ruffle the system. The creative person isn't always accepted by the traditional teacher because he/she has to be dealt with uniquely and can't be treated in the ordinary way. Can you tolerate creativity in your patients? Will you help them learn through exploring, manipulating, questioning, experimenting, testing, and modifying rather than by accepting your word as final authority?

No one knows if creativity has a genetic link or if it is totally a function of the environment. But sex differences do exist in the human brain. Female infants show a somewhat larger area of visual cortex in the right hemisphere of the brain than do male infants. According to J. Wada of The University of British Columbia (25), this fact implies a possible anatomical basis for the female advantage in nonverbal ideation.

The two cerebral hemispheres differ in function. The left hemisphere is almost always dominant for language, logical reasoning, and mathematical calculation. The right hemisphere is nonverbal and processes spatial and visual abstractions, recognition of faces, a sense of one's body image, music, and it may be closer to intuitive or preconscious processes and fantasy (25). A fascinating study of the right hemisphere is found in reference 18.

In a 10-year-study of creative people Getzels and Csikszentmihaly found that some definite factors in a child's environment can encourage the child to become a problem finder (one who is creative) before he/she becomes a problem solver. These factors are (1) being the oldest or only child; (2) having a working mother who delegates responsibility; (3) having parents who support creativity; and (4) going to schools that encourage problem finding (6).

Torrance contends that smothering creativity is an American phenomenon (72). He points out that adults often repress fantasies, hold back learning, and overemphasize sex roles in children. Creativity will emerge if family life and child rearing are organized so that every child has the opportunity to reach his/her potential (67). By the time a child enters school, the foundation for creative development has been laid. Schools will then influence further development.

During their children's elementary years, Americans tend to stress conformity to the peer group, use punitive discipline, orient their children to success, equate divergency with abnormality or delinquency, and make a sharp distinction between work and play. In their high school years, American youth are frequently pressured into striving for popularity, achieving high grades, getting work done on time, and making conventional occupational choices. In college (as well as high school) American students are sometimes forced to overemphasize the acquisition of categorized knowledge, memorization of facts, and standard testing. Thus covering subject matter rather than seeing the interrelationships is often the result. You may recognize this pattern in your own experience. One adult writes that as a child he was fascinated with the circus (6). He spent every possible moment absorbing the aura of its life. Pressure to conform, however, pushed him into the conventional education route and he eventually acquired a Ph.D. in geography and a responsible college faculty position. Still, even with a family of four children to support, he would fantasize and dream about the circus. He is unique because with his family's approval, he quit his job and joined a circus, an unusual turn of events in American culture.

Suggestions to foster creative learning as you teach patients/clients are to

1. Allow opportunity for creative behavior, such as providing for independent learning through the study of appropriate literature or asking questions that require more than recall.
2. Develop your own skills in creative learning according to methods described later in the chapter.*
3. Reward creative achievements by respecting unusual solutions and by not threatening with immediate evaluation before an idea is completely tested.
4. Develop a constructive rather than critical attitude toward information gleaned.
5. Establish creative relationships, especially with children. Permit one thing to lead to another and embark on the unknown; yet provide adequate guidance.
6. Provide for continuity of creative development in problem finding and solution finding (72).

*When almost 600 nonnursing and nursing students at a large state university were surveyed about their perceptions of their creativity, nursing students perceived themselves as significantly less creative (36).

Creativity is *not* synonymous with *permissiveness* or *chaos*. You are the resource, the organizer. Often you will be authoritative. You will say "Sugar elimination will modify your diabetic condition. Omitting egg yolk may help lower your cholesterol. Chewing sugarless gum will cut down on dental caries. Adequate exercise will strengthen those muscles." But how you then help the client work with those facts in the situation will reveal either your authoritarian or your creative teaching manner.

SOME IDEAS TO CONSIDER

In addition to developing a creative teaching manner, you may want to ponder the following ideas concerning the nature of teaching and learning. These ideas originated in various disciplines: psychoanalysis, adult education, language and communication studies, anthropology, and nursing.

Significant Learning

Carl Rogers defines *significant learning* as learning that makes a difference—that affects all parts of a person and influences behavior, course of action, attitude, and personality (57). Rogers substantiates his claim that such learning does take place by citing his experience with psychotherapy. He assumes that it can also take place in an educational setting under certain ideal conditions.

1. The person must clearly perceive the problems and issues that are to be resolved.
2. You, the nurse-teacher, must be openly aware of the attitudes you hold and accept your own feelings.
3. You must accept the person as he/she is and understand his/her feelings.
4. Resources (such as literature about health promotion, crutches, cookbooks, yourself) should be given if they are useful to the person and not an imposition.
5. Evaluation should be conceived as knowing that the client is adequately prepared to solve the problem if he/she so desires, but leaving the person free to choose whether to put forth the required effort (57).

Two college students, both taking an education course and writing papers on learning theories, were overheard in the following conversation:

Did you get your term paper on learning written?

Yes, I'm almost done. I've found one article that expresses exactly what I believe. I'll try to work it in with all the hairy material the prof expects.

(*Significant learning*?)

Pedagogy Versus Andragogy

The saying from the Talmud, "Much have I learned from my teachers, even more from my classmates, but most of all from my students," has special significance in Knowles's theory of adult education. As a person matures, he/she

1. Moves from dependency to a self-directing position.
2. Accumulates experiences that become an increasing resource for learning.
3. Moves in the direction of learning that harmonizes with current developmental tasks.
4. Changes from subject-centered, postponed applications characteristic of children's education to problem-centered, immediate applications of knowledge (29).

Others have also emphasized these guidelines for adult learning.

As a nurse–teacher you may be working with a variety of age groups. Some will be self-directing adults. You can apply these crucial assumptions as you teach adult patients and their family members if you let them help plan and conduct their own learning programs to some extent. Build on and make use of their life experiences to gain greater learning, and be sure learning is appropriate to their developmental tasks. (For example, don't try to get the 40-year-old heart patient to plan his retirement if he still has realistic aspirations for becoming a company vice-president.) Teach what is significant to their particular life problems, not what you think is a good subject. You may need to help them in organizing material, refocusing thinking, reassuring by pointing out what they already know, giving authoritative answers when needed, and giving individual attention to those who do not learn well alone. Keep in mind that the adult learner has many priorities other than learning. Other life responsibilities will greatly affect the ability to learn and the time he or she can spend. The adult learner, however, may use a small portion of time effectively because of having learned how to integrate previous experiences with new learning.

Other factors must be considered for the learner in later maturity. Probably this person will need the reassurance that he/she isn't too old to learn. The person will also need such features as large print and excellent lighting for diminished eyesight; clear, distinct speaking for less acute hearing; and frequent summaries and slower presentation because it may take a little longer to synthesize the material.

Similarly, you must adjust to the children and youth you teach, to their dependency needs, lack of experience, developmental tasks, and lack of sophistication in problem solving. Children lack the seasoned habits of adults and may respond more quickly to a change in pattern. Use a developmental approach (43). You have a special responsibility to children as a teacher of health promotion because eating, exercise, and health practices become routinized early in life. The child who comes to you may have had little health teaching at home or in school. A questionnaire filled out by 910 early elementary classroom teachers (kindergarten through third grade) revealed generally low nutritional-knowledge scores (53). Obviously such teachers cannot teach good nutritional habits to their students.

The child may be inspired to learn through playing games, reading appropriate books or cartoons, or using puppets. Simple drawings, with explanations in the appropriate age level language, may help explain a body part, a procedure, or what a medicine will do in the body. Children also enjoy arts and crafts, cooking, planting, and drama (such as simple role playing). Incorporating any of these activities into health teaching may enhance learning.

Language: Prohibitor in Teaching-Learning

Language, our primary tool for education, can open up new worlds to people or leave them in a state of confusion. Nonverbal behavior is also significant. Communication developed first through the physical movements of people or objects; then through drawings, which represented objects or needs of people; next through giving spoken names to important ideas, concepts, and objects; and finally through establishing written signs to correspond to these names (17).

We sometimes forget that written signs have no physical resemblance to their referents. Two people must have a mutual understanding about the meaning of a word or communication does not occur. We also do not have distinct and separate signs for each observed occurrence. Thus although dwellings can be generally subdivided into houses, apartments, condominiums, and mobile homes, even these words cannot give a unique description of your dwelling. Because we cannot keep producing exact sounds for all different experiences, we have words that have many different meanings, such as *fast*, which can mean a speed, a dye that remains in place, or a certain type of friend. *High* can mean a physical elevation, a degree of alcohol or drug intoxication, a musical pitch, or a kind of religious ceremony; it can mean "grave" or "serious" (as in *high treason*), or "expensive" or "costly." *Reading* a skin test is not the same as *reading* an essay. Furthermore, the mind seems to decode messages in relationship to its own background situation, prejudices, and moods. For example, a person can hear and repeat exactly what you have said without believing a word of it.

Given such possibilities of faulty language communication, even if technical language is adjusted to the client's level and explanations are logically coherent and complete, the patient should have additional understandable experiences about the new concepts to be learned. Comprehension must not be evaluated totally on the basis of language or reading response. Because motion pictures, television images, photographic slides, and pictures look like their referent, and the first two also sound like their referent, these and other (audio) visual aids should be strongly considered as adjuncts to verbal explanations.

Culture: Prohibitor in Teaching-Learning

The preceding ideas on adult education may work well in American majority culture but fail miserably in a culture where authority is unquestioned and where concepts of self-help and audience participation are not valued. For instance, if a married woman from a strict patriarchal system is a patient, you should teach the husband what must be done in order to be effective.

Evidence is lacking to support the claim that more health education alone will improve health (4). Although millions of dollars were spent on an antismoking campaign, total cigarette consumption in the United States actually increased, mostly among teenagers. The nation's major health problems—alcoholism, heart disease, obesity, certain cancers, and accidents—stem from ignorance or irresponsibility on the part of individuals rather than from inadequacies on the part of health providers.

Culture is often the prohibiting factor when people cannot seem to change lifestyles and attitudes that are responsible for illness, disability, and death.

Cultural and subcultural expectations have a powerful effect on behavior—yours, the patient's, and the family's. Accepting what the group believes to be true on the main issues of life is beneficial to all members of society. When one is relieved of the need to make choices, peace of mind and security result. Thus health education to change habits is likely to fail unless social pressures to maintain the old customs are overcome. At the same time, the new proposed behavior cannot cause too much insecurity, uncertainty, or mental stress.

People conform to the expectations of prestigious members of society and prestige may have little to do with money. Thus important persons need to be consulted and given an opportunity to maintain prestige by having a major part in the changing of health habits. Programs are accepted only to the extent that local representatives—priests, teachers, grandparents, shop stewards, doctors, businesspeople, or the mass media—take part in planning and conducting them.

Ritualistic customs or behaviors are usually tied to elementary functions of life—menstruation, feeding, gestation, defecation. Sometimes the ritual is harmful to health, but attempts to change it may cause resistance because time has sanctified the custom. Examples are female circumcision, defecation in open places, and food taboos for pregnant women.

Every culture accepts and absorbs new ideas, provided that they do not conflict with its own fundamental tenets. All new ideas are at first judged according to existing customs and beliefs and then gradually accepted if they mesh sufficiently with what already exists.

Consider the following suggestions in promoting health education and changes in health practices in any culture.

1. Get intimately detailed knowledge of beliefs, attitudes, knowledge, and behavior of the cultural group and evaluate their psychological and social functions. Try to share the feeling of the culture. Avoid being culture-bound: do not automatically reject concepts and patterns different from personal ones.
2. Identify numerous subcultures, for programs based on premises valid for one group may not be successful with another group.
3. Determine leadership patterns within a community or group. Define the decision makers in the family and larger social institutions, the status of various groups within the community, as well as the status of the health worker in comparison to these groups.
4. Remember that every culture is layered: each has certain characteristics that are manifest and others that are latent—certain components that constitute the stated ideal pattern of behavior but that are seldom practiced. Consider and study both levels. Least visible are the values that give direction and meaning to life.
5. Don't make direct attacks on the fundamental beliefs of the group; instead patiently and gradually change ideas by appealing to the group's desire for health and normality. Avoid abrupt change. Use **linkage ideas,** *ideas consistent with both public health and the cultural belief system.* If no common ground exists, you should add on your ideas to the cultural ideas (21).
6. Consider unanticipated consequences of the health education program and estimate how permanent the introduced changes are expected to be. Consider the untoward consequences of the pro-

gram. Positive results from your teaching in one situation may be considered negative in another situation.

7. Beware of the aspiration gap. Expectations of better living or health conditions, once aroused, are likely to rise more rapidly than improvements in the actual life situation. Supplying help and hope runs the risk of intensifying rather than satisfying felt needs, as rising aspirations outrace material gain, causing discontent and disillusionment. Programs of preventive health measures are the most difficult to establish because of the low value on health, the lack of understanding of cause and effect or the reasons for preventive measures, and the existence in local cultures of competitive preventive measures (38).

For the results of a detailed project that tested the survival power of medical ideas across a language-translation barrier, see Hanson and Saunders (21). For insight into over 100 health education programs that focused primarily on low-income and minority groups, see the October 1975, Part Two, Supplement to the *American Journal of Public Health* (63). Also see references 7, 23, 38, and 64.

Chapter 10 also deals extensively with the significance of culture in health promotion.

Other Prohibitors in Teaching-Learning

A nursing student, somewhat dissatisfied with her nursing education, used an analogy to make a point. She compared some of her nursing instructors to delicate flowers who wilted as teachers. She declared that when she taught, she would be like a dandelion—tough, common, almost indestructible, and with functional component parts (5).

The idea is commendable, but caution is needed. Although armed with the best of theory and methods and with respect for the person, you will at times fail to impart positive health habits through teaching knowledge based on scientific information.

You will be dealing in health education with many myths and forms of unconscious resistance. Some people try to undermine their own health as a means of attracting attention or avoiding a hated job. Others, out of desire to belong, will cling to a false diet theory. Some believe the whole body is a mobile dirt factory with a constant need for cleaning. Even health educators, although highly trained formally, are subject to these devices and beliefs. You may need to teach other teachers.

Occasionally situations arise in which significant learning simply cannot occur. Perhaps you remind the patient of her employer, whom she detests. Or if you are a Black female heterosexual health teacher working with a Caucasian male homosexual patient, you may not succeed in teaching him because of prejudice.

In a hospital setting the question of who shall teach, and when, may be impossible to answer. Health professionals cannot decide who should teach about diagnosis—nurse or physician. And if both, how? Aiming primarily for efficiency runs counter to allowing teaching time. The physician suddenly writes the discharge order. No teaching time is available. In some hospitals and health care agencies a health educator is employed. However, most nurses believe that teaching is an integral part of nursing and that no one person should be hired for that role. Instead, nurses need to fulfill the state Nursing Practice Act, and most of the state acts include health teaching as a part of nursing practice.

In one home health agency a nurse was using an extra 15 minutes per home visit when additional teaching time was warranted. She was later told by her supervisor that she would have to "get her patient count up" because the agency had to take in money from a certain number of visits each day in order to "make payroll and other expenses."

Both sides do exist: Time is needed for patient teaching; money is needed to run the health care business. In one hospital both needs were met. The administration created positions specifically described as health teaching capacities; time was committed for this job; and perhaps most significant from a business point of view, third-party payment from insurance was arranged (47).

Receiving payment for organized health teaching can continue to be the trend if you pursue, at a local level, the possibilities. Third-party payment may come from a "for-profit" organization, such as Aetna; from a "not-for-profit" organization, such as Blue Cross; or from Medicare, Medicaid, or Social Security, if nurses work to influence federal legislation.

Teaching can be harmful if goals are unaccepted, inappropriate, misunderstood, or not broken down into manageable steps. If teaching materials are not appropriate, if teaching is not thorough, or if evaluation is not adequate, the patient may be confused, lose self-confidence, and be unable to adapt to his/her health problem (51).

Obviously the hardest look you take must be at yourself. Communication is often easiest with a person of one's own class or status group because each shares similar premises. But what happens when basic premises are dissimilar? Sometimes you fail.

Failure need not be permanently defeating. Sometimes it escalates the maturing process. Thus you should evaluate and revise working principles from your varied experiences in an attempt to produce better results (and to realize when you can't). This is analogous to the step of evaluation in the nursing process.

METHODS OF TEACHING

Techniques of Teaching

Methods or techniques of teaching are nearly as varied as people. A given technique can be effective in one setting and totally inappropriate in another. The key is in planning the technique for the specific situation.

Basically a climate for teaching-learning must be set. All involved must want teaching and learning to occur and anticipate an improved self-image as a result of learning. Time must be set aside for in-service teaching preparation and patient/client teaching. General team or individual goals must be set. Teaching guidelines and audiovisual materials must be available. The actual setting for the teaching-learning must be conducive. For example, learning is difficult in an overcrowded, poorly ventilated room where people are looking at each others' backs or are uncomfortably seated.

Your responsibility is to know your patient/client and the situation. You might write individual teaching guides on your patients that include such items as

1. The nature of the person's disease, including the person's normal functions, pathological changes, and results of the changes.
2. Hospitalization and nursing care measures, such as diagnostic procedures, treatments, medications, fluids, diet, and rehabilitation.
3. Discharge and home care, including diet, fluids, medications, activity, dressings, rest, general hygiene, prophylaxis, special equipment, and suggestions for improvisations.
4. Community agencies and resources (71).
5. Helpful bibliography.

Obviously age, mental and emotional attitudes, family status, and other factors affecting the person's learning should also be included in this guide. With this ongoing information, you can construct a design for teaching that is based on a priority system.

The priority system may be developed by identifying *acute educational needs* when a lack of understanding causes psychosocial anguish or physical danger; *preventive educational needs* when a person is threatened with a condition and doesn't know how to handle it; and *maintenance educational needs* when an alteration in normal functioning demands an ongoing understanding and skill (55).

Use of the nursing care plan as an integral part of teaching is discussed in Chapter 4. Characteristics of an effective leader are described in Chapter 6 and can be applied to the teacher. Just as a work of art calls for unity, continuity, and a certain sense of pace and movement, so does teaching. Your presentation, behavior, knowledge, and concern will each add components to your effectiveness.

Although certain techniques generally work better than others in specific situations, there are no definite rules. *A teaching method represents a way of thinking.* You must choose a method that you can use effectively and that is beneficial to patients/clients.

Table 5-1 depicts some techniques for producing desired behavioral outcomes (29). You can use your creativity to adapt these methods to your specific situations.

Note that you can build skills without imparting a lot of underlying knowledge. Through demonstration and return demonstration, for instance, you can teach a 10-year-old how to take and report a blood pressure reading accurately without having to explain all the underlying physiology of the heart and all the technicalities of the equipment involved. If, however, through role playing followed by group discussion, you are trying to teach someone how to get along in his/her

TABLE 5-1 Some Techniques for Producing Desired Behavioral Outcomes

RATIONALE	TEACHING METHODS
If you wish to:	*Use:*
impart *generalizations* about experience.	lecture, symposium, panel, reading, audiovisual aids, a book-or pamphlet-based discussion.
apply information to experience through insight and *understanding*.	feedback devices, problem-solving discussions, laboratory experimentation, group participation, case problems.
build *skills*.	role playing, drill, coaching, demonstration, and return demonstration.
create new *attitudes*. (Attitudes are learned through repeated reinforcement of a response to a stimulus. If a response different from the original one is given and reinforced over a period of time, a change in attitude occurs, evidenced by a change in behavior in a particular set of circumstances [21]. Eventually the attitude may become a value.)	reverse role playing, experience-sharing discussion, counseling-consultation, environmental support, games designed to produce certain attitudes, and nonverbal exercises which draw out certain attitudes through gestures, posture, and facial expression, positive and negative reinforcement.
change *values* through the rearrangement of the priority of beliefs.	speakers who have adjusted satisfactorily to a certain condition now facing the patient, biographical or autobiographical reading, drama, philosophical or direct-value-placement discussion with provision for reflection.
promote new *interests*.	field trips, audiovisual aids, reading, creative experiences.

family, you will need to teach the underlying principles of group dynamics and how to use them in a situation that is ever changing.

Individual and Group Teaching

Some techniques are best suited for teaching on an individual basis whereas others are best for large groups or several subgroups.

Individual Teaching can be provided through programmed learning, reading material, audiovisual aids, and one-to-one instruction. **Programmed learning** *provides material in carefully planned sequential steps that leads the person to a mastery of the subject.* The material is presented through program instruction books or a **teaching machine,** *a simple manually operated machine or a complex computer.* One frame of information is presented at a time. The learner then tests his/her grasp of the information in the frame by writing a response to a question, usually a multiple-choice type. The book or machine then gives the correct response. If the learner's response was incorrect, the program then presents (or, in the case of a book, directs him/her to turn to) a repetition of the information or a more detailed explanation, depending on the program and his/her response. The advantages of programmed learning include logical presentation, active learner participation, immediate disclosure of correct response, reinforcement of material, and individual pacing (65). For a summary of the state of the art in using computers to aid learning, see Chapter 14 of reference 71.

Another method of giving individual instruction is by providing factual material. The health organizations discussed later in this chapter provide preventive health-teaching literature as part of their programs. Evaluating the benefits gained from these materials is difficult because people who receive the material often do not respond to the organization's request for feedback, even when given a stamped answer form. One study tried to determine the effectiveness of a breast self-examination by seeking the reactions of 383 women one year after they received teaching kits with filmstrip, teaching notes, and commentary; only 41 percent responded. Women in the upper half of the social scale reacted more favorably: 48 percent of them had established an examination pattern (though not necessarily monthly, as the material suggested) (24). The tendency of upper-class persons to read better and to respond more readily to scientific health teaching than lower-class persons seems evident here.

Other factual reading materials include autobiographies of persons with certain disease processes and "how-to" books by persons who have experienced certain health problems directly or indirectly and want to pass along suggestions to others. Fiction also provides valuable insights into physical and mental illness.

With the constant introduction of more sophisticated audiovisual equipment into the teaching-learning area, you can get and adapt these devices to individual learning. A recorder and cassettes explaining preventive measures, disease processes, or specific instructions can be loaned to the client. He/she can stop the cassette at any point and replay necessary portions until satisfied with the learning. "Talking Books" is a program that records information for the visually impaired. Closed-circuit television or videotape setups allow the person to hear and view material. You can be involved in producing teaching cassettes and television or videotape programs.

These methods of individual instruction are only individual to a certain point. Only when the client can check learning with a resource person, ask further questions as necessary, and have help in making personal applications, will learning become significant. That process involves you. The person doesn't learn from a machine alone. These discussions with patients need not be long. The important point is to be available when they do have questions and to convey that any question or problem is worthy of your consideration.

Group Teaching can meet the person's need to achieve status or security through being a group member. Client groups provide a channel through which feelings and needs can be expressed and met, especially if the people have similar problems, such as colostomy or diabetes. Thus you can use the group process to enhance health teaching or for therapy to aid coping with problems. You may also have an opportunity to work with a group that has formed to accomplish some specific goal, such as losing weight, promoting research to find a cure for cancer, or providing guidance to parents with mentally retarded children. In some cases, information is not enough. Social support is also necessary, especially when engaging in a lesser-valued activity—like not eating sugar when society says that dessert is the best part of the meal. One study of hospitalized diabetics, some taught individually and some taught in a group by a nurse specialist, showed that the latter demonstrated as much or more knowledge and skill in urine testing as the former (45).

In another study 25 experimental patients participated in a small group session the night before surgery. They discussed their concerns and fears and learned what to expect and how to aid in their convalescence. A randomly selected matched control group of 25 patients who underwent similar surgery but who received only routine care were compared, after surgery, with the first group. Results showed that extra preparation increased patient participation, decreased tension and anxiety, and led to more rapid postoperative recoveries (60). In a similar study patients with preoperative teaching had a hospitalization of 1.3 days fewer than those who received no teaching (54).

One minister who had visited hundreds of patients on the night before surgery said, "Fear of the unknown is what I continually find. I don't necessarily mean about the outcome of the surgery, although that is involved. I mean they don't even know about the recovery room process. Instead of giving spiritual help, I find myself telling them many details which the nursing staff should have taught. With these important details at their command, I can see their anxiety lessen." Small group sessions could reduce these fears.

Not only should the rather complicated procedures such as surgery and its accompanying routines be explained. Positive results have also been obtained with minor procedures. One group, for example, was told what sensations to expect and then had blood pressure cuffs placed on their arms and the pressure pumped up to 250 mm Hg. Another group was told only of the procedure—that is, "Your blood pressure will be taken." The conclusion was that accurate expectations about sensations do reduce stress, but that patients should be told only about sensations usually experienced, not those rarely experienced (26). Excessively detailed explanations can raise rather than lower anxiety.

If you work with a group, you should initially set a working social climate. People do not automatically start revealing their problems and supporting and helping each other. You must use some introduction technique that focuses on the individual, his/her personality strengths and resources, rather than on a disease or problem. (The person already knows why he/she is there.) Each person can introduce himself if the group is small. If the group is large (25 or more), you can break it up into subgroups of 5 each and allow each subgroup at least 20 minutes to plan a presentation using one of the following creative techniques. In *the inquiring reporter*, one person in each group (or subgroup) is chosen to compose a feature story about the personalities and resources of group members. The person then presents the story to the total group in 3 minutes. In *the living newspaper*, each group picks a type of newspaper feature—a news story, column, book review, or editorial, for example—and presents a 3-minute group description through that format. In *the television variety program*, each group has a 3-minute segment to present its members through interview, skit, song, or comedy. These methods produce immediate ego-involvement, create an atmosphere conducive to participative learning and sharing of problems and resources, and start the spirit of creative inquiry (28). You can think of other introductory techniques for your particular group situation.

Whatever your reasons for teaching the group, you must assess needs and interests, define purposes and objectives, construct a design, and evaluate success. As you teach, rely on many approaches to accomplish your purpose.

A sample of group approaches that you could use follows.

1. *Support groups.* The total group breaks up into subgroups of three or four people. The purpose is for subgroup members to support one another. If one person misses a session or doesn't understand a procedure, the other members of the subgroup are responsible for getting the missing information to that person. Each has a feeling of being active and of being responsible to one another and each can clarify his/her own understanding while teaching someone else.
2. The *whip group.* This is a variation of the support group. One person in each subgroup is designated to interpret the concepts being taught. Misunderstandings can be caught early, for periodic times are designated for interpretation and discussion.
3. *Directive note taking.* The entire group listens to a lecture for 2 or 3 minutes. Then all stop and write notes on what was said. The teacher checks sample summaries to see how well the ideas are getting across. This procedure is repeated until the end of the session.

For a detailed look at the group process, see Chapter 6.

Problem Solving

Another approach to teaching–learning is the problem-solving technique, which is useful with either individuals or groups and is essentially the creative process discussed earlier. Parnes outlines a seven-step creative problem-solving process that can be written out to clarify thinking (51). The person starts with *confronting "the mess,"* acknowledging the predicament and the resultant dissatisfied feelings. Creative efficiency is increased if people understand the psychological process by which they operate. The emotional and irrational factors in peoples' thinking are more urgent than the intellectual and rational (72). People are free to go on more effectively after acknowledging this first step.

The second step is *clarifying the "fuzzy problem,"* writing a factual rather than an emotional explanation of the situation by answering such questions as who, what, when, where, and how. The third step is *fact finding*, writing information the patient would like to have related to the situation described. The fourth step is *problem finding*, listing all the creative-type questions or challenges suggested by the preceding

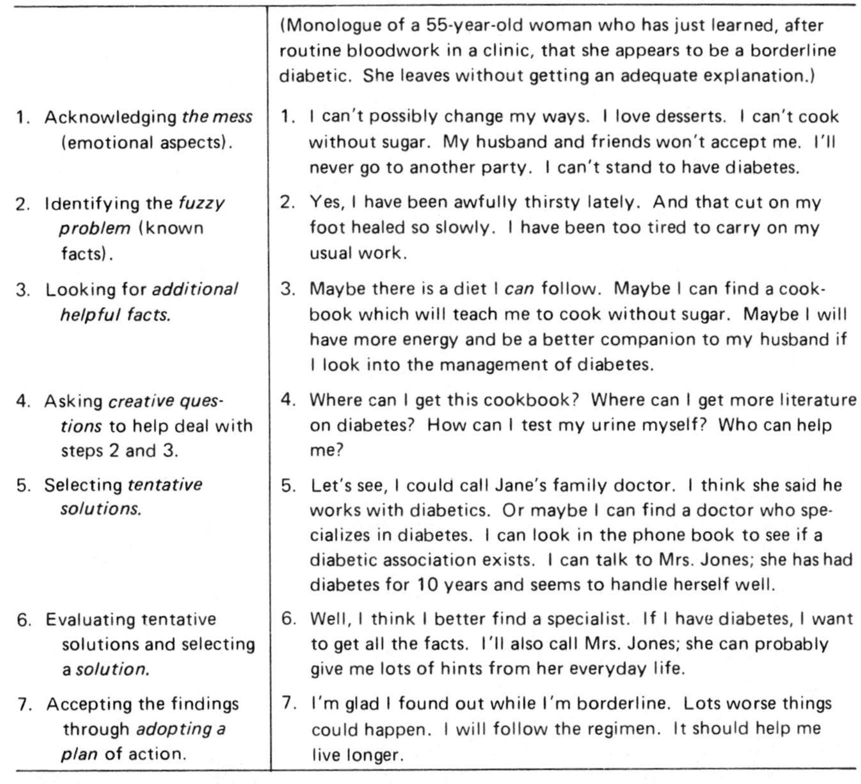

	(Monologue of a 55-year-old woman who has just learned, after routine bloodwork in a clinic, that she appears to be a borderline diabetic. She leaves without getting an adequate explanation.)
1. Acknowledging *the mess* (emotional aspects).	1. I can't possibly change my ways. I love desserts. I can't cook without sugar. My husband and friends won't accept me. I'll never go to another party. I can't stand to have diabetes.
2. Identifying the *fuzzy problem* (known facts).	2. Yes, I have been awfully thirsty lately. And that cut on my foot healed so slowly. I have been too tired to carry on my usual work.
3. Looking for *additional helpful facts.*	3. Maybe there is a diet I *can* follow. Maybe I can find a cookbook which will teach me to cook without sugar. Maybe I will have more energy and be a better companion to my husband if I look into the management of diabetes.
4. Asking *creative questions* to help deal with steps 2 and 3.	4. Where can I get this cookbook? Where can I get more literature on diabetes? How can I test my urine myself? Who can help me?
5. Selecting *tentative solutions.*	5. Let's see, I could call Jane's family doctor. I think she said he works with diabetics. Or maybe I can find a doctor who specializes in diabetes. I can look in the phone book to see if a diabetic association exists. I can talk to Mrs. Jones; she has had diabetes for 10 years and seems to handle herself well.
6. Evaluating tentative solutions and selecting a *solution.*	6. Well, I think I better find a specialist. If I have diabetes, I want to get all the facts. I'll also call Mrs. Jones; she can probably give me lots of hints from her everyday life.
7. Accepting the findings through *adopting a plan* of action.	7. I'm glad I found out while I'm borderline. Lots worse things could happen. I will follow the regimen. It should help me live longer.

FIGURE 5-1 Seven-Step Creative Problem-Solving Process

two steps, such as "How might I . . . ?" and "In what ways might I . . . ?" The fifth step is *idea finding*, or deferred judgment, selecting the most likely ways of solution finding. The sixth step is *solution finding*, in which the best approaches are evaluated; and the seventh step is *acceptance finding*, or adoption of solution. These steps are merely guides to be adapted to personal and group characteristics (see Fig. 5-1).

Some persons are capable of going through these seven steps relying only on their insight. Others can work through the steps themselves but will need you to present the plan to them. And still others will be so engulfed in "the mess" that they will need your careful guidance to move them toward a solution.

Other Approaches

Appropriate visual aids should be used with whatever method is used. Letting people work with their hands as well as their minds is often effective. Groups may make a collage from magazine pictures, for example, foods acceptable to a diabetic versus unacceptable foods; good hygiene versus poor hygiene; elements of health versus elements of illness. Children in an elementary classroom went through numerous magazines, cutting out pictures of people who appeared to be in good health and people who appeared to be in poor health. When all the pictures of unhealthy people were arranged on one poster and all the pictures of healthy people were arranged on another poster, the contrast was startling. This visual confrontation enabled the teacher and students to begin to discuss why these differences existed and to apply the principles to the children's lives.

Clients are also eager to get *handouts*, appropriate visual or written materials that they can keep. Ideally, they will use this material and even pass it on to a relative or friend. You must know each patient's reading ability (or lack of it) and select materials accordingly. Not being able to read is a source of embarrassment to patients. Go over the handout with the person; do not just hand it to him/her.

The *local library* is a useful center for setting up health teaching courses, and it is committed to presenting a variety of programs based on community needs. Additionally, you can use the library's books in your teaching, especially on such subjects as childhood illnesses or sex education. You may even want to use books in the children's library for an elementary presentation of some subjects.

You, as nurse-teacher, can also make use of the local university or college library to keep up to date on educational insights and teaching methods and nursing knowledge. Don't limit yourself to nursing literature.

Teaching *patient/client rights* uses a direct approach either with individual persons or with groups. Although people may have vast resources within themselves, they sometimes do not use them because they have been taught to respect the doctor: "Do not question the doctor's judgment. He/she is too busy to explain." While you and the patient should respect the doctor, the doctor should also respect you and the patient. We question the plumber about the new parts he/she is putting in our sink, ask their cost, and refuse to pay if the work is ineffective but often we fail to question the doctor about medications we take, their cost, or the service fee. And we pay whether satisfied or not.

One study questioned 60 patients in a teaching hospital about the drugs they were taking and concluded that (1) patients have little information about their medications; (2) younger patients know more about their drugs than older ones; and (3) patients who would like more information do not ask (51). Another study confirmed that patients want specific information about their condition (15).

This demand for patient information has been heightened in the last several years by such publications as *How to Choose and Use Your*

Doctor by Dr. Marvin Belsky, *Talk Back to Your Doctor* by Dr. Arthur Levin, and *Managing Your Doctor* by Dr. Arthur Freese (31). All place responsibility on the client to examine potential doctors carefully in terms of reputation, education, affiliations, and thoroughness in procedures (such as taking a patient history). Other articles, such as "Patients' Rights: Choosing a Pharmacist" (61), and "Know Your Medications: Stop Taking Risks!" (16), advocate that the pharmacist provide health services through drug consultations and detailed medical records and that the patient should ask about various drug side effects and the possible danger of improper use.

Table 5-2, based on suggestions from a medical physician, indicates how patients can get specific information from their doctor (46).

TABLE 5-2 Teaching Guide for Client's Rights

FIVE DOs	FIVE DON'Ts
1. When you call the nurse or secretary for an appointment, state your request or problem so the appropriate appointment time can be scheduled.	1. Unless an emergency arises, don't take up extra, unplanned-for time. For example, don't say, "Oh, while I'm here for my ear infection, why don't you do my complete physical."
2. Organize thoughts about your present health status or illness and write them down so you can present pertinent facts to the doctor. These will aid him/her in giving a thorough examination or in making a diagnosis.	2. Don't lie to yourself or to the doctor. Don't let fear cause you to ignore a situation that may need immediate but minimal treatment.
3. Cooperate during the physical exam and allow the doctor to be complete. Don't tell the doctor to skip certain procedures.	3. Don't tell the doctor to give you pills. Don't feel cheated if you don't get medication; many illnesses are minor and self-limiting. Your own observance of a health-promotion regimen may be all you need.
4. Ask your doctor about proper diet, work load, exercise, and rest to help you maintain maximum health. Ask about realistic limitations. If ill, ask your doctor questions about cost of treatment, medication, diagnosis, causes of condition, chances for recovery, or whatever you want to know related to situation. If you have more questions after you leave, write them down and call back for answers. If hospitalized, continue to ask questions about drugs and ongoing treatment.	4. Don't ask for unnecessary hospitalization for x rays or tests because the insurance will pay or because grandma is burdensome. Talk with your doctor about alternate plans that will promote long-range health for everyone involved.
5. Follow instructions after health promotion plan is established. After time, effort, and money are spent, you are the only loser if you refuse to follow suggestions or directions.	5. Don't leave the doctor's office dissatisfied. At least express and explain your feelings. The doctor needs to understand your point of view. Maybe a change can be made or perhaps you need additional information to understand a suggestion or decision.

Evaluation

Evaluation is judging how effective teaching has been. Evaluation is sometimes difficult because clients cannot always be followed long enough to see the results of teaching, and human behavior is so complicated that true changes are hard to measure.

Evaluation can be informal or formal. Informal judgments are made constantly. A patient/client compliments or complains. You react to these judgments. You observe how well a client dresses a wound, irrigates a catheter, or cooks a meal after your demonstration. You may write evaluation notes on the learning ability. By questioning the person's understanding, you are evaluating your teaching. If he/she has learned appropriately—can give explanations and can perform the activities that were taught—the teaching has been adequate. Patients/clients can evaluate their own learning, whether goals were met, and your teaching by using a rating scale or checklist, which further assists your evaluation process.

Every person connected with a teaching-learning program should be involved in evaluating the program. Depending on the specific situation and program, these people might include the participants (patients and teachers); the program director and staff, who can see the program as a whole; the directing committee, who establish objectives and policy; and outside experts, who can be totally objective. Community representatives can supply valuable evaluative information when the teaching is aimed at serving the general public (29).

HOME TEACHING

So often there is no continuity in teaching from health care agency to home. Ideally, all teaching should include the patient's family and its particular circumstances in the plan, but in a setting other than the home the true circumstances often cannot be discerned. When a mother returns to the clinic for the third time with a child who has pneumonia, the doctor and nurses may reprimand her for not taking better care of her child. She may be too proud to say she can only afford to keep one room partially warm, that she doesn't have enough quilts, and that their diet consists mostly of rice.

Sometimes lower-class persons give up before ever starting on a health-promotion plan because they know they cannot afford the fancy equipment or the expensive nutritional supplements recommended by the hospital staff.

The nurse who goes into the home can, in one-half hour, make observations that could never be made under any other circumstances, certainly not in a hospital room. When you enter the home, you see, smell, hear, and feel how the people think and live. Peeling plaster, unpainted walls, holes in the floors, spilled old food underfoot, the smell of urine, piles of dirty clothes, oppressive heat or pervasive cold all give information regarding health (or lack of it). A row of shined shoes, religious articles, a certain painting, photos of children and relatives, framed certificates, rows of books or of store-bought medicine also give valuable information. These are extensions of the personalities. From these observations you can begin realistic health teaching as part of your nursing intervention.

One visiting nurse said her goal was to teach health promotion under existing conditions, to make patients both comfortable and as healthy as possible in their own circumstance. She said that if a patient needed a diet change for heart disease or diabetes, she would ask him to keep a record of everything he ate for three days. Then she would plan an adequate diet around that information. She felt it was futile to change the existing plan drastically, to take away all his favorite foods and add new ones that he didn't like or didn't want to try.

Five Families

The following situations occur in the working day of a visiting nurse. The cases are actual; the names are fictitious. Use the following narrative as a guide to focus on what types of information you can glean and what teaching you can do in the home as opposed to an agency setting.

> Mrs. Taylor has diabetes and because of gangrene has already had one leg removed. She keeps her clinic appointments and always agrees with what the doctor says, but her blood glucose level remains dangerously high. I have been sent to visit Mrs. Taylor to detect the missing link. Why, if she is following instructions, doesn't her blood glucose level diminish? Mrs. Taylor lives in a little clapboard house, the last remaining after an industrial court replaced the community. There is no running water, no inside toilet. But Mrs. Taylor does not complain. This is her home; she will stay here until she dies.
>
> Whenever I visit, Mrs. Taylor is gracious. Yes, she is taking her insulin, following her diet, feeling fine. Still the elevated blood glucose remains. Also, she is gaining weight on a 1200 calorie diet.
>
> After several visits I discern that Mrs. Taylor is telling me what she thinks a nurse wants to hear and is doing something different. I notice that the insulin in the bottle remains at the same level week after week. I see food in the house that is not on her diet. The mystery is solved. I am able to report to the physician; together we will try to convince Mrs. Taylor that taking her

insulin and following her diet are important for her health. Yet, we realize that we cannot force patient compliance.

What would you do?

Mrs. Brown should be a satisfied senior citizen. She lives in a senior citizens' home with every convenience: grocery store, communal dining room, scheduled dances and cultural programs, bus service to shopping centers and appointments, special drivers for special events.

Mrs. Brown has a diagnosis of hypertension and chronic obstructive pulmonary disease. But in the last 12 months her blood pressure has been in normal range and her lungs appear clear. Mrs. Brown has the services of a home health aide, nutritionist, social worker, and registered nurse. Yet she complains! She eats salty foods; she smokes constantly; she says she is going to lose her legs from blood clots; she doesn't like the "old people" in the home (she is 72); the bus leaves for the shopping center too early; the social worker merely chats with her; the girl who drives her to special occasions has a "death trap" car; her doctors don't care.

I discover that Mrs. Brown lost her husband six years ago. He had taken complete care of her needs. She is still grieving this loss.

I ask her psychiatrist, "Is there any need for me to remain on the case?" The psychiatrist says, "If you don't, she will die."

What would you do?

According to medical predictions, Mrs. Dixon was to die. She has inoperable cancer. She has been given all treatment possible. Yet Mrs. Dixon is not dying. She is getting better. Her main wish is to avoid institutionalized care until absolutely necessary. But the only place she can live is with a single daughter whose job keeps her gone days and many evenings. Mrs. Dixon is mentally alert, but her physical weakness keeps her in bed most of the time.

The doctor sends me in to coordinate Mrs. Dixon's care.

What would you do?

I have been asked to visit a man with chronic brain syndrome. The doctor said to insert a feeding tube because the wife reports that her husband "sleeps all the time and won't eat a thing." I discover that Mr. Henry can be aroused and that he says he is hungry. After he eats a bowl of cereal, a dish of cottage cheese, a piece of toast, a bowl of ice cream, and a glass of milk, I begin to suspect that the main problem may be Mrs. Henry, not Mr. Henry! Further investigation reveals that Mrs. Henry is giving her husband a triple dose of sleeping medication and that she doesn't offer him food.

I report the situation to the doctor and order a worker (home health aide, social worker, or myself) from our agency into the home daily to see that

Mr. Henry's basic needs are met. This action is only temporary since daily visits cannot be made indefinitely.

What would you do?

Mrs. Charles has multiple sclerosis. She cannot move her body except for her mouth. She has a catheter for urinary drainage and requires an enema for bowel evacuation. Her husband is out of work and sits and drinks beer all day. Her mother, who is almost blind, is trying to manage the cooking and cleaning. The home health aide and I visit two or three times weekly to give Mrs. Charles what care she gets. There is no money to pay for food and utilities, let alone drugs.

What would you do?

Not everyone wants or needs a nurse in the home, but a lack of followup in home health teaching exists. A routine phone call to patients who have been seen in other circumstances can determine if a home visit would be helpful.

AGENCY TEACHING

Effective teaching often involves making a pertinent referral. Once you understand the health status of the person and of the family and home situation, you can refer the person to the agency that can give the most help. In fact, you should not attempt to provide services in areas where you are not fully trained, especially if expert service is simply a matter of proper referral.

Survey your local community for health-teaching agencies. You should know which services you can expect from these agencies. Larger cities sometimes have community-service directories that give this information. Keep abreast of newly added programs. Don't overlook church and club groups that sponsor or help with health education.

Chapter 2 outlines some basic health agencies. Table 5-3 presents some specific service and educational agencies. These services are not inclusive, and they vary with location. The table does, however, point out the vast resources available.

CURRENT CHALLENGES

Teaching–learning is important at any stage of the wellness–illness continuum, but more emphasis now is given to teaching health promotion and early prevention. You have a brigade of definitions, theories,

TABLE 5-3 Agencies to Utilize in Health Teaching

AGENCY	SERVICES
American Cancer Society	Provides a service director, who will guide family of cancer patient to community resources and drug discounts. Sponsors screening and rehabilitation programs. Gives financial, equipment, transportation, and service aid. Prints literature on different types of cancer, and preventive and early diagnostic measures. Advocates nonsmoking and avoiding overexposure to sun; monthly breast self-examination; regular mouth, proctoscopy, and total health checkups; Pap test.
American Dental Association	Refers patients to dentists. Intervenes between patient and dentist if patient has complaint about treatment. Prints educational material in cartoon form for children and pamphlet form for adults on proper brushing, nutrition, and importance of periodic cleaning by dentist or hygienist. Defines eight areas of specialization in dentistry.
American Diabetes Association	Teaches about all phases of diabetes from detection through treatment. Prints magazines, newsletters, visual aids. Sponsors speakers' bureaus and camps for diabetic children. Provides test kits for detection, nutritionists for proper meal planning, cookbook for home use, scales for food weighing, identification bracelets.
American Heart Association	Supports research. Prints books, pamphlets, and visual aids to teach prevention and care measures. Offers nutritionist services and a cookbook, speakers' bureau. screening projects for adults and children. Offers free education for health workers. Incorporates a course (in at least one city) on the prevention and treatment of heart disease into the college curriculum of future elementary-school teachers.
The Arthritis Foundation	Prints extensive literature on different types of arthritis, those affected, Social Security benefits for arthritics, medication, diet, approved exercises, quackery, homemaker hints, home care programs. Promotes self-help groups. Supports and finances research and fellowship programs.
Visiting Nurse Association	Provides home care and services through registered and licensed practical nurse; home health aides; physical, occupational, and speech therapists; social service workers; nutritionists.

methods, and agencies to assist you in teaching. But before you can teach effectively in the health care or social systems, you must have a wellness rather than a pathological orientation. Health educators should shift their emphasis from pathology that has never been experienced to things the person has done and enjoyed and will be unable to continue to do if health behavior is not implemented (66).

Health behavior *is any activity undertaken by a person who believes self to be well.* Health behavior and self-care have come to be synonymous.

Practicing health behavior or teaching health behavior is not dramatic. One nurse said that teaching proper diet, weight control, the need for rest and sleep, stress reduction, the importance of exercise, cleanliness, periodic health examination, and immunization is so humdrum. Yet these areas of teaching can eliminate much time, effort, and money spent on teaching in later disease stages as well as eliminate suffering for the person.

For example, on a routine blood pressure check, a 33-year-old Black male learned that the reading was 170/110 mm Hg. Blood testing showed high cholesterol and triglyceride levels. He was also 50 pounds overweight. With teaching and monitoring over a period of a year, he avoided high sugar and salt intake, started regular exercise, and subsequently lost 30 pounds. His blood pressure returned to normal limits so that medication was unnecessary.

According to the often-quoted studies of Breslow and Bellac, persons who followed seven common health habits were not only healthier than those who did not but also lived longer. The practices are:

1. Sleep 7 to 8 hours a night.
2. Eat breakfast.
3. Do not eat between meals.
4. Get exercise regularly.
5. Do not drink alcoholic beverages to excess.
6. Do not smoke.
7. Stay within 10 percent of your proper weight.

In a following study several years after the original one, only the third practice—do not eat between meals—seemed less significant than the other six (52).

Providing you have a wellness orientation, you still must deal with the client where he/she is—culturally, socially, and developmentally. Previously the average layperson did not place health in the same level as did the health worker. The layperson generally takes health action only when he/she believes there is susceptibility to a health threat that could have serious effects on the person's life, when he/she knows what actions to take to reduce the health threat, and when the health threat is greater than the action threat (58).

The layperson, however, increasingly knows what action he/she wants to take. Table 5-4 depicts by subject matter some references that

TABLE 5-4 Sources of Self-Help Literature

SUBJECT	TITLE	AUTHOR	PUBLISHER	SYNOPSIS
Physical Health	*Take Care of Yourself: A Consumer's Guide to Medical Care*	Vickery and Fries	Addison-Wesley, 1977	Detailed flowcharts of most common complaints that take people to a doctor's office.
	The Well Body Book	Samuels and Bennett	Random House, 1973	Emphasizes the "feeling side" of physical health. Excellent sections on preventive medicine, relaxation and physical exam.
	Standard First Aid and Personal Safety	American Red Cross	Doubleday & Co., Inc., 1977	Basic primer.
Stress Management	*High Level Wellness*	Ardell	Bantam Books, 1977	Tools for stress reduction.
	Mind as Healer, Mind as Slayer	Pelletier	Delta, 1977	Synthesis of current understanding of stress as cause of disease.
Stress Management/ Relaxation	*90 Days to Self-Health*	Shealy	Dial Press, 1980	Practical program with self-suggestion and visualization techniques.
Exercise/Stretching	*The Aerobic Series*	Cooper	Bantam Books, various	Getting into and staying-in-shape programs.
Exercise/Stretching	*Stretching*	Anderson	Shelter Publications, 1980	Warming-up exercises with help for some particular body area.
Nutrition	*Diet for a Small Planet*	Lappe	Ballentine, 1982	Vegetarian diet with tasty recipes.
Nutrition	*One Bowl: A Simple Concept for Controlling Body Weight*	Gerard	Random House, 1974	Getting in touch with food feelings. Eating as meditation.
Medication/Drugs	*The People's Pharmacy*	Graedon	St. Martins Press, 1977	Prescription and nonprescription drug information for lay people.

TABLE 5-4 (cont.)

SUBJECT	TITLE	AUTHOR	PUBLISHER	SYNOPSIS
	The People's Pharmacy—2	Graedon and Graedon	Avon, 1980	Continuation of above with reader response.
Psychological Self-Care	*The Art of Loving*	Fromm	Harper & Row, 1974	Information on what everyone thinks is a natural art.
	Your Perfect Right	Alberti and Emmons	Impact, 1970	Original classic on assertiveness training.
Parenting	*Mothers and Infants*	Brazelton	Delta, 1969	For new parents, emphasizes the first year of life.
	The Facts of Love	Comfort and Comfort	Crown, 1979	Introduces sexuality to young people.
Faith	*The Meaning of Persons*	Tournier	Harper & Row, 1957	Classic on spiritual, humanistic respect for people.
Grieving	*Living with an Empty Chair: A Guide Through Grief*	Temes	Mandala Books, 1977	Short, readable, useful.
Variety	*Medical Self-Care*	Tom Ferguson, Editor	Medical Self-Care Magazine, P.O. Box 717, Inverness, Calif. 94937	Published quarterly and offers a variety of self-care topics.
	Taking Care	Donald Vickery, President	Center for Consumer Health Education, 380 W. Maple Ave. Suite 301 Vienna, Virginia 22180	Published monthly and offers information designed to enable consumers to take charge of their health.

are available on subjects of concern. You might want to organize a class around various aspects of these topics.

Besides teaching health promotion and prevention measures to lay people, you may need to direct your teaching toward health educators who continue to focus only on the curative process. You may also establish courses to teach schoolteachers, fire fighters, police officers, ambulance attendants or health agency workers—those who are in a direct position to aid in illness or injury prevention and control.

REFERENCES

1. American Cancer Society, St. Louis, public service literature.
2. American Dental Association, St. Louis, public service literature.
3. **Baldonado, Ardelina,** "Creative Teaching-Learning Strategies," *Journal of Continuing Education in Nursing*, 10, no. 3 (1979), 11-16.
4. **Bartleet, Edward E.,** "The Contribution of School Health Education to Community Health Promotion: What Can We Reasonably Expect?" *American Journal of Public Health*, 71, no. 12 (1981), 1384-89.
5. **Bayer, Mary,** "The Red Dandelion," *Nursing Outlook*, 21, no. 1 (1973), 32.
6. **Boas, Charles William,** "The Circus," *Guideposts*, July 1973, pp. 16-19.
7. **Chatham, Margaret, Ann Hofler,** and **Barbara Lynne Knapp,** *Patient Education Handbook*. Bowie, MO: Robert J. Brady Co., 1982.
8. **Cleino, Bettie,** "Teaching Machines and Programmed Learning," *Journal of Nursing Education*, 3, no. 1 (1964), 13-15.
9. **Closurdo, Janette,** "Behavior Modification and the Nursing Process," *Nursing Digest*, 4, no. 4 (1976), 27-31.
10. **Connolly, Arlene F.,** "Theory and Practice in Teaching and Learning for the Adult Learner," *Journal New York State Nurses Association*, 12, no. 1 (1981), 5-11.
11. "Creativity: Questions, Not Answers," *St. Louis Globe-Democrat*, July 19, 1977, Sec. A., p. 3.
12. **deBono, Edward,** *Lateral Thinking: Creativity Step By Step*. New York: Harper & Row, Publishers, 1970.
13. **Dodge, Joan,** "What Patients Should Be Told: Patients' and Nurses' Beliefs," *American Journal of Nursing*, 72, no. 10 (1972), 1852-54.
14. **Edwards, Betty,** *Drawing on the Right Side of the Brain*. Los Angeles: J. P. Tarcher, Inc., 1979.
15. **Fahrer, Lois,** and **Ronnie Berstein,** "Making Patient Education Work," *American Journal of Nursing*, 76, no. 11 (1976), 1798-99.
16. **Galton, Lawrence,** "Know Your Medications: Stop Taking Risks," *Parade*, January 9, 1977, pp. 8-12.
17. **Gardner, C. Hugh,** "Educators' Failure at Communication," *Intellect*, 100, no. 2350 (1973), 486-88.
18. **Guinee, Kathleen K.,** *Teaching and Learning in Nursing*. New York: Macmillan, Inc., 1978.
19. **Guralnik, David, ed.,** *Webster's New World Dictionary of the American Language* (2nd college ed.). New York: The World Publishing Company, 1972.

20. **Hand, Samuel E.,** *A Review of Physiological and Psychological Changes in Aging and Their Implications for Teaching of Adults.* Tallahassee: Florida State Department of Education, 1956.
21. **Hanson, Robert,** and **Lyle Saunders,** *Nurse-Patient Communication: A Manual for Public Health Nurses in Northern New Mexico.* Washington, D.C.: United States Department of Health, Education, and Welfare, 1964, pp. 121–62.
22. **Hartfield, Mary T., Carolyn Cason,** and **Gerald Cason,** "Effects of Information about a Threatening Procedure on Patients' Expectations and Emotional Distress," *Nursing Research,* 31, no. 4 (1982), 202–05.
23. **Hill R.,** *The Strengths of Black Families.* New York: Emerson Hall, 1971.
24. **Hobbs, Patricia,** "Evaluation of a Teaching Programme of Breast Self-Examination," *International Journal of Health Education,* 14 (1971), 189–95.
25. **Hughes, Helen,** "Creativity in Women," *AAUW Journal,* 70, no. 3 (1976), 6–9.
26. **Johnson, Jean E.,** "Effects of Structuring Patients' Expectations on Their Reactions to Threatening Events," *Nursing Research,* 21, no. 6 (1972), 499–503.
27. **Kazin, Alfred,** "The Human Factory," in *A Walker in the City.* New York: Harcourt, Brace and World, Inc., 1951.
28. **Knowles, Malcolm S.,** "Teaching-Learning Teams in Adult Education," in *The Changing College Classroom,* eds., P. Runkel, R. Harrison, and M. Runkel. San Francisco: Jossey-Bass Inc., Publishers, 1969.
29. ———, *The Modern Practice of Adult Education.* New York: Association Press, 1970, pp. 37, 39–40, 225, 271, 294.
30. **Laird, Mona,** "Techniques for Teaching Pre- and Postoperative Patients," *American Journal of Nursing,* 75, no. 8 (1975), 1338–40.
31. "Learning to Choose and Use a Doctor," *St. Louis Globe-Democrat,* September 25, 1975, Sec. A, p. 4.
32. **Levin, Lowell S.,** "Patient Education and Self-Care; How Do They Differ?" *Nursing Outlook,* 26, no. 3 (1978), 170–75.
33. **Lowenfeld, Viktor,** "Creativity: Education's Stepchild," in *A Source Book for Creative Thinking,* eds. Sidney J. Parnes and Harold F. Harding. New York: Charles Scribner's Sons, 1962, pp. 9–17.
34. **Marks, Janet,** and **Margaret Clarke,** "The Hospital Patient and His Knowledge of the Drugs He Is Receiving," *International Nursing Review,* 19, no. 1 (1972), 39–51.
35. **Marks, Vida,** "Health Teaching for Recovering Alcoholic Patients," *American Journal of Nursing,* 80, no. 11 (1980), 2058–61.
36. **Marriner, Ann,** "The Student's Perception of His Creativity," *Nursing Research,* 26, no. 1 (1977), 57–60.
37. **Marshall, Irene A.,** "Creating an Environment for Learning," *Nursing Outlook,* 22, no. 12 (1974), 773–75.
38. **Martinez, R. A.,** *Hispanic Culture and Health Care.* St. Louis, MO: The C. V. Mosby Company, 1978.
39. **McAlister, Alfred, et al.,** "Theory and Action for Health Promotion: Illustrations from the North Karelia Project," *American Journal of Public Health,* 72, no. 1 (1982), 43–50.
40. **McHugh, Norma, Norma J. Christman,** and **Jean E. Johnson,** "Preparatory Information: What Helps and Why," *American Journal of Nursing,* 82, no. 5 (1982), 780–82.

41. **Megenity, Jean Stone,** and **Jack Megenity,** *Patient Teaching: Theories, Techniques and Strategies.* Bowie, MD: Robert J. Brady Co., 1982.
42. **Milio, Nancy,** "Progress in Primary Prevention: The Smoking-Health Issue," *American Journal of Public Health,* 72, no. 5 (1982), 428–29.
43. **Murray, Ruth,** and **Judith Zentner,** *Nursing Assessment and Health Promotion Through the Life Span* (3rd ed.). Englewood Cliffs, NJ: Prentice-Hall, Inc., 1985.
44. **Nappy, Jean,** "Churches as Settings for Teaching Physical Assessment," *American Journal of Nursing,* 82, no. 8 (1982), 1235–36.
45. **Nickerson, Donna,** "Teaching the Hospitalized Diabetic," *American Journal of Nursing,* 72, no. 6 (1972), 935–38.
46. **Nolan, William,** "Rules to Make You a Better Patient," *Today's Health,* 51, no. 4 (1973), 41–42, 66–67.
47. **Nordberg, Beatrice,** and **Lynelle Hine,** "Third-Party Payment for Patient Education," *American Journal of Nursing,* 76, no. 8 (1976), 1269–71.
48. **Norris, C. Gail,** "Characteristics of the Adult Learner and Extended Higher Education for Registered Nurses," *Nursing and Health Care,* 1, no. 2 (1980), 87–93.
49. "Nursing in the Health Care System," *Perspectives for Nursing and Goals of the National League for Nursing 1979–1981.* National League for Nursing, 1979, pp. 9–14.
50. **Pardue, Austin,** "Don't be Frightened by Failure," *Guideposts,* May 1973, p. 26.
51. **Parnes, Sidney J.,** *Creative Behavior Workbook.* New York: Charles Scribner's Sons, 1967.
52. **Pender, Nola J.,** *Health Promotion in Nursing Practice.* Norwalk, CT: Appleton-Century-Crofts, 1982, pp. 150–75.
53. **Peterson, Mary E.,** and **Constance Kies,** "Nutrition, Knowledge, and Attitudes of Early Elementary Teachers," *Journal of Nursing Education,* 11, no. 4 (1972), 11–15.
54. "Preoperative Teaching Found to Shorten Hospitalization," *American Journal of Nursing,* 75, no. 11 (1975), 2078.
55. **Redman, Barbara K.,** "Guidelines for Quality of Care in Patient Education," *Nursing Digest,* 4, no. 4 (1976), 25–26.
56. ———, *The Process of Patient Teaching in Nursing* (2nd ed.). St. Louis: The C. V. Mosby Company, 1972.
57. **Rogers, Carl,** *On Becoming a Person.* Boston: Houghton Mifflin Company, 1961.
58. **Rosenstock, Irvin M.,** "What Research in Motivation Suggests for Public Health," *American Journal of Public Health,* 50, no. 3 (1960), 295–302.
59. **Sarver, Susan,** and **Margaret Howard,** "Planning a Self-Care Unit in an Inpatient Setting," *American Journal of Nursing,* 82, no. 7 (1982), 1112–14.
60. **Schmitt, Florence E.,** and **Powhatan J. Wolldridge,** "Psychological Preparation of Surgical Patients," *Nursing Research,* 22, no. 2 (1973), 108–15.
61. **Schumacher, Florence,** and **Gerald Schumacher,** "Rx for Choosing a Pharmacist," *Family Health,* 9, no. 6 (1977), 48–49.
62. **Seliger, Susan,** "Stress Can Be Good for You," *The New Yorker,* August 2, 1982, pp. 20–24.

63. **Simmons, Jeanette, ed.**, "Making Health Education Work," *American Journal of Public Health*, 65, no. 10 (1975), Part Two.
64. **Spector, R. E.**, *Cultural Diversity in Health and Illness*. New York: Appleton-Century-Crofts, 1979.
65. **Stevens, Barbara J.**, "The Teaching-Learning Process," *Nurse Educator*, 1, no. 3 (1976), 9 ff.
66. **Suchman, Edward**, "Preventive Health Behavior: A Model for Research on Community Health Campaigns," *Journal of Health and Social Behavior*, 8, no. 3 (1967). 197-209.
67. **Sutterly, Cook**, and **Gloria Donnelly**, *Perspectives in Human Development*. Philadelphia: J. B. Lippincott Company, 1973, pp. 181-85.
68. **Tagliacozzo, Renata**, and **Sally Vaughn**, "Stress and Smoking in Hospital Nurses," *American Journal of Public Health*, 72, no. 5 (1982), 441-47.
69. The Arthritis Foundation, St. Louis, public service literature.
70. **Toffler, Alvin**, *Future Shock*. New York: Random House, 1970, pp. 342-67.
71. **Tornyay, Rheba de**, and **Martha A. Thompson**, *Strategies For Teaching Nursing* (2nd ed.). New York: John Wiley & Sons, Inc., 1982.
72. **Torrance, Ellis Paul**, *Creativity*. Washington, D.C.: National Educational Association of the United States, 1963.
73. **Turvey, M. K.**, and **A. M. Marshall**, "The Influence of the Occupational Health Nurse as Educator," *Occupational Health Nursing*, January 1976, pp. 23-25.
74. **Wagner, Edward H.**, "The North Karelia Project: What it Tells Us About the Prevention of Cardiovascular Disease," *American Journal of Public Health*, 72, no. 1 (1982), 51-54.
75. **Walsh, Joseph**, "Dr. Seuss Meets Dr. Freud: Primary Prevention in the Community Library," *American Journal of Public Health*, 67, no. 6 (1977), 561-62.
76. **Wise, Pat**, "Barriers (or Enhancers) to Adult Patient Education," *Journal of Continuing Education in Nursing*, 10, no. 6 (1979), 11-16.
77. **Woolley, Alma S.**, "Reaching and Teaching the Older Student," *Nursing Outlook*, 21, no. 1 (1973), 37-39.
78. **Wu, Ruth**, *Behavior and Illness*. Englewood Cliffs, NJ: Prentice-Hall, Inc., 1973.

Personal Interviews

79. **Bringewatt, Mark**, student of Malcolm Knowles, May 17, 1973.
80. **Byrne, John**, and **Mary McElfresh**, director and educational director, respectively, St. Louis Visiting Nurse Association, July 6, 1973.
81. **Goldberg, Virginia**, program director, St. Louis Heart Association, June 29, 1973.
82. **Morris, Virginia**, and **Verna Andrews**, registered nurses, St. Louis Visiting Nurse Association, July 12, 1973.
83. **Sellars, Ernest**, director, St. Louis Diabetes Association, July 2, 1973.
84. **Zentner, Reid**, cooperative work training coordinator, Alton, Illinois, public school system, May 5, 1973.

6

Group Work in Nursing

Study of this chapter will enable you to

1. Define *group* and *primary* and *secondary* groups.
2. Discuss the historical evolution of group work and the main types of groups currently used by health workers.
3. Describe the purposes of group work with clients.
4. Describe effective leader behaviors.
5. Discuss responsibilities of the group leader in the preplanning phase.
6. Analyze the group as a system.
7. Explore the behavioral characteristics and forces that contribute to group process.
8. List and define task and maintenance functions in a group.
9. Discuss phases of group process, characteristic behaviors of group members, and leader responsibilities in each phase.
10. Describe the role of group members and problems that can be encountered in group work.
11. Explore examples of group work that can be used in health care settings with clients of various ages.
12. Discuss the purposes and formats of various types of groups.

13. Initiate and maintain a group experience for selected clients by using knowledge from this chapter and guidance of a skilled supervisor.
14. Evaluate the effectiveness of your leadership style and your ability to fulfill the leader responsibilities related to each phase of group work.
15. Work with the recorder, observer, and group members to analyze the effectiveness of members in the group.

Group life is as old as mankind. Early groups formed for protection and physical maintenance. Later group formation included such motives as sociability and companionship.

The **group** *is an assembly of people who meet over a period of time for a specified reason.* Such meetings may be fleeting and superficial; they may fulfill belonging and intimacy needs; or they may provide for a range of experiences in between.

TYPES OF GROUPS

In the past 20 years the small group movement has become a treatment fad. Some groups have been well organized and well led; others appear to be "walk-in confrontation meetings" led by people who have no traditional credentials. You can join personal growth laboratories, weekend marathons, encounter groups, and communication workshops, as well as traditional psychotherapy groups. The group movement of the 1970s united normal people in a society that increasingly isolates people from each other. Groups may be formed in educational, practice, or consultational settings. In the past, therapy groups were usually associated with mental health organizations, psychiatrists, psychologists, or social workers. Now we see many self-help treatment groups.

The differences between these various groups are in the sponsoring organizations, philosophical approaches of the leaders, goals, preconceived ideas of attendees, environmental settings, and the skill and interest of the leader(s) and group members. Thus appropriate group behavior becomes relative.

You will work with various groups of people, including professional team members, other personnel, clients, and their families. You may be involved in formal therapy groups or more informal, teaching or growth-promoting groups. You may work with mentally or physically ill persons or those who have a community or social problem. In any case, the group approach can solve several problems: (1) the need to reach more people effectively in a given time and (2) the need for people to get support and understanding from each other as they learn how to handle the problem or situation under consideration.

You may find yourself leading a weekly support group to maintain nonsmoking or a discussion with a dying patient's family. You may lead a team conference with nurses or with other various health professionals to solve a problem. You may lead an on-the-spot discussion with a group of patients concerning the day's activity or you may lead an educational group to teach cardiac patients about their disease. You may lead a therapeutic group to help people deal with personal relationships or a group that assists people to collectively try to solve economical or environmental issues.

Groups are either primary or secondary, depending on the importance of the group to the person. A **primary group** *is like a family; it has considerable influence upon the person*, especially in emotional aspects of growth. In the **secondary group** *people react to each other in a more formalized manner*—for example, as in a labor union. Thus as goals become more specific, as the range of influence narrows, and as formalities increase, the group becomes secondary.

However, most groups that you will be involved with strive to accomplish a goal through support, stimulation, reality testing, insight promotion, and corrective experiences (46). The leadership approaches you use can be divided into three major types:

1. Evocative: To encourage spontaneous expression of feelings in an atmosphere of acceptance and understanding.
2. Directive: To indoctrinate or give advice, with the emphasis on proper attitudes and conduct, using an authoritarian approach.
3. Didactic: To educate through a class or seminar (68).

This chapter focuses on the principles and dynamics of group process in order to help you better understand and work with various groups through the major approaches.

Evolution of Group Work: An Historical Perspective

The study of group function has long been of interest to many philosophers, scientists, sociologists, psychologists, and educators. The first recognized group work in the twentieth century began in 1905 when Joseph Pratt, a physician, gathered together a group of patients with tuberculosis in order to teach them self-care and at the same time elevate their morale and mood. Many leaders and varieties of group techniques have evolved since (46). Table 6-1 summarizes the major group approaches.

TABLE 6-1 Evolution of Group Approaches

DATE	FOUNDER	GROUP METHOD	DESCRIPTION
1912	Joseph Moreno	Psychodrama	Persons express feelings by acting out various roles on a stage. The audience is asked to identify with these roles and make comments and interpretations to the individuals acting the roles.
1920	Trigant Barrow S. H. Foulkes	Group Psychoanalysis	Theories of individual psychoanalysis, including transference and resistance, are applied to a group.
1935		Alcoholics Anonymous	Alcoholics follow 12 steps toward abstinence with group support and admonition and dependence on God.
1937	Abraham Low	Recovery Inc.	Groups of formerly hospitalized psychiatric patients use Abraham Low's *Mental Health Through Will-Training* as a guide to cope with problems of living.
1930-1940	Leo Festinger Kurt Lewin R. White	Group Dynamics	Leaders apply group dynamics theory, emphasizing interaction, expression of feelings, and cohesiveness.
1940	Maxwell Jones	Therapeutic Community	Members consider individual needs in relation to the group needs and use a total health-promoting environment (called milieu) as an agent for treatment. Staff and patients are considered as peers and mutually responsible for therapy and behavioral outcomes.
1950	Martin Buber	Existential Groups (based on the philosophy that a human being is defined only through community and relationships)	Lonely, alienated, isolated people meet to seek meaning in life, gain spontaneity, and share self with others.
1950	W. R. Bion	Tavistock Conference (name taken from Clinic in England)	Focus is upon the group's common problem or tension. A common theme might be trust, rejection, or loss.
1960	Nathan Ackerman Theodore Lidz Carl Whitaker Donald Jackson	Family Dynamics	Communication and functioning of members within a family system are studied in an effort to help the family work together better as a unit.

TABLE 6-1 (cont.)

DATE	FOUNDER	GROUP METHOD	DESCRIPTION
1960		Training Group Movement	The training method helps mental health workers and others become more sensitive, knowledgeable, and capable. (Transactional Analysis, Encounter, Sensitivity, and other groups emphasizing self-awareness and sociability have evolved from this method.)
1960	Eric Berne	Transactional Analysis (T.A.)	Focus is on symbolic reenactment of the past in present relationships. Members' participation is analyzed according to adult, child, and parent roles.
1960	Lawrence Tirnauer	Encounter Group	Personal growth of people is emphasized through a theme-centered, intense process. (Originally developed to enhance growth of mental health professionals.)
1960	Carl Rogers	Basic Encounter	The nondirective approach is used to help the person learn to express feelings and form a relationship in an open atmosphere. The individual within the group is the focus.
1960	Fritz Perls	Gestalt	The focus is on the person within the group, but it considers that person's whole environment. Role playing, personal experimentation, exploration of feelings, fantasies, and dreams, and having the person "in the hot seat" are used to make the person concentrate on problems and help him/her make changes.
1970s and thereafter		Self-Help Groups	Various people organized groups to help clients cope with specific problems, such as leukemia, cancer, stroke, weight control, cessation of smoking.

PURPOSES OF GROUP WORK

Although a one-to-one relationship, as described in Chapter 4, provides many benefits, group work supplements the benefits of such a relationship. Purposes of helpful group work include to:

1. Learn more about others and the environment.
2. Foster awareness of self and personal behavior.
3. Assist development of a sense of identity appropriate to the current life stage, along with increased self-appreciation and self-esteem.
4. Gain more control over life and a greater sense of personal responsibility and satisfaction.
5. Increase enjoyment of socializing through new acquaintances and friendships and encourage involvement to reduce feelings of loneliness or rejection.
6. Learn more about how the personality and behavior appear to others.
7. Recognize more clearly similarities and differences between self and others.
8. Move away from self-centered and dependent behavior; become more responsive to and considerate of feelings, opinions, and ideas of others.
9. Learn how to state feelings and ideas more clearly and to be better understood as well as more understanding of others.
10. Increase basic skills of working in a group by learning new or practicing alternate ways of behaving.
11. Increase general coping abilities and gain practice in handling daily problems.
12. Encourage continuous new learning.

These purposes can be accomplished through the group process. Silver noted improvement in morale, cleanliness, and general behavior after working with 17 psychotic patients (66). Linden worked over a 2-year period with 51 institutionalized women and found that lost values regained importance; hunger for social relationships returned; regression was halted, and an urge to contribute to group cohesion emerged (40). Goldfarb and Turner treated 150 elderly residents in a nursing home; 49 percent improved with an average of 8.5 sessions (27). Nurses also report the effectiveness of group work (11, 12, 14, 22, 52).

Although many studies present groups formed in institutions, facts are also available for community-based groups. In one case, doctors sent overweight patients to a nurse-led group called L.O.S.E. (League of

Sensible Eaters). Through working with, not against, the culture and using group support, the members are able to accept reduced calorie intake and lose the necessary pounds (35).

THE GROUP LEADER

The single most important factor in success or failure of a group is a knowledgeable, skillful leader. To be a leader, you must understand principles of leadership as they apply to group work, behavior and its meaning, the goals and functions of group members, and the phases of group work. There are no automatically effective leaders. You may informally learn how to lead a group by observing another group leader, but formal study with an opportunity to practice under supervision is the best preparation. Just reading this chapter will not be sufficient to enable you to lead a therapy group. The information presented here gives you a basis, however. Moreover, as the leader, you should be relatively free of unreconciled emotional conflicts and able to tolerate intense emotional reactions. Nothing is more ironic than the leader of a creative marriage group getting a fourth divorce!

Characteristics of an Effective Leader

No leader is perfect! But the following characteristics contribute to an effective leader:

1. Conveys security and acceptance of own limits; in turn, accepts others and helps them feel safe.
2. Demonstrates friendliness, empathy, and concern for others.
3. Listens carefully for unspoken as well as verbal messages.
4. Insists on freedom rather than perfection within the group.
5. Is capable of using humor kindly and appropriately.
6. Permits dissent from group members.
7. Does not resort to and does not permit blaming or persecution of members.
8. Does not anticipate immediate release from conflict but strives to cope with and gain meaning from the conflict as part of the resolving process.
9. Does not permit self to be used as a means to an end and does not use others in this manner (manipulation).
10. Does not assume superiority over others (39, 77).

In addition to these characteristics you, as the leader, must have a capacity to love, laugh, and cry. Spontaneity must be tempered with restraint; compassion must be combined with objectivity, and assertiveness must be coupled with the ability to listen.

If the preceding characteristics are present, the leader will show respect to each group member as a unique human being. In turn, the group member will respond to the respect and can achieve his/her greatest growth potential.

Leadership Style

Certainly different leaders have different styles; be aware of the type of leadership you develop and be sensitive enough to observe the result of your methods. Do you lean toward being autocratic, for example, wanting absolute rule? Do you lean toward a laissez-faire attitude, letting people act without interference or direction? Do you lean toward being democratic, trying to treat everyone the same but under established ground rules? One study of the effects of these three styles on group performance found that the democratic style resulted in increased friendliness, group-mindedness, motivation, and originality (76).

Also, the leadership approach may vary, although your basic philosophy about leading groups remains the same. At one meeting you may be abrupt and forceful; at another you may talk in a slow, relaxed manner. Whatever your approach as leader, you will need to maintain your own position, adhere to the set group norms, and avoid giving orders that cannot or will not be obeyed. You will also need to use established channels to give directions, listen attentively to each member and the group as a whole, and demonstrate that you know what you are talking about (1).

As a leader, you may not change the struggles and pain of life, but you can help others cope and live with them.

Responsibilities of the Leader

Desired characteristics and effective style are not enough. You must have a keen sense of responsibility as well. You are accountable for preplanning before the group begins, for careful planning and management through each phase, and for evaluation after termination.

Preplanning is discussed here, and the other responsibilities are discussed with each group phase later in this chapter.

Before making any decisions about the group, you should ask yourself the following questions:

1. What type of group do I want? One that focuses on activity, support, insight, discussion, or reality orientation?

2. How does my agency regard group therapy? Will the group have agency support?
3. What are my strengths and weaknesses? Am I prepared to do group work? How can I learn more about leading groups?
4. Do I need a cotherapist? Do I need this validation or support from another person, another model for the group?
5. Would I benefit from a supervisor or counselor who could help me validate group processes, rethink my leadership style, and help me become more effective in the group experience?
6. How will I choose group members? Should the group be homogeneous with all members having a similar problem? Should the group be heterogeneous, with a variety of problems presented? Can I handle the heterogeneous group that is more lifelike?
7. What are the members' needs? Will I have time and opportunity to interview each member before the first meeting?

If possible, before the first meeting *the leader should orient the selected group members* to the general purpose and plan of the group sessions and expectations of the members. Although this information must be repeated at the first session, the members have some understanding about why they were chosen; they have the right to make the final decision about attending. The first session will be less disorganized if members have received prior information about the group.

You are responsible for physical and structural arrangements. Tentatively decide if sessions should be held daily, once weekly, or on some other basis. Starting time, duration of session, and place should be consistent unless the leader and members wish to make a different decision. Whether the sessions are open or closed often depends on the type of group and kind of clients and agency. In an **open format** *new members are continually added and other members leave.* In a **closed format** *the membership remains the same for the duration of the group.* Visitors to group sessions are usually discouraged; therefore members should not bring family or friends unless specified. The size of the group ideally should be between 8 and 12 people so that everyone will have an opportunity to participate. During the meetings the seating arrangement should allow all members to see each other face to face; a circular arrangement is usually best. Mechanical equipment—for example, movie or slide projector or tape recorders—is used for certain groups. Equipment should be obtained in advance and be in working order.

The group's surrounding area becomes very much a part of the group itself and influences the effectiveness, activity, and life of the group. Such factors as uncomfortable temperature, uncomfortable furniture, disturbing noise, distracting sounds, repugnant odors, and physical discomfort of any kind decrease group efficiency. How the members sit in the group, where the leader sits, how small or large the room is, and whether members are facing one another all influence the group's total functioning (7). Consider the physical and emotional environment and the members' comfort and safety to encourage group growth.

Decide whether to have a group recorder and observer. The **recorder** *takes notes of the session proceedings* in order to provide a summary of content and free members from taking notes. The **observer** *does not participate but analyzes the group process with the leader.* The observer evaluates the group atmosphere, participation of members, effectiveness of the leadership, group cohesiveness and productivity, and general flow of the discussion. These two service team members can validate with you about group process and thus enable the group to function more productively. The need for a recorder and observer will depend on the size, type, and goals of the group and your expertise.

Begin your plan for the specific session. Be as prepared as possible. But once you begin, the best way to become more expert is to plunge ahead. You are human and you will make mistakes, but remember that your humanness will draw you closer to your group.

THE GROUP AS A SYSTEM

Systems theory was discussed in Chapter 1 and the health care system in Chapter 2. The family as a system is described in Chapter 12. Your perspective as group leader will be broadened if you look at your group as a system.

Characteristics of the System

The group has many parts—individual members with unique personalities, needs, ideas, potentials, and limits. In turn, the group as a whole takes on a personality, certain goals, and limits. In the course of development a pattern of communication, general behavior, and a set of norms, beliefs, and values evolve. Parts become differentiated: each member assumes special functions. As a group reaches maturity, it becomes increasingly complex, differentiated, interdependent, and integrated. The group develops its own subculture and identity because of commonly experienced meanings, definitions, norms, and behavior. Yet it also relates to an outer environment. Groups, like organisms, are characterized by a **steady state,** *a sense of balance or equilibrium that is maintained even as the group changes* (1).

Actually, two groups can each be in a steady state but still act differently. One group may emphasize clear, time-related objectives and seek specific results (Weight Watchers), while another group may have diffuse goals, for example, students meeting weekly to talk about feelings related to patient care. To remain in a steady state, however, both of these groups will have two characteristics in common. Each group will have a **consensus**—that is, *members agree on norms and roles.* The group will also have a **goal** *or purpose* (1), such as losing 10 pounds in 2 weeks or learning to speak comfortably in front of others.

Behavioral Aspects of the Group

When a person joins a group, an attempt is made to match the person's needs and the group's offerings. If the needs are met, socialization occurs. The person and group work together as the person gains new acceptance and new friends, learns about other lifestyles, or prepares for a new occupation. The person's fit into the group is on one of three levels: (1) compliance—conforming without believing the group's view, (2) internalization—adopting the group's view because it is already the person's own view, and (3) identification—changing the original beliefs and behavior while taking on the group view (1).

Social control and conflict occur in the system. The group achieves an identity by setting standards or norms, shaping its members' behavior through approval and reinforcement or disapproval, ridicule, exclusion, or punishment (1). Traditionally, for example, Robert's rules have been used in formal meetings to control when and how members speak. If this procedure provides security and order, the group functions well. If, however, someone continually speaks "out of order," conflict is evident. The group's steady state will be in jeopardy unless members can put the offending member in line or reach a compromise.

Structural Aspects of the Group

Each group has a **boundary,** *unwritten rules about how members should act with each other in and outside of the group.* Moreover, the group's boundaries usually include a certain number of people and a specified meeting place and time (1).

Autonomy, *the essence of being separate from other groups,* exists, although the members simultaneously take part in other groups (1).

Role differentiation occurs; *members take on different tasks and are known for these tasks.* These roles usually place members into a **hierarchy,** *a rank of importance* (1). Some roles seem to be standard and persist regardless of who occupies them; for example, there is (1) the scapegoat, the receiver of group hostility; (2) the clown, the giver or butt of humor; (3) the peacemaker, the reducer of conflict; and (4) the idol, the moral or social standard bearer (32).

THE GROUP AS A PROCESS

Group process *refers to the interaction between members and leader(s), each fulfilling certain functions as the group as a whole and individual members proceed through various stages of development.* Each of the facets of group process will be discussed.

Principles of Behavior

All behavior has meaning. Each activity has significance: the sigh or the spoken word, the lack of response or the argumentative response. If you attend only to the obvious and remain unaware of covert behavior, you will not be as helpful to the members. Overinterpretation of every word and gesture can be equally ineffective, even destructive. Choose only certain patterns of behavior—for example, behavior that is bothersome to the group members—to question further or to interpret.

Behavior occurs on two levels simultaneously: behavior is cognitive and affective at the same time. **Cognitive behavior** *refers to understanding the goals intellectually, discussion of facts, issues, and topics about the members or others, and attention to procedural questions* (6). **Affective behavior** *refers to feelings, group morale and participation, influence of members on each other, style of leadership, and degree of conflict, competition, and cooperation* (6). For example, a person may *understand* his/her cardiac condition and list in detail dietary and activity instructions, but *feelings* of fear and vulnerability to further illness and his/her anger about the limitations may interfere with functioning at home. Reactions of the leader and members will influence his/her behavior and feelings.

The cognitive level of behavior is relatively easy to recognize, but you must be more perceptive when observing affective behavior. Ask yourself the following questions in order to analyze affective behavior more effectively.

1. What is the overall feeling generated within the group?
2. What emotions can I detect within myself and the group? Interest, boredom, anger, hopelessness? What are my clues? Voice tone, facial expressions, body posture, gestures?
3. Even though the physical surroundings are conducive to comfort, am I seeing the signs of anxiety described in Chapter 7, such as

blushing, rapid breathing, perspiration, frequent shifting from place to place? (These may also be signs of physical distress).

Dynamic forces exist within a group, although they cannot be seen as easily as the chairs or table in the room. These forces exist within the person (intrapsychic), between people (interpersonal), and in the environment. The feelings, ideas, and defensive maneuvers of the person affect behavior and therefore the entire group. Members affect each other as they avoid, ignore, or support each other. The irritability or concern that members feel for each other and the degree of willingness to listen, share, and compromise can create a group atmosphere that is either unharmonious or smooth. External events cannot be kept outside the group (the sick child, the angry husband, hazardous weather, or difficulties at work). Even room temperature and decor, distracting noise, or the number and appearance of group members affect group behavior.

Here is a list of guidelines related to the group process.

1. You may change the person's attitudes more easily by changing the group's emotional climate than by trying to change the person directly.
2. Groups demand a certain degree of conformity from members. The more **cohesive** (*closeness, sense of belonging to*) the group, the more power it has over the member's behavior. Cohesiveness depends on how the group is meeting the member's needs.
3. Opinions and behaviors that deviate from the rest of the group are likely to be ignored, rejected, or punished by the members.
4. Efforts from people outside the group to cause the member to deviate from group norms will encounter strong resistance from the member.
5. Decisions made by a group obtain greater commitment from the member than arbitrarily imposed decisions from outside the group. The member will not lose face by not following through with his/her verbal decision made in front of the group.
6. People tend to be more effective learners when acting as group members than when acting as individuals.
7. The greater the member's prestige in the eyes of the other members, the greater the influence he/she can exert.
8. The more closely a person's attitudes, values, or behavior fit the group's purpose, the more influence the group will exert on him/her.
9. Group climate or style of group life has an important impact on the personalities of members. The behavior of members may differ greatly from one group to another (16, 73).

Group Goals

All groups are trying to reach at least one **primary goal,** *a target, aim, or long-range task that gives direction.* The primary goal may be to develop a product or an idea or to promote personal maturity, as simple as companionship or as specific as planning a party. In order to reach the main goal(s), the group may set up **secondary goals,** *short-term objectives that must be reached* (42). For example, in planning a party, Mary is in charge of decorations; Henry is in charge of games. Keep in mind that primary and secondary goals change as the group changes. As goals are met, new goals evolve if the group is to stay together.

Group Functions

Two kinds of behavior are seen in every group in order to achieve group goals: task functions and maintenance functions. **Task functions** *are behaviors directed toward selecting and achieving primary and secondary goals of the group.* **Maintenance functions** *are activities that assist and support the welfare, morale, harmony, and relationship of the group* (42, 43).

Task functions, functions that get a job done, include the following behaviors:

1. Initiating activity. The person suggests new ideas or ways to organize the group.
2. Seeking information. The person asks for clarification or facts pertinent to the discussion.
3. Seeking opinion. The person asks for a statement of feelings or ideas.
4. Giving information. The person offers facts in order to push what he/she thinks should become the group's view.
5. Giving opinion. The person states a belief about a suggestion or piece of information based on personal values or experience instead of on facts.
6. Clarifying or elaborating. The person gives examples or develops meanings to help the group envision how a proposed solution might work.
7. Coordinating. The person shows relationships between or pulls together various ideas, suggestions, or activities.
8. Summarizing. The person restates ideas after the group has discussed them.
9. Testing. The person examines the practicality of ideas, makes application of suggested solutions to real situations, and preevaluates. (42, 43).

Maintenance functions, functions that increase feelings of security, include the following behaviors:

1. Encouraging. The person is warm, friendly, responsive to others, praises others and their ideas, and pushes for group solidarity.
2. Expressing group feelings. The person summarizes group feelings and reactions.
3. Harmonizing. The person mediates differences between other members or relieves tensions and conflict through use of humor or pleasantries.
4. Compromising. The person yields, admits error, or moves his/her original position in order to work out a conflict in which he/she is involved.
5. Gatekeeping. The person makes it possible for another member to contribute to the group by calling on him/her or by suggesting a time limit for talking to another. Thus the gatekeeper keeps communication channels open.
6. Setting standards. The person states standards for the group to use in choosing a task, procedure, or solution. The group is reminded to avoid decisions that conflict with group standards (42, 43).

Phases of the Group

The evolution of a group can be traced from formation, to working together, through termination. During each phase the leader will have certain responsibilities. (See Table 6-2.)

Phase I—Formation of the Group takes place when the group is a collection of independent persons with little affection and no real commitment to one another. Every member responds personally to the group experience but often feels isolated or lonely. The group may be perceived as threatening to the person and he/she responds with the usual pattern of behavior to stress, such as aggression, withdrawal, competition, or vacillation (1).

Carl Rogers describes fives steps or patterns that make up the first major phase.

1. *Milling around.* A period of initial frustration; confusion; awkward silence; polite, superficial, or irrelevant conversation; self-preoccupation; and intellectualization. The person may search for status or power, resist authority, pair off, or "gang up" with another.
2. *Resistance to personal expression or exploration.* A few people reveal rather personal attitudes initially, which causes great ambiv-

TABLE 6-2 Leader Responsibilities During Phases of Group Work

FORMATION OR ESTABLISHMENT PHASE	CHANGE OR WORKING PHASE	TERMINATION PHASE
1. Help the group get acquainted by defining/redefining the problem or reason for meeting.	1. Call on the group to clarify, analyze, and summarize problems.	1. Prepare the group for the time of termination and separation.
2. Establish a group *contract, an agreement between leader and members,* after discussion with the members. The contract can be general or specific, depending upon how it is established. (Yalom suggests that the contract covers attendance and completion of group experience.) Confidentiality should be clearly understood.	2. Permit verbal rebellion or expression of negative feelings to help the member gain comfort, insight, and tools for relieving pent-up feelings of anxiety, guilt, and anger. Through this release and mutual sharing of feelings, thoughts, fantasies, and experiences, members become better acquainted with one another and learn to care about each other.	2. Help the group review, summarize, and evaluate experience and growth.
3. Help the group establish ground rules about appropriate behavior.	3. Provide for security of the members and safety of property.	3. Help the group to separate physically and let go emotionally from each other and from you (46, 80).
4. Invite trust gently, allowing distance when necessary.	4. Clarify feelings, encouraging all members to state feelings.	
5. Help members discuss feelings and thoughts about their expectations, misconceptions, or group experiences generally.	5. Help the group to operate with decreasing direction.	
6. Redirect questions so they are answered by members.	6. Encourage involvement, cooperative activity, mutual support.	

TABLE 6-2 (cont.)

FORMATION OR ESTABLISHMENT PHASE	CHANGE OR WORKING PHASE	TERMINATION PHASE
7. Help all members participate, calling on them if necessary.	7. Observe for members who block change or growth within other members. (Discussed further under "Frequent Problems with Group Work".) (46, 80)	
8. Keep members' attention on goals while evaluating group process.		
9. Clarify issues as they arise.		
10. If a recorder and observer are present, assist them in their roles, and clarify their roles to the group (46, 80).		

alence in the other members. Most will not disclose much about themselves.

3. *Description of past feelings.* Expressing feelings unrelated to present problems occurs first and begins to assume a large proportion of the discussion.
4. *Expression of negative feelings.* Anger directed toward the leader or members is usually the first significant expression of feelings. Deeply positive feelings are more difficult and dangerous to express. The member may feel that no one is interested in his/her problem at this early stage.
5. *Expression and exploration of personally meaningful material.* At this point, a member begins to reveal his/her inner self, a painful process to which the group may not yet be receptive (59).

During Phase I the members discuss the structure of the group, what "freedom" means to this group, and how each member interprets what the leader says. Each person struggles for security, to gain equilibrium, and to adapt to the new situation. Agreement among members that feelings, thoughts, and behaviors are to be tolerated is essential for beginning an open discussion and moving toward an identity and a subculture (1).

Phase II—Change Within the Group—The Working Phase occurs when the emphasis shifts from personal needs, goals, and desires to more collective identity. The person's mood changes. The members engage in more genuine conversation. Each member attempts to find a place within the group, the power he/she has, and the expectations of the group. The members gradually become more patient, respectful, and cooperative and are able to plan together. Now the members begin to "crack the facade." Most people want to trust each other, but they still are blocked by fear of rejection, betrayal, and exposure—remnants of past painful experiences. However, now the person begins to risk—to trust. He/she tests by stating real feelings; if the person is not criticized and not laughed at, he/she will feel safe and secure in discussing more negative feelings. Other group members will follow when they see that the atmosphere is accepting, realistic, and perhaps different from past group experiences. Feelings of intimacy and closeness emerge between members; mutual support is felt. As the person receives honest feedback from others about his/her behavior, he/she grows in self-understanding and self-acceptance. Behavior will change in a desired direction. Productivity and progress toward a goal are enhanced. The group might now be called socialized (1, 59, 77).

Phase III—Crisis Within the Group may occur at any time in the life of the group or it may not occur at all (1).

A **crisis** is a *turning point*. If the members are now expressing their deepest negative and positive feelings with honesty, forcefulness, and spontaneity, and if reactions are accepting, the person experiences a turning point toward behavior change. If negative feelings and conflict take the upper hand, however, this can be a turning point toward regression or disintegration of individual members or the group.

Conflict occurs *when there is a discrepancy between what members want from a group experience and what they feel they are obtaining* (1). Group conflict occurs for various reasons.

1. The leader or other members may challenge or harshly confront the person who is honestly discussing feelings. The remainder of the group may then feel more anxious or rejected.
2. Members may seek out each other between group sessions to show concern or share experiences. Too much outside contact causes the group to become nonfunctional.
3. The member may refuse to move toward group goals, which might include talking about personal problems, sharing experiences, being honest, participating in an activity, or changing behavior patterns of lifestyle (59).

When conflict occurs, the group responds in various ways. The nonconpliant member may be forced out; sometimes he/she is dominated by another and is forced to remain quiet. Sometimes alliances form as members speak for or against each other. Ideally, members collectively arrive at a satisfactory compromise or solution that safeguards the common interests of the group and satisfies members' needs. In this case, the solution may be more creative and productive than the one given by any individual member (59). The leader is responsible for helping the group avoid or overcome disruptive forces; all have a responsibility to avoid manipulation or denigration of any member.

Phase IV–Termination should be planned in advance and should be talked about prior to the date. **Termination** *occurs when goals are met or when special circumstances with the leader, members, or agency make further meeting impossible or nonhelpful.* If the group experience has caused the person to feel better about self and has been important, he/she may still feel separation anxiety, loss, rejection, and abandonment even though the stated goal has been reached (1). Members may doubt their ability to carry on without the group. Special attention should be given to this phase. Perhaps members procrastinate with goals because they fear the loss of support from group members to be greater than not achieving the goals. Feelings about separation must be worked through or the person's self-confidence and sense of independence will suffer. In addition, he/she will have difficulty coping with other losses in life. The members should leave the group feeling an increased self-worth and feeling positive about their behavorial change. They acknowledge that they will miss group members and their support, but they feel that they can replace the group activity with other activity.

The group experience is difficult to describe; so much of it is in the realm of feelings. Only a positive group experience can help the person know the warm, safe emotional climate that encourages a deep sharing and hence a broader scope of thinking and attitudinal changes.

GROUP MEMBERS

An effective group cannot exist without effective group members. Each member must have a sense of obligation, dependability, trust, and confidentiality to carry out the maintenance and task functions previously described and to produce optimum results in meeting group and individual goals.

Each group member should prepare carefully before the group meeting so that the person can do his/her own thinking, come to a conclusion, and then speak ideas clearly and concisely. Each member should ask questions if he/she does not understand. The person should speak when he/she has something to say but listen attentively when others are contributing. Observation of the group process and maintenance of an accepting climate are also a responsibility. The group member contributes to guidelines for making decisions and helps to establish conditions under which each member can make unique contributions without probing or manipulation from other members. He/she helps other members to cope with conflict and, in turn, should receive help.

Frequent Problems in Group Work

Group members may not always be able to contribute effectively to the group for a number of personal reasons. Some members may use obstructive maneuvers to block change or growth. Such maneuvers might include angry silence, monopolizing the conversation, being repeatedly late or absent, yawning repeatedly, trying to assume the therapist's role, or constantly changing the subject. Other obstructive behaviors include overreacting to others' statements or hurling verbal abuse, compulsive premature self-revelation, or attempted or actual physical abuse (1). All such destructive behaviors can be categorized under the following individual roles:

1. Aggressor. The person expresses disapproval of other members' feelings, ideas, or behavior; takes credit for others' ideas or shows envy.
2. Blocker. The person opposes without reason, is resistant, stubborn; goes off on a tangent; argues; rejects others' ideas without consideration.
3. Help-seeker. The person tries to get a sympathetic response by expressing insecurity, personal confusion, or self-depreciation without reason or consideration of others' problems.
4. Playboy. The person displays lack of involvement in the group, cynicism, horeseplay, mimicking.
5. Self-confessor. The person uses the group as an audience to express personal points of view, feelings, or themes irrelevant to the group.
6. Dominator. The person asserts authority or superiority by monopolizing or manipulating group members through flattery, interruptions, or by giving directions.
7. Special-interest pleader. The person introduces or supports suggestions related to personal concerns or philosophy.
8. Competitor. The person competes with others to produce the best ideas, talk the most, play the most roles, or gain the leader's favor.
9. Blackmailer. The person intimidates others into going along with personal schemes; threatens that confidential content will be discussed outside the group or that the members will suffer harm in some way if they do not go along (42, 43).

Such behavior may be caused by the person's negative self-concept, inability to communicate appropriately with others, or anxiety in a group situation.

Other forces or behaviors that block change and interfere with the member's effectiveness are resistance, transference, and countertransference (1, 59). **Resistance** *is any psychological maneuver on the part of the group member to avoid self-awareness, personal growth, change, or helpful relationship with the group and other group members.* Feelings of apathy, hostility, or fear may be the cause. Defense mechanisms, such as denial, projection, or isolation, are used. Resistance may result in a person's breaking away from the group or destroying its progress. **Transference** *refers to unconscious attachments directed toward the leader or group members whereby feelings, attitudes, and experiences will be expressed that are appropriate to parental or other authority figures from the past.* The deviant member may strike out at the leader or another member who reminds him/her of a hated boss or relative. Or the member may be overaccepting of what others say because he/she has always acted like the "good" or submissive child with parents and supervisors. On the other hand, the leader may experience **counter-**

transference, *an unconscious or conscious emotional reaction to the individual group members. The leader may respond to certain members as he/she did to others in his past life.* These reactions may be either positive or negative. The leader may treat a member with special privilege because she reminds the leader of a favorite aunt. Or the leader may be either overprotective or too authoritarian.

You must understand these forces. Ask yourself: What am I doing to cause these reactions? What do I feel about individual members? What can I do about these feelings? Transference is inevitable; use it to promote self-understanding. Recognize countertransference and work through the feelings so that you can be objective and not obstructive.

You are responsible for preventing obstructive behavior in the group. You may be able to confront the offending group member about the behavior, but he/she may not be able to understand the behavior or give reasons for it. You may encourage other group members to work with you in eliciting more desirable and group-oriented behavior. Feedback from the group to the person about obstructive behavior may be sufficient. You may need to work with the person in individual counseling to help him/her learn more effective behavior. Sometimes showing the person respect and friendship can meet emotional needs, and compliance, and even make him/her feel a working part of the group. If you work to provide an emotionally safe climate, you will probably reduce the person's needs to behave offensively, and you may reassure the other members so that they can help support the offending member.

EVALUATION

Just as in the nursing process, evaluation is an essential and continuous part of the group process. Evaluation must be done by the leader and group members. Figure 6-1 presents a form that could be used by group members to evaluate their participation in the group.

Here is a list of questions that the leader could use as a means of self-evaluation.

1. Am I successful in reducing the member's anxiety about participating in this group.
   (a) Do I encourage a warm-up period with members before the meeting begins?
   (b) Do I convey warmth, support, and nonthreatening humor?
   (c) Do I arrange for a comfortable meeting environment? Do I allow each member personal space?
   (d) Do I use a matter-of-fact, businesslike approach if the group consists of suspicious or unfriendly members?

Evaluation of myself before group:

Evaluation of where I would like to go:

Long-range goal:

What I can do to achieve this goal:

Evaluation of group goals:

My participation in the group (rate each behavior on the following scale):

1. Always
2. Usually
3. Often
4. Sometimes
5. Never

	1	2	3	4	5
1. Make clear open statements					
2. Paraphrase others' comments					
3. Direct my comments to group members					
4. Encourage others to participate					
5. Listen attentively to other members					
6. Share openly my feelings with the group					
7. Give feedback					
8. Help summarize					
9. Work toward productivity					
10. Validate perceptions					
11. Support others in group					
12. Stay actively involved					

FIGURE 6-1 Group Member Self-Evaluation Form

2. Do I reward participation and promote progress toward group goals by verbal replies, smiling, or nodding my head?
3. During the orientation phase have I conveyed to the members that participation is a group norm? Or do I talk too much and for too long?

4. Do I encourage all members to participate by accepting statements and working them into the group discussion so that they have meaning to the group, making reluctant members feel that their ideas are wanted and needed? Do I prevent talkative members from monopolizing without conveying rejection? Do I keep discussion and activity moving, protecting members from attack but accepting disagreement or conflict if expressed reasonably?
5. Can I keep quiet during pauses so that group members realize their responsibility toward the group discussion?
6. Do I hear ideas and feelings expressed by members and restate them accurately in a more concise, clear form, thus conveying acceptance, attention, respect, and understanding without necessarily agreeing?
7. Am I sensitive to nonverbal communication from group members? Am I aware of and able to respond to sadness, apathy, hostility, or intense concentration?
8. Do I keep the group interested by asking questions that stimulate problem solving, encouraging tasks that are neither too easy nor too hard, clarifying situations, inquiring about feelings, and raising alternative choices? Do I avoid doing all of the work?
9. Did I learn enough about each member before the group started? Have I learned enough to promote a sense of trust and group cohesiveness and to be able to ask pertinent questions about a member's behavior?
10. Do I summarize periodically to move the discussion forward, indicate progress, restate the problem in a new light, or point up differences that exist in the group?
11. Do I receive genuine feedback verbally or do members tell me what they think I want to hear?
12. Do I use every possible opportunity to give the group real power to make choices? Do I recognize that patient groups tend to be more conservative than staff in decisions and can usually be trusted about matters related to them?
13. Do I turn responsibility over to the group as soon as possible and regain it when necessary?
14. Am I being understood by those with different behavior or opinions, conveying respect, providing for their emotional safety, and preventing scapegoating by members? When scapegoating appears, am I comfortable enough to look for and deal with members' feelings of worthlessness, fear of weakness, and fear of similarity to the deviant?
15. Am I contributing to group cohesiveness by encouraging members to make choices, agree on goals and norms and the means to

achieve them, talk out and resolve differences, and review and alter goals as necessary so that the group remains helpful?
16. What is my leadership style?
17. Am I developing and rewarding qualities of leadership among the members? Do I support members who have the ability to draw out others? Do I encourage members to direct statements and questions to each other rather than to me? Am I quiet whenever possible?
18. Is the group moving toward its goal and am I encouraging progress by helping the group remain aware of goals and progress the members are making?
19. Am I flexible enough to revise goals as members progress or circumstances change (70)?

As a group leader, you will probably never to able to answer "yes" to every question on this list. But if your answers progress from "sometimes" to "often" to "usually," you will experience the rewards from observing growth in group members and in realizing your own increasing effectiveness as a group leader.

EXAMPLES OF GROUP WORK

Groups can be formed with all ages. On the following pages are examples of how four different groups might function: the first is a group of second-graders; the second is a group of young adults and middleagers; and the third and fourth groups are in later maturity.

Teaching-Activity Group

The goal of the teaching-activity group is to present specific information, mainly through members' participation in activities. Activity groups can be effective with any age if the activities and goal are centered around the needs of the group and not around the leader. (Unfortunately, in some settings we still see the therapist-leader making the doll or having the party while the bored participants look on.)

One successful teaching-activity group involved a group of second-graders. A mother-nurse became alarmed by her children's increasing desire for sugary foods. Investigation pointed to television as a "big pusher." One Saturday morning the mother watched the shows with her children for 2 hours and noted that 25 out of 50 commercials were for food having a high sugar content. She decided to start neighborhood group sessions.

The sessions with the children were held for 30 minutes once a week and lasted over a 3-month period. The goal was to teach basic nutrition through activity. The children were interested; they were assigned to listen to television commercials and report on them to the group. They cut pictures of the basic four foods out of magazines to make posters. They helped their mothers read label ingredients, wrote poems and songs about various foods, made butter and applesauce, and discussed their growing knowledge weekly. The children remained interested and excited with their own findings and creations and they reported that they were "teaching their parents" about what foods made healthy bodies.

Discussion-Discharge Planning Group

The goal of the discussion group is to encourage communication and learning through involvement with other people. Education is the major objective; however, individual strengths are recognized and support is given to increase self-esteem and self-worth and help the person work through personal problems.

The goal of the discharge group is to retrain institutionalized patients to resume life in the community or to prepare patients to realistically anticipate home life after discharge from the hospital. The members discuss feelings about discharge and they role play some of the real problems associated with the transition to community or home living.

These purposes were combined in one group made up of young adults and middleagers who had new colostomies (a surgical opening in the abdominal wall to which the intestine is attached for elimination.) They met daily for 1-hour sessions during their last five days in the hospital and met weekly for an hour for 3 months after discharge. Sessions were led by an enterotherapist and psychiatric nurse as co-therapists. Subjects discussed included their feelings of damaged self; concerns about sexual function; adapting the irrigation procedure to the home bathroom; odor control; diet; activity; and the purchase, cost, and management of appliances and supplies. The group also learned about helpful organizations, such as the local Cancer Society and Ostomy Club. Family members attended specified sessions with the group members.

After the procedural aspects of care were worked through, considerable time was spent discussing feelings about the diagnosis and prognosis of cancer and the meaning of the ostomy to the self, family, and lifestyle. Gradually through the support of the leaders and each other, the members were able to reintegrate the body image, regain normal sexual functioning, and resume normal roles in the home and community. According to later visiting nurse reports, the good adjustment achieved by the group members and their families was maintained after termination of the group.

Reality Orientation Group

The purpose of reality therapy is to reverse or halt the confusion, disorientation, social withdrawal, and apathy characteristic of residents in institutions (27). Reality orientation also helps the staff recognize that regressive behavior does not necessarily accompany old age and that expecting regression in the elderly and treating the person as an infant will reinforce such behavior.

Reality orientation has three components that should be used simultaneously: (1) a 24-hour daily routine, (2) supplementary classroom experience, and (3) attitude therapy. Every staff-patient contact is used to improve the patient's understanding of person, time, and place. Basic, current, and personal information is repeated as often as necessary to the person. Information about the day, month, year, time, and weather is placed throughout the institution so that residents can readily see the information. Staff members state what they are doing in all activities with the person. Repetition of information and reinforcing the person's correct response are essential (30).

Supplementary Classroom Reality Orientation is a simple form of small group work for severely confused and disoriented persons. A group of four to six residents meet daily for 30 minutes with a staff person who is familiar with their total nursing care plan and needs. The immediate goal is to teach these people basic information and establish group communication in a structured setting. The classroom setting provides for personal attention in a firm, supportive environment. Classroom reality orientation for 6 weeks is effective in reversing signs of memory loss, confusion, and disorientation in patients, including those over 80 years of age (4).

Attitude Therapy is basic to all reality orientation. A consistent attitude and approach maintained by all staff members when they care for the person or lead the group are essential to convey to the resident what is expected of him/her. One or a combination of the following five attitudes is prescribed as part of the treatment: active friendliness, passive friendliness, matter of fact, kind firmness, and no demand (30).

Reality orientation is effective. After one year of treatment patients in several studies markedly improved in behavior by showing more self-pride, greater socialization, improved manners, more interest in radio and television, and more concern about general appearance. Improvement was shown by 76 percent of the regressed patients (23, 30). Reality orientation programs are useful in that some residents improve considerably in behavior; all can be maintained at the functioning level observed on admission to the institution; regression typical of institutionalization is prevented.

Remotivation Group

Remotivation is a simple form of group work that can be used in a nursing home, hospital, or senior center. The goal is to prevent disengagement, increase interest in reality, and increase intellectual ability as the person focuses on simple, objective aspects of everyday life.

Remotivation sessions involve five specific steps:

1. *Creating a Climate of Acceptance.* About 5 minutes are spent greeting each person by name, expressing pleasure at his/her presence, and making encouraging remarks.
2. *Creating a Bridge to the World.* Approximately 15 minutes are spent talking about a topic of general interest that was chosen by the group at the previous session. Each person is encouraged to respond.
3. *Sharing the World We Live In.* Approximately 15 minutes are spent in further developing the topic just discussed and using visual aids.
4. *Appreciating the Work of the World.* Approximately 15 minutes are used to discuss jobs that relate to the topic, how a commodity is produced, and the types of related jobs done by the group members in the past.
5. *Creating a Climate of Appreciation.* Approximately 5 to 10 minutes are spent expressing pleasure in the patients' attendance and in their contributions. Plans are made for the next meeting. This step helps to provide continuity and something to look forward to (48).

The group is usually limited to 12 sessions, one hour per session, with as many as 15 patients in a group. The leader can be an attendant, although a professional nurse leader can add to the depth of such groups. The sessions are held in a comfortable setting; patients sit in a semicircle. The leader maintains a warm, accepting climate and the session is structured in classroom style around the discussion of a specific topic. The topic for the day may be centered around an animal, nature study, a poem, or game—any topic that is of interest to the group. These contacts with reality serve to interest and involve the patient in living again. Nurses working with the elderly have reported a change in life satisfaction after a series of remotivation groups (48).

Sample Session: Fifteen people are escorted into the activity room where tea and cookies are being served. Each person is greeted by name and is welcomed; thus a *climate of acceptance* is created. The leader starts the group by commenting, "Today we are going to talk about picking apples." A poem is read several lines at a time so that each person has a turn. Apples are passed from person to person to see, smell, and touch. Questions are directed to the group with much feedback given after each response. The leader moves around the room touching and talking to individual patients, thus *creating a bridge to the world.* Patients begin to talk more to one another after a session or two. John may recall how he picked apples on his father's farm when he was a child. Mary talks about making apple butter. Cora shapes her favorite recipe for apple pie. Henry states he worked in a canning factory (*sharing the world we live in*). With the leader's guidance, the discussion continues on a related subject: making apple products, commercial or home canning, caring for an orchard. Group members are encouraged to talk about their past experiences or jobs. Pictures or an object such as an apple doll may be passed around the group to elicit response (*appreciating the work of the world*). As patients share the experiences of their lives, today's world becomes less frightening. Interest in living is renewed. The leader comments on the responsiveness of each person, states appreciation to the patients for coming, and reminds each one of the next session. Goodbyes are said: Each person is called by name as he leaves. Patients leave with a feeling of being accepted and restored (*creating a climate of appreciation*).

GROUP PROCESS WITH DIFFERENT AGE GROUPS

As you work with different age groups, you must consider the members' developmental phase. Review of normal development, for example, using the Murray and Zentner text, *Nursing Assessment and Health Promotion Through the Life Span* (53), or other texts, may be necessary. The type of group you establish, the goals, and the activities will differ with the age or developmental era of the members (12, 13, 14).

For example, use touch and play concepts and activities with children to help them learn new information or work through distressing feelings. Adults usually prefer a talking group, but elderly adults will present some special considerations.

Touch is used more with people in later maturity than with young adult, adolescent, or even middle-aged clients. Touch used spontaneously and with affection compensates for the emotional, social, and sensory deprivation felt by the elderly. They will reach out to you; you should be comfortable with touch. They are more likely to tolerate and understand the needs of the person who is different in behavior. The members will be patient as you focus on one member for a time; if they trust you, they know you will also give them attention. Younger groups are more likely to be impatient with you and the deviant member, be sarcastic to one another, or compete to get attention.

Discussion themes center on loss and reminiscing regardless of the type of elderly group you are leading. Younger groups talk more about their present activities and concerns and future aspirations.

Elderly group members who have lived long enough to develop a historical sense are more concerned about world affairs generally than younger persons, who are more concerned with their own problems.

Elderly group members are more tolerant of their leader. You do not need to be a mechanistic answer machine. Time has conditioned them to know that some questions do not have answers. The leader is allowed to be human. They often perceive when you feel ill or are very worried and will be as supportive, warm, and understanding as possible. Elderly people have a need to be needed; they will give as much to you—or more—than you give to them. Little gifts brought to you should be graciously accepted.

Group work can be a growth opportunity for both you and the members. The experience will be stimulating and enjoyable, but it will also be demanding. At times you will feel distressed as you observe and listen, as you experience a member's problems vicariously. Yet you will find great rewards as you provide opportunities for touching, closeness, and sensory and emotional stimulation between the group members and between them and yourself. The group experience can make a real difference in the lives of your clients—and in your life.

REFERENCES

1. **Anderson, Ralph,** and **Irl Carter,** *Human Behavior in the Social Environment.* Chicago: Aldine Publishing Company, 1974.
2. **Armstrong, Shirley,** and **Sheila Rouslin,** *Group Psychotherapy in Nursing Practice.* New York: The Macmillan Company, 1963.
3. **Arnhart, Emelia A.,** "Establishing Group Work in a Psychiatric Unit of a General Hospital," *Journal of Psychiatric Nursing and Mental Health Services,* 13, no. 1 (1975), 5-9.
4. **Baines, J.,** "Effects of Reality Orientation Classroom on Memory Loss, Confusion, and Disorientation in Geriatric Patients," *The Gerontologist,* 14 (1974), 138-42.

5. **Balgopal, P.**, "Variations in Sensitivity Training Groups," *Perspectives in Psychiatric Care*, 11, no. 2 (1973), 80-86.
6. **Blocher, Donald,** *Developmental Counseling.* New York: The Ronald Press Company, 1966.
7. **Bormann, Ernest,** *Discussion and Group Methods: Theory and Practice.* New York: Harper & Row, Publishers, 1969.
8. **Bradford, L.,** and **Dorothy Mial,** "When Is a Group?" *Educational Leadership,* 21 (1963), 147-51.
9. **Britnell, Judith,** and **Karen Mitchell,** "Inpatient Group Psychotherapy for the Elderly," *Journal of Psychiatric Nursing and Mental Health Services,* 19, no. 5 (1981), 19-24.
10. **Browne, Louise,** and **Jennie Ritter,** "Reality Therapy for the Geriatric Psychiatric Patient," *Perspectives in Psychiatric Care,* 10, no. 3 (1972), 135-39.
11. **Burgess, Ann,** and **Aaron Lazare,** "Nursing Management of Feelings, Thoughts, and Behavior," *Journal of Psychiatric Nursing and Mental Health Services,* 10, no. 6 (1972), 7-11.
12. **Burnside, Irene,** "Group Work Among the Aged," *Nursing Outlook,* 17, no. 6 (1969), 68-71.
13. ———, "Group Work with the Aged," *The Gerontologist,* 10 (1970), 241-46.
14. ———, "Overview of Group Work with the Aged," *Journal of Gerontological Nursing,* 2, no. 6 (1976), 14-17.
15. **Butler, Robert,** "Intensive Psychotherapy for the Hospitalized Aged," *Geriatrics,* 15 (1960), 644-53.
16. **Cartwright, D.,** "Achieving Change in People: Some Applications of Group Dynamics Theory," *Human Relations,* 4 (1951), 381-92.
17. **Citrin, Richard,** and **David Dixon,** "Reality Orientation—A Milieu Therapy Used in an Institution for the Aged," *The Gerontologist,* 17, no. 1 (1977), 39-43.
18. **Cohen, Roberta,** "Cognitive Orientation for Patients in Group Psychotherapy," *Perspectives of Psychiatric Care,* 7, no. 2 (1969), 76-79.
19. **Culbert, S. A.,** "The Interpersonal Process of Self-Disclosure: It Takes Two to See One," *Explorations in Applied Behavioral Science.* New York: Renaissance Editors, 1967.
20. **Derbyshire, Robert,** *Practice of Medicine* (Vol. 10). Hagerstown, MD: Harper & Row, Publishers, 1976, Sect. 6.
21. **Durkin, Helen,** *The Group in Depth.* New York: International Universities Press, Inc., 1964.
22. **Ebersole, P.,** "From Despair to Integrity Through Reminiscing with the Aged," in *A.N.A. Clinical Sessions.* New York: Appleton-Century-Crofts, 1975.
23. **Folsom, J.,** "Reality Orientation for the Elderly Mental Patient," *Geriatric Psychiatry,* Spring 1968, pp. 291-307.
24. **Gallese, Lucile,** and **Edna Treuting,** "Help for Rape Victims Through Group Therapy," *Journal of Psychiatric Nursing and Mental Health Services,* 19, no. 8 (1981), 20-21.
25. **Gartner, Audrey,** and **Frank Riessman,** *Self-Help and Mental Health, Hospital and Community Psychiatry,* 33, no. 8 (1982), 631-35.
26. **Goldberg, Carl,** *Encounter: Group Sensitivity Training Experience.* New York: Science House, Inc., 1970.

27. **Goldgarb, A.,** and **H. Turner,** "Psychotherapy of Aged Persons—Utilization and Effectiveness of Brief Therapy," *American Journal of Psychiatry*, 109 (1953), 916–21.
28. **Hargreaves, Anne,** "The Group Culture and Nursing Practice," *American Journal of Nursing*, 67, no. 9 (1967), 1840–46.
29. **Harris, C.,** "The Florida State Hospital Patient Behavior Rating Sheet," in *Behavior Assessment: New Directions in Clinical Psychology*, eds. J. Cone and R. Hawkins. New York: Brunner-Mazel, 1976.
30. **Harris, Clarke,** and **Peter Ivory,** "An Outcome Evaluation of Reality Orientation Therapy with Geriatric Patients in a State Mental Hospital," *The Gerontologist*, 16, no. 6 (1976), 496–503.
31. **Heath, Tony,** "Drama Therapy," *Nursing Times*, 78, no. 6 (1982), 1055–57.
32. **Homans, George C.,** *The Human Group*. New York: Harcourt, Brace & World, Inc., 1950.
33. **Jersild, Elaine,** "Group Therapy for Patient's Spouses," *American Journal of Nursing*, 67, no. 3 (1967), 544–49.
34. **King, Kathleen,** "Reminiscing Psychotherapy with Aging People," *Journal of Psychiatric Nursing and Mental Health Services*, 20, no. 2 (1982), 21–25.
35. **Kopelke, Charlotte,** "Group Education to Reduce Overweight in a Blue Collar Community," *American Journal of Nursing*, 75, no. 11 (1975), 1993–95.
36. **Lazarus, Lawrence W.,** "A Program for the Elderly at a Private Psychiatric Hospital," *The Gerontologist*, 16, no. 2 (1976), 125–31.
37. **Lego, Suzanne,** "Five Functions of the Group Therapist—Twenty Sessions Later," *American Journal of Nursing*, 66, no. 4 (1966), 795–97.
38. **Lewin, Kurt,** "Frontiers in Group Dynamics: Concept, Method and Reality in Social Science; Social Equilibria and Social Change," *Human Relations*, 1 (1947), 5–42.
39. **Lindeman, Edward,** *The Meaning of Adult Education*. Montreal: Harvest House, 1961.
40. **Linden, M.,** "Group Psychotherapy with Institutionalized Senile Women," *International Journal of Group Psychotherapy*, 3 (1953), 150–70.
41. ———, "Transference in Gerontologic Group Psychotherapy," *International Journal of Group Psychotherapy*, 5 (1955), 61–79.
42. **Lippitt, Gordon,** and **Edith Seashore,** *The Leader and Group Effectiveness*. New York: Association Press, 1962.
43. ———, "The Professional Nurse Looks at Group Effectiveness," *Leadership in Nursing Series*. Washington, D.C.: Leadership Resources, Inc., 1966, pp. 14–15.
44. **Luft, Joseph,** *Group Process: An Introduction to Group Dynamics*. Palo Alto, CA: National Press Books, 1970.
45. **Manaster, Al,** "Therapy with the 'Senile' Geriatric Patient," *The International Journal of Group Psychotherapy*, 22 (1972), 250–57.
46. **Marram, Gwen,** *The Group Approach in Nursing Practice*. St. Louis: The C. V. Mosby Company, 1973.
47. **Matheson, Wayne, E.,** "Which Patient for Which Therapeutic Group," *Journal of Psychiatric Nursing and Mental Health Services*, 12, no. 3 (1974), 10–13.
48. **McClelland, Lucille,** *Textbook for Psychiatric Technicians*. St. Louis: The C. V. Mosby Company, 1971.

49. **Meerloo, J.**, "Modes of Psychotherapy in the Aged," *Journal of the American Geriatrics Society*, 9 (1961), 225–34.
50. **Moody, Linda, Virginia Baron,** and **Grace Monk,** "Moving the Past into the Present," *American Journal of Nursing*, 70, no. 11 (1970), 2353–56.
51. **Morrison, Malcolm,** "A Human Relations Approach to Problem Solving," *The Gerontologist*, 16, no. 2 (1976), 185–86.
52. **Mummah, Hazel R.,** "Group Work With Aged Blind Japanese in the Nursing Home and in the Community," *The New Outlook for the Blind*, 69, no. 4 (1975), 160–64.
53. **Murray, Ruth,** and **Judith Zentner,** *Nursing Assessment and Health Promotion Through the Life Span* (3rd ed.). Englewood Cliffs, NJ: Prentice-Hall, Inc., 1985.
54. **Nordmark, Madelyn,** and **Anne Rohweder,** *Scientific Foundations of Nursing* (2nd ed.). Philadelphia: J. B. Lippincott Company, 1967.
55. **Ohlsen, Merle,** *Group Counseling* (2nd ed.). New York: Holt, Rinehart, & Winston, Inc., 1977.
56. **Petty, Beryl, T. Moeller,** and **R. Campbell,** "Support Groups for Elderly Persons in the Community," *The Gerontologist*, 15, no. 6 (1976), 522–28.
57. **Racy, John,** "How a Group Grows," *American Journal of Nursing*, 69, no. 11 (1969), 2396–2402.
58. **Rogers, Carl,** *On Becoming a Person*. Boston: Houghton Mifflin Company, 1961.
59. ———, *Carl Rogers on Encounter Groups*. New York: Harper & Row, Publishers, 1970.
60. ———, "Carl Rogers Describes His Way of Facilitating Encounter Groups," *American Journal of Nursing*, 71, no. 2 (1971), 275–79.
61. **Rouslin, Sheila,** "Relatedness in Group Psychotherapy," *Perspectives in Psychiatric Care*, 11, no. 4 (1973), 165–71.
62. **Scott, M. Louise,** "To Learn to Work with the Elderly," *The American Journal of Nursing*, 73, no. 4 (1973), 662–64.
63. **Servellen, Gwen,** and **Lynn Vohs Dall,** "Group Psychotherapy for Depressed Women," *Journal of Psychiatric Nursing and Mental Health Services*, 19, no. 8 (1981), 25–31.
64. **Shepherd, Clovis,** *Small Groups*. San Francisco: Chandler Publishing Company, 1964.
65. **Shere, E.,** "Group Therapy with the Very Old," in *New Thoughts on Old Age*, ed. R. Kastenbaum. New York: Springer Publishing Company, Inc., 1964.
66. **Silver, A.,** "Group Psychotherapy with Senile Psychotic Patients," *Geriatrics*, 5 (1950), 147–50.
67. **Smith, E. Frances,** "Teaching Group Therapy in an Undergraduate Curriculum," *Perspectives in Psychiatric Care*, 11, no. 2 (1973), 70–74.
68. **Solomon, Philip,** and **Vernon Patch,** *Handbook of Psychiatry*. Los Altos, CA: Lange Medical Publications, 1971.
69. **Sommer, Robert,** "Working Effectively with Groups," *American Journal of Nursing*, 60, no. 2 (1960), 223–26.
70. **Swanson, Mary,** "A Check List for Group Leaders," *Perspectives in Psychiatric Care*, 7, no. 3 (1969), 120–26.

71. **Sweeney, Anita,** and **Elaine Drages,** "Group Therapy—An Analysis of the Orientation Phase," *Journal of Psychiatric Nursing and Mental Health Services,* 6, no. 1 (1968), 20-26.
72. **Thralon, Joan,** and **Charles Watson,** "Remotivation for Geriatric Patients Using Elementary School Students," *Nursing Digest,* 5, no. 4 (1975), 48–49.
73. **Trow, W., S. Zander, W. Morse,** and **D. Jenkins,** "Psychology of Group Behavior: The Class as a Group," *Journal of Educational Psychology,* 41 (1950), 322–88.
74. **Water, Jane,** *Group Guidance, Principles and Practices.* New York: McGraw-Hill Book Company, 1960.
75. **Werner, Jean,** "Relating Group Theory to Nursing Practice," *Perspectives in Psychiatric Care,* 5, no. 6 (1970), 248–61.
76. **White, R.,** and **R. Lippett,** "Leader Behavior and Member Reaction in Three Social Climates," in *Group Dynamics,* eds. D. Cartwright and A. Zander. Evanston, IL: Row Peterson, 1953, Chapter 40.
77. **Wicks, Robert J.,** *Counseling Strategies and Intervention Techniques for the Human Services.* Philadelphia: J. B. Lippincott Company, 1977.
78. **Wolff, K.,** "Group Psychotherapy with Geriatric Patients in a Mental Hospital," *Journal of the American Geriatrics Society,* 5 (1957), 13–19.
79. **Yalom, Irvin,** and **Florence Terrazas,** "Group Therapy for Psychotic Elderly Patients," *American Journal of Nursing,* 68, no. 8 (1968), 1690–98.
80. ———, *The Theory and Practice of Group Psychotherapy.* New York: Basic Books, Inc., 1970.
81. **Yeaworth, Rosalee,** "Learning Through Group Experience," *Nursing Outlook,* 18, no. 6 (1970), 29-32.

7

Application of Adaptation Theory to Nursing

Study of this chapter will help you to

1. Define *adaptation, adjustment*, and key concepts related to adaptation.
2. Discuss the application of adaptation theory and related concepts to nursing.
3. Differentiate between stress and anxiety and describe physiological, cognitive, emotional, and behavioral reactions to stress responses in each stage of the General Adaptation Syndrome.
4. Discuss examples of physiological processes and physical defense mechanisms in the body that are adaptive and factors that influence these adaptive processes.
5. Describe psychological adaptive processes and factors that influence these processes.
6. Differentiate levels of anxiety and physical, cognitive, emotional, and behavioral manifestations at each level.
7. Discuss examples of and factors influencing cultural and social adaptation.
8. Identify adaptive behaviors used in family interaction.
9. List examples of situations or behaviors that interfere with adaptation.

10. Discuss nursing measures that will assist the person or family to adapt to or cope with internal or external changes (physical, emotional, social, cultural).
11. Identify various body rhythms and give examples of body rhythms that maintain adaptation.
12. Describe how biological rhythms are affected during illness.
13. Analyze effects on patient/client care when body rhythms are considered in medical and nursing practice.
14. Discuss nursing measures to assist the person's maintenance of normal biological rhythms during illness.
15. Relate mobility and the effects of exercise to physical, emotional, and social adaptation.
16. Define *immobility* and describe the dimensions of immobility.
17. Discuss the physiological effects of immobility on the various functional areas of the body and related nursing measures to enhance or restore adaptive processes.
18. Describe the effects of emotional or behavioral immobility and nursing measures that enhance or restore psychological adaptation.
19. Work with a patient/client to maintain or restore physiological and emotional adaptation.

A concept that is easily applied to the science and art of nursing is **adaptation.** *Through this process people, either individually or in groups, constructively cope with conditions imposed internally or externally in order to meet their needs.* These new, different, or threatening conditions—stimuli, forces, stressors, pathologies—may be entirely beyond a person's control or may result from the freedom to choose alternatives. The term **adjustment** *refers to minor changes in customary behavior to meet life's problems more effectively.*

Adaptation and life are synonymous; each involves the whole organism. All systems previously described must be adaptive in order to function. Adaptation permits forward movement by reducing or negating the effects of discord, deviance, or adverse forces accompanying change. No adaptation is permanent or static because change is constant. Change or adaptation should be accomplished without excess physical illness, loss of long-range goals or values, psychological disintegration, or disruption of the person's or system's overall social functioning.

The definition of *health* and its related concepts outlined in the first chapter of this book introduced you to the concept of adaptation.

Although adaptation as a concept is not emphasized in other chapters, its implications permeate the book. An appropriate teaching method promotes adaptation. Carrying out the nursing process aids adaptation. Behavior in the phases of crisis is the person's way of adapting. Environmental, cultural, religious, social-class, and family influences are integral factors in adaptation. In each developmental era the person undergoes adaptive changes (52). This chapter explores the application of adaptation to nursing practice.

ADAPTIVE PROCESSES

Although adaptive processes may seem to be strictly physiological, they affect the whole person. Thus the key concepts discussed here regarding these processes in general should be considered in relation to psychological, sociocultural, and family adaptation as well. Nursing implications are related throughout.

Homeokinesis

Homeokinesis *refers to the ability of the organism to preserve its integrity through change and the element of motion* that is characteristic of physiological adaptation. Dynamic, self-regulating processes work to maintain or restore the internal environment to normal. Homeokinesis involves **negative feedback** *in which a deviation in one direction results in a reaction in the opposite direction*. The classic example is the maintenance of a relatively constant environment in the home by means of a control device, a thermostat.

The Body as an Open System

Physiological adaptation may be considered by viewing the body as a complex open system in which a dynamic balance is maintained with the surrounding environment. Each interrelated subsystem (organs, tissues) of the body is an open system made up of additonal subsystems (cells). Levels of organization within and among systems include the cellular, structural, organ-system, and physiological-process aspects (83). To illustrate, the regulation of body temperature involves skin, respiratory, circulatory, and neurological structures. Variations in the degree of adaptation may also occur. Changes in function of one body part mediate change elsewhere. Examples include the carotid sinus reflex that slows the heart rate, thereby reducing blood pressure through decreased vasoconstriction, and eye adaptation to light and dark through pupil dilation and changes in the rods and cones. Increased production of antibodies occurs in response to the presence of foreign protein in the form of a bacterium. And decreased oxygen tension at higher altitudes increases blood hemoglobin content (35).

Basic adaptive responses are sufficiently known to permit prediction of outcomes that relate directly to many aspects of nursing care. Detection of **hyperpyrexia**, an *increased body temperature*, in the patient, for example, will permit you to plan for increased perspiration, resultant dehydration, increased cardiac and respiratory rates, increased surface heat loss, and eventual decreased metabolism, leading to a decreased heat production (47). Plans for fluid replacement, rest, conservation of body heat, and monitoring of vital signs will be some basic components of the febrile patient's care plan. Special skin care will promote adaptation of the integumental system, preventing skin breakdown caused by deprivation of moisture and nutrition to the skin during hyperpyrexia.

Maintaining a Steady State

A person's functioning as an integrated behavioral unit can be viewed on a continuum: at times he/she is operating as a stable integrated unit with consistent, orderly behaviors and at other times as an unstable, ineffective, nonintegrated unit in coping with stimuli. The human is remarkably adaptive.

In the **stable** *or* **steady state** *there is an optimal energy balance between utilization and conservation.* Any disturbance in a system stimulates return to a steady state or **equifinality,** *a characteristic or original state that the organism strives by nature to assume through self-regulatory processes* (46).

All people have a potential for energy imbalance and inappropriate energy allocation. One of the best ways to assess imbalance is to note inconsistency between behaviors: the person says one thing and does another. The apparently calm, friendly patient for instance, may actually be feeling great anxiety, undergoing great energy utilization, and experiencing covert behavioral and physiological instability. Illness is also likely to cause energy imbalance, which indicates that the body's responses are inadequate to its special needs. Illness may be regarded as a life process that is regulating or striving toward normalcy following a disturbance to the system. Recovery is an adaptive response to maintain the body's integrity, a reestablishment of equifinality, the steady or stable state. Chronic disease or disability represents an altered state between usable energy and the steady state. When a person's regulatory processes are all properly functioning, he/she is in a steady adaptive state and can then deal most effectively with whatever situations are presented.

The Adaptation Syndrome

Stress *is a physical and emotional state always present in the person, one influenced by various environmental, psychological, and social factors but uniquely perceived by the person, and intensified in response when environmental change or threat occurs internally or externally and the person must respond.* The manifestations of stress are both overt and covert, purposeful, initially protective, maintaining equilibrium, productivity, and satisfaction to the extent possible (14, 67).

The person's survival depends on constant mediation between environmental demands and adaptive capacities. Various self-regulatory physical and emotional mechanisms are in constant operation, adjusting the body to a changing number and nature of internal and external stressors, agents, or factors causing intensification of the stress state. **Stressors** (*stress agents*) include cold, heat, radiation, infectious organisms, disease processes, mechanical trauma, fever, pain, imagined events, and intense emotional involvement. A moderate amount of stress, when regulatory mechanisms act within limits and few sysmptoms are observable, is constructive. The exaggerated stress state occurs when stressors are excessive or intense, limits of the steady state are exceeded, and the person cannot cope with the stressor's demands. **Distress** *is negative, noxious, unpleasant, damaging stress* (67, 72).

Responses to stress are both local and general. The **Local Adaptation Syndrome**, typified by the inflammatory response, *is the method used to wall off and control effects of physical stressors locally.* When the stressor cannot be handled locally, *the whole body responds to protect itself and ensure survival in the best way possible through the* **General Adaptation Syndrome.** The general body response augments bodily functions that protect the organism from injury, psychological and physical, and suppresses those functions nonessential to life. The General Adaptation Syndrome is characterized by Alarm and Resistance stages and, when body resistance is not maintained, an end stage, Exhaustion (67, 71, 72).

The General Adaptation Syndrome

The **Alarm Stage** *is an instantaneous, short-term, life-preserving, and total sympathetic-nervous-system response* when the person consciously or unconsciously perceives a stressor and feels helpless, insecure, or biologically uncomfortable. This stage is typified by a "fight-or-flight" reaction (67). Perception of the stressor—the alarm reaction—stimulates the anterior pituitary to increase production of adrenocorticotropic hormone (ACTH). The adrenal cortex is stimulated by ACTH to increase production of glucocorticoids, primarily hydrocortisone, or cortisol, and mineralocorticoids, primarily aldosterone. Catecholamine release triggers increased sympathetic nervous system activity, which stimulates production of epinephrine and norepinephrine by the adrenal medulla and release at the adrenergic nerve endings. The alarm reaction also stimulates the posterior pituitary to release increased antidiuretic hormone (70, 72). Generally the person is prepared to act, is more alert, and is able to adapt.

Physiologically, the responses that occur when the sympathetic nervous system is stimulated are shown in Fig. 7-1 (33, 41, 67, 68, 69, 71, 72, 73, 76).

To complicate assessment, there are times when *parts* of the parasympathetic division of the autonomic nervous system are inadvertently stimulated during a stressful state because of proximity of sympathetic and parasympathetic nerve fibers (14, 65). With intensification of stress, opposite behaviors are then observed. They are shown in Fig. 7-2 (33, 67, 68, 69, 70, 71, 72, 73, 76).

The **Stage of Resistance** *is the body's way of adapting, through an adrenocortical response, to the disequilibrium caused by the stessors of life* (67). Because of the adrenocortical response, increased use of body resources, endurance and strength, tissue anabolism, antibody production, hormonal secretion, and changes in blood sugar levels and blood volume sustain the body's fight for preservation. Body response eventually returns to normal.

If biological, psychological, or social stresses, single or in combination, occur over a long period without adequate relief, the Stage of Resistance is maintained. With continued stressors, the person becomes distressed and manifests objective and subjective emotional, intellectual, and physiological responses, as shown in Fig. 7-3 (67, 69, 70, 71, 72, 73).

Be aware of these signs and symptoms (shown in Figure 7-3) in yourself as well as in patients. You will encounter considerable stress in the work of nursing. Identify stressors, especially in situations in which your sense of self is threatened or in which you are made to feel incompetent. Share your feelings and talk about your work experiences with someone whom you trust and who will offer feedback about your coping skills. You will need someone who values you as a person, not just as a worker, who sees you as more than nurse, job, position, or nurturer, and who can help you put stressful work situations into perspective. Strive to develop a sense of being master of your own life and

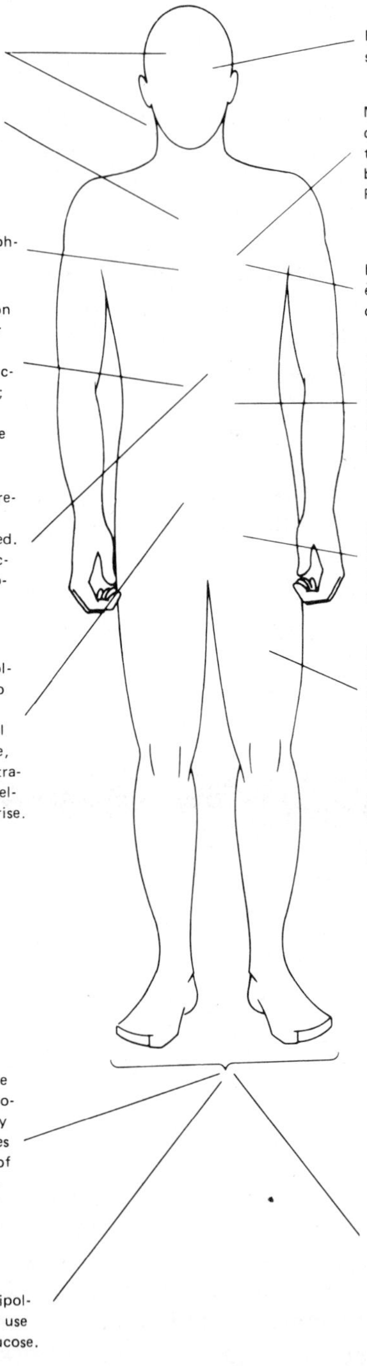

Headache from tense neck & shoulder muscles.

Pupils dilate; use maximum light for vision. Vision initially sharp, later blurred.

Anti-inflammatory responses increase from glucocorticoid production. Defences against inflammation/infection high for short time.

Myocardial rate, strength, and output increased by greater epinephrine production; more blood available throughout body as pulse rate and strength increase. Palpitations or arrhythmias may occur.

Respiratory rate/depth increased as bronchi dilate, due to increased epinephrine; allows adequate oxygenation.

Blood pressure rises when increased norepinephrine produces peripheral vasoconstriction.

Hyperglycemia from glucagon secretion in pancreas causing glycogenolysis; for energy demands after initial hypoglycemia. Increased glucocorticoid production results in gluconeogenesis in liver; body cells have sufficient glucose for stress response. Protein catabolism due to conversion of protein to glucose.

Increased blood clotting due to catecholamine stimulation of increased production of clotting factors. Increased blood viscosity may result in stasis and thrombosis if Alarm Stage persists.

Gastric glandular acid and volume secretion reduced; less essential functions such as digestion and excretion reduced. Intestinal smooth muscles relax, reducing motility. Sphincters contract. Anorexia, constipation, or flatulence may occur.

In urinary bladder, detrusor muscle relaxes and trigone sphincter contracts; micturition inhibited. Or person voids only small amounts but feels urgency.

Salt and water retained by kidneys bolster intravascular blood volume due to increased antidiuretic hormone and aldosterone production and peripheral vasoconstriction; fuller blood pressure, less urinary output, and hemoconcentration result. Sodium chloride in extracellular fluid reduced; potassium levels rise.

Blood supply shunted to brain, heart, and skeletal muscles rather than to periphery due to peripheral vasoconstriction. Skin pale, ashen, cool. Vasoconstriction stimulated by increased secretion of renin by kidney with reduced blood supply to kidney. Renin secretion stimulates production of plasma angiotensinogen; in turn, production of angiotension I and II causes vasoconstriction and increased blood pressure in vital organs.

Muscle tonus increased by epinephrine production; activities may be better coordinated, or rigidity and tremors may occur. Metabolic alterations in muscles with glycogenolysis and reduced use of glucose. Blood lactate and glucose increase.

Metabolism increased up to 150%, providing immediate energy and producing more heat due to catecholamine release. Body temperature may rise. Perspiration. Mild dehydration from increased insensible fluid loss. (Dry lips and mouth occur.) If metabolism remains high, tissue catabolism, insomnia, fatigue, and signs of dehydration such as dry skin, weight loss, and decreased urinary output occur.

Metabolic changes in adipose tissue; lipolysis and release of free fatty acids for use by muscles. Glycerol converted to glucose.

FIGURE 7-1 Alarm Phase, General Adaptation Syndrome: Physiological Responses to Sympathetic Nervous System Stimulation. (From Murray, Ruth and M. Marilyn Huelskoetter, *Psychiatric/Mental Health Nursing: Giving Emotional Care* (Englewood cliffs, N.J.: Prentice-Hall, Inc., 1983), p. 377. © 1983 by Prentice-Hall, Inc. Used with permission.

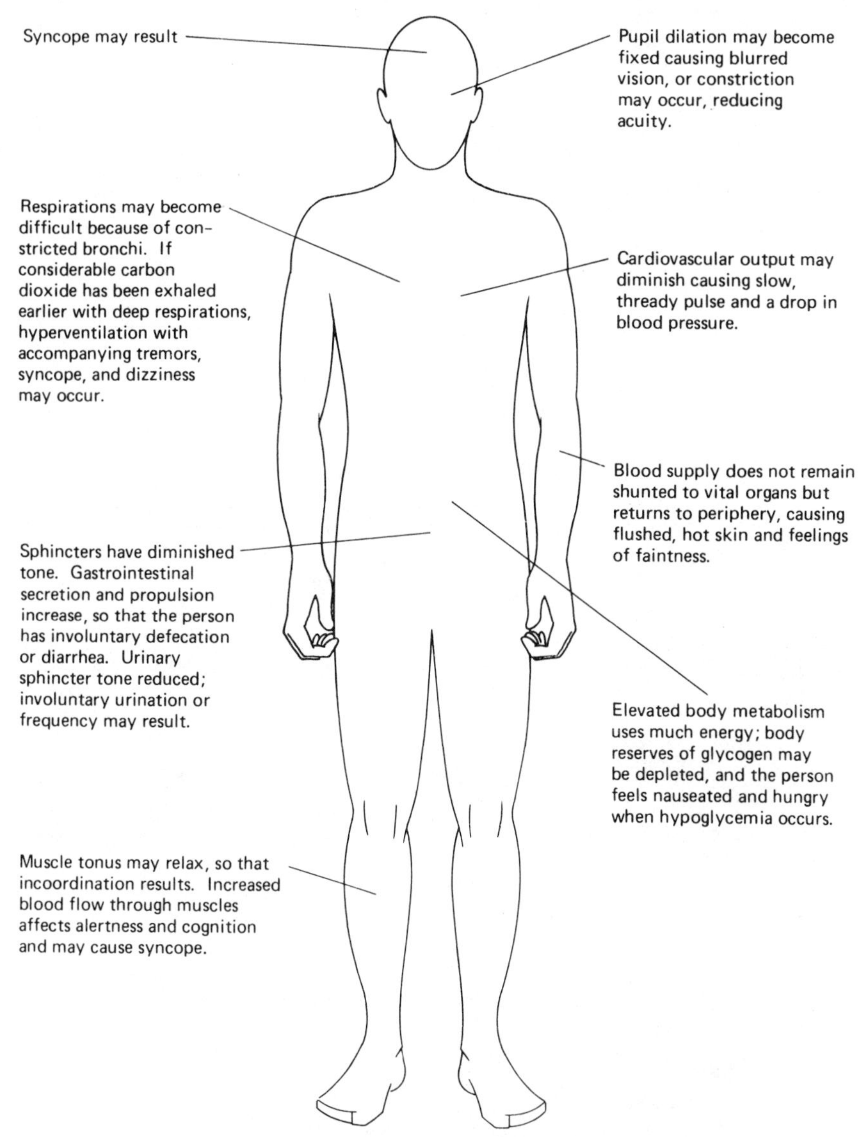

FIGURE 7-2 Alarm Phase, General Adaptation Syndrome: Physiological Responses to Parasympathetic Nervous System Stimulation. (From Murray, Ruth and M. Marilyn Huelskoetter, ***Psychiatric/Mental Health Nursing: Giving Emotional Care*** **(Englewood Cliffs, N.J.: Prentice-Hall, Inc., 1983), p. 378. © 1983 by Prentice-Hall, Inc. Used with permission.)**

circumstances, a feeling that you can exert some control over what happens to you by the way you view yourself and adjust your behavior. When you can cope with your own work-related and other stressors, then you can help patients and their families to be adaptive.

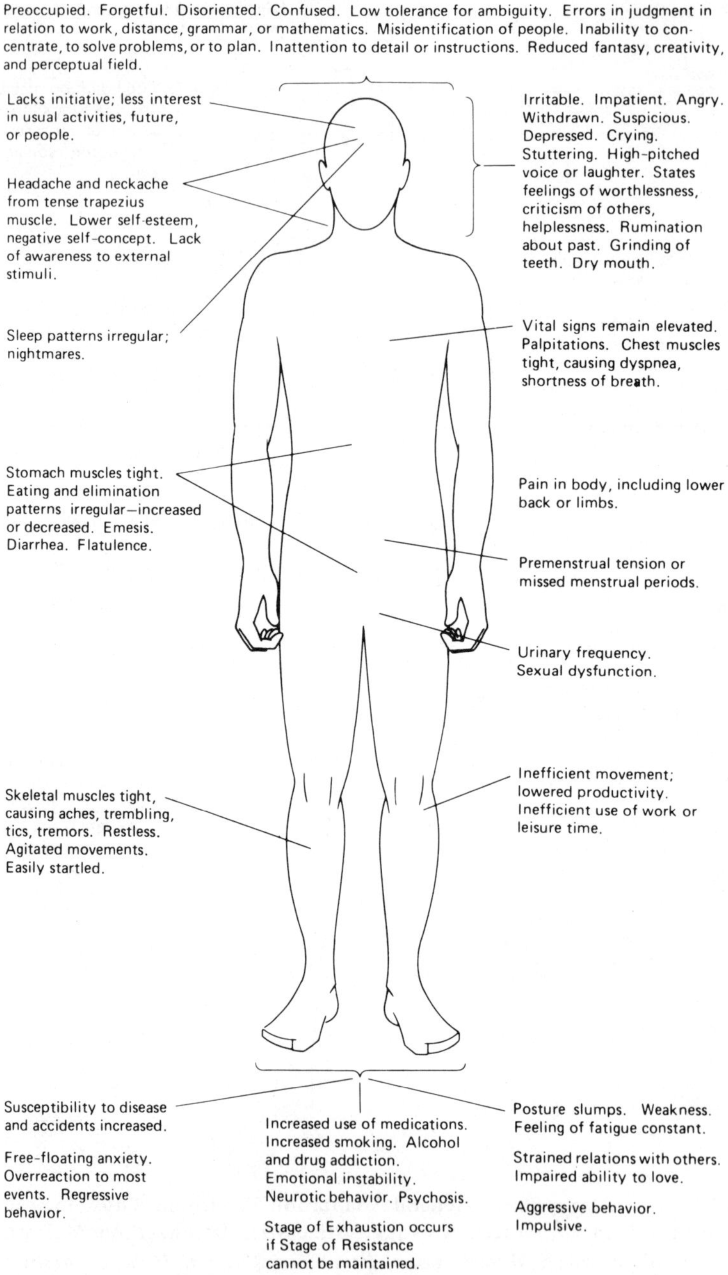

Preoccupied. Forgetful. Disoriented. Confused. Low tolerance for ambiguity. Errors in judgment in relation to work, distance, grammar, or mathematics. Misidentification of people. Inability to concentrate, to solve problems, or to plan. Inattention to detail or instructions. Reduced fantasy, creativity, and perceptual field.

Lacks initiative; less interest in usual activities, future, or people.

Irritable. Impatient. Angry. Withdrawn. Suspicious. Depressed. Crying. Stuttering. High-pitched voice or laughter. States feelings of worthlessness, criticism of others, helplessness. Rumination about past. Grinding of teeth. Dry mouth.

Headache and neckache from tense trapezius muscle. Lower self-esteem, negative self-concept. Lack of awareness to external stimuli.

Sleep patterns irregular; nightmares.

Vital signs remain elevated. Palpitations. Chest muscles tight, causing dyspnea, shortness of breath.

Stomach muscles tight. Eating and elimination patterns irregular—increased or decreased. Emesis. Diarrhea. Flatulence.

Pain in body, including lower back or limbs.

Premenstrual tension or missed menstrual periods.

Urinary frequency. Sexual dysfunction.

Skeletal muscles tight, causing aches, trembling, tics, tremors. Restless. Agitated movements. Easily startled.

Inefficient movement; lowered productivity. Inefficient use of work or leisure time.

Susceptibility to disease and accidents increased.

Free-floating anxiety. Overreaction to most events. Regressive behavior.

Increased use of medications. Increased smoking. Alcohol and drug addiction. Emotional instability. Neurotic behavior. Psychosis.

Stage of Exhaustion occurs if Stage of Resistance cannot be maintained.

Posture slumps. Weakness. Feeling of fatigue constant.

Strained relations with others. Impaired ability to love.

Aggressive behavior. Impulsive.

FIGURE 7-3 Stage of Resistance, General Adaptation Syndrome: Signs of Emotional, Intellectual, and Physiological Distress (From Murray, Ruth and M. Marilyn Huelskoetter, *Psychiatric/Mental Health Nursing: Giving Emotional Care* (Englewood Cliffs, N.J.: Prentice-Hall, Inc., 1983), p. 380. © 1983 by Prentice-Hall, Inc. Used with permission.)

Stress is additive. The repeated or chronic exposure to stress, even when the stressors are of widely differing kinds, including other people and their feelings, ultimately takes a toll on the individual. Reserves of adaptability are used that can't be replaced. Some experience with stressors may aid coping with stress and be protective against stress-induced disease. Certain coping methods, feeling in command of the situation, and strong family and social ties can help a person to suffer less deleterious effects of stress. Breaking ties by separating from the group or a loved one, divorce, mobility, or death, and the resultant sense of loss, rejection, and loneliness predispose to disease and death (51, 70, 72).

The **Stage of Exhaustion** *occurs when the person is unable to continue to adapt to internal and external environmental demands.* Physical or psychic disease or death results because the body can no longer compensate for or correct homeostatic imbalances. Manifestations of this stage are similar to those of the Alarm Stage except that all reactions first intensify and then diminish in response and show no ability to return to an effective level of function. Frequent or prolonged General Adaptation Syndrome response triggers disease through adrenocortical hypertrophy, thymolymphatic atrophy, elevated blood glucose, ulceration of the gastrointestinal tract, reduced tone and fibrosis of tissues, and vasoconstriction (67, 71, 72).

Health care workers are concerned with promoting the Resistance Stage and preventing or reversing the Exhaustion Stage, whether through drugs, bedrest, medical treatments, crisis intervention, psychotherapy, or social action. Ideally, you should identify potential stressors that the person might encounter and determine how to alter the stressors or best support the person's adaptive mechanisms and resources physically, emotionally, and socially, for the person will respond as an entity to the stressors. The relationship of stress to life crises or changes is discussed in Chapter 8 and must be considered whenever you are doing health promotion measures or intervening with the ill person.

PHYSIOLOGICAL ADAPTATION

The processes of homeokinesis, maintenance of a steady state, and the General Adaptation Syndrome just described all affect physiological adaptation.

Adaptation to the Environment

Adaptation enables living organisms to respond to changes in their environment in such a manner that injury or disease is prevented, damage is repaired, or a comfort level for coping with the altered environment is attained. Adaptation assists a person to function within a normal range.

Regulation of Body Core Temperature

Regulation of a relatively constant internal temperature is one of the physiological processes that demonstrates the principle of adaptation (9, 40). Generally the nude body is capable of maintaining the normal body core temperature between 98°F (36.6°C) and 100°F (37.7°) indefinitely when exposed to dry air temperatures ranging from 60°F (21°C) to 130°F (54.4°C). Certain feedback mechanisms in the nervous system provide the regulatory processes necessary to stabilize core temperature and most operate through the temperature-regulating center of the hypothalamus.

The preoptic receptors in the hypothalamus are primarily responsible for detection and response when core temperature is above normal; the peripheral receptors are more important when core temperature is below normal. Signals from the peripheral receptors are transmitted to the hypothalamus, where they are integrated with signals from the preoptic area to provide the final efferent message for control of heat gain and loss. This control center is called the *hypothalamic thermostat* (65).

Sweating begins at 37°C (98.6°F) and increases rapidly as the core temperature rises; it ceases if the temperature falls below that level. Heat production is similarly adaptive, for at any temperature below 37°C (98.6°F) mechanisms that produce heat are activated, notably muscle activity culminating in shivering. Increased heat loss occurs in two ways in response to overheating: (1) by stimulation of sweat glands to increase evaporation and (2) by inhibition of certain sympathetic centers in the posterior hypothalamus, permitting vasodilation of skin vessels (65).

Adaptation to cold is equally efficient. Vasoconstriction in the skin is the first change and it occurs over the entire body, closing off conduction from internal structures and conserving body heat. Sweating is completely checked at 37°C (98.6°F) and evaporative cooling ceases (65).

Heat production occurs through shivering and sympathetic excitation. The primary motor center for shivering is situated in the posterior hypothalamus. It is activated by severe body cooling that sends impulses down the brain stem to the cord to the anterior motor neurons. Skeletal muscle tone is intensified throughout the body; muscle metabolism speeds up, and the rate of heat production is increased as much as 50 percent. Once the muscle tone reaches a crucial point, shivering begins as the result of feedback oscillations of the muscle spindle stretch reflex mechanism. Maximum shivering can raise heat production as much as five times normal (65).

Sympathetic stimulation of circulating norepinephrine and epinephrine in the blood can trigger an immediate rise in the rate of cellular metabolism by requiring greater oxidation of foodstuffs to produce the amount of high-energy phosphates required for normal body functions. This adaptive mechanism for increased heat production is called *chemical thermogenesis*. Although not nearly as effective in adults as in infants, it can increase heat production in infants by as much as 100 percent, a crucial factor for maintaining normal body temperature in the neonate (65).

The comfort we experience at 72° with a relative humidity of 50 percent on a calm day could not be enjoyed if our core temperature of 98.6° fluctuated. When a change in weather occurs, our hypothalamic thermostats signal immediately to hold temperature and other vital functions constant. If our bodies could not cool themselves in an environment of 105° during a summer heat wave, permanent brain damage would transpire within minutes; similarly, a drop of but 9 degrees on a zero day could mean death (57).

Research shows that weather affects humans. Body chemistry changes with the seasons; for example, certain individuals burn extra fats in cold weather. Although the body's overall metabolism conserves and endures, surface capillaries close down, resistance to disease lessens, cardiovascular illnesses occur frequently, and the death rate peaks world-wide in winter (57).

The transitional seasons impose the most stress, especially spring. Switching from winter to summer may trigger such an explosive change in the organism as to almost match the about-face in the weather. Blood acidity rises, cholesterol and sugars climb to high levels; hormones surge. A burst of energy may be felt: the housewife feels impelled to get busy with new tasks and the young man's fancy may indeed turn to thoughts of love (his hair and beard double their rate of growth (57).

Psychiatric admissions mount in the spring and the suicide rate in the United States peaks in March and April. Disruptive weather patterns with their erratic, day-to-day changes may be the cause. One day hot and the next day cold heightens stress as the body strains to adjust. It is speculated that the spring and fall winds, often blowing at an infrasound level (too low to be heard but still affecting the organism), influence the central nervous system. Often named witches' winds because they are associated with illness, traffic collisions and job accidents, crime and mental illness, scientists have studied the Chinook in northwestern United States, the Santa Ana in the Southwest, the Sirocco in

Italy, and the Foehn in Central Europe for the changes in human behavior they seem to induce and the efforts of the body and mind to adapt and cope (57).

Dr. Felix Sulman of the Bioclimatology Unit at Hadassah University Medical Center in Jerusalem has studied the effects of winds on health. He found that 30 percent of the country's population suffers symptoms linked to the seasonal hot wind, the Sharav, and that these symptoms begin a surprising 12 hours before its actual arrival. It was discovered that as the Sharav approaches, the air in its path nearly doubles its content of ions and the ratio of positive to negative ions burgeons dramatically (57). Dr. Sulman concluded that this dramatic disturbance in the balance of the electrically charged molecules produces major changes in the system chemistry of weather-sensitive people. Some generate large amounts of serotonin (a potent vasoconstrictor hormone that carries messages inside the brain), some manifest increased thyroid activity, and others have been found to overproduce adrenalin. Dr. Sulman calls this last effect "adrenalin exhaustion syndrome," for it induces nervous tension, depression, and fatigue. Thus the body sometimes adapts negatively to adverse environmental influences (57).

Mechanisms of Defense

The human body is equipped with various defensive physiologic mechanisms. They help to reduce injury and prevent the invasion of pathogenic microorganisms, thus promoting and maintaining a healthy status. When these mechanisms fail, various disease states result: neoplastic, infectious, viral, toxic, or traumatic.

Some *defensive mechanisms are of a general nature and serve to protect against many types of harmful agents; they are the basis of* **nonspecific resistance.** Other *defensive mechanisms are specific against a certain harmful agent and no other; they are spoken of as* **specific resistance** or **specific immunity** (31).

Nonspecific Resistance. Some principal nonspecific forms of body resistance are the skin, mucous membranes and their secretions, the skull, reflex movements, phagocytosis, inflammation, and interferons.

The first line of defense is the unbroken *skin* and *mucous membranes* that protect the deeper tissues from mechanical and chemical injury and that provide a barrier against the penetration of bacteria. The skin and mucous membranes are constantly in contact with microorganisms. Certain microorganisms that are regularly present on these coverings constitute their normal flora of resident bacteria. When the person's resistance is lowered by injury to the tissues or by a disease process that reduces general resistance, these resident microorganisms, as well as pathogenic microorganisms, flourish (54, 65). Pathogenic microorganisms may gain entry through broken skin or mucous membranes, the respiratory or gastrointestinal tracts, the vagina, or blood vessels, especially the veins. Microorganisms are spread through direct contact, droplet infection (organisms that are sneezed or coughed), food and water, insect and animal bites, or contaminated equipment, such as in intravenous or intramuscular administation of medications.

Reproduction of resident skin flora and the growth of pathogenic microorganisms are minimized by lack of sufficient moisture and the presence of specific antibacterial and antifungal organic acids. A surface film on the skin, which consists of secretions from sebaceous glands and sudoriferous (sweat) glands and of products of *cornification* (the process whereby the epidermis hardens), provides an acid environment and has antibacterial and antifungal properties. These properties enable the film to act as an antiseptic, to neutralize acid and alkali substances, and to interfere with the absorption of toxic agents (30, 54). Because some soaps are highly alkaline, their excessive use should be avoided to prevent the removal of this protective surface film.

The epidermis, which partly consists of a layer of dead cells, serves as another defense mechanism. As the cells of the epidermis die, their protein material undergoes a change. The new protein form is called *keratin*, a tough, fibrous protein that causes the epidermis to become highly resistant to environmental elements, including bacteria, fungi, parasites, and most injurious chemicals (30, 65). If this layer of skin (also called the horny layer) is broken, physical and chemical agents can enter the body (75). So protect yourself and the patient from scratches, cuts, and any breaks in the continuity of the skin.

Mucous membranes line cavities or passageways of the body that communicate to the exterior. These membranes secrete a fluid, *mucus*, which consists of several mucopolysaccharides, inorganic salts, water, and epithelial cells. The membranes and mucus serve to decrease bacterial invasion and lessen the severity of chemical or mechanical trauma (65).

The surface of the stomach is lined with cells that secrete an alkaline fluid containing mucus. A layer of mucus 1.0 to 1.5 mm thick covers the gastric wall and serves as a protective barrier against various forms of chemical and mechanical irritants, such as digestive enzymes, hydrochloric acid, and abrasive foods (65). The parietal cells of the gastric glands secrete a solution that contains hydrochloric acid. This acid environment acts as a barrier to destroy most pathogens that enter the digestive tract. The acid environment of the stomach can be diminished temporarily, however, by such foods as milk and eggs; thus the protective action of the acidity is decreased (31). Remember this when planning or instructing patients in diets that must contain large quantities of milk products and eggs.

Some mucous membranes in the digestive tract secrete substances that have bacteriostatic properties. Those in the intestines, for instance, secrete certain enzymes capable of destroying pathogens (34).

The genitourinary tract is also lined with mucous membranes. Pathogens entering the vagina are usually destroyed by the acid secretions produced by the cells lining this area. Frequent vaginal irrigations, or douches, will lower the acidity in the vagina and therefore lessen the protective function of the mucous membranes there (34).

A ciliated mucous membrane lines the respiratory tract. The external nares are surrounded by fine hairs that block pathogens from entering the nose; pathogens that do enter are trapped by mucus secreted by the cells lining the nasal passageways. Inhaled bacteria escaping these two defense mechanisms are usually blocked by *cilia* (hairlike projections), whose wavelike motions move the pathogens toward the pharynx, where they are swallowed or expectorated (65).

The eye is protected by several defense mechanisms. The skull provides a *bony orbit* that protects the eyeball (as well as the brain and vital centers) from mechanical injury. The *eyelids*, which are lined with a conjunctival membrane, serve as protective coverings for the eyeball. *Eyelashes*, lining the free edges of the lids, act to prevent foreign bodies from entering the eye. Tears or *lacrimal fluid*, secreted by the lacrimal glands, have a lavage action that serves to wash foreign bodies out of the eyes and to dilute irritant meterials. Excessive tear formation occurs any time a foreign particle or other irritant gets in or near the eye. The lacrimal fluid also contains an enzyme, *lysozyme*, which functions to destroy bacteria (31, 65, 75).

Some *reflex* or *voluntary acts* assist the body to rid itself of pathogens. Sneezing and coughing eliminate pathogens from the respiratory tract whereas vomiting and diarrhea help to eliminate them from the gastrointestinal tract. The reflex of blinking renews the tear film over the cornea and prevents the entrance of foreign material. Reflex muscular movement, such as removing the hands from a hot stove or foot from a sharp object, prevents injury.

One of the most important nonspecific mechanisms in the prevention of disease involves leukocytes (wandering cells) and certain phagocytic tissue cells.

Phagocytosis is performed by **phagocytes,** *special cells capable of ingesting and digesting bacteria and dead tissues.* In **phagocytosis** *projections of cytoplasm engulf solid particles external to the cells.* In order to promote phagocytosis, *opsonins* (globin molecules) combine with the bacteria and dead tissues and increase their cohesiveness with the phagocytes. Some pathogens may survive and multiply in the phagocytes, instead of being destroyed, and are transported in the bloodstream from one part of the body to another. Some phagocytes—for example, the stationary macrophages—are capable of forming immune bodies against foreign agents (79).

Phagocytic cells are classified according to size as macrophages and microphages. *Macrophages* are either stationary or mobile. The stationary cells, *tissue histocytes*, are permanently located in the interstitial tissues of the **reticuloendothelial system,** *which is composed of connective-tissue cells widely scattered throughout many vascular and lymph channels*, including the bone marrow, spleen, liver, and lymph nodes. The reticuloendothelial system serves as the primary line of defense after bacteria have invaded the body. The mobile macrophagic cells are *lymphocytes* and *monocytes*, which are formed in the lymph nodes (31, 54).

Microphages are smaller and more numerous than the macrophages, and the phagocytic power per cell is greatly reduced. The microphagic cells are *granulocytes*, which are formed in the bone marrow. After their formation, the granulocytes are transported throughout the body via the blood. Jointly, *the granulocytes, lymphocytes,* and *monocytes are referred to as* **leukocytes,** mobile units of the body's defense system (31, 54, 79).

Any microorganisms that survive the action of the phagocytes trigger a second defense mechanism near the area of the invasion. This response is called the **inflammatory response.** Because inflammation is one of the most common body responses to injury, knowledge of the inflammatory mechanism provides a basis for understanding many infectious and noninfectious diseases.

First, there is an accelerated blood flow to the site because of a dilatation of the adjacent capillaries. This process increases the amount of oxygen and nutrients in the area and produces *redness* and *heat* at the site. An accompanying increase in the permeability of the capillaries causes white blood cells and serum to escape into the surrounding tissues. The accumulated fluid (blood cells and serum) causes area *swelling*, and pressure on the nerve endings produces *pain*. Together the pain and swelling produce *limitation of movement*. Thus the cardinal signs of inflammation are redness, heat, swelling, and limitation of movement. Pain as a subjective symptom results (31, 40, 54).

Phagocytosis occurs with the increased number of localized white blood cells during the inflammatory reaction. The phagocytes engulf and destroy the pathogens. Dead phagocytes, pathogens, tissue cells, and tissue fluid accumulate. This accumulation is known as *pus*. The dead pathogens and tissue cells are eventually carried away by the leukocytes via the blood and lymph. Those in the bloodstream are carried to the spleen, liver, and bone marrow, where the phagocytic cells (macrophages) engulf and digest them. Those in the lymph stream are filtered out by the lymph nodes and ingested by phagocytic cells (31, 54).

An additional *nonspecific resistance to disease that inhibits multiplication of viruses may be found in the form of* **interferon.** Several types of cells in the body secrete the protein interferon. When a cell is infected by a virus, its secretion of interferon increases. Interferon does not benefit the cell that is already infected but causes other cells to enhance their defense posture and increase their resistance to the viral invasion. Interferon is not specific in its action against any particular virus but acts against viruses in general (31, 42, 65, 66). Human-derived interferon has been shown active against some human cancers as well as against human viral diseases. Drug companies, plus several independent research teams, are currently experimenting with methods to produce human interferon from bacteria, a feat that promises to make ample quantities of the substance available for testing against viral infections and cancer (16, 29, 42).

Specific Resistance-Specific Immunity. Specific immune responses are characteristic of vertebrate animals. Immune responses can be viewed in the same way as other adaptive processes in the body—as a stimulus-response sequence. The immune system, often referred to as the third line of defense (the first and second lines of defense being mechanical barriers and the various types of phagocytes), is an important companion to the nonspecific defenses previously described.

The immunological response is initiated by the invasion of the body by foreign molecules. These foreign molecules are known as *antigens.* Antigens stimulate the body to produce either specific proteins, called *antibodies*, or defensive cells that interact with the antigens and make them harmless (54, 66).

The immunological response has two separate components. The cell-mediated component or *cellular immunity* is involved in the body's response to fungi, viruses, tumors, and transplants of foreign tissue. *T lymphocytes* are responsible for mediating cellular immunity. Once stimulated by an antigen, these lymphocytes increase in size and then multiply. Eventually the lymphocytes leave the lymph nodes and make their way to the site of the invasion, where they destroy the invading cells. The sensitized lymphocytes are also capable of stimulating other lymphocytes at the invasion site and enhancing the local inflammatory response. It is hypothesized that the T lymphocytes do not actually produce antibodies (31, 54, 65). The antibody-mediated component or *humoral immunity* is primarily involved in the response to bacterial infections. In humoral immunity *B lymphocytes* become activated by antigens. The B lymphocytes increase in size and differentiate into *plasma cells*; these cells produce large amounts of antibodies that circulate freely in the blood and the lymph. Once formed, the antibodies are contained in serum globulins, especially gamma globulins (54, 65, 66).

Interaction and cooperation between antibody-mediated immune response and cellular-mediated immune response are important in eradicating infections and preventing their recurrence. The immune state, which results in humoral or cellular immunity, may be permanent or transient.

Active immunization *occurs when the body is sensitized by an antigen.* The antibody-mediated and/or cellular-mediated immune responses occur. An active immunity may last from 10 years to a lifetime (54). The first encounter that an individual has with an antigen is characterized by the primary response. Initally there is a lag phase that may last from 20 hours to a few days. During the lag phase little or no response to the antigen occurs. A slow increase in antibody concentration in the body fluids follows and then a gradual decline as the antigen is overcome. With the second encounter with a particular antigen, the antibody concentrations or titers rise rapidly and often reach levels 200 times greater than the concentrations observed during the primary response (66).

Natural acquired active immunity *occurs when the host's body produces antibodies following the invasion of pathogens.* Natural active immunity can be acquired from subclinical forms of disease and from repeated contacts with pathogens not virulent enough to produce disease (40, 54). Chickenpox, mumps, and smallpox usually confer permanent immunity after recovery from a single attack.

Artificial active immunity *occurs after an individual is inoculated with a specific antigen that stimulates the production of antibodies.* The two main agents used for these inoculations are vaccines and toxoids. *Vaccines* are prepared from microorganisms that are living, attenuated, dead, or inactivated. Living vaccines are usually prepared with organisms of lower virulence; attenuated or weakened strains are used in the Bacillus-Calmette-Guerin (BCG) vaccine for tuberculosis. The vaccines for whooping cough and typhoid fever are prepared from dead bacteria and the vaccines for measles and influenza from inactivated viruses. A vaccine can be prepared from a strain that does not produce disease in humans but that compares with the antigenicity of human strains—for example, the use of cowpox vaccines for smallpox vaccinations (54).

Toxoids are prepared from attenuated forms of toxins (poisonous chemical substances produced by certain bacteria). When introduced into the body, attenuated toxins stimulate the production of antitoxins. Toxoids are used to immunize the host to such diseases as diphtheria, scarlet fever, and tetanus (31, 66).

Passive immunization *occurs when the person acquires resistance* *to a disease by receiving antibodies or lymphocytes from an external source*. Passive immunization is immediate, but the duration of its effectiveness is no more than a few weeks. In **natural passive immunity** *antibodies pass from mother to the fetus by way of placental transmission*. This immunization is critical for the survival of the newborn, for significant antibody formation does not appear until a month or two after birth. Cellular-mediated immunity functions are also slow to develop in the newborn. The placental membranes are permeable to maternal immunoglobulins. Thus the newborn has partial immunity to those diseases to which its mother is immune (54). The transmission of antibodies from mother to baby by colostrum and milk secreted by the mammary glands is still being investigated and sources vary in their interpretation of present data (54, 66).

Artificial passive immunity *occurs when immune bodies or antibodies for specific diseases are obtained from other human beings or animals and injected into a person who has been exposed to the same disease and who needs antibodies to prevent the establishment of the disease*. These antibodies provide temporary immunity, allowing the person time to produce his/her own antibodies. Tetanus antitoxin and gamma globulins for hepatitis and German measles provide this form of protection (5).

Transfer of pathogenic microbes can be prevented and controlled through proper personal hygiene habits. Covering the mouth and nose when coughing or sneezing, disposal of contaminated tissues, and control of dust and particulate matter minimize the spread of airborne droplet infection. Thorough handwashing, use of individual equipment, and disinfection and sterilization of equipment prevent direct spread of microorganisms by touching of contaminated areas of articles. Foods and liquids require careful handling by few people so that they do not become sources of infection.

Immunizations and various *medications* (such as antibiotics) also aid the human's natural defenses by producing a desired effect on a particular body system. *Biological rhythms* are also increasingly understood as essential to adaptation. A later section of this chapter discusses this subject in detail.

Motion is synonymous with life and adaptation. When either the internal or the overall mobility of the person is interfered with, adaptation is inadequate. The hazards of immobility and nursing measures for dealing with them are discussed in detail later on in this chapter.

Biofeedback: New Dimensions for the Mind

Bridging the gap between physiological and psychological controls has fascinated people for decades. Despite the wealth of biological and psychological scientific effort devoted to the control of physiological, behavioral, and emotional responses, little has been done to explore the capacity of the individual to hold the reins of control over his own body functions.

Biofeedback, a new and far-reaching discovery, has emerged from biological research. It is a mind-body technique that allows the person to communicate with his/her inner being. It is the feeding back of personal biological information to oneself in order to control voluntarily the autonomic nervous system (10).

Biofeedback permits a person to become familiar with internal functions, such as a moving index of body temperature or a reading of brain waves. As with externally directed behavior, the person is able with practice to learn how to control internal behavior (10). Most people have experienced the doctor's interpreting for them, in an illness-wellness context, the results of physiological tests. If able to read the same information as it is occurring within you, you are using biofeedback.

Biofeedback has two aspects: the actual use of biomedical devices capable of taking a reading of one's physiological activity, such as temperature or heart rate, and the training in which one learns what to do with the devices. The client is linked to the instruments, which are modified to display the body information as visual or auditory signals, by delicate wires or tubes connected to special sensing materials taped to the skin. The body information is carried back to the devices, which continually read the signals reflecting the constantly changing activity within (10). As the client continues to work with biofeedback instrumentation, an association develops between changes in body signals and various subjective feelings that are either consciously or subconsciously recognized. The monitor gives information about the degree of success. Dependence on the instrumentation is temporary. Eventually the person should be able to monitor the fluctuations and thereby exercise some conscious control over physiological adaptation. Once learned, control over a physiological function is retained in the person's memory for a long time (10).

Much success has been demonstrated in the use of biofeedback for the prevention and relief of such medical problems as tension headaches and Raynaud's disease. Work is being done to explore learned control over blood pressure, heart rate, and peripheral vasodilation and vasoconstriction. Control over some aspects of respiratory function could ease the discomforts of persons with obstructive pulmonary disease.

There are intimate interactions between the mind, emotion, and body function. The process of biofeedback is essentially a mental function and it has relevance in most medical, psychological, psychosomatic, and emotional problems.

For centuries Indian fakirs have performed such feats as lying on beds of nails or walking on live coals. In recent studies of such persons EEG readings have shown a preponderance of alpha waves, waves associated with deeply relaxed meditative states in which one is able to turn off distractions and free the mind of all invading thoughts or images. The practice of total relaxation is used in biofeedback training and is an example of a person's adaptive capacity. Proponents of a "relaxation response" method suggest that periods of meditation, in a quiet environment with the mind shifted from external thought to a passive attitude and the body in a comfortable position, will produce a physiological adaptation. This state, tested at a Harvard laboratory, produces significant decreases in oxygen consumption, carbon dioxide elimination, and rate of breathing (6).

Helping patients relax when coping with stress has always been a nursing goal. Research in biofeedback may provide new techniques with which to assist patients in a variety of situations: the preoperative patient in a state of tense anticipation of the unknown; the mother in labor with whom we have already begun to recognize the value of relaxation; and the postsurgical patient whose pain is increased because of tension. The basic principles of biofeedback have become a necessary component in the education of today's nurse. For further reading on this relaxation technique, see references 6, 28, and 45.

PSYCHOLOGICAL ADAPTATION

Whether life offers psychological threat involving loss and suffering or the challenge of goal attainment, adaptational tasks are necessary for psychological growth. The term **coping** is sometimes used to refer to *the psychological way in which a person deals with life's demands and goals* (39).

Key Concepts

Psychological adaptation *refers to intrapsychic organization and behavioral adequacy in attaining appropriate human relationships.* Adaptation is achieved through the personality structure called the **ego,** *that part of the person concerned with the processes of judgment, thinking, memory, perception, discrimination, motor activity in response to perception, understanding, association, communication, control over behavior, and use of adaptive or defensive behaviors* (14, 25). The ego refers to what we commonly think of as the conscious self.

Failure to satisfy basic innate or acquired needs or to reconcile conflicting value systems constitutes **psychological stress.** Stressors may exist in the real world or only be perceived as real by the person. But three basic causes of psychological stress exist: (1) loss of something valuable, (2) injury or threat of injury, physical or emotional, and (3) frustration of drives. Each person's individual perception of events determines the reaction; this fact explains the wide variety of possible responses to a given situation (14, 25, 26).

Adaptive behavior *helps us to adjust to or cope with certain circumstances whereas* **defensive behavior** *causes us to alienate ourselves from certain circumstances or to avoid life's demands and goals.* Patterns for both behaviors originate in the early formative years of childhood when anxiety and discomfort with people are first experienced and are learned without much awareness on our part. By adulthood these patterns are usually fixed, unconscious, and automatic. Current experiences sometimes reactivate feelings and behavior associated with long-forgotten experiences and elicit responses similar to ones that were originally adaptive but may now be inappropriate, useless, or incapacitating. Thus what was once adaptive behavior becomes defensive.

Generally **defensive behavior** *is an exaggerated response to experience used too frequently or for too long duration when a situation is perceived or anticipated as a threat to self* or to a situation inconsistent with the existing self-image (14, 25). The experience is temporarily rendered harmless by being distorted or denied to awareness. A normally active person who sprains an ankle, for instance, may insist on continuing routine activities, denying the implications of the sprained ankle. Such behavior is defensive. To admit the necessity of staying off the sprained ankle is adaptive, for healing is fostered through resting the part.

Adaptive behavior is maximum when the person is feeling a sense of discovery, a purposeful changing of self, or creativity. The adapting person is not necessarily happy, content, or a conformist. But he/she is living constructively and in as much harmony with the culture and others as possible to allow for a balanced satisfaction of needs (14, 25).

The processes or functions of the ego help the person to delay gratification, presume a sense of reality, and feel a sense of mastery or achievement in the world. The ego also mediates among inner demands, needs, impulses, and drives (the *id*) and the internalized prohibitions and rules of society, parents, and outer reality (the *superego*). As the ego becomes stronger in its role as mediator between inner demands and outer reality, more efficient and complex mechanisms are developed for adaptive behavior. Thus the person can adapt emotionally to the physical or social surroundings.

The well-organized, adapting ego can recognize anxiety (feelings) as a signal in a situation and can cope with this situation and feelings. Mechanisms of adjustment are not used too frequently, too intensely, for too long a duration, or too rigidly. The underdeveloped, maladaptive ego has either no organized behavioral mechanisms for response to anxiety or uses the same defensive mechanisms rigidly in every situation, to an excessive degree, for too long a duration. Such a person is vulnerable to small amounts of anxiety and cannot adapt to his/her feelings. Mental illness occurs in such persons (25, 26).

The human psyche is highly versatile in arranging or using adaptive behaviors. Such versatility is fortunate, for the anxious, uncomfortable person thus has many resources to draw on and can use a combination of behaviors. But people generally use only certain mechanisms that work best for them, thus establishing styles of adjustment by which others can predict their behavior. Nevertheless, a common core of needs, drives, patterns of responses, and other psychological phenomena can be identified. Understanding the similarities and general patterns of behavior promotes an understanding of a person's psychological adaptive potential.

Behavioral patterning, *using a cluster of behaviors that have a common goal and are used with predictability and regularity when a person is faced with a similar stimulus or need*, is an adaptive process that minimizes the amount of energy needed to cope with changing surroundings and promotes stability or a steady state (14). Behaviors previously successful are repeated, usually without thinking, so that the myriad of daily routine activities are done automatically. *Nursing Assessment and Health Promotion through the Life Span* explores some of the normal behavioral patterns in each life era (52). The person does not substitute new behaviors unless they are advantageous; and the substitution depends on the source and intensity of stimuli and on a comparison of the satisfaction provided by the established pattern with the predicted satisfaction to be gained by changing behaviors. People vary in the ease with which they can change or adapt.

The interruption of these patterns during illness, whether related to eating, bedtime, work, socialization, or hygiene, constitutes a crisis. You will assess behavioral patterns and help the person cope or adapt to the changed internal environment (illness) and the changed external environment (health care system). Chapters 3, 4, 5, and 8 discuss ways in which you can assist.

The body usually maintains or regains internal constancy through automatic regulatory mechanisms without conscious effort. The person's relationships with others, however, depend on his/her behavior, whether consciously or unconsciously motivated. Therefore the person is usually more concerned about others and the external environment than his/her body unless the malfunctioning body part interferes with daily activity. An illness is of secondary concern to someone who is about to experience a business loss or who feels great occupational obligations, for instance.

One study gathered the life histories of three groups of individuals: (1) expatriate anti-communist Chinese students in New York, (2) American workers who were frequently ill, and (3) American workers who were usually healthy. Results indicated that the healthiest persons were those whose life situations satisfied their particular needs and goals, however they might differ from the population in general. The interviews revealed that clusters of illness tended to occur during significantly stressful periods when the person was striving to adapt to what were perceived to be threatening environmental demands (82). A longitudinal study of discharged Navy men revealed the same relationship between stress-evoking life situations and clusters of illness (58).

Although *stress* and *anxiety* are used interchangeably, the terms are not the same. **Anxiety** *is the psychological response to excessive unchanneled energy resulting from the stress reaction; it is a vague, diffuse feeling of dread, uneasiness, or general discomfort resulting from perception of a threat to the self, real or imagined* (14, 25).

Anxiety is the response to feeling helpless, isolated, alienated from others, insecure, an object rather than a unique, worthwhile person. Anxiety, like stress, is subjective and indirectly observable. Severe anxiety immobilizes the person. But using the energy generated from the stress state (as explained in the discussion of the Adaptation Syndrome) to create a plan of action or goal mobilizes or motivates the person under stress.

The energy aroused by the stress state, manifested in feelings of anxiety, can be dissipated or reduced in intensity by walking, talking, crying, or other physical and social activity. Yet frequently the ill person has limited ways of working off tension.

Certain variables alter the stress state and resultant anxiety: the physical and mental status, age, temperament, health status; the kind, nature, or number of stressors; the duration of exposure; and past experiences and reaction to similar stress.

Manifestations of Anxiety

People use various behaviors to cope with anxiety or to attempt to change a stressful situation. Redistribution of energy is often not consciously recognized; thus a person may be unaware of any behavioral shifts, although others notice them. Certain behavioral changes may be the best the person can do at the time, although they seem inadequate to an objective observer. You must be observant of the responses that may indicate psychological stress.

Table 7-1 summarizes manifestations of the various levels of anxiety (24, 27, 38, 56, 61, 64, 70, 80, 81, 84).

TABLE 7-1 Manifestations and Levels of Anxiety

Level	Area	Manifestations
Mild	Physiological	Tension of needs motivates behavior. Adaptive to variety of internal and external stimuli.
	Cognitive	Attentive, alert, perceptive to variety of stimuli, effective problem solving.
	Emotional	No intense feelings; self-concept not threatened. Use of ego adaptive mechanisms minimal, flexible. Behavior appropriate to situation.
Moderate	Physiological	Some symptoms may be present.
	Cognitive	Perceptual field narrow; responds to directions. Tangible problems solved fairly effectively, at least with direction and support. Selective inattention—focus is on stimuli that do not add to anxiety.
	Emotional	Impatient, irritable, forgetful, demanding, crying, angry. Uses any adaptive mechanism, e.g., rationalization, denial, displacement, to protect from feelings and meaning of behavior.
	(Physiological, cognitive, and emotional changes of Alarm and Resistance Stages. Individual functions in normal pattern, but may not feel as healthy physically or emotionally as usual. Illness may result if feeling persists.)	
Severe	Physiological	Alarm Stage changes intensify, and Stage of Resistance may progress to Stage of Exhaustion.
	Cognitive	Perceptual field narrows; stimuli distorted, focus is on scattered details. Selective inattention prevails. Learning and problem solving ineffective. Clarification or restatement needed repeatedly. Misinterprets statements. Unable to follow directions or remember main points. Unable to plan or make decisions; needs assistance with details. Disorganized. Consciousness and lucidity reduced.
	Emotional	Self-concept threatened; sense of helplessness; mood changes. Behavior erratic, inappropriate, regressive, inefficient. May be aware of inappropriate behavior but unable to improve. Many ego defense mechanisms used; dissociation and amnesia may be used. Disorientation, confusion, suspicion, hallucinations, and delusions may be present.
	(Psychoses or physical illness or injury may result.)	
Panic	Physiological	Severe symptoms of Exhaustion Stage may be ignored.
	Cognitive	Sensory ability and attention reduced so that only object of anxiety noticed.

	May fail to notice specific object of concern or disastrous event but will be preoccupied with trivial detail.
Emotional	Self-concept overwhelmed.
	Ego defense mechanism used, often inappropriately and uncontrollably.
	Behavior focused on finding relief; may scream, cry, pray, thrash limbs, run, hit others, hurt self.
	Often easily distracted; cannot attend or concentrate.
	No learning, problem solving, decision making, or realistic judgments.
	May become immobilized, assume fetal position, become mute, or be unresponsive to directions. Needs protection.
(Psychoses may occur.)	

The General Adaptation Syndrome described earlier can be modified to assess psychological adaptation. In the *Alarm Stage* the person has an increased ability to perceive data, comprehend relationships, and do problem solving. He/she feels mildly anxious but can cope with the situation. Should the feelings of alarm persist, the degree of anxiety heightens and other types of psychic behavior that are less adaptive may be evoked: irritability, anger, demanding, denial, withdrawal, crying, hypersensitivity to noise and confusion, hallucinations, loquaciousness, silence, and eventual panic if the stimuli are overwhelming. Exposure to intense psychological stimuli can cause death.

During the *Resistance Stage* psychological adaptive mechanisms include the behaviors typical of moderate anxiety. The person has a narrowed perceptual field but the ability to focus on a delineated subject or situation while shutting out irrelevant distractions. He/she can comprehend relationships; has a strong feeling of persistence; shows stereotyped, rigid behavior; but does problem solving to attack a problem directly. Various ego-adaptive mechanisms may be used, though not excessively—for example, sublimation, reaction formation, rationalization, selective inattention, displacement, or overcompensation. The Resistance Stage involves some deliberative change of behavior as the person gains control of self, others, or the inanimate environment.

Should the person's attempts at coping with the feelings involved in a situation be unsuccessful, the *Stage of Exhaustion* would be manifested by physical or mental illness (neurosis, psychosis). Now the person gives up coping attempts or uses inappropriate or ineffective behavior. Without help, the person might indeed become chronically ill or even die.

Intervention for the person passing through these stages is crisis intervention, discussed in Chapter 8; relevant techniques of therapeutic communication are discussed in Chapter 3.

You can practice some of the following ways to adapt to stress as well as teach these methods to others.

1. Identify stressful aspects of your lifestyle to reduce frequency of the stress response or to avoid stressors when possible.
2. Analyze what is making you tense or anxious and try to lessen the stressfulness of the situation.
3. Develop spiritual and philosophical resources by talking to others who are wiser than you and by using literature and prayer.
4. Keep something as the central core of your life and being, as your shelter or haven—for example, a religious, philosophical, moral, or ethical belief; a special place in your home to relax; a specific time for doing certain pleasurable activities; or a person who is a confidant and friend.
5. Try to slow your hectic pace. Do one thing at a time.
6. Use temporary avoidance of identified stressors at times for regaining strength, energy, and ideas about fun in order to cope.
7. Assume a more passive attitude toward irritating or frustrating events. Consciously work to remain calm or avoid the problem until you are in a better emotional condition to cope with it.
8. Determine ways to enjoy selected stressors as a challenge by adjusting personal philosophy or behavior patterns.
9. Accept the love and support from others, their encouragement and suggestions; be willing to receive help.
10. Set aside time for relaxation each day. You may want to try relaxation techniques, such as transcendental meditation, yoga, biofeedback, or the relaxation response, or seek sources of joy and humor.
11. Talk about your feelings with friends, family, or a counselor to gain objectivity about the problem, validate ideas and potential solutions, and affirm what you need and want to do.
12. Accept things you cannot change. Do not expect too much from others. Accept your own normal irritation, anger, or crying.
13. Try to correct aspects of your life that cause stress or worry or change a role that doesn't suit you.
14. Don't push yourself beyond your limits of achievement or expect too much of yourself. Be satisfied with less while you do your best.
15. Use physical exercise and recreation to work off the energy of anxiety and to relieve tension. Find a fulfilling hobby or try doing something helpful for someone. Books and audiotapes are available describing relaxation techniques and recreational activities or hobbies.
16. Use visualization, imagery, or faith to affirm the answer to the problem until the solution is reached.

TABLE 7-2 Various Thought Strategies to Handle Stress and Their Rationale

MENTAL RESPONSE	DEFINITION AND RATIONALE
1. Use of knowledge	Learn causes of stress and ways to prevent or manage situation.
2. Objectivity (reality orientation)	Sort out, compare, and validate events, ideas, and emotions to get a total perspective and better understanding on basis of facts, not just feelings; maintain realistic perception.
3. Analysis	Study logically and systematically the component parts of a situation to arrive at realistic explanations and answers; manage part if not all of situation.
4. Concentration (mental self-control)	Deliberately set aside thoughts and feelings unrelated to the situation to master tension, save energy, find answers, and make necessary decisions for the task at hand.
5. Planning	Think through situation prior to action to release tension, promote problem solving, and avoid unnecessary use of energy, error, and consequent frustration.
6. Fantasize (daydream)	Visualize release of tension and successful achievement rather than dwelling on fear of failure, in order to plan strategy, ensure goal-directed action, cope with stressors, and relieve tension.
7. Rehearsal	Fantasize or anticipate event or another's response prior to stressful event in order to practice coping mentally or behaviorally and to gain confidence in ability to manage.
8. Substitution of thoughts and emotions	State ideas and feelings that are different than real ones in order to avoid adding to stressful situation or to meet demands of the situation.
9. Suppression	Hold thoughts and emotions in abeyance or momentarily forget, in order to wait until it is more timely to change behavior, attack a problem, or implement a solution.
10. Valuing	Establish or reaffirm religious or sociocultural values to foster sense of balance and relaxation in face of stressors.
11. Empathy	Imagine how others in the situation are feeling so that behavior can take these feelings into account.
12. Humor	Point out inconsistencies in situation, laugh at self, and use past feelings, ideas, and behavior in order to be playful, keep objective distance from a problem, reduce anxiety, maintain self-identity, enrich solution, and add enjoyment to life.
13. Tolerance of ambiguity	Function in a way that lays the basis for eventual effective solutions when the situation is so complex that it cannot be fully understood or clear choices cannot be made now (28, 45, 64).

(From Murray, Ruth and M. Marilyn Huelskoetter, *Psychiatric/Mental Health Nursing; Giving Emotional Care,* © 1983, pp. 410-411. Reprinted with permission of Prentice-Hall, Inc., Englewood Cliffs, N.J.

17. Use conscious cognitive coping responses, such as those described in Table 7-2.
18. Seek psychotherapy if stress keeps you from functioning at your full capacity.
19. Carry out health promotion measures described in Chapter 1.
20. Realize that stressors are inevitable and can be handled and that some are necessary for survival, learning, development, and self-actualization.

ANTHROPOLOGICAL ADAPTATION

A culture makes adaptation possible through its ideas, inventions, and customs. Together with physiological adaptive processes, culture is a powerful force. The human, for example, is able to live in a wide variety of climates because the body has adjusted gradually to permit survival. People also heat and cool the environment for comfort, control predators and parasites, and domesticate animals and plants for personal needs. We have constructed a variety of lifestyles and patterns of social relationships to guarantee our survival and to free ourselves from the limits of physical environments. Prescribed cultural norms are the most effective adaptive mechanisms that humans use: they affect physical, social, and mental well-being; aid adaptation to diverse situations, environments, and recurring problems; and teach about other environments to which we may have to adapt. In addition, some adaptive modifications are achieved through genetic, physiological, and constitutional capacities that have been transmitted for generations through natural selection or cultural conditioning. Physical mutation may also promote permanent changes in a group if it enables the person to compete successfully and live, promoting adaptation.

Different forms of physical or cultural selection are as follows:

1. Survival of the fittest, in which persons who cannot cope or who have dysfunctional mutant genes are most subject to an inability to reproduce or to early death. This condition is most intense when resources are scarce or competition is intense.
2. Modification of the environment to help the person with a condition that interferes with optimum health. An example is treatment of diabetes, inherited by a recessive gene, which permits a normal life span and adaptation in other spheres.
3. Cultural changes that strive to make the person diversified. Mass uniformity prevents adaptation to changing and diverse environments. Persons living in different regions of the same culture, for example, often live differently in some respects while adhering to the overall value system.

4. Cultural conditioning or teaching the person how best to survive in the environment and life situation (21).

Culture allows diversity within a framework of uniformity (customs, traditions). Today cultural differences are being recognized as factors to be dealt with in nursing practice, especially in the United States with its pluralistic society. Nursing care plans in America, however, often fail to recognize the special care requirements of patients from diverse sociocultural backgrounds and have instead a strong reference to Anglo-American values. Lack of diversity in your thoughts and actions prevents your adaptation to the patient as a person as well as your aiding that individual's adaptation to the illness state. Unit II provides information to widen your understanding in this respect.

SOCIAL ADAPTATION

People need other people to become and remain socialized; consequently, **social adaptation**, *adjusting the self to a group*, is essential. Sensory-deprivation experiments indicate that a continual flow of changing sensory stimuli is necessary for a person's mental health. The infant needs stimulation through touch from another human being. Withholding caresses and normal human contact or similar emotional deprivation utimately results directly or indirectly in physical as well as mental deterioration.

In developing, a person learns to accept symbolic rather than actual touch until the mere act of verbal recognition serves the purpose. The fact that people recognize one another's presence, and thereby offer the social contact necessary for the preservation of health, is more important than what is said.

Sensory stimulation that keeps certain parts of the brain active appears necessary in order to maintain a normal waking state. This need to be recharged by stimulation, especially by social contact, may be regarded as one of the biological origins of group formation. The fear of loneliness (or of lack of social stimulation) is one reason why people are willing to resign part of their individual desires in favor of group consensus while at the same time developing a high proficiency in getting as many satisfactions as possible from socialization (82).

Through social adaptation the human being receives spiritual and emotional nourishment, obtains responses to love and creativity, and attains power and prestige. Threats to the ability to perform in these areas produce the everyday stresses that can cause disability and disease (82).

RESPONSES TO SOCIAL CHANGE

It is imposssible to generalize about social adaptation or to define it as social striving or obtaining cultural goals. The individual's response must be considered objectively. Persons who are comfortable in a social climate of brotherly love and unworldliness, for example, would find it hard to survive or be happy in a competitive world.

The human being adheres to societal expectations, and social behavior evolves from assuming particular social roles. Behavior toward others is prescribed by **social norms,** *rules that define and prescribe performance and attitudes for persons in particular social positions.* There is a certain assumed degree of stability about norms so that each person knows what to expect from others. How norms are lived depends on the person's concept of his/her role and the adaptive reactions of others as well as personal adaptive abilities. If mutual expectations are not met, adaptation to a situation is difficult (55).

Social change is rampant in today's world. Unsuccessful social adaptation to rapid change can contribute to illness, such as ulcers, heart disease, or arthritis. Illness, in turn, may force more social adaptations on the person (25).

Modern individuals are increasingly exposed to stresses of a symbolic nature. For this reason, goals and values determine the response of the whole being toward health or disease. As time evolved, values and goals became a way of life, and the person's performance has reflected the worth of chosen values. In both social and bodily health we have often been more maladapted than not, more sick than well.

Modern Western civilization requires the use of traditional adaptations, as well as new ones, to cope in a changing society. Conflict between the pressures of one's past and pressures newly encountered cause problems for those who change environments, whether the new one be another country, a different work climate, or a new social position. The social and cultural pressures that a person feels, the psychological drive, and innate abilities all influence his/her interpretation of and response to illness (25).

The only stable thing in life is change. The human mind has created social change, ongoing and relentless. Reason has aided us in adaptation, but it has also created challenges. Power beyond the dreams of the past has built a scientific technology that protects us from the elements and from other destructive forces in the environment, but with this life has come new hazards of injury, death, and changes in the air breathed and the food eaten.

Illnesses related to modern technology and to social relationships are gaining attention. Society requires that people live together without destroying each other; differences in people and ideologies must be tolerated for survival. Adaptations fraught with stress accompany these developments. You will need to view the person in the context of biological tendencies, learned patterns of response, and the pressures, both tangible and intangible, to which he/she is exposed. Your assessment of the person must include a search for the forces that arouse, and the mechanisms that regulate, adaptive efforts (82).

Toffler has confronted us with the concept of "future shock," a force he predicts will ensure adaptational breakdown unless people can come to grips with rapid social change. Toffler describes the frequent shifting of families from one place to another, alterations in bureaucratic structures that may speedily engulf the worker in change, and diversity of options and continuing novelty in many life situations. The disposable, transient culture makes it difficult for people to establish roots or pass on culture as a guideline to future generations (78).

Because of the "future shock syndrome," the risk of illness can be predicted from the amount of change present (78). If a person is in the equivalent of the Alarm Stage continually, body defenses weaken. Extreme examples of persons caught in rapidly changing environments are the combat soldier, the flood victim, the culturally dislocated traveler. Other examples include the aged who are uprooted and the person who moves from a rural to an urban environment.

The principles of crisis therapy discussed in Chapter 8 will be useful in helping people adapt to social change. You must constantly adjust to new surroundings, or create new ones, in order to remain adaptive. In nursing you adjust in the work environment to changing client groups and the patient adjusts to the sick role and health care system and workers. You can also develop for yourself and teach others about adaptive behaviors to overcome the stress of constantly changing life, for to deny that change is occurring is to distort reality. Change will seem easier if you are the one initiating at least part of the change. At times you can purposefully focus on one aspect of a situation; eventually, however, awareness must expand to include the total situation.

Find a place for temporary isolation, a retreat where you can shut out the noise and where you can maintain the same environment and routine. Equally indispensable is a set of values, religious, ethical, or philosophical, that will serve as guiding principles in a variety of situations.

FAMILY ADAPTATION

Adaptive responses in the family, *a social system, represent the means by which it maintains an internal equilibrium so that it can fulfill purposes and tasks, deal with stress and crisis, and allow for growth of individual members.* Some capacity for functioning may be sacrificed in order to control conflict and aid work as a unit. But the best functioning family keeps anxiety and conflict within tolerable limits and maintains a balance between effects of the past and new experiences (48). Just as other social systems adapt, so must the family system.

Ideally, the family achieves equilibrium by talking over problems and finding solutions together. Humor, nonsense, shared work, and leisure all help relieve tension. The family members know that certain freedoms exist within their confines that are not available elsewhere. Yet even the most stable family will briefly use the following behaviors to cope with stress, which, in turn, promotes more stress. However, these mechanisms are not overused in healthy families (48).

Adaptive Mechanisms in Family Life

Family conflict can be avoided or minimized through scapegoating, coalitions, withdrawal of emotional ties, fighting, use of family myths, reaction formation, compromise, or designation of a family healer. Two or more of these mechanisms may be used within the same family. If these mechanisms are used exclusively, however, they become defensive and are unlikely to promote resolution of the conflict so that the same issue will arise repeatedly (48).

Scapegoating or Blaming involves labeling one member as the cause of the family trouble and is expressed in the attitude, "If it weren't for you. . . ." Or one member may offer himself as a scapegoat to end an argument by saying, "It's all my fault." Such labeling controls the conflict and reduces anxiety, but it prevents communication that can get at the root of the problem. Growth toward resolution of the problem is prohibited.

Coalitions or Alliances may form when some family members side together against other members. Antagonisms and anger result. Eventually the losing party tries to get control.

Withdrawal of Emotional Ties, loosening the family unit, and reducing communication may be used to handle conflict, but then the family becomes rigid and mechanized. Family members are also likely to seek affection outside the family so that the home becomes a hotel with everyone superficially nice. In some families there is no show of emotion, for such emotion signifies loss of control or giving in to unacceptable impulses.

Repetitive Fighting through verbal abuse, physical battles, loud complaints, curses, or accusations may be used to relieve tension and allow some harmony until the next round. The fight may have the same theme each time stress hits the family. The healthy family allows some "blowing up" as release from everyday frustrations, but it does not make a major case out of every minor incident or temporary disagreement.

Family Myths or Traditional Beliefs can be used to overcome anxieties and maintain control over others. Such statements are as follows: "Children are seen, not heard." "We can't survive if you leave home." "Talking about feelings will cause loss of love." In contrast the healthy family members encourage growth and creativity rather than rigid control.

Reaction Formation is seen in a family in which there is superficial harmony or togetherness. Traumatic ideas are repressed and transformed into the opposite behavior. Everybody smiles but nobody loves. No one admits to having any difficulties. Great tension is felt because true feelings are not expressed.

Resignation or Compromise may provide temporary harmony when someone gives up or suppresses the need for assertion, affection, or emotional expression in order to keep peace. The surface calm eventually explodes when unmet needs can no longer be successfully suppressed.

Designation of One Person as Family Healer or Umpire involves using a "wise one" (most often in the extended family), or a minister, storekeeper, bartender, or druggist to arrange a reconciliation between dissenting parties. Part of the dynamics sometimes underlying the helper role is that the referee gets great satisfaction from finding someone worse off than self. The healer feels a sense of heightened self-esteem or omnipotence. A variant of the healer role is that of family "protector." Here one person takes on all the stresses in order to save other members stress or conflict. One person ends up fighting the battles for everyone else in the family.

You may find yourself in the role of family healer. Help the family to develop harmonious ways of coping and avoid the protector or omnipotent role.

INADEQUATE ADAPTATION

Disturbances in adaptation (nonconstructive behavior) result in illness or various disorders—physically, emotionally, socially. Some behaviors that are adaptive for a time become defensive or inadequate if used for prolonged periods. Illness or sensory distortions may, in turn, cause or further enhance disturbed adaptation. Inadequate adaptation may occur when there is

1. Failure to sense change, present or coming; selective focusing on the here-and-now.
2. Adherence to values or beliefs no longer considered valid by the social environment.
3. Undue commitment to unrealistic, immoral, unethical, or inhumane goals.
4. Use of adaptive mechanisms no longer appropriate.
5. Resistance to rational change.
6. Presence of physical disease or disability.
7. Sensory distortion or deprivation.
8. Failure to discriminate because of thought disturbances or organic problems.
9. Severe anxiety feelings.
10. Overspecialization, limiting one's ability to adapt to new and changing circumstances.
11. Focusing on the involved body part or only one aspect of a situation rather than the entire body or situation (50).

Yet *apparently maladaptive behavior should be considered as the best that the person is capable of at that time*. So-called deviant behavior may actually be adaptive and may eventually promote constructive change in or for the person or group. Adaptive deviance is seen in the client who demands control over herself and his/her treatment, for example, or in the nonconformist nurse who views a situation from a different perspective, acts accordingly, and improves nursing care as a result. Also, inadequate behavior in one person may permit others in a group to function appropriately as a result. When a person is sick, the symptoms and problems may inadvertently preserve family equilibrium by drawing attention away from family conflicts. The sick member may be designated the scapegoat or patient even though other family members are more socially or emotionally ill.

IMPLICATIONS FOR NURSING

Adaptation is a concept that can provide a unifying structure for nursing practice. It can link together the mass of information considered necessary to professional nursing practice. It helps you see how various factors affecting the person do not exist in isolation but in a multidimensional whole. It helps you more accurately predict and more effectively help each person adapt to a crisis, illness, or disability.

If you are in a leadership position, teach your coworkers to report signs and symptoms of adaptational failure, such as restlessness, withdrawal, rigidity in behavior, or inability to make a decision, just as they would note a disease symptom. Your knowledge of the patient's *accustomed* adaptive pattern, obtained through a nursing history, will help you formulate a plan of care to meet special needs. Assess needs, ways of coping, and the predominant stimuli affecting that person. If inadequate adaptation is occurring, attempt to modify or manipulate the stimuli to make a positive response possible. Adjusting the physical environment or using methods of purposeful communication is a way to enhance adaptation.

You can use adaptation theory as an independent nurse practitioner. You might be available in a community to promote adaptation where circumstances are making harmful demands—where a disease has broken out or a natural disaster occurred. Or you might do health teaching, diet counseling, support before surgery, discharge planning, and health maintenance among those persons in the community who have health problems in varying degrees.

Whatever the setting in which you practice, your assessments must be based on scientific knowledge, combined with an appreciation of the individual's behavioral responses. There are three basic forms of nursing intervention: (1) support and maintain adaptive behaviors, (2) teach and counsel in order to provide the person with additional or alternative behaviors that would enhance adaptation, and (3) modify physiological, emotional and behavioral patterns to reduce dysfunction (3). When your intervention influences adaptation favorably and promotes social well-being, it is *therapeutic*. If you cannot alter the course of adaptation and your best efforts only maintain the status quo or a slow downhill course, you are acting in a *supportive* role (36).

Adaptation as a concept is applicable to the nurse as well as the patient/client for you will have to adapt to a new and different perspective and lifestyle as you involve yourself actively in the profession. You may feel threatened at times by the challenges. An understanding of yourself and your adaptive capacities will help you to keep faith in yourself and your ability to cope, adapt, learn, grow. You will become more comfortable with change and challenge, recognizing that they are part of normal adult living.

So far this chapter has considered the concept of adaptation in its broadest sense. The two sections forming the rest of the chapter deal with matters crucial to adaptation: the maintenance of biological rhythms and the hazards of immobility. Related nursing responsibilities are also discussed in each section.

REFERENCES

1. **Alexander, Franz,** "The Development of Psychosomatic Medicine," in *New Dimensons in Psychosomatic Medicine*, ed. C. W. Wahl. Boston: Little, Brown & Company, 1964.
2. **Antonovsky, A.,** *Health, Stress and Coping*. San Francisco: Jossey-Bass, Inc., Publishers, 1979.
3. **Auger, Jeanine,** *Behavioral Systems and Nursing*. Englewood Cliffs, NJ: Prentice-Hall, Inc., 1976.
4. **Beland, Irene,** ed., *Clinical Nursing: Pathophysiological and Psychosocial Approaches* (4th ed.). New York: Macmillan, Inc., 1981.
5. **Benenson, Abram,** *Control of Communicable Diseases in Man* (12th ed.). Washington, D.C.: American Public Health Association, Inc., 1975.
6. **Benson, Herbert,** and **Miriam Z. Klipper,** *The Relaxation Response*. New York: Avon Books, 1976.
7. **Bergersen, Betty S.,** "Adaptation as a Unifying Theory," in *Theoretical Issues in Professional Nursing*, ed. Juanita F. Murphy. New York: Appleton-Century-Crofts, 1971.
8. **Brock, Thomas,** and **Katherine Brock,** *Basic Microbiology with Applications*. Englewood Cliffs, NJ: Prentice-Hall, Inc., 1978.
9. **Brock, Lord, J. M. Skinner,** and **J. T. Manders,** "Observations on Peripheral and Central Temperatures with Particular Reference to the Occurrence of Vasoconstriction," *The British Journal of Surgery*, 62, no. 8 (1975), 589–95.
10. **Brown, Barbara B.,** *New Mind, New Body*. New York: Bantam Books, 1975.
11. **Brunner, Lillian,** and **Doris Suddarth,** *Textbook of Medical Surgical Nursing* (4th ed.). Philadelphia: J. B. Lippincott Company, 1980.
12. **Burd, Shirley F.,** "A Psychological Approach to Adaptation," in *Theoretical Issues in Professional Nursing*, ed. Juanita F. Murphy. New York: Appleton-Century-Crofts, 1971.
13. **Burnes, A. J.,** and **S. J. Roen,** "Social Roles and Adaptation to the Community," *Community Mental Health Journal*, 3 (1967), 156.
14. **Byrne, M.,** and **L. Thompson,** *Key Concepts for the Study and Practice of Nursing*. St. Louis: The C. V. Mosby Company, 1972.
15. **Clark, Carolyn,** "Reframing," *American Journal of Nursing*, 77, no. 5 (1977), 840–41.
16. **Clark, Matt,** and **Sharon Begley,** "The Making of a Miracle Drug," *Newsweek*, January 28, 1980, pp. 82–83.
17. **Coelho, George, David Hamburg,** and **John Adams,** *Coping and Adaptation*. New York: Basic Books, Inc., 1974.
18. **Collins, K.,** and **J. Weiner,** *Human Adaptability: A History and Compendium of Research in the International Biological Programme*. London: Taylor and Francis Publishers, 1977.
19. **Conroy, R. T. W. L.,** and **J. N. Mills,** *Human Circadian Rhythms*. London: J. & A. Churchill, 1970.
20. **Coulter, P.,** and **M. J. Brower,** "Parallel Experience: An Interview Technique," *American Journal of Nursing*, 68, no. 5 (1968), 1028.

21. **Dobzhansky, T.**, "Man and Natural Selection," in *Man in Adaptation: The Biosocial Background*, ed. Y. A. Cohen. Chicago: Aldine Publishing Company, 1968, pp. 37–48.
22. **Dubos, René**, *Man Adapting*. New Haven: Yale University Press, 1965.
23. **Edholm, O.**, *Man: Hot and Cold*. London: Edward Arnold Publishers, Ltd., 1978.
24. **Eisendorfer, Carl**, "Anxiety in the Aged," in *Phenomenology and Treatment of Anxiety*, eds. W. Fann et al. New York: Spectrum Publications, Inc., 1979, pp. 43–49.
25. **Engel, G.**, *Psychological Development in Health and Disease*. Philadelphia: W. B. Saunders Company, 1962.
26. **Evans, Frances Monet Carter**, *Psychosocial Nursing: Theory and Practice in Hospital and Community Mental Health*. New York: Macmillan, Inc., 1971.
27. **Fink, Max**, "Anxiety, Anxiolytics, and the Human EEG," in *Phenomenology and Treatment of Anxiety*, eds. W. Fann et al. New York: Spectrum Publications, Inc., 1979, pp. 237–50.
28. **Flynn, Patricia**, *Holistic Health: The Art and Science of Care*. Bowie, MD: Robert J. Brady Co., 1980.
29. **Freese, Arthur**, "Only $100 Trillion a Gram: Interferon Has a Future!" *Science Digest*, 87, no. 4 (1980), 49–53.
30. **Frobisher, Martin**, and **R. Fuerst**, *Microbiology in Health and Disease*. Philadelphia: W. B. Saunders Company, 1973.
31. **Fuerst, Robert**, *Microbiology in Health and Disease* (14th ed.). Philadelphia: W. B. Saunders Company, 1978.
32. **Heath, D.**, *Man at High Altitude: The Pathophysiology of Acclimatization and Adaptation*. Edinburgh: Churchill Livingstone, 1977.
33. **Horowitz, Mardi**, *Stress Response Syndromes*. New York: Jason Aronson, Inc., 1976.
34. **Johnston, Dorothy**, and **Gail Hood**, *Total Patient Care: Foundations and Practice* (2nd ed.). St. Louis: The C. V. Mosby Company, 1976.
35. **Langley, L. L**, *Homeostasis*. New York: Reinhold Book Corporation, 1965.
36. **Levine, M.**, "Adaptation and Assessment: A Rationale for Nursing Intervention," *American Journal of Nursing*, 66, no. 11 (1966), 2450–53.
37. **Levinson, D. J.**, "Role, Personality, and Social Structure in the Organizational Setting," *Journal of Abnormal Psychology*, 58 (1959), 170.
38. **Lief, Harold**, "Anxiety, Sexual Dysfunction, and Therapy," in *Phenomenology and Treatment of Anxiety*, eds. W. Fann et al. New York: Spectrum Publications, Inc., 1979, pp. 311–24.
39. **Lipowski, Z. J.**, "Physical Illness, the Individual, and the Coping Process," *Psychiatry in Medicine*, 1, no. 4 (1970), 91–102.
40. **Luckman, Joan**, and **Karen Sorensen**, eds., *Medical-Surgical Nursing: A Psychophysiologic Approach* (2nd ed.). Philadelphia: W. B. Saunders Company, 1980.
41. **Marcinek, Margaret**, "Stress in the Surgical Patient," *American Journal of Nursing*, 77, no. 11 (1977), 1809–11.
42. **Marshall, Eliot**, "Gambling on Interferon," *Science*, 216, no. 4550 (1982), 1078–79.

43. **Maykoski, Kathleen, Marilyn Rubin,** and **Sr. Agnita Day,** "Effect of Cigarette Smoking on Postural Muscle Tremor," *Nursing Research*, 25, no. 1 (1976), 39-43.
44. **McAdams, Constance,** "Interferon: The Penicillin of the Future?" *American Journal of Nursing*, 80, no. 4 (1980), 714-18.
45. **McKay, Matthew, Martha Davis,** and **Patrick Fanning,** *Thoughts and Feelings: The Art of Cognitive Stress Intervention.* Richmond, CA: New Harbinger Publications, 1981.
46. **McKay, Rose,** "Theories, Models, and Systems for Nursing," *Nursing Research*, 18, no. 5 (1969), 393-99.
47. **McLeod, Dorothy L.,** "Physiological Model," in *Theoretical Issues in Professional Nursing*, ed. Juanita F. Murphy. New York: Appleton-Century-Crofts, 1971.
48. **Messer, Alfred,** *The Individual in His Family, An Adaptational Study.* Springfield, IL: Charles C Thomas, Publisher, 1970.
49. **Moos, R. H.,** *Human Adaptation: Coping with Life Crises.* Lexington, MA: D. C. Heath & Company, 1976.
50. **Murphy, Juanita,** ed., *Theoretical Issues in Professional Nursing.* New York: Appleton-Century-Crofts, 1971.
51. **Murray, Ruth,** and **M. Marilyn Huelskoetter,** *Psychiatric/Mental Health Nursing: Giving Emotional Care.* Englewood Cliffs, NJ: Prentice-Hall, Inc., 1983.
52. **Murray, Ruth,** and **Judith Zentner,** *Nursing Assessment and Health Promotion through the Life Span* (3rd ed.). Englewood Cliffs, NJ: Prentice-Hall, Inc., 1985.
53. National Institute of Mental Health, *Biological Rhythms in Psychiatry and Medicine.* Washington, D.C.: United States Department of Health, Education, and Welfare, 1970.
54. **Norton, Cynthia Friend,** *Microbiology.* Reading, MA: Addison-Wesley Publishing Co., Inc., 1981.
55. **Parsons, T.,** *Structure and Process in Modern Societies.* Glencoe, IL: The Free Press, 1960.
56. **Peplau, Hildegarde,** *Interpersonal Relations in Nursing.* New York: G. P. Putnam's Sons, 1952.
57. **Ponte, Lowell,** "How a Change in the Weather Changes You," *Reader's Digest*, March 1982, pp. 55-62.
58. **Rahe, Richard H., Joseph D. McKean, Jr.,** and **Ransom J. Arthur,** "A Longitudinal Study of Life-Change and Illness Patterns," *Journal of Psychosomatic Research*, 10 (1967), 355-66.
59. **Reres, Mary,** "Coping with Stress in Nursing," *The American Nurse*, 9, no. 9 (1977), 4.
60. **Richter, Curt,** *Biological Clocks in Medicine and Psychiatry.* Springfield, IL: Charles C Thomas, 1965.
61. **Roessler, Robert,** and **Jerry Lester,** "Vocal Patterns in Anxiety," in *Phenomenology and Treatment of Anxiety*, eds. W. Fann et al. New York: Spectrum Publications, Inc., 1979, pp. 225-35.
62. **Roy, Sr. Callista,** *Introduction to Nursing: An Adaptation Model.* Englewood Cliffs, NJ: Prentice-Hall, Inc., 1976.

63. **Samuels, Mike,** and **Hal Bennett,** *The Well Body Book*. New York: Random House, Inc., 1973.
64. **Saranson, Irvin,** and **Barbara Saranson,** *Abnormal Psychology: The Problem of AdaptiveBehavior* (3rd ed.). Englewood Cliffs, NJ: Prentice-Hall, Inc., 1980.
65. **Selkurt, Ewald,** ed., *Basic Physiology for the Health Sciences* (2nd ed.). Boston: Little, Brown & Company, 1982.
66. **Settlemire, Thomas,** and **William Hughes,** *Microbiology for Health Students*. Reston, VA: Reston Publishing Company, 1978.
67. **Seyle, Hans,** *The Stress of Life*. New York: McGraw-Hill Book Company, 1956.
68. _____, "Stress Syndrome," *American Journal of Nursing*, 65, no. 3 (1965), 97-99.
69. _____, *Stress without Distress*. Philadelphia: J. B. Lippincott Company, 1974.
70. _____, "Implications of Stress Concept," *New York State Journal of Medicine*, October 1975, pp. 2139–45.
71. _____, *The Stress of Life* (rev. ed). New York: McGraw-Hill Book Company, 1976.
72. _____, "Forty Years of Stress Research: Principal Remaining Problems and Misconceptions," *Canadian Medical Association Journal*, 115 (July 3, 1976), 53-56.
73. _____, "Stress and the Reduction of Distress," *Primary Cardiology*, 5, no. 8 (1979), 22-30.
74. **Shafer, Kathleen, Janet Sawyer, Audrey McCluskey, Edna Beck,** and **Wilma Phipps,** *Medical-Surgical Nursing* (7th ed.). St. Louis: The C. V. Mosby Company, 1980.
75. **Smith, Alice Lorraine,** *Microbiology and Pathology*. St. Louis: The C. V. Mosby Company, 1976.
76. **Stephenson, Carol,** "Stress in Critically Ill Patients," *American Journal of Nursing*, 77, no. 11 (1977), 1806-9.
77. **Stewart, E.,** "To Lessen Pain: Relaxation and Rhythmic Breathing," *American Journal of Nursing*, 76, no. 6 (1976), 958-59.
78. **Toffler, Alvin,** *Future Shock*. New York: Random House, Inc., 1970.
79. **Vander, Arthur, James Sherman,** and **Dorothy Luciano,** *Human Physiology: The Mechanisms of Body Function* (3rd ed.). New York: McGraw-Hill Book Company, 1980.
80. **Williams, Cindy,** and **Thomas Holmes,** "Life Change, Human Adaptation, and Onset of Illness," in *Clinical Practice in Psychosocial Nursing: Assessment and Intervention*, eds. Dianne Longo and Reg Williams. New York: Appleton-Century-Crofts, 1978, pp. 69-85.
81. **Williams, R., et al.,** "Disturbed Sleep and Anxiety," in *Phenomenology and Treatment of Anxiety*, eds. W. Fann et al. New York: Spectrum Publications, Inc., 1979, pp. 211-23.
82. **Wolf, Stewart,** and **Helen Goodell,** eds., *Stress and Disease*. Springfield, IL: Charles C Thomas, Publisher, 1968.
83. **Yamamoto, William S.,** "Homeostasis, Continuity, and Feedback," in *Physiological Controls and Regulations*, eds. William S. Yamamoto and John R. Brobeck. Philadelphia: W. S. Saunders Company, 1965.

84. **Zung, William,** "Assessment of Anxiety Disorder: Qualitative and Quantitative Approaches," in *Phenomenology and Treatment of Anxiety*, eds. W. Fann et al. New York: Spectrum Publications, Inc., 1979, pp. 1-17.

Section I

RELATIONSHIP OF BIOLOGICAL RHYTHMS TO MAINTENANCE OF ADAPTATION

DEFINITIONS

Self-sustaining, repetitive, rhythmic patterns found in plants, animals, and man are termed **biological rhythms.** Biological rhythms are found throughout our external and internal environment and are basic to our adaptation and survival. Biological rhythms may be exogenous or endogenous.

Exogenous rhythms *depend on the rhythm of external evironmental events*, such as seasonal variations, lunar revolution, or night-and-day cycle, which function as time givers. These events help to synchronize internal rhythms with external environmental stimuli and establish an internal time pattern or biological clock.

Endogenous rhythms arise *within the organism*, such as sleep-wake and sleep-dream cycles. Endogenous and exogenous rhythms are usually synchronized. Many internal rhythms do not readily alter their repetitive patterns, however, even when the external stimuli are removed. For instance, when a person shifts to sleeping by day and waking at night, as frequently happens with nurses, a transient or temporary desynchronization occurs. Body temperature and adrenal hormone levels are usually low during the sleep cycle. With the shift in sleep and walking, the person is awake and making demands on the body during the usual sleep period. Three weeks may be needed before internal rhythms adapt to shift. A similar period of desynchronization occurs when a person makes a flight crossing time zones (30, 50, 51).

Within any 24-hour period, physiological and psychological functions reach maximum and minimum limits. When a physiological function approaches a high or low limit, the body's feedback mechanisms attempt to counterregulate the action. *This form of endogenous rhythm that reoccurs in a cyclic pattern within a 20- to 28-hour period is a* **circadian rhythm.** Body temperature, blood pressure, urine production, and hormone, blood sugar, hemoglobin, and amino acid levels demonstrate this rhythmic pattern. Similar variations or rhythms in the levels of alertness, fatigue, tenseness, and irritability can also be demonstrated.

CIRCADIAN RHYTHMS IN WELLNESS

Rhythms occur throughout the life cycle of each individual. From the time of birth different body structures and functions develop circadian rhythmicity at different rates.

Development of Rhythmicity

Pediatric researchers and physiologists have contributed to the timetable of physiologic rhythms in infancy. Their research has revealed the following information.

1. The only circadian rhythm recorded in the first weeks of life is the periodicity of electric skin resistance; resistance is high in the morning and low at night.
2. The infant's sleep-wakefulness patterns begin to take on adult circadian regularity by the third week of life with periods of wakefulness occurring most often during the early morning hours and about 5 P.M.
3. Normal-term infants display a 40- to 50-minute sleep cycle with approximately one-half of the cycle spent in a REM state.
4. At the end of the fifth and sixth months of life, body temperature, heart rate, and urine volume excretion show high peaks in the daytime hours and lows at night during sleep.
5. Almost all body functions have assumed circadian characteristics with a day-night fluctuation near the adult pattern by the ninth month of life.
6. Urine excretion levels of phosphate, creatine, creatinine, and chloride show a day-night difference by 16 to 22 months of age.
7. Human growth hormone secretion for infants peaks during REM sleep.
8. Periodicity in blood sugar level and blood pressure patterns were demonstrated by the age of 7 (2, 14, 40).

Decline of Rhythmicity

The aging process is generally described as an inevitable gradual decline; after maturity there is reported to be a slow but steady deterioration of efficient body function. Research has shown that the internal time is at least partly influenced by neural and metabolic processes. With normal aging, oxygen consumption during activity decreases by about 50 percent and kidney function decreases. The change in metabolism and altered circulation of electrolytes, oxygen, creatinine, and urea nitrogen all influence the energy supply, activity capacity, and invisible rhythms (18, 20, 44).

Mental Efficiency, Performance, and Circadian Rhythms

Circadian rhythms develop throughout the life cycle. Mental efficiency and performance have been related to rhythm in body temperature and catecholamine excretion in the adult.

In human beings the body temperature rises and drops by approximately 2 degrees over each 24-hour period. The body temperature begins to decline about 10 P.M., is lowest on awaking, gradually rises during the morning, levels off in the afternoon, and then drops again in the evening. The level of adrenocortical hormone secretion appears correlated with body temperature rhythms and the individual's state of alertness and wakefulness. The level of adrenocortical hormones rises early in the morning, peaks around the time we typically awaken, and then drops to a low point by late evening (23, 47, 53). Usually the best mental and physical performances coincide with peak temperature and the least desirable performances tend to coincide with intervals of lowest body temperature. In addition, studies have shown that the lowest excretory rates of epinephrine in day-active people correlate with the time of maximum fatigue and poorest performance (30, 53).

Studies have also shown that the daytime performance on verbal and spatial matching tasks does not remain constant but fluctuates cyclically within a 90- to 100-minute period. When performance improves in one task, the individual's skill decreases in another (28). Researchers have theorized that many disasters were the result of failure to consider human biology. For example, at the nuclear accident at Three Mile Island, the three young men in the control area worked on a shift system called slow rotation—days for a week, evenings for a week, and late nights for a week. Such a rotation causes a desynchronization of circadian rhythms that alters performance levels. The President's investigating commission stated that during the first two hours of the accident the operators ignored and failed to recognize the significance of several items that should have warned them that they had an open valve and an accident related to loss of coolant (23).

CIRCADIAN RHYTHMS IN ILLNESS

Data confirms an interrelationship between circadian rhythm and mental or physical illness. Also, the pattern of living taught by the culture affects body rhythms. Epidemiological research continues to seek further correlations among these factors. A few examples of how circadian rhythms influence illness are presented next. (For a more extensive discussion, refer to references 5, 7, 10, 29, 42, 51, and 53, listed at the end of Section 1.)

Diagnostic Cues

Observing the integration of the body's rhythms (or lack of such integration) can be used to determine the person's health status. Diagnosis and treatment of some illnesses can be determined from the study of circadian rhythms or biological time. In some instances, the illness alters the pattern of circadian rhythm. Other illnesses show exaggerated or decreased symptoms at a particular biological time. Blood pressure and temperature values, laboratory findings, and biopsy specimens for cell study differ according to the biological time of day. For instance, growth hormone levels in the blood are highest during the night hours; therefore routine blood values taken at 8 A.M. will not give a total picture. The percentage of red blood cells drops about 4½ percent late at night; a decrease in red blood cells of 5 percent prompts blood transfusions in some hospitals. Ambiguous laboratory findings, the need for repeated medical tests, and the potential for unnecessary medical therapies can be avoided if the person's normal biological rhythms are considered first.

Rhythmic time cycles appear to influence many aspects of human life. Births and deaths occur more frequently at night and during the early morning. Persons with ulcers and allergies suffer more in the spring; allergic responses, including asthmatic attacks, occur more frequently at night and in the early morning hours. There are certain yearly peaks in the number of suicides, psychotic episodes, and accidents. Eventually knowledge about circadian rhythms and biological time may serve as a major tool in preventive health programs.

Depression

A definite relationship is seen between health and the rhythmicity of depressed people. Altered biochemical rhythms, diurnal (daytime) mood swings, and altered sleep cycles have been noted. Researchers have hypothesized that abnormalities of sleep patterns in some types of depression are due to abnormal internal phase relationships of circadian rhythms. The circadian rhythm of REM sleep may occur abnormally early (52). * Depressed persons usually experience insomnia or periods of predawn wakefulness. Their sleep cycles are shortened and

*See Murray and Zentner, *Nursing Assessment and Health Promotion Through the Life Span*, Chapter 8, for a discussion of the adult sleep-wake cycle.

fragmented and they are easily disturbed by environmental changes. Successful treatment frequently comes in the form of antidepressant drugs that can slow biological clocks (that is, lithium carbonate) or speed biological clocks (that is imipramine) (4).

Various mental functions and the emotion, behaviors, and autonomic responses associated with them depend on certain chemicals secreted at the synapses of the neurons in specific pathways of the brain. Several brain neurotransmitters (norepinephrine, dopamine, serotonin, and acetylcholine) undergo cyclic changes in amount of chemical present. These fluctuations are thought to be related to factors concerned with periodicity and emotion (28, 31, 48, 53).

Cancer

Cells in almost every tissue of our body divide or reproduce in a circadian rhythm. Normal cells show intervals of accelerated reproductive activity. In human beings, for example, skin and liver cells are more active at night. Cancer cells do not reproduce at the same rate as normal cells; abnormal mitosis (cell-reproduction) rhythms and, in many instances, a complete lack of circadian rhythm have been reported.

Research suggests that people who are desynchronized or constantly consuming foods and drugs that change the phase of their circadian rhythms may be a high risk group for cancer (53). Health teaching should include the need to decrease the intake of coffee, tea, and certain barbiturates that may be carcinogens.

Successful treatment of cancer with radiation relies on the fact that x-ray therapy diminishes the noncircadian mitosis of cancer cells. Research has indicated that an animal's resistance to cancer drugs is high at one time and low at another (23, 42). Optimum effectiveness of drug therapy can be achieved by changing the drug dosage and time of administration to coincide with the low in the cycle of resistance.

Adrenal Hormone Production

The blood and urine concentrations of adrenocorticosteroid hormones in persons on schedules of diurnal activity and nocturnal sleep drop at night and rise to highest levels in early morning. The course of the adrenal cycle may also be followed by measuring the eosinophil (white blood cell) level; eosinophils decrease as the blood level of adrenal hormones increases.

Light is probably the synchronizer of the adrenocorticosteroid rhythm. This factor has implications for people who are night workers or who have varying degrees of blindness. Because adrenal hormones control other circadian rhythms within the body, knowledge of their cycle is important in the study and treatment of numerous conditions.

Low blood levels of adrenal hormones affect the nervous system and cause a person to be more sensitive to sounds, tastes, and smell. Sensory acuity reaches its maximum at the time of lowest steroid levels. A sudden drop in acuity occurs in the early morning as steroid levels begin to rise. A person is therefore better able to detect taste, smell, or sound at the end of the day. Daily fatigue from lack of sleep and neurologically related symptoms associated with adrenal insufficiency (Addison's disease) may be related to low levels of adrenal hormones.

Adrenal rhythm is also important in handling certain allergies. Sensitivity to histamine follows a circadian rhythm: It peaks about the time of evening or night when adrenocorticosteroids are reaching their lowest levels. Nasal congestion from hayfever, skin reactions from drug sensitivity, and breathing crises in asthma patients occur more frequently during the evening or night (42, 53). Suggest to individuals with hayfever and asthma that they do their gardening and weeding in the morning when their adrenocorticosteroid levels are at their highest.

Rhythm Alteration by Drugs

Circadian rhythms can be altered by drugs. Actinomycin-D (an antibiotic) can alter the rhythms of synthesis within the cell's DNA (deoxyribonucleic acid) and RNA (ribonucleic acid) molecules. This shift in rhythm may, in turn, alter the circadian rhythm of some central nervous system functions. Such barbiturates as sodium pentobarbital and sodium thiomylal may also shift circadian rhythms. These drugs suppress the normal rhythm of adrenal hormones, which may account for some of the hangover effect, mental blunting, and confusion that frequently accompany their use (5, 36).

Some drugs may be given deliberately to produce altered circadian rhythms. Certain enzyme inhibitors are being used experimentally to shift the circadian activity-sleep cycle. Other drugs, tricyclic antidepressants, extend the period of the sleep cycle. Methylated xanthines (theophylline in tea, caffeine in coffee) can advance or retard the biological clock, depending on the phase of the rhythm in which they are taken (4, 23, 31, 42). Attempts are also being made to discover if certain adrenal hormones will lessen the period of transient desynchronization that occurs when a person enters a different time zone (51).

IMPLICATIONS FOR NURSING

Altered Rhythms Resulting from Hospital Environment

Because our cyclic functioning is synchronized with environmental stimuli, physiological disequilibrium or maladaption occurs whenever we are confronted with environmental or schedule changes. Transient desychronization may occur whenever a person is exposed to the hospital or nursing home stimuli. New noise levels, lighting patterns, schedules for eating, sleeping, and personal hygiene, and unfamiliar persons intruding on the person's privacy may all contribute to this desynchronization. Disturbed mental and physical well-being and increased subjective fatigue reflect the conflict between the internal time pattern and external events. Several days are usually required before the person adapts to the environment and thereby regains synchronization—normal biological rhythms.

You can control some external factors, such as meals, baths, and various tests, make them more nearly similar to the patient's normal (outside) routine, and lessen the stress to which the patient is subjected. Obtaining and using a nursing history is one method of lessening this stress.

A nursing history is directed at getting information about the patient's pre-illness or prehospitalization patterns for sleep, rest, food and fluid intake, elimination, and personal hygiene (see Fig. 7-4). You can ask the following questions: Do you consider yourself a "day" person or a "night" person? Do you feel cheerful when you first wake up? If you feel irritable when you first wake up, how long does this last? Do you have a time of day when you feel that you function best? How do you feel when travel or hospitalization causes you to change your habits (49)? Once this information has been obtained, nursing actions can be initiated that support the patient's established daily patterns and possibly prevent total disruption of body rhythms during hospitalization.

After the patient has been hospitalized for a few days, certain objective data are available that will assist you in determining a rough estimate of the person's circadian patterns. The routine graphic record supplies information about the patient's vital signs. Using this source, you might be able to identify peaks and lows in blood pressure, pulse, or temperature curves. Such a graph could also reveal if the three functions vary together, as in the case of most individuals, or if there is some desynchrony present. Also, an intake and output record that shows both the time and the amount voided will aid in determining the patient's daily urinary-excretory pattern. If the patient is not on intake and output, you might ask that he/she keep an output record for a few days so that biological rhythms can be assessed (49).

Circadian Rhythm Log

In addition to the postadmission nursing history, a daily log of sleep and waking hours, meal times, hunger periods, voiding and defecation patterns, diurnal moods, and other circadian rhythms recorded for 28

FIGURE 7-4 History of Pre-Illness Patterns

Patient's Name: Sociocultural data:

Diagnosis:

Admitting Date ____________________ Date of History____________________

History obtained by____________________

Habits of Daily Living:

1. Food habits: Diet:
   A. Meal patterns: Time Usual Foods
      Breakfast
      Lunch
      Dinner
      Snacks
   B. Food dislikes:
   C. Food allergies:
   D. Foods which disagree or cause discomfort:

2. Fluid habits:
   A. Fluid preferences:
   B. Fluid dislikes:
   C. Usual amount of fluid intake prior to illness:

3. Sleep habits:
   A. Usual bedtime?
   B. Usual number of hours of sleep?
   C. Get up during the night?
   D. Nap habits?
   E. Number of pillows desired?
   F. Number of blankets desired?
   G. If unable to sleep at home, what things do you do that help you fall asleep?

4. General hygiene:
   A. Bathing preference: Usual time
      Tub __________ __________
      Shower__________ __________
   B. Care of teeth: Usual time of cleaning
      Natural __________ __________
      Dentures__________ __________

FIGURE 7-4 (cont.)

5. Elimination:
   A. Usual bowel habits:
      Frequency ________ Time ____________
   B. Bowel irregularities:
      Constipation? _______ Diarrhea? __________
      What usually helps regularity?
   C. Urinary habits:
      Frequency of voiding:
      Bladder irregularities:

Any questions from the patient:

Observations made during history-taking:

---

days prior to hospitalization can help determine the person's cyclic patterns. Diagnostic tests and certain forms of medical and nursing therapy can then be appropriately prescribed by using the person's own baseline rhythms measurements. Determination of each patient's rhythms before, during, and after hospitalization or illness will eventually be possible when more simplified, economical, and accurate measurement devices are available.

You can also establish your own circadian patterns to help you to gain insight into physical feelings and behaviors. You can use this information to plan your days to advantage. You might choose to cope with the most difficult patient assignment during the time of peak mental and physical performance, for example.

Drug Response and Administration

Drug effectiveness can be altered by the time of day that the particular drug is administered. Aspirin administered at 7 A.M. will remain 22 hours in the body; aspirin administered at 7 P.M. will last 17 hours. Some antihistamines last only 6 to 8 hours if taken at night but are effective 15 to 17 hours when taken at 7 A.M. Digitalis (a cardiac glycoside) is several times more effective when administered in the early morning than when administered at other times. The dosage of analgesics needed to relieve pain during the evening or dark hours is more than that needed during the daytime. Sensitivity to pain increases in the evening (51, 53).

People respond differently to drugs. Recent research indicates that the effectiveness of most drugs is influenced by the individual's biological clock. A drug taken at one time acts differently than the same drug, in the same dose, taken a few hours later or earlier. The action of the drug is affected by the person's physiological functions at the time of administration (31, 53).

Circadian rhythms are also important factors in determining drug toxicity. A distinct 24-hour rhythm of vulnerability or resistance to drugs has been identified. Before setting a drug's toxic level, both the person's biological clock and the drug dosage must be considered. At present, problems exist in determining toxicity levels. Federal research guidelines do not consider the circadian rhythms of the animals being tested. Noctural animals are tested in the daytime; animals are tested before they have had time to adjust to a new laboratory environment; animals are tested in light and dark cycles that are not regulated; and animals whose feeding schedules are not fixed and recorded are tested. All these factors can cause altered rhythms in animals and altered vulnerability or resistance to the drug being tested (23, 32). For example, when rats were given a nearly lethal dose of amphetamine at one time in their circadian cycle, 6 percent of them died. At another time in the cycle 78 percent died (23).

One area of **chronopharmacology** *(study of cellular rhythms in relationship to drug therapy)* that has been researched extensively is the relationship of adrenocortical function and corticosteroid drug administration. The secretion of corticosteroids by the adrenal cortex has a 24-hour rhythm, with the highest corticosteroid values expected after the usual time of awakening. When corticosteroids are administered either daily or on alternate days, adrenal suppression and possibly growth disturbance can be minimized by timing to the circadian crest in adrenocortical function (46). Morning doses of prednisolone (a glucocorticosteroid) are less likely to cause alterations in the rhythmic pattern of urinary excretion than twice-daily divided doses or a single dose in the late evening (42).

Without the aid of suitable measurement devices, it is impossible to determine a person's biological clock. Drug administration is therefore usually based on other factors. Most medications are given before or after meals, at bedtime, or at the convenience of nursing personnel and patients. In the future, as knowledge of the internal clock increases, you, the nurse, will find yourself altering drug administration times to suit the person's biological time. Perhaps you will be in charge of a master computer that, after analyzing information about each person's biological clock, will send the appropriate medication dose at the appropriate time.

Vital Signs Routine

A person's internal and skin temperature each shows a systematic rise and fall over a 24-hour period, a cycle difficult to alter in normal adults. Body temperature usually peaks between 4 P.M. and 6 P.M. and reaches its lowest point around 4 A.M. in people who are active by day and sleep at night. When the internal temperature is normally peaking, other body functions, such as pulse rate, blood pressure, and cardiac output (volume of blood pumped by the heart), are also changing. Pulse rate is high when the temperature is highest and drops during the night. The human heart rate will vary as much as 20 or 30 beats per minute in 24 hours. Blood pressure shows a marked fall during the first hour of sleep, followed by a gradual rise during the remaining time, with a peak between 5 and 7 P.M. Cardiac output reaches minimum levels between 2 and 4 A.M., the period of lowest temperature findings (10, 23, 51, 53).

The existence of a normal rhythm temperature pattern has been known for almost 200 years. Verification of blood pressure, pulse, and cardiac output rhythms has been demonstrated. Yet this knowledge has not been applied by hospital personnel when establishing time schedules for routine measurements of body temperature, pulse, and blood pressure. In most hospitals the schedule is based on factors of tradition or convenience, such as the time of shift change. Because the primary reason for checking these measurements is to detect the presence of an elevation, the procedure should be done at the time when maximum levels occur (2, 23, 53). The implications for nursing practice include the importance of establishing routines for temperature measurements with circadian rhythms in mind, considering the time of day when evaluating temperature measurements, and considering the person's preadmission rest and activity routine.

Work Schedule

Nurses as well as many industrial and law-enforcement personnel are frequently required to change shifts every week or month. Shift workers who rotate reportedly are more subject to anorexia, digestive disturbances, restless sleep patterns, lowered work quality, and more errors and accidents. Rotating shift assignments are thus relevant to these workers' health and quality of work performance (16, 53). Altering the sleep-wake sequence requires time for the person to make adjustments and regain synchrony.

If shift rotation cannot be eliminated, then individuals should be required to rotate no more frequently than once a month. Consistently working at night allows a person to acquire a new sleep-wake rhythm. Therefore night work should be made more attractive to persons who can adapt to the shift and are willing to remain on it permanently. Those who cannot adapt should be exempt from rotation.

Health teaching of any rotating-shift worker concerning the possible consequences of such a routine should not be overlooked. Night workers on medications should be made aware that the effects of medications may vary somewhat from those they usually experience when working days. The susceptibility to various degrees of drug metabolism occurs thoughout the day but even more so when a person is experiencing jet lag or the early phase of shift rotation. Individuals with chronic illness, such as diabetes, epilepsy, hypertension and cardiac problems, must consider these factors when they plan their medication regimen.

REFERENCES

1. **Aschoff, Juergen,** "Circadian Systems in Man and Their Implications," *Hospital Practice*, 11, no. 5 (1976), 51-57.
2. **Bassler, Sandra Furman,** "The Origins and Development of Biological Rhythms," *Nursing Clinics of North America*, 11, no. 4 (1976), 575-81.
3. **Binkley, Sue,** "A Timekeeping Enzyme in the Pineal Gland," *Scientific American*, 240, no. 4 (1979), 66-71.
4. **Buchsbaum, Monte,** "The Chemistry of Brain Clocks," *Psychology Today*, 12, no. 10 (1979), 124.
5. **Bunning, Erwin,** *The Physiological Clock* (3rd ed.). New York: Springer-Verlag, Inc., 1973.
6. **Carney, Leo,** and **Richard Hill,** "Human Tear pH: Diurnal Variations," *Archives of Ophthalmology*, 94, no. 5 (1976), 821-24.
7. **Colquhoun, W. P.** ed., *Biological Rhythms and Human Performance.* New York: Academic Press, Inc., 1971.
8. ———, *Aspects of Human Efficiency: Diurnal Rhythm and Loss of Sleep.* New York: Crane, Russak & Co., Inc., 1972.
9. **Conlee, R. K., M. J. Rennie,** and **W. W. Winder,** "Skeletal Muscle Glycogen Content: Diurnal Variation and Effects of Fasting," *American Journal of Physiology*, 231, no. 2 (1976), 614-18.
10. **Conroy, R. T. W. L.,** and **J. N. Mills,** *Human Circadian Rhythms.* London: J. & A. Churchill, 1970.
11. **Crossman, B.,** "Circadian Rhythms and Renal Transplants," *Nursing Times*, 76, no. 32 (1980), 1395-98.
12. **Czeisler, Charles, Elliot Weitzman, Martin Moore-Ede, Janet Zimmerman,** and **Richard Knauer,** "Human Sleep: Its Duration and Organization Depend on Its Circadian Phase," *Science*, 210, no. 4475 (1980), 1264-67.
13. ———, **Martin Moore-Ede,** and **Richard M. Coleman,** "Rotating Shift Work Schedules that Disrupt Sleep Are Improved by Applying Circadian Principles," *Science*, 217, no. 30 (1982), 460-63.

14. **Deters, Gladys,** "Circadian Rhythm Phenomenon," *American Journal of Maternal-Child Nursing*, 5, no. 4 (1980), 249–51.
15. **Farrell, Barbara,** and **Margaret Allen,** "Physiologic/Psychologic Changes Reported by USAF Female Flight Nurses During Flying Duties," *Nursing Research*, 22, no. 1 (1973), 31–36.
16. **Felton, Geraldine,** and **Mary Patterson,** "Shift Rotation Is Against Nature," *American Journal of Nursing*, 71, no. 4 (1971), 760–63.
17. **Ferin, Michel, Franz Halberg, Ralph Richart,** and **Raymond L. Vande Wiele,** eds., *Biorhythms and Human Reproduction*. New York: John Wiley & Sons, Inc., 1974.
18. **Gedda, Luigi,** and **Dianni Brenci,** *Chronogenetics: The Inheritance of Biological Time*. Springfield, IL: Charles C Thomas, Publisher, 1978.
19. **Halberg, Franz, E. Johnson, W. Nelson, W. Runge,** and **R. Sothern,** "Autorhythmometry: Procedures for Physiologic Self-Measurements and Their Analysis," *The Physiology Teacher*, 1, no. 4 (1972), 1–11.
20. **Hall, LaVonne,** "Circadian Rhythms: Implications for Geriatric Rehabilitation," *Nursing Clinics of North America*, 11, no. 4 (1976), 631–38.
21. **Hayter, Jean,** "The Rhythm of Sleep," *American Journal of Nursing*, 80, no. 3 (1980), 457–61.
22. **Hedlund, Laurence, John Franz,** and **Alexander Kenny,** eds., *Biological Rhythms and Endocrine Function*. New York: Plenum Press, 1975.
23. **Hilts, Philip,** "The Clock Within," *Science '80*, 1, no. 8 (1980), 61–67.
24. **Hoskins, Carol Noll,** "Level of Activation, Body Temperature and Interpersonal Conflict in Family Relationships," *Nursing Research*, 28, no. 3 (1979), 154–60.
25. ———, "Chronobiology and Health," *Nursing Outlook*, 29, no. 10 (1981), 572–76.
26. **Kicey, Carolyn Adams,** "Catecholamines and Depression: A Physiological Theory of Depression," *American Journal of Nursing*, 74, no. 11 (1974), 2018–20.
27. **Klaus, Marshall,** and **John Kennell,** *Maternal-Infant Bonding*. St. Louis: The C. V. Mosby Company, 1976.
28. **Klein, Raymond,** and **Roseanne Armitage,** "Rhythms in Human Performance: 1½-Hour Oscillations in Cognitive Style," *Science*, 204 (June 22, 1979), 1326–28.
29. **Krieger, Dorothy,** ed., *Endocrine Rhythms*. New York: Raven Press, 1979.
30. **Lanuza, Dorothy,** "Circadian Rhythms of Mental Efficiency and Performance," *Nursing Clinics of North America*, 11, no. 4 (1976), 583–94.
31. **Leff, David,** "Chronobiologists Tell Clinicians–Think Circadian," *Medical World News*, July 23, 1979, pp. 44–53.
32. **Luce, Gay Gaer,** *Body Time: Physiological Rhythms and Social Stress*. New York: Pantheon Books, 1971.
33. **McGovern, John P., Michael H. Smolensky,** and **Alain Reinberg,** *Chronobiology in Allergy and Immunology*. Springfield, IL: Charles C Thomas, Publisher, 1977.
34. **McIntoch, Tracy, David A. Lothrop, Austin Lee, Benjamin T. Jackson, Donald Nabseth,** and **Richard H. Egdahl,** "Circadian Rhythm of Cortisol Is

Altered in Postsurgical Patients," *Journal of Clinical Endocrinology and Metabolism*, 53, no. 1 (1981), 117-21.

35. **Miles, L. E. M., D. M. Raynal,** and **M. A. Wilson,** "Blind Man Living in Normal Society Has Circadian Rhythms of 24.9 Hours," *Science*, 198, no. 4315 (1977), 421-23.
36. **Mills, John,** ed., *Biological Aspects of Circadian Rhythms*. New York: Plenum Press, 1973.
37. **Natalini, John,** "The Human Body as a Biological Clock," *American Journal of Nursing*, 77, no. 7 (1977), 1130-32.
38. **Nolten, Wolfrom, Marshall D. Lindheimer, Patricia A. Rueckert, Suzanne Oparil,** and **Edward N. Ehrlich,** "Diurnal Patterns and Regulations of Cortisol Secretion in Pregnancy," *Journal of Clinical Endocrinology and Metabolism*, 51, no. 3 (1980), 466-71.
39. **O'Dell, Margaret,** "Human Biorhythmology: Implications for Nursing Practice," *Nursing Forum*. 14, no. 1 (1975), 43-47.
40. **Palmer, J. D.,** *An Introduction to Biological Rhythms*. New York: Academic Press, Inc., 1976.
41. **Pflug, B., R. Erikson,** and **A. Johnsson,** "Depression and Daily Temperature," *Acta Psychiatrica Scandinavica*, 54, no. 4 (1976), 254-66.
42. **Reinberg, A.,** and **F. Halberg,** eds., *Chronopharmacology*. Oxford: Pergamon Press, 1979.
43. **Rubin, Zick,** "Seasonal Rhythms in Behavior," *Psychology Today*, 13, no. 7, (1979), 12 ff.
44. **Samis, Harvey,** and **Salvatore Capobianco,** *Aging and Biological Rhythms*. New York: Plenum Press, 1978.
45. **Saunders, David,** *An Introduction to Biological Rhythms*. New York: John Wiley & Sons, Inc., 1977.
46. **Smolensky, M. H.,** and **A. Reinberg,** "The Chronotherapy of Corticosteroids: Practical Application of Chronobiologic Findings to Nursing," *Nursing Clinics of North America*, 11, no. 4 (1976), 609-19.
47. **Sorensen, Karen,** and **Joan Luckmann,** *Basic Nursing: A Psychophysiologic Approach*. Philadelphia: W. B. Saunders Company, 1979.
48. **Stephens, Gwen,** "Periodicity in Mood, Affect, and Instinctual Behavior," *Nursing Clinics of North America*, 11, no. 4 (1976), 595-607.
49. **Tom, Cheryl,** Nursing Assessment of Biological Rhythms," *Nursing Clinics of North America*, 11, no. 4 (1976), 621-30.
50. ______, and **Dorothy Lanuza,** "Symposium on Biological Rhythms: Introduction," *Nursing Clinics of North America*, 11, no. 4 (1976), 569-73.
51. United States Department of Health, Education, and Welfare, Public Health Service, *Biological Rhythms in Psychiatry and Medicine*. Chevy Chase, MD: National Institute of Mental Health, 1970.
52. **Wehr, Thomas, Anna Wirz-Justice, Frederick Goodwin, Wallace Duncan,** and **J. Christian Gillin,** "Phase Advance of the Circadian Sleep-Wake Cycle as an Antidepressant," *Science*, 206 (November 9, 1979), 710-13.
53. **Weston, Lee,** *Body Rhythm: The Circadian Rhythms Within You*. New York: Harcourt Brace Jovanovich, 1979.

Section II

RELATIONSHIP OF MOBILITY AND BODY MECHANICS TO MAINTENANCE OF ADAPTATION

Motion in the living organism is the perpetual force of adaptation and is therefore synonymous with life. Our degree of mobility determines our adaptive capacity at the cellular, systemic, and structural levels, as well as the degree to which we can make psychosocial adjustments.

If we can comprehend the body's adaptation to strenuous physical activity, we can more fully understand the hazards of immobility and formulate a plan of nursing care to combat its deleterious effects. In any exercise program, whether designed for the healthy individual or for the patient in need of rehabilitation, Edington states that the planning must be based on the following concepts.

1. Exercising is a function of the type of demands made on the body.
2. Specific exercises call forth particular biological effects.
3. The type of exercise will determine its source of energy.
4. Training or conditioning is the result of adaptive processes elicited by regular exercise.
5. Fatigue and exhaustion occur when the body is unable to meet the demands of exercise (8).

Exercise can be classified according to the speed of muscular activity, the resistance to movement, and the time span or duration. The conditioning of any part of the body can be achieved through regular and frequent exercise that stimulates subcellular mechanisms to bring about a trained state. The body is set up so that the specific exercise causes muscle cells to adapt in such a way as to be better prepared to protect themselves against the stress of the exercise. This ongoing process achieves the successful conditioning desired. It is believed that this adaptation within the cells takes place during the recovery phase (8).

During the stress of exercise short-term adaptation is taking place in the cell by inactive chemicals becoming active. Long-term adaptation is taking place in the cell by an increase in the amount of chemicals, mainly proteins. Together this adaptation resists fatigue and conditioning is experienced. So our resistance to fatigue is increased by the body's ability to strengthen muscle cells that are vulnerable to certain exercises (8).

To understand exercise fully, we must be aware of the functional structure of the muscle cells. Performance depends on the efficiency of cell function, whether muscle, brain, endocrine, blood, or any other cell. The interaction of the cell components determines the functional response of each cell. Cell membrane provides cellular and subcellular specificity. The processing of information is done by the nucleus; the cell's energy source is the mitochondrion; contractile elements give the muscle cells the ability to contract. Each component is essential for muscle cell function (8).

Muscles contract due to an intricate blending of neural innervation, a concentration of calcium and contractile proteins in the cells, and the production of energy. Muscles shorten when energy produces an interaction between actin and myosin muscle proteins. Relaxation occurs as the neural stimulation is withdrawn and calcium removed. During excessive exercise demands efficient communication links between subcellular compartments are necessary, for these compartments are selectively altered by specific exercises. This alteration causes the exercise capability to vary, which in turn selectively alters the training adaptation. Thus training adaptations are specific to the exercise conditions (8).

Muscles derive energy from the oxidation of food by way of three biological pathways: fatty acids, glucose, and oxygen. Chemical bonds are broken. Carbon dioxide is released and hydrogen atoms are transported to the mitochondria, where they combine to form water. Energy is then provided to form ATP (adenosine triphosphate) and this energy-capturing molecule is transported to the cells, where it is enzymatically broken down and its energy surrendered. For longer lasting activities—more than a few seconds—carbohydrate is needed for energy. Through a complex breakdown, intramuscular glycogen is converted to a nonoxidative formation of ATP molecules for more prolonged response (8).

Strenuous exercise requiring power induces a remarkable adaptation. Glycolysis increases markedly, as does the concentrates of alpha-glycerol phosphate and lactate in the muscle. These are dead-end molecules, for they cannot be metabolized during strenuous muscle activity. When the exercise ceases, however, the alpha-glycerol molecules can be reconverted to lactate or further metabolized to CO_2 and water. The lactate itself can be used to form CO_2 and water or be transported to the liver where two lactate molecules can then be converted to a glucose molecule and either stored as glycogen or released for transport by the blood to the muscle (the Cori cycle) (8).

The chief enzymatic systems that produce oxidative metabolism are involved with glycolysis, fatty acid oxidation, the citric acid or Krebs cycle, and the electron transport system (8).

It would be impossible to explain fully in this book the many intracacies of the mechanisms of motion in the human body. The responses discussed represent examples of adaptation in the cell during muscle activity. Another example worth mentioning is sensory feedback, which involves the action of a sensory nerve either facilitating or inhibiting a motor neuron as it continually alters the load put on the muscle spindle. This factor is important in the regulation of muscle tension, the strength of muscle output, and the speed of skilled movements (8).

The benefits of exercise done regularly are quickly lost by inactivity. In 2 or 3 weeks lack of exercise will cause a 20 percent loss of conditioning previously obtained over a long period. In a month of inactivity the loss may be as high as 50 percent. Always it requires a longer period of time to regain conditioning than to lose it. Exercise should not be skipped for more than a few days (5).

DIMENSIONS OF IMMOBILITY

Immobility, *prescribed or unavoidable restriction of movement in any sphere of a person's life*, must be viewed in a broad context. Even normal physiological or psychosocial experiences have their dimensions of immobility. A new student adjusting to college life, for example, feels a certain restriction of free movement compared to the ease with which he/she could function in the former school environment. Similarly, pregnancy imposes varying degrees of physical, psychological, and social adaptation restrictive of free movement.

The dimensions of immobility can be identified as area, cause, extent, direction, duration, sequelae, and volition (6). Nursing care based on these dimensions will provide support and promote adaptive responses when health is threatened.

Area. A person may be immobilized in any one or in several areas or facets of life: physical, social, intellectual, or psychological. Physical immobility is not confined to loss of musculoskeletal function, the application of casts, or the use of traction. It may be restriction of movement for an elderly person who cannot go out to shop because there are too many stairs to climb, a lack of transportation, or no one to help carry a heavy load. Social immobility can occur in a number of ways. The widow may find that her ability to lead the life to which she has been accustomed is restricted because as a single woman she no longer fits into her group of friends. The person who migrates from one country or region to another may have difficulty establishing friendships. Intellectual immobility exists for those limited by a lack of mental development. Psychological restrictions can arise from maladaptation to stress. Physiological processes may be slowed or made nonfunctional by disease or injury.

Cause. Factors within the person or in the environment may cause limited mobility. Disease states are generally considered as causes of immobility, but the therapy used in the treatment of the disease, such as traction or a cast, could be more immobilizing than the illness itself.

Extent. Immobility will vary in intensity at different times for a given person. Also, two people may have basically the same injury and treatment plan but may recover at different rates; this difference often reflects how each perceives the disability. Therefore the extent of the immobility is relative.

Direction. Only in death is there no potential for change. In the living organism immobility undergoes directional shifts as adaptation occurs. The interplay of organ systems, cell metabolism, and body defenses and the influence of psychosocial factors mediate the direction of change toward improvement or regression.

Duration. The length of time during which degrees of immobility will occur under certain describable circumstances is predictable to some extent. The physician is able to predict the number of days that must elapse before sutures may be safely removed. The nurse plans for the possible duration of the patient's immobility in many ways: How frequently and for how long will it be necessary to check the obstetrical patient's fundus? When will the postoperative patient be able to help with his bath? What plans should be made for teaching the new diabetic or the new colostomy patient the ways in which each can take care of self at home?

Sequelae. Maladaptive responses stemming from a primary disease process or disability may extend the duration of immobility or change its direction. Effective preventive measures designed to avoid harmful side effects must be part of every nursing care plan. You will need to predict the probable hazards associated with the particular area and degree of immobility with which you are dealing in order to avoid or minimize unfavorable effects.

Volition (Use of Will). The patient with a fractured bone, an abdominal incision, or arthritic joints may need help in accepting nursing care that provides necessary mobility within prescribed limits, especially when movement or a change in position causes pain. On the other hand, when a disability occurs that is not accompanied by sufficient discomfort to limit mobility, the patient may not easily accept prescriptions for needed rest and restricted activity. In either case, patient teaching should help shorten, or at least not prolong, the person's period of forced immobility.

A person experiencing social or psychological immobility may also have lack of volition. You can help strengthen the person's will by recognizing his/her status, giving encouragement whenever possible, and making suggestions to increase self-motivation.

EFFECTS OF IMMOBILITY ON FUNCTIONAL AREAS

Cardiovascular Function

The adequate exchange of respiratory gases and metabolic substances depends on the efficiency of the cardiovascular system, including the heart, arteries, venous channels, and lymph vessels. Physical immobility produces three critical changes in the adaptive ability of this system to carry blood to and from capillaries: in (1) vasomotor control, (2) blood return to the heart, and (3) venous stasis (3, 13).

Orthostatic hypotension *is the inability of the autonomic nervous system to adapt readily to a sudden change from a recumbent to an upright position.* Equalization of the blood supply throughout the body is affected adversely during prolonged bedrest. The valves within the veins require muscle action to assist them in opening to permit venous return of blood to the heart. Without adequate muscle contraction, tone is lost, muscles lose strength, and venous blood tends to pool in the lower extremities. The decrease in neurovascular reflex control of blood vessels during bedrest may be caused by the lower pressure, higher flow, and increased diameter of vessels in the supine position (3).

Although rest is considered an essential factor in the treatment of disease, a second major change in cardiovascular performance resulting from immobility has been identified. The heart suffers an increased work load in the resting supine position, resulting from the altered distribution of blood throughout the body. Gravity provides downward pressure in the erect position. When it is relieved by lying down, the circulating blood volume is increased, placing an additional load on the right side of the heart as more blood returns from the periphery to the heart (3).

Periodically the patient on bedrest is required to exert strain on the heart in what is known as the *Valsalva maneuver*. This is the act of fixing the thorax, holding one's breath, and thereby forcing pressure against the closed glottis—the action one takes when straining to defecate. Intrathoracic pressure is increased and prevents venous blood from entering the large vessels. When the breath is expired, a sudden drop in the intrathoracic pressure occurs, resulting in a rush of blood to the heart. This maneuver may be used by a bedfast patient as often as 20 to 30 times per hour as he/she uses the arms and the muscles of the upper trunk to change position in bed (13).

Thrombus formation is the third hazard associated with cardiovascular functions during immobility. Venous stasis occurs, leading to hypercoagulability of the blood. External pressure is exerted by the patient's position, the bedding, or both. Bed patients are often dehydrated, which contributes to an increased viscosity of the blood and may, in turn, lead to clotting. Also, the blood level of calcium is increased during rest. The calcium may combine with material from platelets to form thrombin (a precursor for the conversion of fibrinogen to fibrin), producing hypercoagulability (13).

The intima of blood vessels may be easily damaged by maintaining one position for a prolonged time, especially if one extremity rests on the other. Platelets will then form a matrix over the damaged area and may form a clot.

Range-of-motion exercises to assist in venous flow and the restoration or maintenance of muscle tone will be important to your care of any patient on bedrest. Consult a nursing fundamentals text for specific information on doing range-of-motion exercises. Self-care should be encouraged as much as possible within the limits set by the medical regimen. Frequent changes in position should be required, especially for providing a change from horizontal to vertical whenever possible. Patient teaching should help the patient learn how to move in bed with a minimum of effort; an overbed trapeze can be provided for this purpose.

One of the best examples of nursing support for adaptation is that of preventing constipation. Positioning the patient in a well-supported position on the bedpan or commode helps to relieve the strain that might otherwise put too much work load on the heart.

Respiratory Function

Certain adaptive responses are compensatory during immobility: basal metabolism decreases, cells require less oxygen for synthesis of proteins, and less carbon dioxide is produced as a by-product of cell metabolism. In addition, the rate of respiration decreases, there is less movement of secretions, and oxygen-carbon dioxide balance is altered (13).

Added to the compensatory decrease in respiration during periods of bedrest are a number of factors that are significant for nursing care. Chest expansion may be adversely affected. The bed may splint the chest by its pressure, especially if the patient maintains one position too long. Some postures may compress the thorax. Abdominal distention or a tight binder or dressing may prevent the normal descent of the diaphragm during inspiration. Drugs that depress the central nervous system will affect the respiratory center in the medulla, motor areas of the cerebral cortex, and the cells of the spinal cord.

Pooling of secretions follows respiratory embarrassment. Inflammation of the trachea and the bronchial tree leads to a further decrease in the ability to use normal cleansing mechanisms, such as coughing and deep breathing. Stagnant secretions provide a receptive medium for the growth of microorganisms, thereby increasing the chances of threatening sequelae.

Lack of respiratory movement and the pooling of secretions result in oxygen-carbon dioxide imbalance. The first adaptational response resulting from increased accumulation of carbon dioxide in the blood is temporary stimulation of the respiratory centers. Continuous stimulation causes the aortic and carotid bodies to react against the stimulus and overadaptation to excessive stimulation causes the respiratory centers to become depressed. Respiratory acidosis follows and may lead to cardiac failure unless reversed.

Nursing measures for prevention of functional respiratory disabilities are those that preserve the patient's ability to breathe. They begin with astute observation of respirations—their rate, depth, and quality. The way in which a patient uses muscles to breathe is important. The person may be using neck muscles to supply force. Position may give a clue to difficulty in breathing, or he/she may speak in partial, clipped sentences, indicating an inability to inspire sufficient air. Listen to the breathing and then use a stethoscope to ausculate breath sounds to provide a basis for accurate reporting of signs and symptoms.

Turning, coughing, and deep breathing are among the simplest and yet most effective methods for preserving the immobilized patient's respiratory function. Teaching the patient how to do these regularly and encouraging self-care as the disability permits will provide support for cardiopulmonary functions, which, in turn, promotes healthy adaptive responses in other systems.

Nutrition and Elimination

Because immobility reduces the energy requirements of cells and slows metabolic processes, gastrointestinal function is impaired, affecting both the ingestion of food and the elimination of wastes (3, 13).

At prolonged rest, nitrogen balance in the human is reversed to a negative state. Anabolic and catabolic activities are not equal—the balance is upset: catabolism is increased and protein loss is accompanied by mechanical and psychological disturbances in gastrointestinal functions as the desire for food diminishes.

Anorexia results in a loss of nutrients and is likely to prolong whatever disease process or dysfunction caused the immobilization in the first place. Although loss of appetite is an adaptive mechanism in response to decreased metabolic requirements, sufficient nutrients for basal metabolism and for compensation of catabolic losses must be maintained if healing is to take place.

Adequate amounts of the Basic 4 food groups served in small, frequent feedings may help encourage the person to eat. Individual preferences and cultural variations in food habits may need to be considered and food should be appetizing and served appropriately hot or cold. Food becomes a source of comfort for the immobilized person, a symbol of the caring of others, a welcome break in the day's routine.

Elimination is the other significant gastrointestinal function affected by prolonged rest. The combination of smooth and skeletal muscle activity with complex reflex action provides for successful defecation. Loss may occur in any of these mechanisms. Lack of muscle tone occurring during immobility is reflected in a weakening of the abdominal muscles needed for the expulsion of stool. Dehydration may cause fecal material to be dry and hard. Suppression of the urge to defecate often occurs. The patient is in an unfamiliar environment; privacy is minimal; the usual pattern of living has been disrupted. Often the person must assume an unnatural position to defecate. If the gastrocolic reflex that moves the fecal contents from the sigmoid into the rectum is ignored repeatedly, it will become less strong until it possibly disappears altogether and chronic constipation develops.

Fecal impaction can and does frequently occur in immobilized persons, regardless of age, unless nursing intervention has been preventive rather than curative. Increased fluid intake, a daily serving of prune juice in anticipation of prolonged bedrest, and preservation of muscle tone are measures that will prevent constipation and mechanical intervention. The addition of fiber foods, such as bran cereals, whole wheat breads, nuts, and raw vegetables, is helpful in maintaining bowel tone. Teach immobilized patients to select menus that will include not only essential nutrients but also foods that supply bulk and roughage as tolerated. The elderly patient with a stroke or fractured hip, the patient in casts or traction regardless of age, or anyone confined to bed for an extended period for any reason are all people for whom an early assessment of bowel habits and a preventive plan of care are essential.

Patient teaching is important because many persons do not understand what constitutes a normal bowel pattern. Misconceptions about the frequency, amount, and characteristics of a normal stool must be clarified. What is normal for one person will not be for another. The idea that a daily bowel movement is necessary for all people may need to be explored with the patient, for cultural groups vary in their emphasis on this and other body functions. It is not the frequency of defecation but its characteristics that determine healthy gastrointestinal function. If the stool is soft, formed, and easily expelled, the frequency is not significant. Evacuation twice a week in sufficient amounts and of soft consistency is considered normal bowel function in the immobilized patient (13).

Many pharmaceutical stool softeners are available for patients who may need help in getting a bowel pattern established, but the use of laxatives and enemas should be discouraged. In any bowel-training program, the patient's habits prior to immobility should be investigated and incorporated into the plan. Peristalsis sufficient to move bowel contents into the rectum usually occurs most strongly after breakfast. Therefore, following that meal, the patient should be encouraged to use the bedpan, commode, or lavatory, allowing about 15 minutes for the process. Sometimes digital stimulation of the anal sphincter or the use of a suppository may be helpful in establishing this pattern.

If an acceptable pattern for defecation has not been established and a fecal impaction occurs, the cardinal symptom will be the frequent passing of liquid fecal material from around the impacted stool. When this situation is suspected, a rectal examination should be done; if there is an impaction, it must be dislodged and removed by gentle digital manipulation. An oil-retention enema given above the mass an hour prior to digital removal will prevent undue discomfort for the patient. Cleansing enemas are usually used following removal of the impaction. Health teaching to promote an improved intestinal tone through diet, increased fluid intake, and activity is essential to prevent a recurrence.

Locomotion

Maintenance of structural stability is essential for the person's adaptation to the environment. Integrity of osseous (bony) structures, efficiency of muscle action, and an intact integument (skin) are the first lines of defense against physical trauma. Muscles, bones, and skin are coordinated with the nervous system to produce the complex process of locomotion. The element of stress is important to motor function. Without the normal stresses and strains of daily activity, strength is depleted as bones lose their solidity and muscles become too atonic to support the weight of the body and move its parts with ease. Cell nutrition suffers because the muscle pump activity cannot be maintained for adequate circulation of blood.

Immobility contributes to three major complications of musculoskeletal deterioration and they are manifested in tissue changes and dysfunction of bones, muscles, and skin. Each complication contributes to the other (13).

Osteoporosis is one of the deteriorative processes resulting from immobility. Adaptive mechanisms and a balance of energy exchange are continually striving to maintain optimum strength in osseous tissue. A bone is a living structure. Its growth and development are built on a vital matrix that carries the calcium necessary to give it strength and solidarity. Counterforces are constantly breaking down and replacing this matrix and its calcium throughout the life of the bone (13).

Osteoblasts *are cells that form the bony matrix.* Their function depends on the stresses and strains of movement; without this stimulus, they cease forming new bone. Meanwhile, the **osteoclasts,** *cells that have the opposing function of absorbing and removing osseous tissue from the bone,* continue their destructive process. Decalcification occurs; phosphorus and nitrogen are removed; and *as this demineralization progresses, the bone becomes porous, producing a condition known as* **osteoporosis.**

Weight bearing, which is unnoticed by normal, active persons, becomes painful for the person with osteoporosis. Bones may compress and become deformed and they are easily fractured. Demineralization of bone cannot be diagnosed by x ray until approximately 50 percent of the calcium is lost. Patients with this condition, in which there has been a gradual onset, are usually beyond middle age. They may have a great deal of generalized pain on bearing weight and become less mobile as the disease progresses. This situation leads to further complications, with muscles losing tone from disuse and the skin becoming susceptible to pressure from prolonged rest in one position.

The significance of osteoporosis is that it can occur in a relatively short time in any person, regardless of age, during prolonged periods of immobility. Nursing measures for prevention or decrease of mineral loss must be those directed toward maintenance of weight bearing and muscle strengthening. Stress on bones can be provided through exercises and the use of weight-bearing equipment, such as a tilt bed or oscillating bed. If walking is difficult or limited, having the patient use a walker or parallel bars at regular intervals may be prescribed. One of the best nursing interventions is to encourage the patient to participate in his/her own care, to stretch, to reach, to exercise against resistance to the maximum ability.

Dr. Herta Spencer of Loyola University's Stritch School of Medicine calls osteoporosis "the most common systemic bone disorder in the

United States." She estimates that 15 million Americans are afflicted with it, most of them women. In addition to splitting hips, it annually causes 500,000 fractures of the spine, ribs, wrists, and other bones (10).

Calcium, the mineral from which the body builds bone, is often lacking in the adult diet. Bones and teeth are 99 percent of the calcium in our bodies; the other 1 percent is essential for controlling nerve impulse, muscle contraction, heart rhythm, and blood coagulation. Calcium is continually used up and then replenished by the foods that we eat. If the normal daily intake supply is depleted, the body must dip into its bone reserve.

If the bone reservoir is tapped excessively over a period of years due to a chronically low intake of calcium, the bones lose their density and become fragile. A minor slip may cause a fractured hip or vertebrae may collapse simply from carrying the body weight in a normal upright position. (Often the hip fracture causes the fall rather than the other way around.)

Much of this trauma can be alleviated by a few simple precautions. First, sufficent calcium must be ingested daily—at least 800 mg. either in the form of 3 cups of milk or 3 ounces of Swiss cheese or the equivalent. Some biophysicists argue that it should be increased to as much as 1200 to 1500 mg a day. Secondly, regular exercise is critical. Several years ago a selected group of menopausal women were studied at Nassau County Medical Center, New York, and the Medical Research Center, Brookhaven National Laboratory. When half were made to exercise for 1 hour three times a week over a period of time, their body calcium increased by an average of 20 grams; meanwhile, it decreased in every one of the other sedentary women (10). A 77-year old woman member of the Brookhaven group continues to spend four mornings a week in a group exercise program. She walks on a treadmill, pedals a stationary bicycle, and gently works out with barbells. She no longer experiences the pain she once suffered as a result of her osteoporosis (10).

Contractures of the muscles is the second deteriorating process. Prolonged disuse of any muscle produces **atrophy,** *the wasting away of muscle tissue*; the size of the muscle decreases and its strength ebbs. If weakness prevents the full range of muscle contraction or if there is *imbalance between the strength of opposing muscles,* **contracture** can occur: the weak muscle cannot contract adequately and its antagonist exerts an opposing pull, thereby flexing part of an extremity in a fixed, sometimes irreversible, position.

Proper body alignment in an anatomically correct position is important during bedrest and is the first step toward increased mobility and preservation of function. A firm mattress and perhaps a bed board are necessary when there is to be a prolonged stay in bed. The use of a properly placed footboard will prevent footdrop by assisting the patient to use the muscles of the lower legs. The board must be placed so that it rests firmly against the patient's feet and does not require him/her to stretch to reach it.

Frequent and regularly scheduled changes of position combined with full range-of-motion exercises for all unaffected joints are essential. Again, the patient and family should be taught how to help in these exercises so that they may participate together in care.

Skin breakdown also occurs frequently with osteoporosis or contracture formation and is the third deteriorative process.

The Integument

The moving and turning just referred to are directly related to the maintenance of skin integrity. Ordinarily a person who sleeps or rests in bed turns and moves, changing position and avoiding pressure on any one area for very long. This shifting about occurs frequently even during sleep. The movement preserves the integument from assault that might deprive skin areas of an adequate blood supply over a period of time and thus cause breakdown.

Persons who are aged, paralyzed, obese, or immobilized because of disability are all prone to skin breakdown. Either the sensation is not keen enough to warn of pressure or there is a lack of ability to turn without aid because of weight, weakness, or the pressure of restrictive mechanical devices. If no assistance is given to provide mobility, the skin suffers in two ways: (1) muscle disuse decreases the circulatory exchanges in the soft tissues and (2) the constant pressure obstructs the flow of blood to the part. **Ischemia,** or *local anemia* of the area, develops, which leads to necrosis and ulceration. This is the classic decubitus ulcer that is so insidious in its onset and so difficult to heal. In addition to the threat of skin breakdown due to immobility per se, there is the danger of malnutrition in the bedfast patient because of being in negative nitrogen balance. Unless the skin receives adequate nourishment, it cannot survive the effects of constant pressure and embarrassment of its blood supply, a fact that emphasizes the interrelationship of the body's functional areas (3, 13, 14).

Nursing intervention is the primary preventive therapy in this area. Skin breakdown can and must be prevented through nursing, not medical, care. The development of an open area caused by pressure is unnecessary today. The responsibility for initiating prophylactic measures rests with you. In addition to frequent position changes, gentle massage over bony prominences, range-of-motion exercises, and mechanical aids may be used. An alternating-pressure mattress, a flotation mattress with its gel foam pad that protects the sacral area, oscillating beds, tilt boards, or even a simple measure, such as a sheepskin under the hips, can be used to protect the skin.

Position change must be accompanied by close inspection and meticulous care of the skin. The patient's linen should be dry and wrinkle-free at all times. Keep the skin clean and use an emollient lotion to keep it pliant. Make sure that the lotion you use is thoroughly absorbed, or the excess removed, to prevent maceration of skin by too much moisture.

In essence, prevention ensures an intact musculoskeletal system in the immobile patient. Provide as much movement as possible. Use anatomical positioning that avoids pressure points for long periods. Encourage the patient to participate in self-care. Use patient teaching for optimum nutrition. And base your intervention on careful assessments of skin and muscle tone so that the direction of adaptation will be toward full function.

Urinary Excretion

Figure 7-5 shows that free drainage of urine from the calycses of the kidney to the bladder for excretion through the urethra is designed, in the human, for the upright position. When a person is supine, urine must leave the kidney against an upward gradient. Hence mobility for the bedfast patient preserves urinary function. Any stasis of urine in the renal pelvis for even a few days may lead to infection or the formation of **renal calculi,** *urinary tract stones* (3).

Protein breakdown, bone demineralization, and loss of muscle tone during prolonged immobility contribute to marked changes in urinary excretion. The nephron continues to be selective of constituents in the blood, excreting those in excess and preserving those in deficit. Minerals and salts are in excess in blood plasma as a result of bedrest and so the nephron increases excretion of them. These particles become ideal nuclei for the formation of renal calculi. Their precipitation is favored by stasis, alkaline urine, decreased volume of urine, and bacterial invasion (3, 13).

Nursing intervention can prevent urine stasis through frequently changing the patient's position and avoiding a supine position for too long a period of time. An alkaline urine occurs during bedrest because of a lack of muscular activity; acid end-products decrease and the urine pH rises. Acid-ash between-meal snacks, such as cranberry juice or cereals, can help overcome this condition and should be a part of every immobilized patient's care plan.

Forcing fluids is perhaps the simplest and most effective means for preserving urinary function; yet it is often overlooked or given only lip

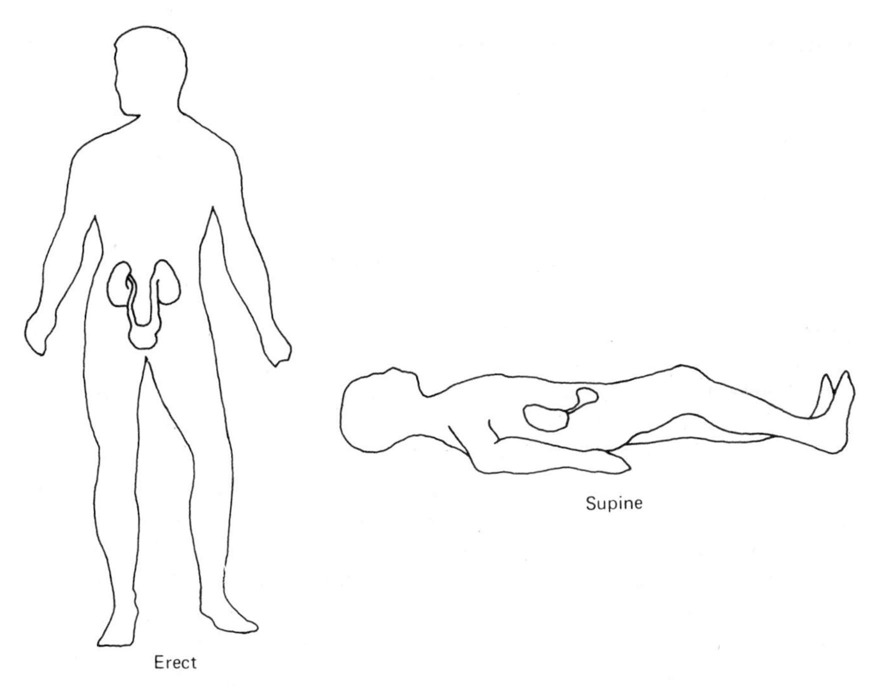

FIGURE 7-5 Urinary Drainage Related to Position

service. Keeping a pitcher of water at the bedside and changing it faithfully is likely to be considered adequate provision of fluid intake, but unless you actually assist the patient in drinking the water, it will do no good. This assistance is different for every patient. It may mean keeping the water within easy reach or pouring it when strength is diminished. But two actions are essential: (1) *offer the water frequently* as you encourage its use and (2) *carry out effective teaching* as to its importance for body fluids as well as urinary excretion.

Prevention of urinary tract infection depends on nursing measures. Indwelling catheters should be used only when other measures to keep the patient dry and the bladder empty have failed. During their use meticulous perineal care and cleansing of the catheter where it emerges from the meatus must be done at least once daily.

Metabolic Processes

The functional changes resulting from prolonged rest include the following: a decreased metabolic rate, tissue atrophy, protein catabolism, bone demineralization, altered exchange of nutrients and vital substances between the intracellular and extracellular compartments, fluid and electrolyte imbalance, and changes in gastrointestinal motility (13).

Some changes resulting from immobility have been discussed: the decreased metabolic rate, protein breakdown, threat of renal calculi, decreased muscular use, and loss of stress to the skeletal system. Another important effect of bedrest is the loss of heat by conduction and radiation because of the pressure of the bed and its linens. Blood vessels are dilated in the supine position, and because much of the body's surface is covered with bedclothes, perspiration increases. This factor adds to the fluid loss and with perspiration the essential electrolytes, sodium, potassium, and chloride are lost.

Diurnal patterns are closely bound to metabolic response. Activity of body functions, such as temperature, hormone secretion, and renal regulation, is at its best during a person's waking hours; during sleep most body functions are reduced to a minimum. If a person is supine for long periods, whether asleep or awake, these physiological functions will decline to a minimal output.

Metabolic homeostasis is preserved through the nursing measures discussed in relation to all the functional body systems: around-the-clock exercise and movement, increased fluid intake, acid-ash foods, attention to nutritional and elimination needs, care and stimulation of the integument, and interventions that conserve heat loss and cardiac output.

Psychosocial Aspects

Ego identity is distorted by immobility. The integrated personality that a person develops through socialization and the meanings he/she assigns to situations are threatened when restriction of free movement occurs (13).

Learning and motivation are affected and problem solving becomes less direct when a person is isolated or immobile. Drives, expectations, and emotional responses are altered: the first two are diminished and the last are expressed in behaviors not typical of the person's usual pattern. Withdrawal, apathy, aggressiveness, or regression may occur where no such behavior previously existed. Lack of self-determination in activities changes behavior.

The immobilized person views the environment, including people, from a different physical position; the feedback relied on to tell who and what he/she is may seem unfamiliar. The person may incorporate the apparatus of hospitalization into his/her body image. Thus traction equipment, casts, intravenous or any other tubing attached or inserted may alter self-perception.

Changes in the way that sensory stimuli are perceived occur because the sensory processes are slowed during prolonged bedrest or isolation. Form and substance, weight, pressure, and temperature may be perceived differently. Time is now ordered by others' activities. Direction often means one place—where the person is. There is no east, west, north, or south.

The social institutions of the family, education, religion, work, and recreation ordinarily define a person's roles. During immobility roles are reversed, changed, or eliminated according to the restrictions imposed. In American culture, youth, vigor, upward mobility, and energy expenditure are stressed as desirable attributes. During prolonged disability the loss of or diminished capacity for these highly valued goals is interpreted by the patient, and sometimes by those with whom he/she associates, as a loss of personal worth. It is no wonder that under such circumstances a person develops behavior patterns misunderstood by and unacceptable to others.

Nursing intervention for psychosocial adaptation should concentrate on helping the patient move from dependence to independence, providing sensory stimuli, promoting adjustment to a temporary or permanent body image threat, orienting him/her to time and place, and giving support during necessary role change.

Through your astute assessment, you can make a systematic and complete care plan that can be used by the entire staff. A clock and a calendar are necessary to a patient's orientation to reality, for even the short-term patient often misjudges the passage of time. Describing location of the room in relation to the points of the compass and in relation to other parts of the unit can be extremely helpful. You might move the patient's bed to a courtyard or lounge when long-term disability precludes being moved on a cart or using a wheelchair. In this way, the patient's environment is extended, and he/she experiences increased sensory input.

Patient teaching is essential for psychosocial as well as physical adaptation to immobility. Explain procedures and equipment to the patient and teach him/her ways of participating in self-care and of making use of increased leisure time. Work with the family or friends to help stabilize the patient's societal roles. Encourage loved ones to treat the patient with the same respect as in the past. As soon as possible the person should be allowed to participate in the same decisions and role expectation that the family assigned to him/her before illness.

Immobilization disability is one of today's major health hazards. Mobility supports autoregulatory processes. Through patient teaching and intervention based on scientific rationale, you can help each patient and family experiencing some immobility to adapt as fully as possible.

REFERENCES

1. **Beeson, Paul B.,** and **Walsh McDermott,** eds., *Cecil-Loeb Textbook of Medicine*. Philadelphia: W. B. Saunders Company, 1971.
2. **Bolaskas, Arthur,** *Body Life*, New York: Grosset & Dunlap, Inc., 1977.
3. **Browse, N. L.,** *Physiology and Pathology of Bedrest*. Springfield, IL: Charles C Thomas, Publisher, 1965.
4. **Brunner, Lillian Sholtis,** et al., *Medical-Surgical Nursing* (2nd ed.). Philadelphia: J. B. Lippincott Company, 1970.
5. **Canter, Robert C.,** *Health Maintenance Through Physical Conditioning*. Littleton, MA: PSG Publishing Company, Inc., 1981.
6. **Carnevali, Doris,** and **Susan Brueckner,** "Immobilization: Reassessment of a Concept," *American Journal of Nursing*, 70, no. 7 (1970), 1502–7.
7. **Daniels, Lucille,** *Therapeutic Exercises for Body Alignment and Function*. Philadelphia: W. B. Saunders Company, 1977.
8. **Edington, D. W.,** and **V. R. Edgerton,** *The Biology of Physical Activity*. Boston: Houghton Mifflin Company, 1976.
9. **Feldenkrais, Moshe,** *Awareness Through Movement: Health Exercises for Personal Growth*. New York: Harper & Row, Publishers, Inc., 1977.
10. **Galton, Lawrence,** "How You Can Prevent Brittle Bones," *The Arizona Star*, Tucson, AZ, November 23, 1982, "Parade" section, pp. 19–21.
11. **Margaria, Rodolfo,** *Biomedics and Energetics of Muscular Exercise*. Oxford: Clarendon Press, 1976.
12. **Metz, Edith A.,** "Development of a Standardized Test of Cognitive Aspects of Efficient Body Movement for Technical and Professional Nursing Students," *Nursing Research Conference*, 5 (1969), 196–207.
13. **Olson, Edith V.,** "The Hazards of Immobility," *American Journal of Nursing*, 67, no. 4 (1967), 779–97.
14. **Wessels, Norman K.,** "How Living Cells Change Shape," *Scientific American*, 225, no. 4 (1971), 77–82.
15. **Winters, Margaret Campbell,** *Protective Body Mechanics in Daily Life and in Nursing*. Philadelphia: W. B. Saunders Company, 1955.
16. **Works, Roberta F.,** "Hints on Lifting and Pulling," *American Journal of Nursing*, 72, no. 2 (1972), 260–61.

8

Crisis Intervention: A Therapy Technique

Study of this chapter will help you to

1. Differentiate between crisis and stress.
2. Identify the types of crises and give examples of each.
3. Describe factors that influence coping with and the outcome of a crisis.
4. List the phases of crisis and discuss normal behavioral responses in each phase.
5. Compare and contrast reactions of a family, group, or community to a crisis or disaster.
6. Discuss examples of behavior that indicate a crisis was not adequately resolved, including psychophysiological illness.
7. Discuss the necessity of integrating crisis theory into your philosophy of care.
8. Relate the steps of the nursing process to crisis therapy.
9. Modify principles of crisis intervention for use in telephone intervention.
10. Discuss suicidal behavior in relation to crises.
11. Assess and counsel the person in a suicidal crisis.
12. Work with survivors after intentional death of a loved one.

13. Define *loss*, *grief*, and *mourning* and discuss the crisis of separation and loss as a part of life.
14. Describe the sequence of reactions and behaviors typical of the grief syndrome and mourning process.
15. List factors influencing the mourning process.
16. Explore your role in helping the person who has experienced loss.
17. Apply principles of crisis intervention with the client who has been a victim of physical assault.
18. Discuss factors contributing to the person's definition of and susceptibility to illness.
19. Identify the sick role and behaviors typical of the sick role.
20. Compare the reactions of the person who is ill at home to those of someone hospitalized for illness.
21. List and discuss the stages of illness and tasks of convalescence.
22. Define and discuss the characteristics of and reactions to impaired role behavior.
23. Discuss reactions of the family to impaired role or to chronic illness or disability.
24. Explore how you can help a person and family resolve the crises of suicide, illness, disability, or loss, or assault.
25. Assess and care for a patient and family in a crisis.

> I remember all the feelings in my first semester of college. I never thought I'd make it! I was mad at my teachers. Then I realized it wasn't my teachers. It was me! In retrospect, realizing that I was in a crisis helps me understand what I was living through.

Crisis theory provides nursing with a theoretical model of the processes of adaptation that follow certain kinds of stressful, disquieting, unmanageable events in the person's life. Its usefulness lies in its systematic organization of events that appear haphazard and unpredictable and in its potential to guide you when working with people in crisis.

DEFINITIONS AND CHARACTERISTICS

Crisis *is any transient situation that requires the reorganization of one's psychological structure and behavior, that causes a sudden alteration in the person's expectation of self, and that cannot be handled with the usual coping mechanisms* (20, 37).

The person's ordinary behavior is no longer successful emotionally, intellectually, or physically. Old habits are disturbed and the person feels motivated to try new responses in order to cope with the situation at hand. Even if the person's behavior is inadequate or inappropriate to the present situation and may differ from normal, it should not be considered pathological. The crisis may also reactivate old unresolved crises or conflicts, which imposes an additional burden to be resolved. The crisis is a turning point, however, and with its resultant mobilization of energy is a second chance to correct earlier maladaptations or faulty problem solving. The time of crisis serves as a catalyst or opportunity for growth emotionally. There is a realignment of behavior that, if all goes well, will lead to a state of equilibrium or behavior that is more mature than the previous status. On the other hand, because of the stress involved and the felt threat to equilibrium, the person is also more vulnerable to regression and mental or physical illness. The outcome—either increased maturity or illness—depends on how the person handles the situation and on the help that others give. Encountering and resolving a crisis are normal processes that each of us faces many times during life.

Stress, defined and discussed earlier, must be differentiated from *crisis*. **Stress** *is the everyday wear and tear on the body, the effects of the rate at which you live at any moment, positive and negative, physical, emotional, or mental* (111). All living organisms are constantly under stress, and anything, pleasant or unpleasant, that speeds up the intensity of life causes a temporary increase in stress or in the wear and tear on the body. A painful blow or a passionate kiss can be equally stressful, for example. Stress does not consist merely of damage but also of the adaptation to damage, and it can be positive and life promoting. During a stressful period the person can use normal coping mechanisms. The temporary upsets in equilibrium are solved by previously learned coping techniques and various mechanisms of tension discharge, such as talking. Stress, however, has a great potential for reducing the person's level of mental health, whereas crisis has a great potential for raising it. Yet both may have either a positive or negative outcome (103, 111).

Not all persons facing the same hazardous event are in a state of crisis. But certain events or situations are viewed as a crisis by everyone in that some behavioral adjustment must be made by anyone facing that situation. Research by Holmes and Rahe has shown that the number and seriousness of certain types of life changes or crises recently encountered increase the person's chance of facing other crises, including illness or accidental injury (52). Crises also vary in degree; a situation may be perceived as major, moderate, or minimal in the degree of discomfort caused and the amount of behavioral change demanded.

Crisis in the person's life can be considered from the standpoint of adaptation theory discussed in Chapter 7. The total person responds to crisis in ways that affect adaptation or higher levels of integration of total body function. The response to crisis is also a way of adapting. Crisis, and one's reaction to it, affects physiological, intellectual, emotional, social, and cultural aspects of the person's life as well as of the family unit.

TYPES OF CRISES

Two types of crises affect the person and family systems: (1) developmental, maturational, or normative and (2) situational or accidental (1).

Developmental Crisis

Developmental crises *are transition points, the periods that everyone experiences in the process of biopsychosocial growth and development and that are accompanied by changes in thoughts, feelings, and abilities.* These are times in development when new relationships are formed and old relationships take on new aspects. Others have new expectations of the person and certain physical, emotional, intellectual, and social tasks must be accomplished so that the person can move to the next phase of development. The onset of the developmental or maturational crisis is gradual because it occurs as the person moves from one stage of growth and development to another; the crisis does not last for the entire era, however.

Why does normal development leave the person vulnerable to crisis? Spiegel's description of role theory is helpful for understanding (116).

Role *is a goal-directed pattern of behavior learned within one's cultural setting and carried out by the person in the social group or situation because both the person and the group expect this behavior.* No role exists in isolation. It is always patterned to dovetail with or complement the role of another. When one person changes role, the role partners—other persons in the system—undergo reciprocal role or behavioral changes. The times of maturational or developmental crisis are mainly periods of many role changes, although they may be slow and gradual and vary from one culture or class to another. A maturational crises occurs when the person is unable to make role changes appropriate to a new level of maturity. The stressful events are the social and biological pressures on the individual to see the self in a new and different role and act accordingly (116).

There are three main reasons why someone may be unable to make the role changes necessary to prevent a maturational crisis:

1. The person's inability to picture the self in a new role. Roles are learned; adequate role models may not exist.
2. The person may be unable to make role changes because of a lack

of intrapersonal resources—for example, inadequate communication skills, realization that with life passing it is not possible to achieve certain goals, or inability to realize alternatives to the present lifestyle.

3. Refusal by others in the social system to see the person in a different role. When the adolescent tries to move from childhood to the adult role, for instance, the parent may persist in keeping him/her in the child role (116).

The primary developmental crises are entry into school, puberty, leaving home, engagement, marriage, pregnancy, childbirth, middle age, menopause, retirement, and facing the death of others and of the self.

Situational Crisis

The **situational crisis** *is an external event or situation—one not necessarily a part of normal living and often sudden, unexpected, and unfortunate—that is too threatening to the person's immediate resources or ability to cope and that requires a change in behavior.* The self-concept is threatened. The person feels overwhelmed and helpless. There is a threat or danger to life goals; tension and anxiety are evoked; unresolved problems and crises from the past are reawakened. The amount of time taken for healthy or unhealthy adaption to occur may take as little as 1 to 6 weeks, or as long as 6 months or a year, depending on the situation, its meaning to the person, and the inner resources and outer support system available. A situational crisis may occur at the same time as a developmental crisis (95).

Situational crises include natural disasters, such as a hurricane, tornado, or flood; loss through separation, divorce from, or death of a loved one; losing one's job, money, or valued possessions; and a change in job. Illness or hospitalization, a power struggle on the job, a promotion or sudden change in role responsibilities, or a forced geographical relocation are other examples. Suicide attempts and violence, such as rape or being a victim of crime, can also be classified as this type of crisis (26).

FACTORS INFLUENCING THE OUTCOME OF CRISIS

Various factors influence how someone reacts to and copes with crisis situations (20, 37):

1. *The person's perception of the event.* If the event or its consequences conflict with the value system or wishes for the future, the situation is defined as hazardous. The perception of the event is reality for the person regardless of how others might define

reality and determines behavior. To illustrate, two persons live through the disaster of a flood. One loses a house and all possessions; the other loses a boat, but everything else is intact. Yet the latter may react with greater shock, denial, anger, or depression than the person who loses a home and possessions because of their different perceptions—the meaning to each of the loss.

2. *The physical and emotional status* of the person, degree of health, amount of energy present, age, genetic endowment, and biological rhythms.
3. *The coping techniques or mechanisms and the level of personal maturity*. If adaptive capacities are already strained, or if the stress is overwhelming, the person will cling to old habits and the behavior will probably be inappropriate to the task at hand. The person who has met developmental tasks all along will adapt more easily in any crisis.
4. *Previous experiences with similar situations*. The person must learn to cope with stress and change. If someone resolved past crises by distorting reality or withdrawing, then when similar crises arise, the person must attempt to cope with a new situation while burdened with prior failure. Crises of any kind are often cumulative in effect. The most recent crisis revives the denial, depression, anger, or maladaptation that was left unsettled or unresolved from past crises.
5. *The objectively realistic aspects of the current situation*, such as personal or material losses, and the number of life crisis changes encountered in the past year.
6. *Cultural influences*. How the person is trained and socialized in the home to solve problems and meet crisis situations, expectations of how the social group will be supportive during crisis, and the method established by the social system to provide help all influence present behavior.
7. *The availability and response of family and close friends or other helping resources*, including professional persons. The less readily available the person's environmental or emotional support systems are to decrease stress or buttress coping responses, the more hazardous he/she will define the event. The family system, by its influence on development of self-concept and maturity, can increase or decrease vulnerability to crisis. When someone's involvement with others is concentrated on only a few family members—as, for example, in the nuclear versus the extended family support system—vulnerability is increased. The reaction to crisis is also increased in today's mobile, urbanized society because traditional support systems of long-term family and friends have been disrupted. Thus the professional person is more likely to be needed and sought. Even a small amount of influence exerted by a signi-

ficant person can be enough to decide the outcome for mental health and against mental illness. Sustained mental health, however, is chiefly a result of a life history of successfully resolving crises. The family, like the individual, may be **crisis prone**, *vulnerable to situational or developmental crises that occur frequently and have a cumulative effect.*

The crisis-prone person or family often demonstrates the following characteristics:

1. Rapid encountering of one stressful situation after another, with inadequate time to adjust to or cope with any one situation.
2. A history of inadequate coping skills.
3. Lack of communication skills or inability to ask for help because of emotional isolation from others.
4. Feelings about solving problems alone because of loss of persons or things that were viewed as supportive or because of feelings of racial or ethnic prejudice, demoralization, or alienation.
5. Inadequate family, social, religious, economic, or employment supportive resources.

Frequent illness or accidents, legal problems, or abuse of alcohol or other drugs may also increase the risk of other crises (50, 90).

Crisis effects are reduced by

1. Anticipating and preparing for the so-called unpredictable events, such as change of developmental stages, natural disasters, or death.
2. Redefining or changing goals when something seems insurmountable.
3. Developing communication skills and a support system.
4. Seeking help to work through each crisis and unresolved past crises (50, 90).

PHASES OF CRISIS

All crises require a sudden and then later restructuring of biopsychosocial integration before normal function can be maintained. The phases involved are shock, followed closely by general realization of the crisis; then defensive retreat; acknowledgment; and, finally, adaptation or resolution (20, 37).

In the Initial, Impact, or Shock Phase the person briefly realizes the seriousness and threat of the situation and then feels a high level of stress, helplessness, anxiety, chaos, and possibly panic. He/she feels overwhelmed and depersonalized. Self-esteem is threatened, and thinking and behavior are disorganized. The person is unable to plan, to reason logically, or to understand the situation. Judgment is impaired. Habitual or automatic problem-solving behaviors are used without success, although the person cannot perceive any inadequacy. He/she may suffer physical illness or injury and either focus attention on them or completely ignore the physical status. Socially the person is unable to function appropriately, becoming withdrawn, docile, or perhaps hyperactive and chaotic. Basic needs cannot be met without help.

The shock phase usually lasts a short time, perhaps a few hours or a day or two. The reactions of the alarm stage of the stress syndrome discussed in Chapter 7 cannot be tolerated for too long. On either perceiving or being told what has happened, the person copes with the realization of the sudden discontinuity in life through the second phase, defensive retreat.

In Defensive Retreat the person tries previously successful ways of solving problems and adjusting, but tension and discomfort are not reduced and the situation is not alleviated. He/she feels increasingly upset and ineffective. At the first try the problem is directly approached, but the behavior does not work. Then he/she may try to redefine the problem (usually unrealistically), avoid the problem, or seek the support of others. Generally the person retreats into the self, avoiding reality, denying, fantasizing about what could be done or how well he/she once handled problems. The person may become disoriented, indifferent, apathetic, or euphoric. Usually because of repression, the person will claim to feel all right and will not perceive the anxiety and ineffective behavior. Changes suggested by others are resisted; a rigid manner of thinking and expressing the same ideas over and over are common. Behavior is ineffective and disorganized; daily activities cannot be carried out. The person cannot devise alternate courses of action and cannot predict accurately the effects of behavior. Physical symptoms are generally minimal; the person may feel better than usual. Socially the person may be withdrawn or superficial and hyperactive and unable to maintain social roles adequately. The phase of defensive retreat may last for a brief or prolonged period, depending on circumstances.

Denial is a mechanism used in defensive retreat and involves use of three other mental mechanisms:

1. Rationalization about discomfort or symptoms and the cause of the situation (for example, the person with chest pain says that it is indigestion).
2. Displacement of dangerous, disquieting, uncomfortable informa-

tion onto the health team or family, often in the form of demands or complaints.
3. Projection of personal feelings of inadequacy onto others, saying how inept or neglectful others are.

The purposes of these mechanisms are to protect the self from painful information.

The Third Phase, Recoil or Acknowledgment, begins when the facts can no longer be denied. The person realizes the objective reality of the situation and slowly begins to redefine it, attempting to do problem solving. Tension and anxiety again rise. Reality may seem harsh; and depression, agitation, apathy, self-hate, low self-esteem, and the process of mourning occur. The person's coping abilities and self-concept may disintegrate before energy can be directed toward coping. Thinking may at first be disorganized, but gradually the person can make appropriate plans and find solutions for the situation by trial and error. Physically he/she may feel well or tension may be somaticized. The person will give up certain goals as unattainable. The person will recognize that he/she has been a social burden and make plans to resume former roles to the degree possible.

The Fourth Phase, Resolution or Adaptation and Change, occurs when the person perceives the crisis situation in a positive way and integrates the painful event into the new self. Problem solving is successful and feelings about the event are expressed. A new sense of worth, a firm identity, a gradual increase in satisfaction in mastering the situation, and a gradual lowering of anxiety result. Thinking and planning are organized; appropriate resources and abilities are used. Physically the person is functioning at the optimum level. Socially he/she resumes status and roles and repatterns behavior to cope and thus avoid future similar crises. In order to integrate the crisis into the personality, the person must develop a different concept of self and the lifestyle. The person does not feel bitter about the event encountered or changes made.

At this point the person should be at a higher level of maturity and adaptation than earlier: He/she has acquired new coping mechanisms.

Resolving the crisis is made more difficult by the negative influences discussed earlier and by additional hardships or complications caused by the crisis itself. Ineffective mastery or problem solving or lack of expression of feelings associated with the crisis may cause a restricted level of funtioning in one or all spheres of the personality. The problem may be repressed and permanently denied and unresolved or major disorganization such as neurosis, psychosis, socially maladjusted behavior, or chronic physical disability, may occur.

These are the predictable phases of crisis; however, each stage is not sharply demarcated. One stage may merge into another or certain behaviors may not appear at all, particularly in developmental crisis in which the person's functioning may be appropriate in one sphere but less so in another aspect of the personality. In addition, the person may be at the beginning of one phase and then return to the previous phase behaviorally. Thus the person may demonstrate some behaviors indicative of one phase—such as defensive retreat—and simultaneously demonstrate a few behaviors of shock or acknowledgment.

Family Reactions

The family unit undergoes essentially the same phases of crisis and manifests similar reactions as the designated client, although the intensity and timing may differ.

If the source of trouble is from within the family, it is usually perceived as more distressing than an external source of trouble, for internal problems reflect lack of harmony and inadequacy in the members. Shock and defensive retreat reactions may be more pronounced during times of internal trouble. As acknowledgment of reality occurs, there is a strong tendency to scapegoat family members to restore family balance. Crisis events for the family include the developmental and situational crisis previously discussed (90, 95).

Group or Community Reactions

A social group or entire neighborhood may feel the impact of an individual or family in crisis.

The community is also affected by natural disasters, such as a flood, tornado, hurricane, or blizzard; by disasters resulting from advances in our civilization, such as chemical or radiation spills and electrical blackouts; and by disasters for which humans are responsible, such as fire or war.

Community reactions to any of these disasters are influenced by the following factors (6, 26, 48, 51, 54, 79, 90, 95):

1. Element of surprise versus preparedness. If warnings are not given about an impending crisis—or if warnings are given without an action plan—panic, shock, denial, and defensive retreat are more likely to occur.
2. Separation of family members. Children are especially affected

by separation; the family should be evacuated from a disaster area as a unit.

3. Availability of outside help.
4. Leadership. Someone must make decisions and give directions. Usually the police, Red Cross and Civil Defense workers, National Guard, military, or professionals in a community are seen as authoritative persons. Coordination of the activities of all these groups is essential to deliver services and avoid chaos.
5. Communication. Public information centers must be established to avoid rumor, provide reassurance and direction, and ensure that all citizens get information about coping measures, evacuation, reconstruction, rehabilitation, and available financial aid. Otherwise citizens will later be bitter and suspicious when some learn that others benefited more than they did.
6. Measures taken to help reorientation. Communication networks lay the foundation for re-identification of individuals into family and social groups and for registration of survivors.
7. Presence of plans for individuals and social institutions to cope with disaster, including evacuation of a population from a stricken area if necessary. Emergency plans focus on the following concerns:
   (a) Preservation of life and health through rescue, triage, inoculation, and treatment of the injured.
   (b) Conservation and distribution of resources, such as shelter, water, food, and blankets.
   (c) Conservation of public order by police surveillance to prevent looting and further accidents or injuries.
   (d) Maintenance of moral through dispatching health and welfare workers to the disaster scene.
   (e) Administration of health services.

Communities in crisis have characteristics in common with individuals in crisis. The most immediate social consequence of a disaster is disruption of normal social patterns and services; the community is socially paralyzed (90).

In a major disaster about 75 to 90 percent of the victims will be in shock, followed by the phase of defensive retreat, in response to warnings of disaster, orders of evacuation, destruction of homes, and disruption of water, electricity, heat, food supplies, communication, traffic, and transportation. Also, there is potential inability of the health agencies to care for the injured and ill because of manpower and supply shortages or damage. In addition to individual reactions, an atmosphere of tension, fear, confusion, and suspicion exists; facts are distorted and rumors are rampant. Normal functioning is reduced as businesses, vital services, schools, and recreational areas may be closed. Although some people are in shock or denial, there will be a few who take advantage of the chaos to loot and steal and a few businesses may profiteer (26, 48, 57, 79, 90).

Response to external emergencies is often quicker than the response to internal stresses or crises. About 10 to 25 percent of the victims remain reality oriented, calm, and able to develop and implement a plan of action; such people often are those with advanced training. But these crisis workers may react with at least brief periods of shock and defensive retreat after most of the immediate work is done (48, 51, 90).

When reality is acknowledged, people in the community at first become more cohesive as they help each other; then individual problems become the focus. People find shelter, look for someone to be with, want to be cared for, express a sense of loss through crying and talking, and share with others how they managed to survive. During this time, depending on the amount of damage, anger and frustration are keenly felt as the person evaluates the damage and feels robbed of possessions that have been worked for thoughout life. The older, dependent, or incapacitated person may become seriously ill or die because he/she feels unable to start all over again. If loved ones were killed, grief and mourning for them, as well as for lost possessions, result. Guilt reactions as a result of being unable to save the loved one, of being spared death, and of relief at being alive are common. Reactive depression, anxiety reactions, regression, dreams, suicidal thoughts, physical illness, psychotic episodes, and neurotic reactions occur and may last for several months or a year after the disaster. The more severe the disaster, the longer these reactions last. Some people's psyches may be permanently damaged. Older people who suffer a disaster are statistically more likely to die within the year following the disaster. Also, psychological effects are more severe and slower to resolve when survivors perceive the disaster as a result of human callousness or error rather than as an act of God or nature (26, 48, 51, 76, 79, 90).

Resolution occurs in individuals as previously described and is related to the individual's psychological health before the crisis as well as to the kind of help given to the family unit during the disaster, the kind of crisis and extent of damage, and the ability of the community to repair damage and return to normal function. Perhaps the best sign of community resolution is a well-developed disaster plan of action, one that can be implemented in the event of another crisis, and community-wide education for individual and family preparedness for disaster.

Other references on community disasters with guidelines for coping are found in references 36 and 54.

INEFFECTIVE RESOLUTION OF CRISIS

If there is no adaptive resolution or change in behavior to cope with the crisis, maladaptive or ineffective reactions occur as an attempt at resolution. There may be a delayed reaction in that the crisis event and its consequences are presently denied and repressed. A reaction is eventually precipitated when a future crisis occurs that recalls the buried feelings and that then renders the person ineffective in functioning. Various other reactions of distorted or inappropriate behavior may occur, although neurosis, psychosis, or socially ineffective behavior occur only in a small percentage of people. The person may be euphoric if denial is prolonged. In the crisis of death of a loved one the person may prolong identification with the deceased by developing symptoms like those in the last illness of the deceased. And eventually the organic pathological changes specific for the disease may occur (22, 72, 99). Sometimes such illness occurs on the anniversary of the loss. Or the aggrieved person may develop a different disease, caused by the **mind-body relationship**—*in which physiological changes result because of the effects of emotional states on body parts and which eventually cause organ damage* (99). (*Illness resulting from the effects of the emotional state is also called* **psychosomatic illness.**)

A study by Rees and Lutkins shows a relationship between loss and the development of psychosomatic symptoms. Bereaved relatives are found to have a higher mortality rate during the first year of mourning, a rate that increased further for widowed persons. The risk of the close relative dying from the effects of anxiety, hostility, and guilt during that first year was significantly increased when the loved one had died at some place other than home (99).

A study by Parkes shows that medical office consultations for psychiatric symptoms and chronic somatic conditions, such as arthritis, increased by 63 percent the first six months after loss of a husband. Thereafter the rate of consultation decreased, but it still remained higher than the premourning period. The aged particularly express grief reactions through somatic symptoms: persons over 64 years had even higher rates of doctors' office visits. The psychic state may contribute to a number of disease processes through increasing biological vulnerability (99).

Personality significantly mitigates the illness-providing effects of stressful life events. Two groups of executives had comparably high degrees of stress over a 3-year interval as measured by the Holmes and Rahe schedule of recent life events. One group suffered high stress without becoming ill; the other reported becoming sick after an encounter with stressful life events. Illness was predictably related to personality.

In comparison with high-stress, high-illness executives, high-stress, low-illness executives show more control, commitment to the job, and interest in change as a challenge rather than change as stress (67). Individuals with a high need for power who are inhibited in expressing feelings are more likely than others to report severe illnesses, apparently related to chronic overactivity of the sympathetic nervous system, with above-average epinephrine excretion and lower concentrations of immunoglobins (80).

Sudden death has occurred in persons who feel depressed, helpless, hopeless, acutely anxious, or angry following a crisis situation, apparently from disequilibrium in the hormonal and autonomic nervous systems (59, 69, 89). The phenomenon needs further study.

Maladaptation may include expressing hostility for an excessively prolonged time against authority figures—doctors, nurses, police officers, parents, or teachers. Prolonged sadness, apathy, lack of initiative, irritability, suspicion, and withdrawing from others because of internalized anger or shock can be equally detrimental to relationships with others and to overall conduct. Feelings of isolation, worthlessness, hopelessness, and guilt may become magnified to the point of inducing suicide attempts. Then, again, the person may suppress his/her own personality, taking on traits of the lost person.

The person who stays compulsively busy or is ritualistic may become ineffective in attempts to cope. Alcohol, drugs, or excessive eating may become a crutch or escape when activity no longer provides adequate tension release.

The person may engage in action detrimental to the self economically or socially through excessive generosity or foolish financial dealings (which represent self-punishment) or through delinquency. The latter invites apprehension, punishment, and, at times, someone else making the decisions.

After loss of a loved one, the person through extreme denial, may continue to act as though the lost person is still alive and present. The survivor, for instance, may continue to set a place at the table for the deceased or keep all the possessions of the lost one. Or the person may acknowledge the death but deny the significance of the loss emotionally or intellectually. He/she may not take care of business matters because the deceased person was the person who previously did so.

You have an opportunity to help prevent maladaptive resolution through appropriate crisis intervention. When assessing the person in any illness situation, determine if the problems and needs could be the result of an earlier crisis that is now causing symptoms or inappropriate behavior.

Working with someone who has maladaptive behavior can be a slow process. You should not expect too much of yourself or the other, for in your disappointment and frustration you may withdraw from him/her, thus preventing crisis resolution. Recognize your strengths and limitations and decide whether the person can use help beyond what you can offer. Accept the fact that because this person is unique, available knowledge and techniques may not be of sufficient help. On the other hand, a possibility of failure should not preclude an attempt to help.

Provide an environment in which the person can experience the phases of recovery from any maladaptive behavior or illness. Help him/her reminisce about what he/she used to do, express fear, look forward optimistically but realistically to the future, and use appropriate rehabilitative measures.

THE NURSING PROCESS AND CRISIS INTERVENTION

You will encounter crises in a variety of settings: the emergency room, recovery room, coronary-care unit, surgical intensive-care unit, industrial or school dispensary, and the obstetrical, pediatric, and psychiatric units. In most of these settings you will collaborate with the physician and other health team members. In the mental or neighborhood health center you may function as primary therapist within agency policy or with other health team members. You may be the sole therapist in telephone crisis work.

Your philosophy of care must include the concept of crisis. The person in crisis is at a turning point and ready for great changes in a relatively short period of time because of the tension, pain, and disequilibrium associated with crisis. These feelings motivate efforts to alter the situation. Distress creates an openness to assistance and change. The person expects expert help and perceives the nurse as an expert. A minimal amount of support and help can influence the outcome of a crisis significantly.

Crisis therapy is based on the theory that aid during crisis will help the person to adapt in a healthy manner. The minimal goal of therapy is psychological resolution of the immediate crisis and the restoration of coping mechanisms to at least the level of functioning that existed before the crisis event. The maximal goal is to bring about a change in behavior that is more mature than that of the precrisis level. Crisis work involves reinstating earlier stress-reducing behavior or developing new adaptive techniques. Underlying these goals is the assumption that the person seeking help has unused resources that, with minimum assistance, can be called on to function effectively in everyday living.

Factors influencing the course of crisis therapy are as follows:

1. Attitude of the therapist and the value placed on crisis work.
2. Use of time, in that assessment is done as quickly as possible to define accurately the nature of the crisis, identify the person's response to the event, and devise a course of action for resolving the crisis.
3. Use of nontraditional treatment practices, for appointment time and place are determined by the degree of stress and impaired functioning that the person is experiencing, the skill of the therapist, and the number and kind of resources in the community available to assist the person.
4. Differences between the value systems of the therapist and the individual concerned. The therapist must be open to what constitutes a problem for another. The person's lifestyle and values may be foreign to or in conflict with those of the therapist, but the person needs acceptance in order to maintain a basic lifestyle and value system.

Assessment

Collecting information must be systematic and yet flexible, rapid enough to interrupt the crisis, but thorough enough to define the problem and phase of crisis and identify and achieve the desired outcomes.

The following factors should be assessed: the anxiety level and feelings of the person; ego functioning (perception, judgment, memory, problem solving); presence of symptoms; whether the person is suicidal or homicidal; and usual living patterns, work arrangements, and interpersonal and social situation. Nonverbal behavior and the consistency between verbal and nonverbal behavior must be noted. The person does not always mean what is said and will not always act in a way that directly expresses true feelings. If the person cannot identify the problem because of disorganized thinking, focus attention on what was occurring just prior to the situation and onset of symptoms. Constructing a sequence of events aids reorientation.

After determining the extent of the problem, focus the person's perception on the event—for example, the illness or loss. What does this situation mean to him/her? How does he/she see its effect on the future? Is the event seen realistically? What hardships have been created by the crisis—for example, job loss due to depression or mental illness, which, in turn, causes financial and family problems and loss of self-esteem?

Ascertain if the person is suicidal or plans to kill another person. If so, try to learn how and when. If the intention is carefully planned and details are specific, hospitalization and psychiatric evaluation must be arranged to protect the person and others.

Your next questions should be directed to the availability of help and supportive others or the extent of isolation from significant relationships. What is the person's relationship with supportive other? Crisis intervention is sharply limited in time. The more persons who are helping, the better. Then, too, when crisis therapy is terminated, if helpful others are involved, they can continue to give support to the person. Assess the adaptive capacities of the others involved in the situation who have not sought help but who might also be experiencing crises. If no helpful resources are available, you become a temporary support system while helping the person to establish a relationship with a person or group in the community or work setting.

Ascertain what the person usually does when confronted with an unsolvable problem. What are the coping skills? Has anything like this happened before? What was done to decrease tension? If the person is trying the same method now and it is not working, what *would* decrease stress symptoms? Any past activity that proved successful could be tried again. Determine strengths and not just problems and limitations.

Through assessment you can determine why this situation is a crisis to this person, why he/she is unable to alter lifestyle to cope with the situation, and what in the lifestyle can be altered so that the crisis can be resolved.

Planning Intervention

As you study the data collected in the preceding manner, the person should also be actively involved in seeking a potential solution. You cannot solve the problem for the person; you can only help that individual to help the self.

The problem should be clarified and the immediate situation put in focus. The plan for intervention is determined by assessing the nature of the crisis (whether acute or chronically recurring), the reactions of others significant to the person, and the strengths and resources of all persons involved. The plan for intervention must extend beyond the person to others involved less directly in the crisis. To understand the person's adaptive capacity in comparison to precrisis adaptation, some attention must be paid both to past experience and to current personal and environmental resources.

Several alternate solutions should be explored. Positive guidelines for action should be given to the person before leaving each session, including the first one, so that alternate solutions can be tested. This step permits evaluation of coping behavior at each successive session so that additional solutions can be sought if necessary.

Intervention

Some help can be provided during the first interview by clarifying the problem with the person and encouraging verbalization of feelings. Getting a hold on a problem by talking it through is the first step in problem solving. The person can begin to recognize what this situation means, how to cope with it, and what or who can help. The resultant increase in self-confidence motivates further coping behavior.

Use primary, secondary, or tertiary preventive intervention, depending on the person and the crisis (20).

Primary prevention, *or preventing a crisis,* can be achieved by helping the person work through developmental periods or anticipated situations.

The anticipation of life crises is an important concept in health promotion and so has broad implications in nursing. If able to prepare for what is potentially in store, the person will be less vulnerable to physical or mental illness, as shown in studies by Janis on the "work of worrying" or anticipatory grieving. The more thorough the thinking, planning, or "work of worry" before a crisis, the more adequate is the subsequent adjustment and the less severe is the impact felt. Persons with either excessively high or excessively low levels of fear or worry, however, are ineffective in preparing for crisis. The high-level worrier feels so much fear that something bad will happen that it is impossible to effectively plan ahead. The low-level worrier does not adequately contemplate impending stress and feels anger and resentment when it comes. The moderately worrisome person can express tension physically, emotionally, and verbally, but maintains self-control and thus rationally plans and adjusts behavior to the situation (60).

You can help the person do the "work of worry" or anticipatory grieving in the following ways: through premarital counseling to increase the chance of healthy resolution of stressful marital events and the achievement of appropriate developmental tasks; teaching and counseling in prenatal classes to prepare for childbirth and child care; talking with a mother whose child will soon enter school or be married; preretirement counseling to help the person plan ahead to meet the problems and developmental tasks associated with retirement; counseling the family of a terminally ill patient; and talking preoperatively with the person who is undergoing major surgery and body-image changes. Can you think of other situations in which primary prevention can promote health?

Preventive intervention is not designed to cause major changes in the maturity of personality structure of the person but rather to maintain the usual level of functioning of equilibrium. The intervention for health promotion described by Murray and Zentner (91) is thus most likely to work with well persons.

Secondary prevention *involves early identification of the crisis so the person can avoid maladaptive behavior.* The person is helped to adapt to the crisis, thereby reducing the intensity and duration of reaction to it. He/she is quickly given support, encouraged to use energies and available resources constructively, and helped to understand that his/her feelings and behavior are a normal response to the situation.

Examples of secondary prevention in crisis therapy are working with women who have not resolved the crisis of motherhood and extending help to the person who is mourning the loss of a significant person, object, or role.

Tertiary prevention *is aimed at preventing further decompensation or impairment, after the person has partially resolved a crisis, so that he/she can continue to live a useful role in the community.* The person's behavior may initially interfere with rehabilitation. When able to resolve the meaning or implications of the crisis and feelings about it, the person will be able to become involved in rehabilitation. Progress depends strongly on the counseling role of the nurse and on continuity in the nurse–client relationship. Through this kind of intervention, the person may eventually rework the crisis and become more effective behaviorally. Examples of tertiary prevention are group therapy with chronically ill or disabled persons to help them cope with their health problems, counseling to help a person work through delayed mourning, and remotivation techniques to prevent further disengagement in the aged [outlined by Murray and Zentner (91)].

Crisis therapy is basically brief and specific to the present situation and involves placing attainable goals directly before the person. Thus the principles of crisis intervention are relevant to all people, including those concerned primarily with the here-and-now, who prefer brief, concrete intervention, and who seek assistance for specific problems.

The person or family in crisis becomes more susceptible to the influence of significant others. A little help directed purposefully and with the right timing is more effective than greater help given at a period of less emotional accessibility. View yourself as intervening in a social system, into a network of relationships, and not as a single resource to the person. Use the skills of other health team members—the doctor, social worker, chaplain, psychologist, and occupational therapist—either directly or for consultation.

Principles of Intervention, discussed next, can be accomplished by using your knowledge of crisis theory, therapeutic communication (discussed in Chapter 3), and establishment of a nurse–client relationship (discussed in Chapter 4).

Show acceptance of the person and establish a positive, concerned relationship so that he/she feels a sense of hope, self-worth, and lessened anxiety.

During crisis you are often confronted by an angry, bitter, or accusatory person or family who berate you, other health team members, or the agency for negligence. Keep two points in mind: their statements may be accurate and justified or that may be the only way they can cope with their own aggression, helplessness, or guilt at the time. Provide the best care possible, show genuine concern, and do not become verbally involved in the dispute. Do not take the behavior personally if it does not apply to you.

Help the person confront the crisis by talking about present feelings of denial, anger, guilt, or grief. Catharsis lowers tension, clarifies the problem, promotes comprehension of the reality and consequences of the situation, and mobilizes energy for constructive action.

Help the person confront the crisis in amounts or "doses" that can be managed, being cautious not to soften the impact of the event too much. The reality of the situation must be kept in the foreground, although periods of relief from facing the whole situation are needed. Help the person first gain an intellectual understanding of the crisis; then encourage an emotional understanding and adjustment. In this way, he/she can more objectively handle the real situation.

Recognize denial as a normal reaction. Cope with personal feelings about the person's behavior and situation; observe such behavior objectively; avoid reinforcing denial; and gently represent reality. Work with other resource persons for information, collaboration, maintenance of support, and representation of reality.

Explain to the person the relationship between the crisis situation and the present behavior and feelings. People feel less overwhelmed and better able to manage when they understand that the feelings are normal in the context of crisis.

Help the person find facts, for facts are less awesome than speculations or fantasies about the situation or the unknown.

Explore past life occurrences only in relation to the existing crisis, particularly if feelings aroused in past crises have been unresolved and are influencing present behavior. The present experience can produce defensive behaviors used in the past that are no longer useful.

Avoid giving false reassurance. Acknowledge the validity of fears and other feelings. Show faith in the person's ability to manage, but do not reduce motivation to cope and adapt by saying that everything will be fine.

Do not encourage the person to blame others for the crisis event, for this process avoids the truth, reduces motivation to take responsibility for personal behavior, and discourages adaptation. Listen initially to rationalizations; then raise doubt about such statements through questioning.

Anticipate that people facing loss may behave in a grossly maladaptive way and need to be treated with tact, patience, warmth, and empathy, as well as encouraged to express feelings without feeling guilty about doing so. Set limits on behavior that would be destructive to the person or to others.

Explore coping mechanisms to assist the person in examining alternate ways of coping and in seeking and using new behaviors or alternate ways of satisfying needs. Help him/her to learn or relearn basic social skills as necessary and to fit the personality to the demands presented by the crisis.

Strengthen or reinforce previously learned behavior patterns that can be effective but are not presently being used.

Clarify and reemphasize responsibility for personal behavior, decisions, and way of life. For example, the person in crisis from illness and hospitalization should be assisted in learning the patient role. Thus, any uncertainty about expectations for self and others is replaced by the feeling of being a participating member of the treatment team. Therefore orientation to the hospital division's policies and routines, the room (and roommate, if any), personnel, diagnostic procedures, and preoperative and postoperative care is necessary. When aware of the possible outcomes of the illness, the person can make decisions about present care goals and future health needs. When he/she knows what to expect from the health team members, behavior can be adaptive. Health care workers can be resources to improve the health status.

Help the person establish necessary social relationships and change personal behavior accordingly. If someone has lost or is otherwise removed from all significant persons, as might be true for the elderly or new immigrants, introduce the person to new people to help fill the void and obtain support and gratification.

Assist the person in seeking and accepting help. By acknowledging that trouble exists, he/she is more likely to use personal resources and the help offered by others. If necessary, encourage acceptance of help with the everyday tasks of living and mobilization of inner strengths as well as concerned others in the environment.

Although you work with a person or family in crisis therapy, some crises may upset an entire community, such as natural disasters. Use of support systems and role redistribution is then more complex.

Crisis Resolution and Anticipatory Planning terminate crisis intervention. Crisis work is then reviewed and the accomplishments of the person in working through the predicament should be emphasized. Adaptive coping mechanisms and appropriate behavior that the person has successfully used should be reinforced. Positive changes in behavior should be summarized to allow reexperiencing and reconfirming the progress made. Give assistance as needed in making realistic plans for the future and discuss with the person ways in which the present experience may help in coping with future crises. The person should leave with self-confidence in managing his/her life and with the awareness that assistance will be available in the future if necessary.

Evaluation. In order to continue to do effective crisis intervention, the step of evaluation in the nursing process must be carried out as discussed in Chapter 4.

A Case Study

Consider the following case. Some of the details are omitted, but the significance of crisis intervention is obvious.

> The police in a Midwestern city of 60,000 picked up a 15-year-old boy for burglary. The Juvenile Department learned this was the boy's first offense and wanted to help avoid a future offense. A juvenile officer contacted the boy's school about his attendance and general conduct; both were reported to be within normal limits. The juvenile officer then asked the school principal to send the boy to the school counselor for psychological testing.
>
> The principal first asked the school nurse to make a home visit. He asked her to gather as much information as possible about the boy's emotional health and background. Then proper referral would be made for psychological testing.
>
> The school nurse found the mother and the rest of the family in an acute situational crisis. The husband had recently left his wife and four children. There was no hope of reconciliation. There was little food and almost no money. Additionally, each child was in developmental crisis. The oldest, the boy who had burglarized, was expected to take over the father's role. He was having a struggle just being an adolescent. But he had stolen to get money for the family. The next oldest child, a 12-year-old girl just entering puberty, was having personal problems at school. She had been especially close to her father and now cried much of the time about his departure. The 5-year-old was having difficulty adjusting to kindergarten. The 1-year-old baby had just learned to walk and was unusually active and demanding, possibly because of the emotional state in the home.
>
> The nurse acted rapidly. She saw the opportunity for intervention at the secondary prevention level. The mother was somewhat apathetic and appeared to be in the defensive-retreat phase of crisis. But she soon responded to the concern and warmth of the nurse, who listened attentively to the story.
>
> The nurse decided that their need for food and money was primary. She

transported the mother first to the Emergency City Aid Department, which provided temporary supplies and cash, and then to the Welfare Department to arrange for more permanent aid. The next day she contacted the Big Sister program at a local college to secure a "big sister" for the 12-year-old girl. The college student was majoring in counseling; so with an understanding of the situation, she was able to give immediate companionship and support. The nurse notified the kindergarten teacher of the 5-year-old's family situation.

After the results were received from the recommended psychological testing, the nurse sent the 15-year-old boy to Project Alter, an organization with staff specially trained to help alter lawbreaking tendencies in adolescents. The organization worked with other community agencies to set up a network of supportive help for the boy.

Because of this immediate help, the mother was able to move quickly to the third stage of crisis acknowledgment. She could now begin crisis resolution and anticipatory planning while giving more attention to the 1-year-old child.

The key figure in this case is the *nurse* who made a quick and valid assessment. She intervened effectively because she understood crisis therapy and because she knew her community's resources. She would evaluate her crisis intervention after resolution of the crisis.

CRISIS INTERVENTION BY TELEPHONE

The ringing clinic telephone is answered. A tremulous young female voice asks "Do you do pregnancy tests without informing parents?"

In the emergency department the nurse is called to the phone because a panicky male voice has inquired, "If ya' hit up Thorazine will it break down in the bloodstream?"

The voice on the other end of the line on a nursing division phone is saying, "You were so nice to me there. You were the only ones who cared. Thanks for trying but it's no use." The speech of the caller is heavily slurred.

Such situations emphasize the need for the telephone counseling skills in nurses who have been taught primarily to rely on face-to-face encounter (45, 66, 73, 100).

Telephone Crisis Centers

Telephone crisis centers are potentially within the reach of everyone in the United States. There are now hot lines for concerns including but not limited to abuse (child, adult, or substance); divorce counseling; gay life difficulties; loneliness; rape; youth run-away or crisis situations; sexual information and counsel; middle-age crises; and outreach to the desperate, depressed, and suicidal. Experience and research both indicate that the telephone is a valuable tool of preventive psychotherapy.

Typically a telephone crisis center operates with a small salaried professional and clerical staff aided by a much larger group of volunteers trained and supervised in doing telephone crisis work. Nurses are often well represented in telephone crisis centers.

Telephone hot lines usually provide training specific to their own particular goals and related to their own particular problem calls. You may want to gain the training and experience a specific telephone counseling center can offer. You will also want to be informed about other telephone crisis lines that are locally accessible. Learn about their services and skills, the training and supervision provided for the crisis workers, and their biases. Is their service prompt, responsive, and reliable? What information and referral services can they provide you as a practitioner? Become well acquainted with the strengths and limitations of crisis lines that your clients may use.

Characteristics of Telephone Therapy

Unique qualities of telephone therapy are (1) client in control, (2) anonymity of client, (3) geographic and personal barriers between client and therapist, and (4) anonymity of the therapist (134).

Such variables can create considerable anxiety, anger, and a sense of helplessness in you. The caller can hang up at any point when he/she feels too threatened. You are without your institutional supports and cannot physically do anything to control an impulsive or hysterical client. You are operating on reduced cues—only those that you can hear. Ironically, these feelings and factors are a basis for identification with the caller's needs. The caller, too, may well feel anxious, angry, and helpless. He/she must depend on you not to terminate the call without being helpful. Usual support systems are lacking. The caller needs to trust you in spite of having reduced cues as to whether you are trustworthy.

The therapist's anonymity in most crisis phone calls can enhance crisis work (34). The caller may decide that you are older and parental or that you are young and romantic. This projection of traits may enable him/her to confide in you. The caller's illusions need not be shattered unless they lead to unrealistic expectations, which you gently but honestly clarify.

Assessment by Telephone

If the caller has just swallowed an overdose of pills, be immediately concerned and interested so that the caller can trust you enough to reveal name and location. *Trust* is the key goal. Listen to the slurred speech and tolerate a wavering level of consciousness. It is self-restraining, difficult, but essential to say initially "Tell me what has happened that you feel you want to stop living," rather than "Tell me who you are and where you are."An open phone line dropped to the floor when the unconsciousness comes can still be traced. A hung-up phone cannot! The highly ambivalent caller will usually provide some means for you to help once he/she senses your concern. You might then say, "I can feel the wish of some part of you to give life another chance. That part of you is fighting hard for your life. I want to get help to you. Tell me how to find you."

When you hear overt panic and hysteria in the caller who has attempted suicide, you can be more direct and say, "I'm sending someone over to take you to an emergency room. Tell me the address where you are now." You can work out arrangements to send a relative, ambulance, or police, depending on the situation. You do all decision making that the caller cannot do, but none that he/she can do.

As you try to discover who the person is, you might say, "Even though my name is Elaine Glenn, people usually call me Lanie. What is your name?" (You may want to use a professional name or alias to keep from being reached via a listed home phone number.) With a caller still reluctant to give a name, you may want to suggest, "We'd find it easier to talk if we used names. Since our conversation is confidential, you can give me a name to call you."

The caller often chooses the phone as a means of self-revelation because he/she feels the problem is embarrassing or even contemptible. Thus your restraint in conveying judgment is essential. If able to present the difficulties to you and find acceptance via phone, the caller may take the next step and accept a referral for face-to-face therapy or emergency treatment.

In one crisis situation the caller described to the nurse how earlier in the day she had rented a motel room while she could be sure there was a vacancy. Late in the evening the caller returned to the motel room and swallowed an indeterminate number of barbiturate sleeping capsules. Some 30 minutes later as her suicidal ambivalence increased, she left the motel room and went to a phone booth to place her call. Her speech became thicker as she talked. The caller was upset over the loss of a boyfriend she hoped to marry and thereby regain custody of her two children who had been placed in foster care. As the nurse helped her consider alternative mechanisms for regaining custody, the caller agreed to go to an emergency room but insisted vehemently that she drive herself there! "My car's got a dented front fender already. I just won't go off and leave it here." The nurse was able to determine the make and year of the car. When she could not persuade the caller to accept other arrangements, the nurse planned with the caller the best route to an emergency room. As soon as the call was terminated, the nurse telephoned the local police to tell them of the situation, describing the car and its anticipated route, although the exact motel was unknown. The police interceded and succeeded in getting the caller and her car to the emergency room. The caller was admitted to the hospital.

In assessing the caller who is depressed, bitter, or overwhelmed by crisis, determine the degree of suicide risk by asking direct questions. Ask questions that determine the extent of clinical depression, extent of drug and alcohol use, family history of suicide or depression, history of previous suicidal thoughts or attempts, and information about any current suicidal plan, such as details of the suicidal plan, the lethality potential of the plan, and available means for carrying through with the plan. Ask what the caller has ingested. How much? The person's weight, height, age. What the caller expects to happen. Who is nearby to help. Address and phone number of caller's location. Contrary to a common fear that asking about suicide will give the client the idea of suicide, your questions about suicide may provide a helpful catharsis and prevent a suicide attempt (32, 90).

Suicide or suicidal behaviors are always a potential response to crisis. Many caregivers are either uninformed or poorly prepared emotionally and educationally to respond helpfully in such cases. They tend to classify all suicidal attempts as manipulative or as indications that a seriously suicidal person will ultimately succeed anyhow. It *is* difficult to see the merits of suicide prevention unless you maintain a respect for the dignity of life, see prior suicide attempters discover a joyous life after recovering from a critical attempt, or see attempters get to the source of problems when you address "suicidal gestures" as help-seeking behavior rather than manipulation. Much has been learned in the past 20 years about assessing the potential suicide. You can recognize who many of these clients are and offer referrals or consultation with mental health professionals. Table 8-1 shows the scope of suicide as one of our most pressing national health problems and specific points for assessment (7, 8, 38, 51, 113, 131).

If you learn of a specific, potentially lethal plan, you should take immediate preventive action. The variables of depression, current suicide plan, previous suicide attempts, and abusive use of alcohol or drugs are all highly significant in determining suicidal risk (91, 105, 106, 107). In these situations, you help the caller to obtain an emergency psychiatric evaluation. Take steps to ensure that the caller is not alone and inform caring friends or relatives of the caller's suicidal intent and its seriousness. Table 8-2 summarizes intervention principles when a caller reports having ingested an overdose of a lethal substance (7, 8, 38, 51, 112, 113, 131).

TABLE 8-1 Suicide as a National Health Problem

1. Suicide is now the ninth cause of death in the United States.
2. Suicide is the second cause of death in the 15- to 24-year-old age group.
3. The annual suicide rate has been increasing for all age groups under 40, as well as for both sexes and minority groups, such as Blacks and American Indians.
4. In the United States 30,000 to 40,000 people commit suicide each year.
5. Almost a quarter of a million suicide attempts occur each year.
6. More than one-third of those who make attempts eventually succeed in suicide.
7. Men are three times more successful than women in committing suicide; more often using highly lethal methods, such as guns, hanging, and lethal gases; perhaps they are more culturally conditioned not to communicate emotional distress.
8. Women attempt suicide three times more often than men; perhaps are just as suicidal, but their most frequent method (chemical overdose) allows more rescue potential.
9. The suicidal client often acknowledges multiple depressive symptoms. These signs include depressed mood, feelings of guilt and worthlessness, lack of self-esteem and self-confidence, irritability, indecisiveness, difficulty concentrating, loss of energy and interest, fears, insomnia, anorexia, headaches, constipation, and other somatic symptoms. Depression is often manifested in children or adolescents by truancy, school phobias, hyperactivity, acting-out behavior, or physical illness.
10. The suicidal client often feels isolated, rejected, misunderstood, deeply hopeless, and overwhelmed. This client does not perceive that things can be all right again.
11. Suicidal thinking while intoxicated may lead to suicidal behavior. Judgment decreases and impulsiveness increases when the brain is anesthetized by intoxicants.
12. Poor impulse control increases the likelihood of suicidal behavior occurring with less than usual provocation. This is particularly the case with children, adolescents, the personality disordered, the psychotic, and the intoxicated.

The Technique of Crisis Intervention by Telephone

Progress is made as you help the caller consider strengths and resources, develop a plan of problem resolution, and take steps toward adaptation. You help the caller convert a problem statement into a *process* of effective problem solving.

Telephone intervention may involve only a single call in which you are a reflective sounding board while the caller reaches an appropriate plan of action. Or the intervention may involve a succession of four or five phone calls in which the caller increasingly moves toward effective action.

The principles of crisis intervention do not change because you are talking by phone instead of sitting face to face. The therapeutic communication methods identified in Chapter 3 remain the same. Silence may still be thoughtful, expectant, anxious, or resistive. But the silence may *feel* much longer when you cannot look at the silent person for cues. Do you hear even a sigh? Do you hear sounds of movement, such as the creak of a chair when someone shifts weight in it? Do you hear the inhale and pushed exhale of a tense drag on a cigarette?

In response to silence you can state your aural observations: "I

TABLE 8-2 Intervention Principles When a Suicide Action Seems Imminent or Has Just Been Made

1. Maintain contact. Keep the phone line open. Decrease alienation and isolation. Extend sincere interest. Do not be aloof. Do not be so casual as to offend self-respect and dignity. Confirm the appropriateness and courage involved in the suicidal person's seeking and receiving help.
2. Help the client see that he/she has at least a fluctuating wish to live if only things could be different. Help the person realize that choices more meaningful than suicide can be explored. Let the person know that you are in favor of him/her choosing life and exploring once again whether "things" can be better.
3. Explore whether there are ways to help the client feel a sense of closeness and importance to a significant *living* other.
4. Clarify the client's point of view on major problems. Develop with the client one very concrete action that can be immediately taken to alleviate some of the stress of the experienced problems.
5. Verbally support and reinforce any capacities for impulse control that the client manifests.
6. When the client trusts you as competent and helpful, express to the client certain strengths and competencies that you see the client as possessing.
7. Plan with the client a series of actions that can be taken. Help him/her realize that these actions can be done only one step at a time.
8. Mobilize the intervention plan. Arrange with the client to use relatives, police, ambulance, emergency services, or mental health resources as indicated. Arrange for overdose containers to be taken to the emergency department, if possible, after suicide attempt.
9. Arrange to stay in touch with the client until the suicidal crisis is significantly alleviated.
10. Don't promise what you cannot deliver. Take care of yourself. The suicidal person may also be a homicidal person.
11. If you are working with a frequent attempter, a primary psychotherapist should be involved. Plans and responsibilities need to be developed with that psychotherapist.
12. Refer and follow up until a successful referral is being used.

heard your sigh. I wonder what you are thinking?" "It sounds as though you are shifting your weight. Was my last question uncomfortable to consider?" "You're quiet. It feels to me as though you may be thinking about something important and trying to decide whether or not to tell me."

Even into a dead silence that is becoming uncomfortably long you can offer, "I'm still here. I'm interested in knowing what's troubling you." You need to clarify your own silences, feelings, and reactions verbally. Because the caller cannot see your thoughtful, furrowed brow, you need to say, "I'm thinking about what you've told me and wondering what alternatives you've already considered." The person *can hear* if your vocal cords tighten in mounting frustration and needs you to clarify the source of the frustration.

Occasionally a telephone caller will find that he/she cannot deal with even the amount of exposure created by dialing the phone. You may hear the click of the phone being hung up and fear that you have failed. Perhaps you have not failed. Perhaps you have succeeded. The caller may have reached a caring, empathetic voice while prepared to find disinterest and rejection. On finding the opposite situation, the caller may hang up and reflect on whether to expose self further. The first contact with you enhances the chance of calling back for further help.

In many situations, the telephone contact cannot provide sufficient therapy. Plan instead to be a bridge between the person in crisis and the appropriate referral source. You might say, "You have family concerns which are very frustrating to you. You deserve an intense effort on someone's part to help you work out solutions. I can't do that in this call. I believe you can get this help at (name, address, phone, hours of service, and the fee range of referral resources nearby). Referrals are most likely to be accepted if they are located nearby and within the economic status of the caller.

Avoid doing an oversell of referrals. Be optimistic when you give a referral, but also add that you would like to hear from the caller again if this referral isn't helpful once he/she gives it a fair try.

Very often the caller is not seeking information for self but for a loved one. Then you will indirectly provide health information, assessment guidelines, and information on available treatment resources to the person in crisis (96). In an emergency situation, however, you should make every attempt to talk directly with the subject whom the caller has in mind.

Evaluation

Frequently in phone counseling you must base your self-evaluation on a single phone encounter. Only occasionally will you know whether your intervention was the turning point toward effective resolution. Yet by examining and practicing the skills used in telephone crisis work, you can develop confidence. Role playing done sitting back to back with your peers can help you develop skills of telephone therapy as they react and analyze your verbal statements and tone of voice.

At one time, a "holler" to a neighbor and a back fence "conference" provided emergency crisis intervention. Today the telephone can do the same. You can use it as one more tool in expanded nursing care.

CARE OF THE HOSPITALIZED SUICIDE ATTEMPTER

If you have successfully referred the suicide attempter into the health care system, the next challenge is working with the person immediately afterward.

The client who regains consciousness after a suicide attempt may severely test your attitudes and beliefs about suicidal behavior. A wide range of behaviors may be seen: anger and dismay at still being alive, euphoria, denial, apathy, belligerence—in fact, almost any behavior seen in the first three phases of active crisis. Because these clients are in active crisis as well as psychological pain, they are unable at this point to make an informed and rational choice about their "right to die"—in the authors' opinion. Your role is to see alternatives and hope for the client when he/she cannot.

Here are some general guidelines to follow.

1. A current suicidal assessment should be recorded and communicated.
2. Detailed data on the actual attempt, steps the attempter took to avoid discovery, *the attempter's notion of the toxicity of the drug, likelihood of rescue*, and so on need to be recorded. (Too often we base our conclusions about intent on *our* notions of toxicity, rescue, and so forth.)
3. Be aware that the behavior that you see immediately postattempt may be highly altered by the physiological effects of the attempt or the psychological effects of rescue and may tell you almost nothing about the psychological status of the client prior to the attempt.
4. Observe and interact! Don't leave a vulnerable client more isolated than he/she was prior to hospitalization. Simply offer your quiet presence at frequent intervals if that is all the client can tolerate.
5. Accept the attempter's perception of his/her life situation as valid for him/her at that point in time.
6. Attend to the family and significant others. Are they in a phase of crisis? Minimizing or denying the event? Seemingly suicidogenic or helpful?

THE CRISIS OF SEPARATION AND LOSS

The crisis of separation and loss can be either developmental or situational in origin and both may occur simultaneously.

Life—A Series of Losses

Loss and the universal reaction to loss, grief, and mourning are experienced by everyone at some time in their lives and frequently you are the one most involved with and available to the person who is experiencing loss.

As one's interdependence with others grows, the likelihood increases that separation, loss of something valuable, or death of a loved one will induce a crisis. The capacity to have warm and loving relationships also leaves one vulnerable to sadness, despair, and grief. The more one has emotionally invested in what is lost, the greater the threat felt to the self.

Every person is also subjected to separations or losses that are subtle and may not be recognized. Any crisis, developmental or situational, involves some degree of loss. If nothing else, there is a loss through change in old behavior patterns and the addition of different coping mechanisms. The process of achieving independence in psychosocial development in the course of normal upbringing involves a whole series of separations. The way these early separations are dealt with affects how later separations and loss, including death, will be resolved. Examples of loss situations, either partial or total, temporary or permanent, throughout the life span include the following ones (6, 12, 13, 22, 29, 47, 57, 88, 95, 98, 103, 133):

1. Period of weaning in infancy; learning to wait.
2. First haircut, even when it involves pride and anticipation.
3. Period of increasing locomotion, exploration, and bowel and bladder control and resultant loss of dependency.
4. Loss of baby teeth, baby possessions, toys, clothes, or pets during development.
5. Change in the body, body image, and self-attitude with ongoing growth and development.
6. Change in body size and shape and in feelings accompanying pregnancy and childbirth; loss of body part or function, external or internal, through accident, illness, or aging.
7. Departure of children from the home when they go to school or marry.
8. Menopause and loss of childbearing functions.
9. Loss of hearing, vision, memory, strength, and other changes and losses associated with old age.
10. Changes and losses in relationships with others as the person moves from childhood to adulthood–loss of friends and lovers; separation from or death of family members; changes in residence, occupation, or place of business; promotions and graduations.
11. Losses that have symbolic meanings, such as the loss of a symptom that attracted others' attention, a loss or change that necessitates a change in body image, or "loss of face," honor, or prestige.
12. Loss of home due to natural disaster or relocation projects; loss of possessions or money.
13. Loss experienced with divorce or incapacitation of a loved one.

Thus the person brings to any major crisis a backlog of experience that predisposes either successful integration of a personal tragedy or failure to absorb another loss or change. The significance of the present reaction may become clear only when you understand the person's earlier separations and losses.

Definitions

Loss can be defined as *giving up external or internal supports required by the person to satisfy basic needs.* In regard to loss, the term **object** *may mean a person, thing, relationship, or situation.*

Grief *is a sequence of subjective states, a special intense form of sorrow caused by loss, either through separation or death of a loved person or loss of an object that is felt to be a part of the self or that provides psychological gratification. Grief is the emotion involved in the work of mourning.* Absence of what is lost is felt as a gap in one's sense of continuity and self-concept.

Grief reaction differs from depression in that cognitive disorders, such as gross distortion of events, are not normally present in grief; also, the reaction is more directly proportional to the amount of loss. In depression, the feeling of sadness and self-depreciation affects the person physically, intellectually, cognitively, emotionally, socially, and spiritually; it is out of proportion to the apparent situation and it is more greatly influenced by developmental and symbolic changes (5).

Mourning *is a broad range of reactions, a psychological process that follows either loss of a significant or valued object or person or realization that such a loss could occur. It is the process whereby the person seeks to disengage self from an emotionally demanding relationship and reinvest emotionally in a new and productive relationship.*

Grief and the Mourning Process

A review of the grief syndrome described by Lindemann and the stages of grief and mourning described by Engel help us understand the dynamics involved when any crisis results in a grief and mourning reaction (34, 76).

On becoming aware of the loss, the person is likely to feel somatic distress and an altered sensorium. The somatic symptoms last from 20 minutes to a few days and may include shortness of breath, choking, sighing, hyperventilation, chills, tremors, fatigue, anorexia, tightness in the throat, emptiness in the abdomen, and loss of strength. The altered sensorium exists during the stages of shock and disbelief or defensive retreat. Included may be feelings of unreality, emotional distance from people, intense preoccupation with the image or occasional hallucination of the lost object or person, helplessness, loneliness, and disorganization. In spite of apparent intellectual and verbalized acceptance of the loss, the implications of the loss are not comprehended. The person may overtly behave as if nothing happened or may be unable to carry out ordinary activities of living, lacking energy, organization, and initiative in doing daily tasks. The person may at times seem out of contact with reality and express feelings of despair and anguish as the reality of loss penetrates awareness.

Increased preoccupation with the lost object a heightened desire to talk about the loss, a search for evidence of failure "to do right," verbal self-accusation, and ambivalence toward the lost object become manifested with increasing awareness of loss.

The greater the ambivalence felt toward the lost object or person, the greater are the feelings of guilt and shame. With any love relationship, the person will also at times feel anger or dislike toward, or desire to be rid of, the person, along with love feelings toward him/her. In addition, the grieving person may feel angry at the lost (deceased, divorced, or separated) person for having left him/her. Guilt and anger feelings, a normal part of grieving, are frequently displaced onto others: the doctor, nurse, employer, family member, or God. If guilt is not resolved, self-blame for the loss and preoccupation with it, with future losses, or with his/her own death will occur. Unsuccessful attempts at expiating guilt and anger may be made by blindly identifying with the lost object, by quickly seeking a substitute relationship or object, by absorbing oneself in work, by overindulging in alcohol or drugs, or by literally fleeing from the situation. The person may fear going crazy because of felt despair, helplessness, hopelessness, and guilt. Early crisis therapy can reduce the intensity of some of these reactions.

Crying (the intensity of which depends on the culture) helps to express some anguish and is a form of communication that engenders support from others. In the United States loss through death is one situation in which adult tears, even in the male, are acceptable and cause no loss of respect.

The Importance of Ceremonies. Restitution for or adaptation to the loss, the actual work of mourning, is assisted by religious, cultural, or legal ceremonies (93).

The funeral ceremony, for instance, with the gathering of people who share the loss of the dead person and who either need or can give support to the grieving survivors, serves several purposes. It helps to emphasize the reality of the death, to minimize the expression of anger, and to expiate guilt. In addition, support is sought from a more powerful figure (God, Allah). Emphasis is placed on the possibility of life and reunion after death in some religions, and the process of identification with the deceased is initiated. Through the ceremony, the person *symbolically* expresses triumph over death and denies fear of death. The shared fellowship of a meal before or after the funeral, common in some subcultures, symbolically expresses return to life through the oral incorporation of eating and talking. The ceremony is the public way of adapting to the loss. But the persons closest to the deceased will continue to suffer for some time after the ceremony.

Other ceremonies dealing with separation or loss and involving the work of mourning may not be as extensive, obvious, or sad as a funeral. Each culture, however, provides ways to help the person acknowledge separation or loss. In fact, some ceremonies are joyous occasions, for the loss or separation means leaving behind old ways and behavior and being promoted or progressing to a new stage of life or adopting new behavior. Consider the baptism or circumcision; the birthday or graduation party; the first communion, confirmation, or Bar Mitzvah; the engagement or baby shower; and the retirement party. Although varying in degree of over expression and intensity of feeling, each represents essentially what the funeral represents after the death of a loved one.

Stages in the Mourning Process. Resolving loss, whether the death of a loved one or the loss of a significant object, status, or job, involves a number of steps (22, 34, 76, 98, 99).

The loss is first felt as a defect in the psychic self as the mourner becomes aware of innumerable ways in which he/she was dependent on the lost object as a source of gratification, for a feeling of well-being, for effective functioning, and for a sense of self. The mourner is not ready to accept a new object in place of the old one, although passively and transiently he/she may accept a more dependent relationship with remaining objects, roles, or persons.

The mourner becomes increasingly aware of his/her own body. In addition to developing symptoms that are a normal part of grieving, the person may develop symptoms similar to those suffered by a deceased loved person. This identification process maintains a tie with the deceased loved one and appeases some of the guilt felt for harboring earlier aggressive or angry feelings toward the dead person. How such symptoms are expressed depends on the person's constitutional factors as well as on past learning about which symptoms are most likely to get attention or to be defined as illness by the self and others.

The person is preoccupied with the lost object; there is a strong wish to have a continuing experience with the lost object. The mourner frequently talks about that which is lost, the pleasant memories and events associated with it. Constantly talking about the loss and its meaning is one way of reinforcing reality as well as of expiating guilt through repeated self-assurance that all possible action was taken to prevent the loss. This repetitious talking continues until the person forms a mental image almost completely devoid of negative characteristics of the lost object to replace that which no longer exists in the real world. This process of idealization follows the difficult and painful experience of alternating guilt, remorse, fear, and regret for real or fantasized past acts of hostility, neglect, and lack of appreciation, or even for personal responsibility for the loss or death.

Through identification following idealization, the mourner consciously adopts some of the behavior and admired qualities of the dead person. He/she changes interests in the direction of activities formerly enjoyed by the lost loved one, adopts that person's goals and ideals, or even takes on certain mannerisms of the deceased. As this final identification is accomplished, preoccupation with the deceased, ambivalence, guilt, and sadness decrease and thoughts return to life. If strong guilt is present, the person is more likely to take on undesirable characteristics, including the last disease symptoms, of the deceased. This negative identity may lead later to seeking a substitute relationship or object, absorbing self in work, overindulging in alcohol or drugs, literally fleeing from the situation by moving to another location, or psychopathology, especially depression.

Feelings are gradually withdrawn from the lost object. A yearning to be with the lost person is replaced by a wish to renew life. The person gradually unlearns old ways of living and learns new life patterns. The lost object becomes detached from the person and is enshrined in the form of a memory, memorial, or monument. At first the person's renewed concern for others may be directed toward other mourners or other persons in crisis. It is easier to feel closeness with someone who has experienced a similar loss.

Finally, the person becomes interested in new objects and relationships and allows self new pleasures and enjoyments. At first the replacements must be very much like the former object, but eventually new relationships are formed and objects acquired that are equally or even more satisfying.

Acceptance–the Successful Work of Mourning–may take 6 to 12 months. Complete resolution of or adaptation to the crisis of loss is indicated by the ability to remember comfortably and realistically both the pleasures and disappointments of the lost relationship. When the mourning process is adaptive or successful, the person is capable of carrying on life with new relationships without mental or physical illness.

This syndrome of feelings, thoughts, and behavior, although varying somewhat in sequence or intensity from person to person, is characteristic of grief and mourning. Resolution of mourning is delayed whenever the person confronts a chronic situation, such as birth of a defective child. Acute grief is manifested at birth of the child (or onset of the situation), but mourning is drawn out as long as the child lives (or the situation continues) (58).

Factors Influencing the Outcome of Mourning

In addition to the factors that affect the resolution of any crisis mentioned earlier, the duration of reaction and manner in which the person adjusts to the changed social environment after loss also depend on the following factors (21, 29, 47, 57, 82, 89, 95, 98, 99, 118, 124):

1. Degree of dependency for support from the lost object. The greater the dependency, the more difficult is emancipation from the lost object and resolution of loss.
2. Degree of ambivalence toward the lost object. Because ambivalence in a relationship determines the amount of felt guilt, this emotion slows the process of idealization, identification, and reinvestment of emotional energy in new objects.
3. Preparation for loss ("anticipatory grieving"), whether the loss was expected or had only been briefly thought of some time in the past.
4. Number and nature of other relationships. If prior to loss, the person derived satisfaction from a variety of other objects, persons, or roles, he/she now has more bases of support and can more readily form new relationships.
5. Age of the mourner or the deceased person. The death of a young person generally has a more profound effect on mourners than the death of an aged person in U.S. culture. There is the feeling of great social loss for the young person who has had inadequate time to fulfill him/herself. Among mourners, children generally have less capacity for resolving loss than adults because of their relative inexperience with crises and abstract thinking.
6. Changes in the pattern of living necessitated by loss of a person, money, job, pet, valuable possessions, role, or status.
7. Social and cultural roles of the mourners as defined by society. Mourning dress, fasting, and sacrifice are indefinitely prescribed in our culture. The role of mourner may also conflict with other roles—for example, with masculine or wage-earner role. Society makes little provision for replacement of the loss or for the discharge of hostility and guilt created by loss.

In general, obstacles to the normal progression of grieving arise when the person tries to avoid the intense distress connected with the grief experience and the expression of related emotions.

Nursing Process for the Person Experiencing Loss

The nurse's role with the person experiencing any kind of significant loss is essentially the same as with the person and family experiencing the greatest loss, death. For a thorough account of these nursing measures, see Murray and Zentner's chapter on death as the last developmental stage (91).

Reactions to loss are not always obvious. In assessing the patient who is admitted for a medical or surgical illness following a serious loss, direct your assessment and intervention to the mourning process as well as to the illness. Recognize the necessity of grief work for this person to achieve an optimum level of wellness.

The principles of crisis intervention described earlier and the concepts of primary, secondary, and tertiary prevention are applicable to the person experiencing loss.

You can help the person finish the mourning process by giving support during disengagement from the significant object and the seeking of new and rewarding relationships and patterns of living. The person cannot be hurried through mourning to resolution of the crisis. Encouragement and a time and place to talk, weep, and resolve grief are needed. The person will need help in developing a philosophy about life to the point where he/she can again tolerate stress, changing behavior to meet the situation rather than using behavioral mechanisms excessively to protect self from reality. Encourage the person to do what he/she can for self. Help him/her experiment with new modes of living and behaving and with new relationships. At times you may be a source of anxiety to this person as you attempt to encourage change and growth, but your simultaneous support will aid resolution.

The person who has been in mourning for some time may exhibit inappropriate behavior. Denial, feelings of emptiness, self-depreciation, anger at self and others, self-pity, somatic complaints, hopelessness, and helplessness may be expressed. Although such behavior may be disturbing, this person needs respect and acceptance from you and others before he/she can again respect self and accept the life situation.

THE CRISIS OF PHYSICAL ASSAULT OR RAPE

To be helpful to the assaulted victim, you must understand that the significant event is that the victim *perceives self* as having been violated (49). A sense of control of the body and destiny becomes part of our psyches once we successfully master the independence strivings of early childhood. Few events can so overwhelmingly and suddenly undermine that essential sense of body integrity as being the victim of bodily or sexual assault. For example, D. K. Ipema identifies loss of choice as a central issue facing rape and other assault victims (56, 90).

Reports of clinical studies of rape victims seemingly date back only a decade or so to that of Sutherland and Scherl in 1970 (119). Later references add information and also describe the silent rape reaction (15, 16, 17, 18). There is an even greater lack of clinical information in considering male victims of sexual abuse, although male victims suffer reactions similar to female victims. Further, any of the following persons may feel like violated victims: the wife forced into sexual submission by her husband, the youngster intimidated into "sexual play" by older children or into an incestuous act, or the adolescent (male or female) psychologically coerced by another into sexual activity not freely willed. Their needs may be similar if not identical to those of rape victims. The following intervention principles along with crisis intervention principles previously described, will apply to the victim of assault:

1. Emotional cartharsis
2. Exploring self-blame
3. Active support and encouragement on a short-term basis
4. Assistance in identifying the situational supports available (90)

In counseling the sexually assaulted victim, try to get your own biases out of the way and *hear* what that individual's experience *was for her/him*. Put aside your beliefs, such as the victim's role in inviting or encouraging the assault. Avoid vicariously fabricating in your own mind what the experience must have been like. The client will need you to provide opportunities for sorting through her/his own conflicting reactions, whether they are vengeful rage, guilt regarding some element of satisfaction, crippling anxiety in the face of such vulnerability, or some combination of all these and more (90). Emergency care of rape victims involves very specific kinds of assistance. Refer to references 11, 53, 90, 114, 117, and 132 for information on emergency care. You may also contact your local rape or crisis center.

Notman and Nadelson help us consider some special factors that are relevant when the sexual assault victims are children or adolescents (93). Rape as the first sexual experience may leave a victim quite confused about the relationship between sexuality, violence, and humiliation. To be sexually assaulted during the years of independence strivings can leave a victim anxious that desired independence is not a safe pursuit. Adolescents have to deal with peer group issues. School phobia and truancy may result (90).

Parents may feel guilt that they did not somehow protect the child or adolescent. They have a need to blame someone, whether attacker, child, or themselves. Sexual assault may be the proverbial straw in a family where members are already crippled by a general inability to discuss sexuality. Acute family crisis may result. Parents, who are anxious about sexuality may react defensively to a fear that their child provoked the assault (90).

Consider indications for concurrent counseling of any male(s) significant to the rape victim (40). At a time when appropriate support to the victim is so indispensable you may first need to help the significant male(s) deal with feelings of rage, impotence, or doubts related to cultural myths, as well as individual defenses.

Rape Prevention

Frequently rape prevention is not possible. Victims may only have a choice between submission or survival. They may react with paralyzing fear, especially when weapons or physical brutality are involved. The victim is usually at a disadvantage in terms of physical strength. "Fighting back" requires not only physical self-defense skills but also a psychological overcoming of cultural inhibitions (14, 90). Rapists typically are opportunists and generally preselect a victim, or type of victim, and an environment conducive to their success.

Some women increase their odds of avoiding rape by massive security arrangements for their apartments or homes. Some feel safer by remaining aloof, unfriendly, and doing nothing that may draw attention to themselves. Some refuse to give or accept help from strangers. Some potential victims avoid actual rape by not showing intimidation or submissive behavior. By striving for a cool, problem-solving mentality, the person may sometimes realize possibilities for escape. It is important to be prudent, discrete, and self-directed. When all that fails, most of us would endure physical abuse to preserve life (90).

ILLNESS: A SITUATIONAL CRISIS

In order to further relate crisis theory to nursing practice, the most common type of family crisis, illness, is discussed. Chapter 1 furnished a basis for the discussion in this section.

Illness may be defined as *an experience, manifesting itself through observable or felt changes in the body, that interferes with the person's capacity to carry out minimum functions appropriate to the customary status* (137).

The sensory quality of the illness experience is the result of nerve receptors. Exteroceptors include the organs of reception for visual, gustatory, olfactory, and auditory sensations. Interoceptors include organs of reception for sensations of pain, touch, pressure, warmth, and cold. Proprioceptors respond to impulses for tension, position, and movement. Illness can be experienced as a change in the intensity, extension, preciseness, or duration of sensation from any of these receptors, accompanying various pathological states (137).

Influences on Illness Susceptibility

In addition to the influences on health and illness discussed in Chapter 1, the difference in illness susceptibility from person to person may arise either from differences in perception and evaluation of the environment or from innate constitutional differences, or both. There is usually a relationship between the frequency of a person's illness episodes and the manner in which life situations are perceived. Those who see their life experiences as challenging, demanding, and conflict-laden suffer more disturbances of bodily processes, mood, thought, and behavior. Susceptibility to illness may also be influenced by actions taken to avoid illness and by age, for adaptive defenses are not well developed in the very young and are less effective in the very old. Developmental level also influences perception and response to environmental demands (34).

Every person is active in a number of social roles that place various demands on the person and call for shifts and flexibility in attitude and behavior. At times, however, the kinds and nature of the roles in which the person is involved are demanding or stressful to the point of contributing to illness. The occupational role is important, for example, a farmer, nurse, steel-mill worker, or office clerk all are predisposed to different types of illness.

The family contributes not only to genetic predisposition but also to the actual etiology of specific diseases through the transmission of social values, the socialization process of the child, and the family pattern of daily living and behavior.

Because health is a multidimensional concept involving varying degrees of feelings, performance, and symptoms, the family places a certain value on health as well as a definition, often unspoken, of what they consider to be illness. For the person from a low socioeconomic background, symptoms are important only if they interfere with everyday functions and work. Therefore such a person goes to the doctor only when severely ill. Perhaps only after the symptoms are corrected does he/she admit the extent of illness, for previously the pressure to earn a living wage kept him/her going. Some people value health so highly that they are acutely aware of many body sensations and any unusual ones are considered symptoms of illness and reported promptly to the doctor. While the latter value system can signal hypochondria, it is also the system that permits early diagnosis and a greater degree of health promotion. The family attitude toward money and spending directly affects its value on health. For some, the new car or television set is more important than the elective surgery or treatment that can be postponed.

The definition of illness is learned by the child through family values. For example, if the father is a construction worker who uses his back muscles considerably on the job, he and his wife are likely to express concern verbally and nonverbally when he suffers backache. His back represents a job, status, money, and masculinity to him. The child perceives the situation; later, if he/she feels uncomfortable, backache may be the complaint. He/she soon learns such a complaint will get the parents' attention because of their value on this part of the anatomy. Backache is defined as illness in this family whereas other symptoms or signs of equal or greater intensity or potential severity may go unattended. The child is likely to keep this orientation into adulthood. Similarly, the pianist, minister, and editor will emphasize their hands, voice, and eyes, respectively. Such attitudes should be recognized and worked with in health teaching and care. Just telling the person which symptoms are regarded as a threat to health is useless. The person's behavior depends on a personal definition of illness.

The family pattern of living and the socialization of family members are influential in contributing to and defining illness—for example, through eating and rest habits, housing and sanitation standards, leisure-time pursuits and hobbies. The family that places a high value on food or that has learned to use food for tension release is more likely to contain obese members who develop illnesses related to obesity. The athletic family is more likely to suffer sprains, bruises, and fractures. A tension-filled family life may contribute to mental illness and indirectly to physical illness or socially malajusted behavior.

Research increasingly shows that the mind-body relationship is a key factor in many illnesses (33). The emotional status and personality of the person affect physiological processes. (Refer to Chapter 7 for a review of the stress syndrome.)

Organic changes and various diseases that occur as a result of stress and emotional factors include peptic ulcers, ulcerative colitis, hypertension, cardiovascular disease, migraine headache, diabetes, asthma and other allergic conditions, eczema and other skin rashes, arthritis, muscle and joint conditions, insomnia, premenstrual tension, and menstrual disorders. Some of these diseases can predispose to more serious conditions; for example, hypertension can predispose to heart failure, cerebral vascular accident, or renal damage. It is also possible that most illnesses, including cancer, infections, the common cold, gingivitis, and dental caries, have their basis in psychological factors. Various references at the end of the chapter describe these psychophysiological illnesses and their effects in adults. Children, as well as adults, may suffer psychosomatic illnesses (10, 25, 31, 33, 34, 39, 55, 67, 69, 87, 108, 109, 115, 128, 129, 130, 136).

The site and types of symptoms do not necessarily remain the same in the person over time. A symptom may have different effects for the same person at different times in life and in different family, group, or cultural circumstances. The Theory of Somatic Weakness explains why emotional stress affects each person differently, or some not at all. Genetic inheritance, previous illness in a body organ, prior strain of a body system, and learned behavior responses all influence which organ-body system will be vulnerable to symptoms or disease when the person experiences distress. A person is more likely to develop a psychosomatic disorder if there is a previous family history of such a disorder. Or a person may develop a psychosomatic disorder by observing and learning a pattern from another family member with the same disorder (136, 137).

Factors Determining the Definition of Illness

People in our society perceive illness as an obstacle to goal achievement, an interruption in the rhythm of life, a personal crisis, a frustration of normal life patterns and enjoyments, a disruption in social relations, or a punishment for misdeeds (137). Thus illness is considered a deviant role because the culture enforces an unusually high level of activity, independence, and responsibility on the person. Illness is closely related in people's minds to the role of childhood dependency. Moreover, resorting too frequently to illness as an escape poses a threat to the stability of social systems. Thus the institutionalized role of illness involves important mechanisms of social control: During illness certain behaviors are expected of the sick person and his/her caretakers.

Being ill involves more than being admitted to a health center or visiting the doctor. When you first see the person during the diagnostic process, the disease may be at midpoint. The diagnosis or definition of illness does not usually occur until after the symptoms are felt and described by the person to someone, usually in the family; both the person and family agree that he/she is ill; and a course of action is planned.

The person recognizes self as ill from the cues given by the illness, such as uncomfortable sensations, or the statements, facial expressions, or actions of others. Recognition of illness is usually made when present cues are seen to agree with past experience. In the absence of familiar cues the person may fail to recognize illness or become so apprehensive that he/she denies it. Even familiar cues may cause sufficient anxiety so that the person denies them and the illness experience (137).

In one study of 563 patients psychosocial factors were found to influence the amount of time that elapsed between the first sign or symptom of cancer and the search for medical help. Detection of cancer through routine physical examination ensured the least delay. In self-discovered signs of cancer worry about the condition reduced delay time more than pain, incapacity, or other factors. Patients of higher social class sought help significantly earlier than the less privileged. Persons who openly used the word *cancer* had less delay than those who used the word *tumor* or another euphemism. Delay in seeking help appears to be conscious and deliberate rather than caused by failure to perceive the neoplasm or comprehend its consequences (46).

Whether the family or others validate the person's definition of illness depends on their pattern of interaction with and expectations of him/her and their past experience with being ill. Does he/she "cry wolf" too often? Malinger? Act "like a baby"? Such interpretations are likely to cause the family to prod the person to persevere in his/her independent, healthy role. The person's role within the family is also crucial. The breadwinner of the family may feel that he/she cannot afford to recognize illness unless it is severe enough to interfere with ability to work.

So the family can either accept or reject the person as ill. In turn, the person will accept or reject the family definition of the situation, depending on how he/she feels. If he/she continues to define self as ill, help is sought. When he/she declares self to be ill, the sick role is entered.

The person's course of action is dependent on previous illness and health care experience, the kinds of help traditionally sought by the family, the knowledgeability about illness and the health care system, value system, religion, and a variety of other factors. Such factors include the nature, visibility, seriousness, and intensity of the illness; the body part involved; the extent to which symptoms interfere with daily patterns of living; the anticipated consequences of the illness; the person's tolerance for abnormality; the tendency to be concerned about self; and the availability, cost, and convenience of treatment facilities. Social class, culture, age, sex, and occupational status are additional determinants of this behavior (137).

The person may seek help for the illness from any one of a number of resources: a family member, neighbor, local pharmacist, chiropractic or osteopathic physician, a medical "quack," soothsayer, religious advisor, herbalist, midwife, nurse, or medical doctor.

Perhaps the best way to ensure that a patient/client will seek a qualified health care worker in any *future* crisis of illness is to treat and care for him/her in a way that is perceived as helpful in the *present* crisis.

The Sick Role

Illness forces the person to assume an unaccustomed social posture called the *sick role* by Parsons and Lederer (71, 96). In the sick role one comes in contact with the caretakers–doctors, nurses, or other health workers–whose jobs are defined by society. In addition, society defines who is sick and who is well. What is considered illness in one culture is not so considered in another.

In the sick role the person has declared self to be in a position in which he/she must be taken care of. Society and the health care system reinforce that he/she is not competent to care for self. He/she cannot do–and supposedly does not know–what needs to be done. Thus a person must follow the orders of others and let others make decisions for and about the self. The sick role frees the person from responsibility for the illness, but it carries the obligation to cooperate with caretakers and to get well. Medical workers get frustrated, angry, or judgmental when it appears that the person will not or cannot get well. While "working" to return to an independent, healthy status, society frees the person from ordinary duties, obligations, and responsibilities. Thus the sick person's two rights are (1) exemption from usual responsibilities and (2) absolution of blame for illness. Three obligations are to (1) view illness as undesirable, (2) want to get well, and (3) seek competent help from and cooperate with caretakers.

Although some health care professionals approach the ill person as a client rather than as a patient–seeking the person's point of view about care rather than being authoritarian–the health care system as a whole treats the ill person (patient) as a child or an object rather than as someone capable of self-care and decision making.

Certain Adaptive Behaviors normally unacceptable to society are common during illness and are considered helpful in promoting rest and recovery. By accepting illness, the structure of the person's world becomes simpler and more constricted. The person becomes somewhat dependent and regressed because of the unpleasant sensations, physical weakness, and helplessness caused by the illness; because of society's expectations; or from egocentricity, feelings of helplessness and concerns about body functions and routines administered for his/her welfare. Withdrawal into self rather than interest in others, a focus on the present rather than on the past or the future, and a reduced ability to concentrate and to think abstractly are all typical behaviors of the sick person. Routines may seem too burdensome so that daily activities, such as taking a bath and personal grooming, may be avoided, if possible, by the sick person. Through social, emotional, and physical regression and in compliance with the medical plan, the sick person redistributes energies to encourage the healing process.

The patient is simultaneously in a position of great power and of extreme weakness. This combination of domination and dependence provokes a difficult inner conflict, a certain ambivalence similar to what young children feel at times. The patient in essence loves the authority figure (the nurse or doctor) for taking care of him/her while simultaneously feeling angry toward the medical worker for being powerful while he/she is essentially helpless.

Certain Deviant or Maladaptive Behaviors in the sick role may occur and be so labeled by the medical team because the behaviors do not assist the person in getting physically well or regaining independence. Someone who uses illness for secondary gain, attention, escape from responsibility, control, or manipulation of others in the environment will not move through the sick role to return to health at the expected pace or in the expected way.

The health team also considers the ill person as deviant if he/she is unable to accept the dependent sick role. Often this pattern occurs when the person has unresolved dependency-independency conflicts. The patient may fear becoming dependent or may actually long to be dependent and feel guilty about this urge. Strongly independent behavior, such as protracted denial of illness, unwarranted physical activity, or refusal to cooperate with health care workers, may be a signal of such inner conflicts. Recognize, however, that in some cultures the ill person may refuse a dependent role because of expectations of self and others (127). On the other hand, excessive dependency, using illness as a refuge, and refusing to engage in self-care activities within one's strength limitations are as detrimental to getting well as is excessively independent behavior.

The patient may hinder progress by becoming apathetic or uninterested in recovering. Overly compliant, submissive, docile behavior should not be mistaken for cooperation with the treatment plan. Rather, the person's feelings of powerlessness and hopelessness, the lack of initiative and enthusiasm, signs of physical and emotional depression, or an apparent retreat as if waiting for death appear to diminish natural body responses for recovery (137).

In addition, any maladaptive response noted in this chapter's discussion of crisis may occur and can hinder progress to recovery, at least from the point of view of the medical team.

The Culture of Illness

Although the prescribed medical care may be identical, a person acts and is treated differently whether sick at home or sick in the hospital. In the home the person is in a familiar environment; it is possible to retain a sense of dignity, rights, and privileges and to insist on being treated on one's own terms. The sick one is reinforced by family and friends, who accord special concessions. These prerogatives are generally disregarded when the sick person enters a hospital in the U.S. health care system.

Hospitalization *may be defined as confinement of a person to an institution, away from the family, for a varying amount of time. Its purposes may be diagnosis; care or treatment that is palliative, rehabilitative, or curative in nature; or restoration of the person to a previous state, such as return to a nonpregnant state after delivery.*

Upon hospitalization, the individual is stripped of personal possessions. Gone are familiar surroundings that afford a sense of security. Instead there are various strange, disquieting, and bothersome odors, noises, and sights. At home the health care worker rings the bell and waits for the door to open. In the hospital the patient rings the bell and waits for a nurse to come. At home the doctor is on call, the nurse is a visitor, and relatives belong. In the hospital the patient is admitted and discharged, the health care workers perform their duties, and relatives are the visitors. At home everyone present acknowledges the patient's wishes. In the hospital all health care workers are in a distinct position to grant or withhold small and very precious favors from the patient, often depending on their personal judgment of the latter and his/her behavior (123).

Reactions to Hospitalization

In the best of settings the person is overwhelmed by many strange, foreboding, conflicting, or frightening feelings. In spite of the many people around, he/she feels isolated and lonely. In fact, lack of privacy, with the intrusion of these many workers into the room, often unannounced, is a frequent complaint. Compartmentalization of care, bureaucracy, and other characteristics of the hospital within the health care system discussed in Chapter 2 combine to strip the person of individuality and identity. He/she is robbed unnecessarily of decision-making power, a sense of responsibility, and significant communication by a rigid schedule, ritualistic routines, and staff who appear to hurry, won't answer questions, talk too fast, or use words not understood. Moreover, the body rhythms are disrupted.

The hospital often means separation from valued person, objects, and activities. It may seem to be a place where one is sent in retaliation for inappropriate behavior or at least a place that inflicts undesirable controls and forced conformity. There is endless waiting and the feeling of boredom, aimlessness, and sameness every day. On the other hand, some people may consider the hospital more as a source of relief. It may seem a secure place, with its emergency equipment and trained concerned personnel, where basic needs can be met without effort of the self. For still others, the hospital is a place to go to die (137).

Health team members should consider some of the possible undesirable side effects of hospitalization on the patient:

1. Enforced dependency on strange authority figures.
2. Dramatic changes in the physical environment.
3. Disruption of daily routines and preferences.
4. Separation from family.
5. Different behavioral expectations imposed by the sick role.
6. Forced adjustment to an interaction with a variety of strangers at a highly vulnerable time.
7. Depersonalization, loss of privacy and freedom, and fostered regression.
8. Increased anxiety from all of these effects, which may cause further physical and mental changes and further impede progression toward wellness.

Thus illness, especially if it necessitates hospitalization, is a crisis. The person is moving from familiar into strange territory and the usual patterns of behavior are not adequate to cope in the strange situation. The crisis becomes greater in its impact when, as a result of the illness, the person must thereafter live with a chronic debilitating or disabling condition or when a structure or function of the body has been altered.

Stages of Illness

The crisis of illness does not occur as an isolated event in the life of the person. The psychological states that occur during illness do not represent a change or difference in the person as much as temporary adaptive behaviors that maintain or promote restoration of the presickness self. The reactions to illness must be understood in terms of the person's prior personality organization. Thus adopting the sick role and going through the phases of crisis during the stages of illness are maladaptive only when the person is *not* sick by commonly accepted standards.

The stages of illness described by Janis, and listed next, fit into the phases of crisis described earlier (60).

Transition from Health to Illness, the First Stage, lasts from the time the person first considers that he/she might be ill until he/she and others acknowledge that the person is ill. During this period the person may show signs of emotional shock if the illness is acute or severe and the disruption to normal life is considerable. Then denial is used, at least briefly, to minimize or ignore the symptoms. If denial is strong, the person has a feeling that nothing can happen to him/her, that he/she never felt better, and he/she may engage in more than the usual amount of activity. Denial is usually impossible to maintain for a prolonged time because of pressure from others, feelings of extreme discomfort, or manifestation of more symptoms when the person tries to maintain normal behavior.

Acceptance of Illness, the Second Stage, occurs when the person feels the reality and impact of the illness, acknowledges the illness, seeks validation from significant others, seeks help from a caretaker, and enters into the sick role with all the related behaviors previously described. During illness the person may go through a mourning process for loss of body function or structure, even if such loss is temporary. During this time the person has many worries–job, finances, ability of the family to manage without him or her, fidelity of the spouse, child care, and loss of status. The patient may become aggressive or haughty, displacing anger on others, even though feeling weak or inadequate. Or the person may be passive in order to control fears and anger.

The stigma, embarrassment, or shame felt because of illness begins to be worked through, along with the emasculating or defeminizing effects felt as part of the illness. Feelings of rejection, of being abandoned, and self-pity gradually diminish.

Different body parts and certain body functions may have great significance to the person. If altered by illness or the treatment plan, the distortion in body image that occurs must be resolved before the patient can enter the last stage of illness, convalescence. Gradually the coping mechanisms are reorganized and perception becomes more realistic.

Convalescence, the Last Stage, is analogous to the adaptation or resolution phase of crisis. Now the person returns to health. Or, in the case in which there is a permanent disability and no further physical improvement is possible, convalescence marks a gradual increase in satisfying experiences. The person's new sense of worth and reduced anxiety enable him/her again to use those abilities typical of health. This period is like moving from adolescence to adulthood. The person is reassessing the meaning of life and is becoming increasingly independent, stable, outward looking, and involved in decision making (92).

There are many variations in convalescence. Physical convalescence frequently occurs before emotional convalescence or resolution of the illness. The person's level of maturity, the kind of crisis intervention given, and the environment in which the person must function combine to determine progress. If others encourage constructive activity instead of passive, less adaptive behavior, the person can more easily resolve feelings about having been ill. Then, again, health may represent more of a threat than illness due to the pressures of life. If illness justifies irresponsible behavior, provides an escape from obligations, or satisfies emotional or financial needs, then the person may actively (although perhaps unconsciously) resist convalescence.

Tasks of Convalescence

Certain tasks must be accomplished, in addition to solving the practical problems of returning home from the hospital, in order to go from illness to full emotional and physical health. The minor adaptations in the physical environment of the home and in the daily routine can usually be easily made. Then the family and friends expect the newly discharged patient to be grateful for recovery and for what they have done for him/her, to be cheerful about rejoining loved ones, and to be eager to return to the usual way of life. However, they may soon find the person is unable to live up to these expectations.

Before resuming the usual activities and making the transition back to health, the person must first accomplish the three tasks of convalescence described by Norris (92). Only then will crisis be resolved.

Reassessment of Life's Meaning is one of the primary tasks for the convalescing patient. He/she thinks about life goals, purposes, and perhaps even the meaning of death and redirects energies toward developing a full potential for living.

Reintegration of Body Image becomes a second major task after the acute phase of illness, when the patient is less concerned about any threat to life. Scarring, deformity, impaired functioning, or removal of valued organs must be dealt with and integrated into the self. The person must work through feeling dependent, "dirty," repulsive, unattractive, or possibly totally unacceptable to certain others. Moreover, he/she may not feel the same even if there has been no actual change in body structure or function.

Moving from the dependent patient role to independent adult status takes time and help. The person must feel self-interest, assertiveness, and persistence. Independence cannot be demanded; it is the result of work, usually between the nurse who views the person as a unique individual and a client and the person who trusts the nurse as a caregiver.

Resolution of Role Changes or Reversals that have occurred during the illness is a third major task and must be worked out within the patient and in relation to family members. After illness, there are no prescribed behaviors for convalescence, but the person usually does not fully assume normal responsibilities for some time. Seeing the family members carry out some of his/her responsibilities may be difficult and family members themselves usually look forward to a return to the normal pattern of living with less burden.

Added to the problems of continued role changes are the mood swings and other unpredictable responses to the convalescing person—behavior that may be very unlike the pre-illness personality. Some distance still exists between the convalescing person and the rest of activities going on around him/her.

Today the sick person normally returns home early in the illness for convalescence or rehabilitation. Before the person's discharge, you must learn if there is a family to help with care or at least a place to go, whether transportation to get home is available, and how the person will manage within specific limits, such as restrictions on mobility or diet. Every ill person comes from a culture and a community and returns to the same. Do not make assumptions; instead ask about the situation so that realistic plans can be made. If you listen and use nondirective interviewing techniques, you can help the person and family reexamine their lives, marshal their strengths, and focus their energies on convalescence.

The person who has a fatal illness will not truly convalesce and yet may enjoy periods of essentially good physical health. The reaction of the person who is terminally ill must be understood in terms of numerous and sometimes conflicting factors, taking into account previous relationships and previous experiences with crisis, particularly illness and loss. There must be an understanding of the significance of family, social group, occupation, and religion as well as of the other sources of love, comfort, and support. The person's self-concept and body image, ability to recognize and cope with reality, and responses to dependency, pain, and uncertainty will influence the overall reaction. Other crucial factors are the nature of the specific illness; the organ or body system affected, along with its symbolic as well as real significance to the person; the type of treatment required; and the degree of functional loss and disfigurement.

Impaired Role Behavior Related to Illness

Following illness or surgery, the person may not regain complete health; he/she may remain chronically ill. The person then reaches a state where he/she gets neither better nor worse but is no longer viewed by self or by society as being ill. He/she may even be disabled by a condition that imposes a restriction on activity and provokes social prejudice and stigma (136). Examples of such conditions include blindness, deafness, and cases in which some body part or function is congenitally or surgically absent or malfunctioning. The disability may or may not be obvious, but the person considers self well most of the time. He/she has emotionally resolved the crisis that surrounded the disability; limited ability to carry on usual roles and responsibilities remains. For the disabled person who is not experiencing illness, social pressures serve to aid in maintaining normal behavior within the limits of his/her potential. This situation is called *impaired role behavior* (43).

The behavior of the person depends on his/her perception of the disability as well as on the perceptions of others. Some persons who are chronically ill or congenitally or surgically disabled will remain in the sick role indefinitely. Such persons have not resolved the crisis of illness; the person with impaired role behavior has.

Characteristics of Impaired Role Behavior differ from those of the sick role. Thomas suggests that **impaired role behavior** *is an extension of the sick role. The disabled person, however, is not considered by society to be exempt from normal behavior or responsibilities within the limits of the condition.* He/she is expected, as far as possible, to improve or modify the life situation in the light of his/her disability, to make the most of remaining capabilities to overcome the disability, and to accept limits realistically. The person is then considered rehabilitated and no longer in the sick role (122).

The behavioral responses of the disabled person also depend on his/her feelings of being accepted or rejected. Schutz describes the basic human need to be included rather than excluded from others, to feel lovable, worthwhile, significant, competent, and responsible. The disabled person desires and needs to have some close relationships with nondisabled persons and needs to be accepted by others for what he or she is, in spite of the disability (110).

Disability often forces the person to modify the self-concept and self-image. New and different body sensations, changed appearance or body functions, and changed or reduced abilities challenge the person's self-confidence. He/she may feel shame, worthlessness, and inferiority, often to a degree not justified by the condition. Negative responses from others intensify low self-esteem and a negative self-image results, for everyone learns to incorporate the image that others have of him/her into the self-concept.

The disabled person is expected to learn to adjust and respond to being dependent on the aid of others to complete tasks or meet his/her needs, in spite of our cultural emphasis on self-reliance and independence. The person is expected to share in the management of the medical condition and be involved in decisions regarding treatment and care. He/she will be asked to explain the disability to others, often revealing considerable personal information, and accept that he/she is an object of curiosity medically and socially. The person recognizes that through these explanations he/she is helping to reduce social stigma, pity, and prejudice, and this will eventually permit greater opportunities to realize his/her potentialities.

The primary reason for considering impaired role behavior is that some people are neither ill—and therefore governed by sick-role norms—nor healthy in the usual sense. The well-adjusted disabled person views the self as physically or psychosocially restricted rather than ill.

In contrast, not accepting one's disability and its attendant limitations results in behavior that interferes with maintenance of health, prevention of further illness, and performance of social roles. Such a person is considered deviant in his/her behavior in that he/she remains in the sick role.

Although acute illness causes worry about outcome of the disease, financial status, and staying abreast of the demands of daily living, family reactions to disability or chronic illness is even more complex.

Family reactions may include a sense of shame, lowered self-esteem, and a sense of family instability as roles and responsibilities are shifted. Members may blame each other for the condition. A sense of depression or grief may be constantly present because the ill or disabled person cannot achieve certain developmental tasks. Family members may fear that they will not be able to meet care demands or financial obligations. Anger may be verbalized or indirectly expressed to the ill person or among family members because of the burdens and stresses encountered. The uncertain future may cause a feeling of hopelessness. Further, family members may feel guilty about their feelings toward the ill person, and yet resent the life changes caused by the chronic illness in the family. References 41, 44, 65, 74, 75, 90, 95, and 109 give additional information about family reactions.

Nursing Responsibility

The Nursing Process and Principles Described Earlier in this chapter and in Chapter 4 are applicable to the care of the sick person and the family. The principles of crisis intervention, combined with the necessary physical care, will help the person reach maximum potential.

Reactions of the Nurse to Loss, Disability, and Intentional Death. Just as patients and families experience various emotional reactions, the stress of being a health care provider can also provoke anxiety. You may identify with the client because of age, sex, disease type, or professional or cultural background. Perhaps you are in a health care field as a counterphobic reaction, as a way to deal with your fears and anxieties related to illness. You may also become very attached to the client and feel a sense of loss on discharge or death. Concerns about failure in doing the job correctly, causing damage to the client and receiving criticism from colleagues, are common sources of anxiety. Anticipating stressors and their effects, and realizing that you are not the only nurse who feels anxious, is an important step in coping with your anxiety and other unpleasant emotions (90).

You are a model of health to your clients. If you cannot cope effectively with stressors, you will not be effective.

The Meaning of the Illness and Related Care Determine Behavior. Diagnostic and treatment activities that the ill person encounters can be classified into four categories, according to the amount of threat perceived in each activity:

1. Intrusion or forceful entry into a body orifice, such as in an enema, catheterization, irrigation, gastric intubation, or injection.
2. Invasion of privacy, as in a probing interview, a vaginal, or rectal examination, or undue exposure of the body during care.
3. Threat of pain, suffering, or annihilation, such as presented by surgery or any other care procedure that threatens to distort, alter, or destroy the person's body image.
4. Little or no threat, as in taking routine vital signs or bedmaking (135).

Because these activities carry certain meanings, you can predict with some degree of certainty the person's behavior. For example, surgery may have any or all of the following meanings to a patient: pain; the unknown; fear of not being told the truth; mutilation and changes in the body image caused by incisions and removals; fear of death; disruption of life plans, including occupational and recreational; and fear of loss of control under anesthesia (61).

Establishing a Frame of Reference is helpful in preparing the person for diagnostic, treatment, or care measures. If he/she can compare a familiar event or sensation to the event about to be experienced, the event will seem less strange. He/she will feel less threatened and more in control of the situation and illness can be better tolerated and perceived more realistically. Of course, the frame of reference must have meaning for the individual. For example, a breast biopsy could be compared to the removal of a mole. If a procedure is going to hurt, the sensation should be described to the person—for example, as feeling like the pain of a burn from a hot stove, a needle prick, a toothache, or abdominal pressure from having overeaten. A patient/client usually will not engage in a comparison of the sensation or experience of illness without prompting; his/her main concern is to get relief from it.

If the person has been prepared intellectually to expect certain consequences, such as the possible outcome of a diagnostic procedure or the complexity of a tentative treatment plan, the emotional reaction will be less disorganized when he/she learns that the possibilities have become reality. He/she needs help in thinking about the possibilities of what might happen so that he/she can use certain behavioral mechanisms that aid coping with potential and actual danger. Behavior will become more cooperative with the health care team, whereas when the person's perception of the diagnostic or treatment plan is anxiety laden and negative, behavior is likely to be negative and uncooperative (61, 62). You will be the health team member best qualified to do this preparation.

Consider the Less Obvious but Equally Important Needs of Patients, such as esthetic needs. Eliminate or at least control unpleasant sights, sounds, and odors whenever possible. Consider the likes and dislikes of the person and the family. Let the family or individual make decisions about "the little things that count" as long as they do not interfere with the treatment plan. Help the person maintain identity by using the proper title and name. Encourage bringing some personal possessions from home and instruct the person and family about hospital routines and policies in order to reduce feelings of strangeness, isolation, and powerlessness. Flexible visiting hours can reduce loneliness and anxiety related to separation from loved ones.

As a nurse, you will coordinate various activities of other health care workers as well as perform the unique functions of care called *nursing*. Often you are the only caregiver prepared to understand the total person and his/her many unique needs while engaging in a therapeutic process with the patient.

The Tasks of Convalescence can best be accomplished when patient, family, and nurse collaborate, with the patient doing most of the work. Promote realistic adaptation by explaining the meaning of the crisis of illness and the tasks of convalescence. With shorter hospitalization the rule today, some resolution of feelings traditionally accomplished in the hospital must now be done at home. Be supportive and accepting and help both family and individual prepare for the tasks of convalescence to be managed at home after discharge. This preparation is as important as the discharge planning that helps the person make necessary physical adaptations or learn self-care. The person may never be able to do the latter satisfactorily if he/she is given no help with the former or has unrealistic expectations about treatment outcomes.

Therapeutic communication is essential in helping the person resolve convalescence. Pick up verbal cues. Reflect pertinent statements. Do not feel you must give answers. Encourage him/her to talk about thoughts and feelings so that he/she will arrive at personal answers and decisions.

Much of the physical care given in the hospital, such as bathing, changing dressings, guiding range-of-motion exercises, and positioning, could be done with greater thought directed toward helping the person acquaint self with and accept the changed body. Preserve and emphasize his/her strengths, but do not ignore or minimize problems. Realistic, pertinent teaching is essential for the person to adapt to a changed body. Further information on assessment of and intervention for an adult with a changed body image is discussed by Murray and Zentner (91). Recognize the signs of independence and promote it—without forcing the person to be independent before he/she is ready.

Final discharge planning and preparing for termination of the nurse–client relationship should be started long before the day of discharge. When you and the person jointly work through feelings about termination, both of you feel less cheated or rejected when he/she leaves the hospital.

You can evaluate the effectiveness of care and preparation for convalescence best through follow-up home visits or interviews with the person and family on their return to the clinic or doctor's office. Convalescence and the crisis of illness have been resolved when the person can talk about illness or surgery with equanimity and acceptance. Convalescence is not resolved when the person needs to talk continuously about the illness experience or states that he/she "never did get over it!" You can help to prevent or minimize such responses.

By intervening as a crisis therapist, you are involved in promoting the health of the person and family in the present situation as well as in future crises. In turn, the health and functioning of the community are indirectly enhanced. Thus a number of systems are positively affected.

REFERENCES

1. **Aguilera, D.,** and **J. Messick,** *Crisis Intervention: Theory and Methodology* (4th ed.). St. Louis: The C. V. Mosby Company, 1982.
2. **Baumann, Barbara,** "Diversities in Conception of Health and Physical Fitness," *Journal of Health and Human Behavior*, 2 (1961), 39–46.

3. ——, and **G. Kassenbaum**, "Dimensions of the Sick Role in Chronic Illness," *Journal of Health and Human Behavior*, 6, no. 1 (1965), 16-27.
4. **Baziak, Anna**, and **Robert Dentan**, "The Language of the Hospital and Its Effect on the Patient," in *Social Interaction and Patient Care*, eds. J. Skipper and R. Leonard. Philadelphia: J. B. Lippincott Company, 1965, pp. 272-77.
5. **Beck, Aaron**, "Etiologies of Depression," in *The Medical Management of Depression*, eds. Denis Hill and Leo Hollister. New York: Lakeside Laboratories, 1970, pp. 17-20.
6. **Benoliel, Jeanne**, "Assessment of Loss and Grief," *Journal of Thanatology*, 1, no. 3 (1971), 182-93,
7. **Berent, Irving**, *The Algebra of Suicide*. New York: Human Sciences Press, Inc., 1981.
8. **Berman, Alan L.**, ed., *Proceedings Fourteenth Annual Meeting American Association of Suicidology*. Albuquerque, New Mexico, 1981.
9. **Billings, Carolyn**, "Emotional First Aid," *American Journal of Nursing*, 80, no. 11 (1980), 2006-9.
10. **Bonami, M.**, "Overt and Covert Personality Traits Associated with Coronary Health Disease," *British Journal of Medical Psychology*, 52, no. 1 (1979), 77-84.
11. **Braen, G. Richard**, *The Rape Examination*. Chicago: Abbott Laboratories, 1976.
12. **Broden, Alexander**, "Reaction to Loss in the Aged," in *Loss and Grief: Psychological Management in Medical Practice*, eds. B. Schoenberg, A. Carr, D. Peretz, and A. Kutscher. New York: Columbia University Press, 1970, pp. 199-217.
13 **Brown, H. F.**, **V. Burdette**, and **C. Liddell**, "The Crisis of Relocation," in *Crisis Intervention: Selected Readings*, ed. H. Parad. New York: Family Service Association of America, 1965, pp. 248-60.
14. **Brownmiller, Susan**, *Against Our Will: Men, Women, and Rape*. New York: Simon & Schuster, Inc., 1975.
15. **Burgess, Ann**, and **Lynda Holmstrom**, "The Rape Victim in the Emergency Ward," *American Journal of Nursing*, 73, no. 10 (1973), 1740-45.
16. ——, "Rape Trauma Syndrome," *American Journal of Psychiatry*, 131, no. 9 (1974), 981-86.
17. ——, *Rape: Victims of Crisis*. Bowie, MD: Robert J. Brady Company, 1974.
18. ——, *Rape: Crisis and Recovery*. Bowie, MD: Robert J. Brady Company, 1979.
19. **Cain, Albert C.**, ed., *Survivors of Suicide*. Springfield, IL: Charles C Thomas, Publisher, 1972.
20. **Caplan, Gerald**, *Principles of Preventive Psychiatry*. New York: Basic Books, Inc., 1964.
21. **Carlson, C.**, "Grief and Mourning," in *Behavioral Concepts and Nursing Intervention*: coord. C. Carlson. Philadelphia: J. B. Lippincott Company, 1970, pp. 95-116.
22. **Carr, A.**, and **B. Schoenberg**, "Object Loss and Somatic Symptom Formation," in *Loss and Grief: Psychological Management in Medical Practice*, eds. B. Schoenberg, A. Carr, D. Peretz, and A. Kutscher. New York: Columbia University Press, 1970, pp. 36-48.

23. **Castleman, Michael,** "If Your Lover Gets Raped," *Medical Self-Help*, 8 (Spring 1980), 22–25.
24. **Chiles, John,** "A Practice Therapeutic Use of the Telephone," *American Journal of Psychiatry*, 131, no. 9 (1974), 1030–31.
25. **Chut, A.,** et al., "Reduction of Plasma Triglyceride Concentration by Acute Stress in Man," *Metabolism*, 28, no. 5 (1979), 553–61.
26. **Ciuca, R., C. Downie,** and **M. Morris,** "When a Disaster Strikes, How Do You Meet Emotional Needs?" *American Journal of Nursing*, 77, no. 3 (1977), 454–56.
27. **Clark, Terri,** "Counseling Victims of Rape," *American Journal of Nursing*, 76, no. 12 (1976), 1964–66.
28. **Cohen, Raquel,** and **Frederick Ahearn, Jr.,** *Handbook for Mental Health Care of Disaster Victims*. Baltimore: The Johns Hopkins University Press, 1981.
29. **Constantino, Rose,** "Bereavement Crisis Intervention for Widows in Grief and Mourning," *Nursing Research*, 30, no. 6 (1981), 351–53.
30. **DeMott, Benjamin,** "The Pro-Incest Lobby," *Psychology Today*, March 1980, pp. 11–18.
31. **Dimsdale, J.,** et al., "The Risk of Type A Mediated Coronary Artery Disease in Different Populations," *Psychosomatic Medicine*, 42, no. 1 (1980), 55–62.
32. **Diran, Margaret,** "You Can Prevent Suicide," *Nursing '76*, 6, no. 1. (1976), 60–64.
33. **Dorfman, W.,** "Psychosomatic Medicine: Some Past and Current Concepts," *Psychotherapy and Psychosomatics*, 31, nos. 1–4 (1979), 33–37.
34. **Engel, George,** *Psychological Development in Health and Disease*. Philadelphia: W. B. Saunders Company, 1962.
35. **Fabrega, H., Jr.,** "The Ethnography of Illness," *Social Science and Medicine*, 13, no. 5 (1979), 565–79.
36. **Ferguson, Tom,** "Coping with Disaster," *Medical Self-Care*, 19 (Winter 1982), pp. 32–37.
37. **Fink, Stephen,** "Crisis and Motivation: A Theoretical Model," *Archives of Physical Medicine and Rehabilitation*, 48, no. 11 (1967), 592–97.
38. **Freese, Arthur S.,** *Adolescent Suicide: Mental Health Challenge*, Pamphlet No. 569. New York: Public Affairs Committee, Inc., 1979.
39. **Friedman, M.,** and **R. H. Rosenman,** *Type A Behavior and Your Heart*. London: Wildwood House, 1974.
40. **Ginnetti, John, Jr.,** Counseling the Man in the Rape Victim's Life," *Nursing '79*, 9, no. 7 (1979), 43.
41. **Glaser, Anselm,** *Chronic Illness and the Quality of Life*. St. Louis: C. V. Mosby Company, 1975.
42. **Goldberg, Evelyn L.,** "Depression and Suicide Ideation in the Young Adult," *American Journal of Psychiatry*, 138, no. 1 (1981), 35–40.
43. **Gordon, Gerald,** *Role Theory and Illness*. New Haven, CT: College and University Press, 1966.
44. **Grace, Helen,** "Symposium on Crisis Intervention," *Nursing Clinics of North America*, 9, no. 1 (1974), 1–96.
45. **Greene, Robert,** and **Frank Mullen,** "A Crisis Telephone Service in a Nonmetropolitan Area," *Hospital and Community Psychiatry*, 24, no. 2 (1973), 94–97.

46. **Hackett, T., N. Cassem,** and **J. Raker,** "Patient Delay in Cancer," *New England Journal of Medicine*, 289 (July 5, 1973), 14–20.
47. **Hall, Joanne,** and **Barbara Weaver,** *Nursing of Families in Crisis.* Philadelphia: J. B. Lippincott Company, 1974.
48. **Hargreaves, Anne,** "Coping with Disaster," *American Journal of Nursing*, 80, no. 4 (1980), 683.
49. **Hilberman, Elaine,** *The Rape Victim.* New York: Basic Books, Inc., 1976.
50. **Hoff, Lee Ann,** *People in Crisis: Understanding and Helping.* Reading, MA: Addison-Wesley Publishing Co., Inc., 1978.
51. ——, and **Marcia Resing,** "Was This Suicide Preventable?" *American Journal of Nursing*, 82, no. 7 (1982), 1107–11.
52. **Holmes, T.,** and **R. Rahe,** "The Social Readjustment Rating Scale," *Journal of Psychosomatic Medicine*, 11, no. 8 (1967), 213–17.
53. **Holstrom, Lynda,** and **Ann Burgess,** "Assessing Trauma in the Rape Victim," *American Journal of Nursing*, 75, no. 8 (1975), 1288–91.
54. *How to Survive an Earthquake.* Available from CHES of California, 1933 Lombardy Drive, LaCanada, CA 91011.
55. **Hull, D.,** "Migration, Adaptation, and Illness: A Review," *Social Science and Medicine*, 13, no. 1 (1979), 25–36.
56. **Ipema, Donna K.,** "Rape: The Process of Recovery," *Nursing Research*, 28, no. 5 (1979), 272–75.
57. **Jackson, Edgar,** *Understanding Grief.* New York: Abington Press, 1967.
58. **Jackson, Pat,** "Chronic Grief," *American Journal of Nursing*, 74, no. 7 (1974), 1288–91.
59. **Jaco, E. Gartly,** ed., *Patients, Physicians, and Illness* (2nd ed.). New York: The Free Press, 1972.
60. **Janis, Irving,** *Psychological Stress.* New York: John Wiley & Sons, Inc., 1958.
61. **Johnson, Dorothy,** "Powerlessness: A Significant Determinant in Patient Behavior," *Journal of Nursing Education*, 6, no. 2 (1967), 39–44.
62. **Johnson, Jean,** "Effects of Restructuring Patients' Expectations on Their Reactions to Threatening Events," *Nursing Research*, 21, no. 6 (1972), 499–504.
63. **Joselson, Maurice,** and **Ruth Joselson,** "Do Perceptual Changes Occur in Crisis? A Case Study," *Journal of Psychiatric Nursing and Mental Health Services*, 10, no. 5 (1972), 6–10.
64. **Kasl, Stanislav,** and **Sidney Cobb,** "Health Behavior, Illness Behavior, and Sick Role Behavior," *Archives of Environmental Health*, 12 (1966), 531–41.
65. **Keining, Sr. Mary Martha,** "Denial of Illness," in *Behavioral Concepts and Nursing Intervention*, coord. C. Carlson. Philadelphia: J. B. Lippincott Company, 1970, pp. 9–28.
66. **King, Glen,** "How to Handle Hotline Calls," *MH* (formerly *Mental Hygiene*), 58, no. 4 (1974), 10–13.
67. **Kobasa, S.,** "Stressful Life Events, Personality and Health: An Inquiry into Hardiness," *Journal of Personal and Social Psychology*, 37 (1979), 1–11.
68. **Krouse, Helene,** and **John Krouse,** "Cancer as Crisis: The Critical Elements of Adjustment," *Nursing Research*, 31, no. 2 (1982), 96–101.
69. **Langone, John,** "When Hopelessness Kills," *Discover*, October 1980, p. 116.

70. **Larson, Virginia,** "What Hospitalization Means to Patients," *American Journal of Nursing*, 61, no. 5 (1961), 44.
71. **Lederer, Henry,** "How the Sick View Their World," *Journal of Social Issues*, 8 (1952), 4-15.
72. **Lee, J.,** "Emotional Reactions to Trauma," *Nursing Clinics of North America*, 5, no. 4 (1970), 577-87.
73. **Lester, David,** and **Gene Brockopp,** eds., *Crisis Intervention and Counseling by Telephone*. Springfield, IL: Charles C Thomas, 1973.
74. **Levinstein, S.,** "The Psychological Management of the Patient with Chronic Illness and His Family," *South African Medical Journal*, 57, no. 10 (1980), 361-62.
75. **Levy, N.,** "The Chronically Ill Patient," *Psychiatric Quarterly*, 51, no. 3 (1979), 189-97.
76. **Lindemann, Eric,** "Symptomology and Management of Acute Grief," *American Journal of Psychiatry*, 101 (1944), 141-48.
77. **Lorber, Judith,** "Good Patients and Problem Patients: Conformity and Deviance in a General Hospital," *Journal of Health and Social Behavior*, 16 (June 1975), 213-25.
78. **Mailick, M.,** "The Impact of Severe Illness on the Individual and Family: An Overview," *Social Work and Health Care*, 5, no. 2 (1979), 117-28.
79. **Maxwell, Christopher,** "Hospital Organizational Response to the Nuclear Accident at Three Mile Island: Implications for Future-Oriented Disaster Planning," *American Journal of Public Health*, 72, no. 3 (1982), 275-76.
80. **McClelland, D.,** et al., "Stressed Power Motivation, Sympathetic Activation, Immune Function, and Illness," *Journal of Human Stress*, 6, no. 2 (1980), 11-19.
81. **McDonald, J. M.,** *Rape: Offenders and Their Victims*. Springfield, IL: Charles C Thomas, 1971.
82. **McDaniels, James,** *Physical Disability and Human Behavior.* New York: Pergamon Press, 1969.
83. **McIntire, Matilda,** and **Carl Angle,** eds., *Suicide Attempts in Children and Youth*. Hagerstown, MD: Harper & Row, Publishers, 1980, Chapter 1.
84. **Mechanic, D.,** "The Concept of Illness Behavior," *Journal of Chronic Diseases*, 15 (1962), 184-94.
85. **Mendez, Lois, Rosalee Yeaworth, Janet York,** and **Trena Goodwin,** "Factors Influencing Adolescent's Perceptions of Life Change Events," *Nursing Research*, 29, no. 6 (1980), 384-88.
86. **Messick, Janice,** "Crisis Intervention Concepts: Implications for Nursing Practices," *Journal of Nursing and Mental Health Services*, 10, no. 5 (1972), 3-5.
87. **Moos, R.,** and **G. Solomon,** "Psychologic Comparisons between Women with Rheumatoid Arthritis and Their Nonarthritic Sisters: II. Content Analysis of Interviews," *Psychosomatic Medicine*, 27 (1965), 150-64.
88. **Muhlenkamp, Ann, Lucille Gress,** and **May Flood,** "Perception of Life Change Events by the Elderly," *Nursing Research*, 24, no. 12 (1975), 109-13.
89. **Murphy, Shirley,** "Learned Helplessness: From Concept to Comprehension," *Perspectives in Psychiatric Care*, 20, no. 1 (1982), 27-32.
90. **Murray, Ruth,** and **M. Marilyn Huelskoetter,** *Psychiatric/Mental Health Nursing: Giving Emotional Care*. Englewood Cliffs, NJ: Prentice-Hall, Inc., 1983.

91. ——, and **Judith Zentner,** *Nursing Assessment and Health Promotion Through the Life Span* (3rd ed.). Englewood Cliffs, NJ: Prentice-Hall, Inc., 1985.
92. **Norris, Catherine,** "The Work of Getting Well," *American Journal of Nursing*, 69, no. 10 (1969), 2118-21.
93. **Notman, M. T.,** and **C. C. Nadelson,** "The Rape Victim: Psychodynamic Considerations," *American Journal of Psychiatry*, 133, no. 4 (1976), 408-13.
94. **Papa, Lorraine,** "Responses to Life Events as Predictors of Suicidal Behavior. *Nursing Research*, 29, no. 6 (1980), 362-69.
95. **Parad, H.,** ed., *Crisis Intervention: Selected Readings*. New York: Family Service Association of America, 1965.
96. **Parsons, Talcott,** "Definitions of Health and Illness in the Light of American Values and Social Structure," in *Patients, Physicians and Illness* (2nd ed.), ed. E. G. Jaco. New York: The Free Press, 1972.
97. **Pederson, Andreas,** and **Haroutun Babigian,** "Providing Mental Health Information Through a 24-Hour Telephone Service," *Hospital and Community Psychiatry*, 23, no. 5 (1972), 139-41.
98. **Peretz, David,** "Development, Object-Relationships, and Loss," in *Loss and Grief: Psychological Management in Medical Practice*, eds. B. Schoenberg, A. Carr, D. Peretz, and A. Kutscher. New York: Columbia University Press, 1970, pp. 3-19.
99. ——, "Reaction to Loss," in *Loss and Grief: Psychological Management in Medical Practice*, eds. B. Schoenberg, A. Carr, D. Peretz, and A. Kutscher. New York: Columbia University Press, 1970, pp. 20-35.
100. Personal experience and communication with Staff and Training Committee, (1967-1977), Life Crisis Services, Inc., Gwen Harvey, Director, 7438 Forsyth, Suite 210, St. Louis, MO 63105.
101. **Pond, H.,** "Parental Attitudes toward Children with a Chronic Medical Disorder: Special Reference to Diabetes Mellitus," *Diabetes Care*, 2, no. 5 (1979), 425-31.
102. **Rahe, R.,** and **A. Arthur,** "Life-Change Patterns Surrounding Illness Perception," *Journal of Psychosomatic Research*, 11, no. 3 (1968), 341-45.
103. **Rapaport, Lydia,** "The State of Crisis: Some Theoretical Considerations," in *Crisis Intervention: Selected Readings*, ed. Howard Parad. New York: Family Service Association of America, 1965.
104. **Reeves, Robert,** "The Hospital Chaplain Looks at Grief," in *Loss and Grief: Psychological Management in Medical Practice*, eds. B. Schoenberg, A. Carr, D. Peretz and A. Kutscher. New York: Columbia University Press, 1970, pp. 362-72.
105. **Resnik, H. L. P., Joseph Sweeney,** and **Audrey Resnik,** "Telephone: A Lifeline for Potential Suicides," *RN*, 37, no. 10 (1974), 1-2 ff.
106. **Robins, Eli,** et al., "The Communication of Suicidal Intent: A Study of 134 Consecutive Cases of Successful (Completed) Suicide," *The American Journal of Psychiatry*, 115, no. 8 (1959), 724-33.
107. ——, "Some Clinical Considerations in the Prevention of Suicide Based on a Study of 134 Successful Suicides," *The American Journal of Public Health*, 49, no. 7 (1959), 888-89.
108. **Rosenman, R.,** and **M. Chesney,** "The Relationship of Type A Behavior

Pattern to Coronary Heart Disease," *Acta Nerv Super*, 22, no. 1 (1980), 1-45.

109. **Satterwhite, B.**, "Impact of Chronic Illness on Child and Family: An Overview Based on Five Surveys with Implications for Management," *Interpersonal Journal of Rehabilitation Research*, 1, no. 1 (1978), 7-17.
110. **Schutz, William**, *FIRO: A Three Dimensional Theory of Interpersonal Behavior*. New York: Holt, Rinehart & Winston, Inc., 1960.
111. **Selye, Hans**, "The Stress Syndrome," *American Journal of Nursing*, 65, no. 3 (1965), 97-99.
112. **Shneidman, Edwin**, "Psychotherapy with Suicidal Patients," *Suicide and Life-Threatening Behavior*, 11, no. 4 (1981), 341-49.
113. ——, *Voices of Death*. New York: Harper & Row, Publishers, 1980.
114. **Silverman, Daniel**, "First Do No More Harm: Female Rape Victims and the Male Counselor," *American Journal of Orthopsychiatry*, 47, no. 1 (1977), 91-96.
115. **Sparacino, Jack, Don Ronchi, Marilyn Brenner, James Kuhn**, and **Arthur Flesch**, "Psychological Correlates of Blood Pressure: A Closer Examination of Hostility, Anxiety, and Engagement," *Nursing Research*, 31, no. 3 (1982), 143-49.
116. **Spiegel, John**, "The Resolution of Role Conflict Within the Family," in *A Modern Introduction to the Family*, eds. Norman Bell and Ezra Vogel. Glencoe, IL: The Free Press, 1963.
117. **Sredl, Darlene, Catherine Klenke**, and **Mario Rojkind**, "Offering the Rape Victim Real Help," *Nursing '79*, 9, no. 7 (July 1979), 38-43.
118. **Steiner, Jerome**, "Group Function Within the Mourning Process," *Archives of the Foundation of Thanatology*, 2, no. 2 (1970), 80-82.
119. **Sutherland, S.**, and **D. Scherl**, "Patterns of Response among Victims of Rape," *American Journal of Orthopsychiatry*, 40, no. 3 (1970), 503-11.
120. **Tarnower, William**, "Psychological Needs of the Hospitalized Patient," *Nursing Outlook*, 13, no. 7 (1965), 28-30.
121. "The Sick Poor," *American Journal of Nursing*, 69, no. 11 (1969), 2424-54.
122. **Thomas, Edwin**, "Problems of Disability from the Perspective of Role Theory," *Journal of Health and Human Behavior*, 7, no. 1 (1966), 2-14.
123. **Ujhely, Gertrude**, "What Is Realistic Emotional Support?" *American Journal of Nursing*, 63, no. 7 (1963), 758-62.
124. ——, "Grief and Depression: Implications for Preventive and Therapeutic Care," *Nursing Forum*, 5, no. 2 (1966), 23-25.
125. **Venokur, A.**, and **M. Seiger**, "Desirable Versus Undesirable Life Events: Their Relationship to Stress and Mental Distress," *Journal of Personal and Social Psychology*, 32, no. 8 (1975), 329-37.
126. **Vincent, Pauline**, "The Sick Role in Patient Care," *American Journal of Nursing*, 75, no. 7 (1975), 1172-73.
127. **Vincent, R.**, "Factors Influencing Patient Non-Compliance: A Theoretical Approach," *Nursing Research*, 20, no. 6 (1971), 509-16.
128. **Waldron, I.**, "Type A Behavior Pattern and Coronary Heart Disease in Men and Women," *Social Science and Medicine*, 128 (1978), 167-70.

129. ———, et al., "The Coronary-Prone Behavior Pattern in Employed Men and Women," *Journal of Human Stress*, 3 (1977), 2–18.
130. ———, "Type A Behavior Pattern: Relationship to Variation in Blood Pressure, Parental Characteristics, and Academic and Social Activities of Students," *Journal of Human Stress*, 6, no. 1 (1980), 16–27.
131. **Wekstein, Louis,** *Handbook of Suicidology*. New York: Brunner/Mazel, Inc., 1979.
132. **Welch, Mary Scott,** "Rape and the Trauma of Inadequate Care," *Nursing Digest*, 5, no. 1 (Spring 1977), 50–52.
133. **Williams, Florence,** "Intervention in Maturational Crisis," *Perspectives in Psychiatric Care*, 9, no. 6 (1971), 240–46.
134. **Williams, Tim,** and **John Douds,** *Crisis Intervention and Counseling by Telephone*, eds. David Lester and Gene Brockopp. Springfield, IL: Charles C Thomas, 1973.
135. **Wise, Doreen,** "Crisis Intervention Before Cardiac Surgery," *American Journal of Nursing*, 76, no. 8 (1976), 1316–18.
136. **Wright, Beatrice,** *Physical Disability: A Psychological Approach*. New York: Harper & Row, Publishers, 1960.
137. **Wu, Ruth,** *Behavior and Illness*. Englewood Cliffs, NJ: Prentice-Hall, Inc., 1973.

UNIT II *FACTORS INFLUENCING HEALTH IN A PLURALISTIC SOCIETY*

9

The Person's Relationship to the Environment

Study of this chapter will help you to

1. Explore the scope of environmental pollution, both outdoor and indoor, and the interrelationship of the different kinds of pollution with one another and with people.
2. Observe sources of air pollution in your community and identify resulting hazards to human health.
3. List types of water pollution and describe resultant health problems.
4. Describe substances that cause soil pollution and the effect of these substances on the food web as well as on other facets of health.
5. Discuss the types of food pollution and ways to prevent food contamination.
6. Listen to noise pollution in various settings and discuss its long-term effects on health.
7. Contrast the different types of surface pollution and resultant health problems.
8. Discuss health hazards that are encountered by workers and the major effects of these contaminants.

9. Discuss and practice ways that, as a citizen, you can reduce environmental pollution.
10. Discuss your professional responsibility in assessing for illness caused by environmental pollutants and in taking general intervention measures.
11. Demonstrate an ability to help establish a therapeutic milieu for a patient/client.

Often the physical environment in which we live is taken for granted, overlooked as a direct influence on people and their health, although ecology is a well-publicized subject. You may wonder why a unit discussing major influences on the developing person and that person's health begins with a chapter about humans and their environment. Yet where we live and the condition of that area—its air, water, and soil—determine to a great extent how we live, what we eat, the agents of disease to which we are exposed, our state of health, and our ability to adapt.

Some environmental factors, both external and internal, that affect health status are discussed in Chapter 1. This chapter focuses primarily on noxious agents in the external environment to which many people in the United States are exposed, agents that are detrimental to health. Because of the interdependence of people, only those living in isolated rural areas escape the unpleasant effects of our urban, technologically advanced society. Yet even the isolated few may encounter some kind of environmental pollution, whether through groundwater contaminated from afar, food shipped into the area, or smog blown from a nearby city.

Nursing in the past was concerned primarily with the patient's immediate environment in the hospital or home. Today the nursing process is increasingly extended to include assessment of and intervention measures directed toward promoting a healthy environment for the person and family, well or ill. Understanding some specific environmental health problems, their sources and effects, will enable you to work both as a citizen and as a professional nurse to help prevent or correct those problems.

HISTORICAL PERSPECTIVE

The natural components of the environment were once considered dangerous. In most instances, people dealt successfully with any environmental problems encountered. In their quest to conquer nature early people discovered fire and the wheel. Fire was essential to survival; but with its advent, natural or manmade sparks and pollutants were sent into the atmosphere—the beginning of environmental pollution.

The fire and the wheel played major roles in the early civilization and industrialization of the world. With the Industrial Revolution came many technological advances that gave people increased power and comforts. These advances also introduced artificial, chemical, and physical hazards into the environment. Soon after the start of the Industrial Revolution, the population of cities grew; disease spread with the crowding of people, and food distribution became more complex. It became apparent that the natural components of the environment were not as dangerous as the manmade components.

Antipollution legislation in the United States can be traced back to the early 1900s. In 1906 the first federal Food and Drug Act was passed, and in 1914 drinking water standards were enacted to serve as guides for water supplied on interstate carriers. Congress passed the federal Water Pollution Control Act in 1948. Most of these legislative moves were poorly funded and supported, however, and so had little effect on growing pollution problems. Finally in the early 1960s Congress began taking a firm and leading role in combating environmental pollution. The Clean Air and Solid Waste Disposal Act of 1965 and the Clean Water Restoration Act of 1966 are examples of this attempt to fight pollution (33, 66). The United States Environmental Protection Agency (EPA) was created in 1970 to consolidate, strengthen, and coordinate federal efforts. The Toxic Substances Control Act of 1976 was the first attempt to provide comprehensive regulation of potentially dangerous chemical substances. The EPA was given the power to control the introduction, production, distribution, and use of any chemical compound that might be harmful to an individual's health or the environment (37, 39).

Throughout the 1970s existing laws were strengthened and new laws enacted to give EPA the mandate and means to accomplish national goals. With the advent of the 1980s, however, the agency began to reverse some earlier decisions and to delay implementation of some of their requirements (71, 72, 73, 88, 118). At present, the agency appears to be in a state of transition with many political, industrial, and environmental groups attempting to influence its decisions.

The entire environment has been and is a vital part of our existence. Human skill in manipulating the environment has produced tremendous benefits; but none has been without a price, the high price of pollution. Pollution of our environment is not only a health threat but also offends esthetic, spiritual, social, and philosophic values. Environmental pollution is a complex, significant problem requiring multiple solutions (see Fig. 9-1).

The following discussion is divided into categories of air, water, soil, food, noise, and surface pollution. Keep in mind, however, that these categories overlap. To illustrate, when a person inhales harmful particles from the soil that have become airborne, soil pollution becomes air pollution. And soil or surface pollution becomes water or food pollution if these harmful particles are swept into the water, consumed first by fish and then by people.

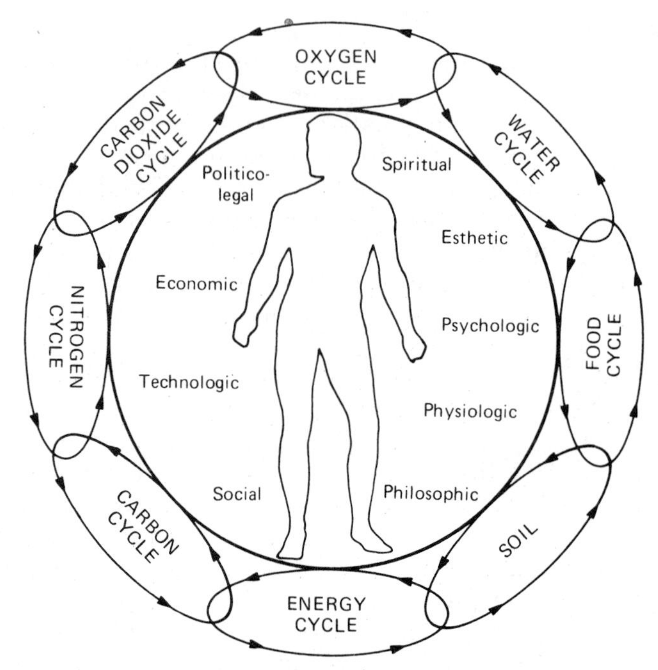

FIGURE 9-1 The Person's Interrelationship with the Environment

AIR POLLUTION

> . . . This most excellent canopy, the air, look you, this brave o'erhanging firmament, this majestical roof fretted with golden fire—why, it appears no other thing to me than a foul and pestilent congregation of vapors.
>
> *Hamlet* (II, ii, 311-315)

Problems of Air Pollution

Air pollution "aerial garbage," is not a new problem. Natural processes, such as forest fires and volcanic eruptions, or burning cities set afire during war, have long contaminated the air. Smog and the byproducts of coal burning have long been recognized as irritating disturbances plaguing many areas and clouding the skies. As long ago as 1272 King Edward I of England issued an edict forbidding the use of a certain coal that was making London's air smoky and sooty.

Air and water pollution act interchangeably; together they present a world problem. All people on the earth share the oceans and the air. Significant local pollution of either can greatly affect distant areas, especially if the oceans cannot, by the processes of precipitation, oxidation, and absorption, cleanse the atmosphere before harmful effects occur. Given enough time, the ocean can cleanse the atmosphere. But if the amount of pollution exceeds the ocean's capacity to neutralize the waste, then the harmful effects are dispersed into the atmosphere and we realize the effects by breathing contaminated air (5).

Sources of Air Pollution

The five most common pollutants found in the air are suspended particles, sulfur oxides nitrogen oxides, hydrocarbons, and carbon monoxide. The sources of air pollution vary; more than 8000 air monitors across the country measure and record air pollution levels. The 1977 Report of the EPA's National Air Quality division gives the following percentages: (123)

	SUSPENDED PARTICLES	SULFUR OXIDES	NITROGEN OXIDES	HYDROCARBONS	CARBON MONOXIDE
Transportation (cars, trucks)	9%	3%	40%	41%	83%
Fuel combustion	39	82	56	5	1
Industrial processes	43	15	4	36	8
Solid-waste disposal	3			2	3
Miscellaneous (forest fires, agriculture)	6			16	5

A major cause of air contamination is imperfect combustion. **Perfect combustion** exists only in the chemistry books and is *the result of hydrogen and carbon uniting completely with oxygen, thereby relinquishing heat, water vapor, light, and carbon dioxide to the air.* **Imperfect combustion** refers to *the additional liberation of carbon monoxide, sulfur oxides, and nitrogen oxides into the air.* Car exhausts in heavy traffic produce a significant amount of **carbon monoxide,** *a colorless and odorless poisonous gas produced during the incomplete combustion of carbon.* This gas combines with the hemoglobin of red blood cells in place of oxygen and can produce a **hypoxic state,** *a decreased amount of oxygen* in the body. The severity of this state depends on the ratio of carbon monoxide to oxygen in the air inhaled. The deficiency of oxygen in the blood caused by carbon monoxide primarily affects respiration and the function of the brain and heart.

Carbon monoxide in high concentrations can cause death: in small amounts it can cause dizziness, headache, fatigue, and impaired perception and thinking. Carbon monoxide pollution can be especially dangerous for persons who suffer from heart disease, respiratory disease, or anemia, for they already have a physiologically impaired oxygen-carrying capacity (138, 143), and for the fetus because it can cause retardation of growth and brain development.

Sulfur oxides *are poisonous gases that come from factories and power plants that burn coal or oil-containing sulfur*, eventually producing dangerous sulfur dioxide. *Sulfur dioxide combines with water to form* **sulfuric acid (H_2SO_4),** *a heavy, corrosive, oily, colorless liquid* that irritates the sensitive mucous membranes of the eyes, nose, and throat and injures the mucous membrane that lines the lungs and the delicate structures accessory to the lung tissue. Besides directly affecting our health, sulfur dioxide and its byproduct, sulfuric acid, indirectly jeopardize health by damaging plant life and contributing to rust on metals. In the process of trying to control these harmful effects through technological means, a new industrial pollution is sometimes created. Rust-proof cans may contain some elements that contaminate the environment, for instance, and they also add to waste-disposal problems.

Other gaseous end products from burning fuels are the nitrogen oxides, especially nitrogen dioxide. While this gas hovers in the air, producing an unpleasant, characteristic odor, it causes irritation to the mucous membranes and creates a haze that destroys the view and blocks out necessary and helpful rays from the sun.

Another air contaminant is **particulate matter,** *minute particles, such as dust, dirt, air, smoke, and fly ash.* Particulate matter, suspended in vapors and fumes, may hover for annoying and dangerous periods of time, depending on atmospheric conditions. These pollutants may soil surfaces, scatter or distribute light rays unevenly, and most dangerously, enter the lungs of people breathing the air. The severity of the lungs' response depends on the percentage of particulate matter or fumes and vapors in the air mixture and on preexisting lung disease.

Breathing in asbestos particles released into the atmosphere from certain construction industries and from the wearing of brake lining and clutch facings in cars can cause cancer. Asbestos is also widely used for fire-proofing and insulating homes and public and private buildings. When the asbestos material becomes damaged or starts to deteriorate, asbestos fibers are released into the air (137, 143). Inhaled beryllium, used in making metal alloys, also is known to cause a debilitating form of lung infection (140). Cigarette smoke has been identified as an air pollutant, causing increased carbon monoxide content in the blood. In addition, numerous other chemicals make up the particulate matter in tobacco smoke. Tobacco smoke can produce cardiovascular, respiratory, and other symptoms in nonsmokers as well as smokers.

Second-hand smoke can produce cancer in the nonsmoker as well as smokers. Sufficient exposure to any type of particulate pollution may lead to pulmonary emphysema (143, 146) (a condition in which the alveoli of the lungs become distended or ruptured).

Unlike the other forms of pollutants mentioned, ozone is not emitted directly by specific sources. **Ozone** (*triatomic oxygen* O_3) *is a pungent, colorless, toxic gas*. In the upper atmosphere ozone forms a protective barrier that prevents excessive ultraviolet light from reaching the earth. In the lower atmosphere ozone is *formed in the air by chemical reactions between nitrogen oxides and hydrocarbons* (*volatile organic compounds*), such as the vapors of gasoline and chemical solvents. These reactions are stimulated by sunlight and produce a type of *photochemical smog*. Photochemical smog was first noted in the Los Angeles area. Since then, it has been observed frequently in many other cities. Ozone reaches peak levels in most parts of the country during the summer. Ozone severely irritates the mucous membranes of the nose and throat. Normal functioning of the lungs is impaired and the ability to perform physical exercise is reduced. Individuals with chronic lung disease are more severely affected. Ozone also irritates the eyes (123, 134, 138).

The EPA has developed the Pollutant Standards Index (PSI) as a means of reporting daily air pollution concentrations. The PSI converts the pollutant concentrations measured in a community's air to a number on a scale of 0 to 500. Intervals on the PSI scale are related to the potential health effects of the daily measured concentrations of the five major pollutants previously described. The intervals and terms used to describe the air quality levels are as follows: 0 to 50, good; above 50, moderate; above 100, unhealthful; 200 to 299, very unhealthful; 300 and above, hazardous (126). When the pollution index is over 100, individuals with existing heart or respiratory ailments should reduce physical exertion and outdoor activity.

Four additional air pollution problems should be mentioned: depletion of the upper atmosphere ozone layer, increasing levels of atmospheric carbon dioxide, acid rain, and radioactive substances. As noted, a small layer of ozone surrounds the earth and blocks much of the ultraviolet radiation from reaching the earth's surface. The ozone layer is in danger of being depleted by the continued use of fluorocarbons (freon) and chlorofluoromethanes that release chlorine into the stratosphere to combine with ozone. The continued use of fluorocarbon-propelled aerosol products and supersonic transport planes would add to that danger (118). In Caucasians short-wavelength ultraviolet sunlight is thought to cause melanoma and nonmelanoma skin cancer that would increase in incidence if there were a reduction of the ozone layer (26, 115).

The *atmospheric content of carbon dioxide* has increased by 15 percent in the past century. CO_2 is added to the atmosphere by burning fossil fuels and clearing forests. The increased level of atmospheric CO_2 alters the heat balance of the earth. Areas of the world are becoming warmer and wetter. Such changes might eventually result in polar ice caps melting, flooding of large coastal plains areas, and disrupting agriculture with altered food production (47, 99).

Acid rain *is the end product of chemical reactions that begin when sulfur dioxide and nitrogen oxides enter the atmosphere from coal-, oil-, and gas-burning power plants, iron and copper smelters, and automobile exhausts.* These gases undergo changes and eventually react with moisture to form sulfuric acid and nitric acid. One-half to two-thirds of the pollution falls as acid rain or snow; some of the remainder is deposited as sulfate or nitrate particles that combine with dew and mist to form dilute acids (35). Most of northeastern United States and parts of Ontario, Quebec, Nova Scotia, and Newfoundland, as well as portions of the upper Midwest, the Rocky Mountains, and the West Coast, now receive strongly acidic precipitation (30, 31, 47, 148). The full effect on the environment is not understood as yet. Certain freshwater ecosystems are particularly sensitive to acid; fish, frogs, and certain aquatic plants die. Acid rain may actually increase the yield of several crops, such as corn and tomatoes (35, 65). It will be years before the full effect of acid precipitation is known. At present, the only solution is to decrease the emissions of sulfur and nitrogen oxide to the atmosphere.

Radioactive substances are produced by mining and processing radioactive ore and by nuclear-fission and radiation procedures used in industry, medicine, and research. Pollution from radioactive materials poses a serious threat to our ability to reproduce and to our gene structure. It is also related to an increase in leukemia, as demonstrated in persons working with radioactive materials over long periods without adequate safeguards and in survivors of Hiroshima and Nagasaki. A small fraction, 1 to 3 percent, of all cancers in the general population is attributable to natural radiation. Occupational irradiation produces an increase of less than 1 percent over the natural incidence (7, 141).

All forms of air pollution are physically irritating and present a potential hazard to our long-range health either by direct harm to the mucous membranes of the respiratory tract or by the indirect effects of continuously breathing contaminated air. Only in becoming aware of these factors as personal health threats will we seriously consider alternatives to using two or three cars, seek to know the serious hazards in our jobs, and become concerned about houses downwind from an industrial site or the amount of ultraviolet light we receive.

The citizen's role is a collective one. Consistent public concern to maintain standards and federal regulations must continue if we are to maintain the excellent effects of existing programs.

Indoor Air Pollution

Recent air samplings in new energy-efficient homes have shown that many pollutants are more concentrated indoors than out. Nitrogen dioxide and carbon monoxide accumulate when gas stoves and heaters are burning. **Radon,** a *natural radioactive gas produced by the decay of radium*, seeps into basements through cracked floors and diffuses out of brick and concrete building materials. Formaldehyde escapes into the air from foam insulation, particle board, and furniture made of plywood. Formaldehyde gas in newly insulated homes has reached concentrations high enough to cause dizziness, rashes, nosebleeds, and vomiting. Indoor radon may be contributing to thousands of lung cancer cases each year (32). Particles, such as dust, soot, ash, or cigarette smoke, may be inhaled into the lungs.

Indoor air pollution can be controlled by several measures: proper venting of gas stoves and heaters, painting over materials that emit radon and formaldehyde, and daily airing of the house.

WATER POLLUTION

Pollution of the water from the natural processes of aquatic animal and plant life, combined with man-made waste, constitutes another hazard to the delicate state of human health. Man-made water pollution has two major origins, *point sources* and *nonpoint sources*. Point sources are those that discharge pollutants from a well-defined place, such as outlet pipes of sewage treatment plants and factories. Nonpoint sources consist of runoff from city streets, construction sites, farms, and mines (140). The water pollutant list is long: phosphates in laundry detergents; acid contamination from mine drainage; and industrial effluent of toxins, acids, radioactive substances, and mineral particles, such as mercury. Increasingly obvious causes are salinization of water from evaporation in the arid West, land erosion, heat from industrial processes, and oil spills (102).

Types of Water Pollution

Water pollutants causing much of the problem can be categorized as common sewage, infection-causing organisms, nutrients, synthetic chemicals, inorganic chemicals, sediment, or heat. The common denominator of major water pollutants is called biologic oxygen demand (BOD), which is the amount of free oxygen that extraneous substances absorb from water.

Common Sewage, traditional waste from domestic and industrial sources, is a significant problem because oxygen is required to render this waste harmless. This waste thus uses up oxygen needed by aquatic plant and animal life. With increasing amounts of sewage, the problem is even more serious because of the inability of the water to deal successfully with the waste. When bacteria in the water can no longer decompose the waste, widespread aquatic death results. Waste will then accumulate, and the water will become useless as a personal or industrial resource.

Infection-Causing Organisms pollute water when sewage carrying these bacteria enter a river or stream. A human or animal drinking this water can become ill. Microbiology and pharmacology have done a great deal in helping prevent and treat such diseases by identifying the responsible microorganisms and developing appropriate vaccines and antibiotics. Occasionally a whole community or area may be negatively affected, however, because of a gross error that contaminates a large body of water with diseased microbes. These microbes may spread infectious hepatitis or typhoid fever, especially in rural and urban fringe areas where population density is high and public utilities are limited.

Nutrients that nourish plant life, especially phosphates and nitrates, are produced by sewage, industrial wastes, and soil erosion. These nutrients are not easily removed by treatment centers because they do not respond to the usual biological processes. Moreover, treatment centers may inadvertently change these substances into a more usable mineral form that stimulates excessive plant growth. This growth, in turn, becomes a problem by interfering with treatment processes, marring the landscape, producing an unpleasant odor and taste in the water, and disturbing the normal food web in a body of water. Because humans depend on many lower forms of life for food, this process could eventually affect their well-being if it occurred on a large scale. (See Fig. 9-2.)

Synthetic Chemicals that are used in everyday household chores, especially chemicals found in detergents, pesticides, and other cleaning agents, affect the water. They may be poisonous to aquatic life even in small proportions. When resistant to local treatment measures, they can produce an unpleasant taste and odor in the water. The extent of the long-term problem is not known, but the possibility of human

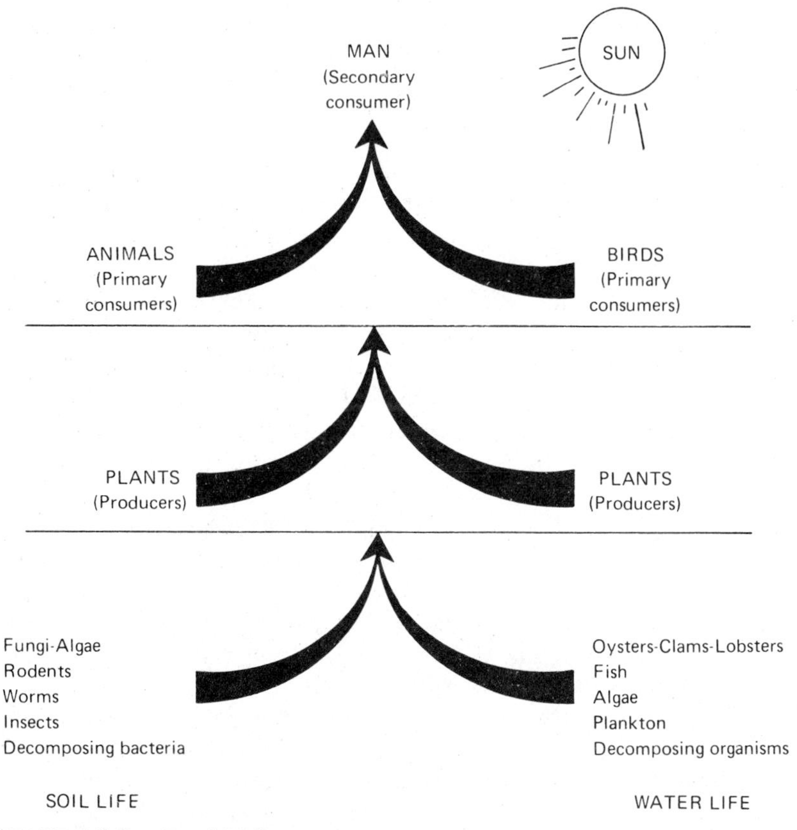

FIGURE 9-2 Food Web

poisoning over a long period by the consumption of small doses of these chemicals taken in drinking water cannot be ignored. This problem is discussed later in the chapter.

Inorganic Chemicals or mineral substances from mining or manufacturing processes can destroy land animals (including people) and aquatic life when ingested. Industries sometimes improperly and illegally empty large quantities of toxic materials into sources of local water supply. This group of pollutants corrodes water-treatment equipment and makes waste treatment an even more expensive problem.

Sediment—particles of earth, such as dirt and sand—consists of pollutants that are becoming a problem because of the magnitude of its debris. Sediment causes a nuisance and a hazard by covering food sources for aquatic life (and thereby eventually reducing sources for other life), by filling streams, and by preventing natural reservoirs from filling during rainy seasons. Resultant floods destroy animal and plant life and property and can cause epidemics of such water-borne diseases as typhoid and salmonellosis. Because of its sheer volume, sediment also increases the cost of water treatment.

Heat becomes a problem because it reduces the ability of the water to absorb oxygen. If significant amounts of water are heated through industrial use, the water becomes less efficient in providing oxygen for aquatic life and in assimilating waste. Even more dangerous, the ecological balance of lakes and rivers can be permanently upset through prolonged alteration of water temperature. The food that people eat either comes directly from water or has fed on aquatic life somewhere in the food web. Faced with an expanding world population, we must increasingly be aware of the significance of every organism in the food web (Fig. 9-2) and its relationship to us.

One of the most frightening results of water pollution is the threat to the oceans. The collective discharges of the world's nations and the practice of ocean dumping of sewage sludge may permanently pollute the oceans. The Ocean Dumping Act was amended in 1977 so that ocean dumping would not be allowed after December 31, 1981. Yet ocean dumping of solid, semisolid, or liquid waste generated by municipal wastewater treatment plants not only continues but is also increasing. When the act was amended in the 1970s, most people were concerned about the environment. In the 1980s, the major concern has become the cost of enforcing environmental standards. Continued research on the effects of deep ocean dumping and the development of a waste management plan for coastal areas and pretreatment techniques that reduce the danger of sewage sludge should be continued before major investments in other forms of disposal are made (119).

Problems in Water Purification

The natural water purification process involves the action of bacteria using oxygen to decompose organic matter. If too much waste is dumped into a given body of water, this natural cleansing process cannot take place, or at least does not take place fast enough. Further, once the water in the underground aquifer is contaminated, it is nearly impossible to guarantee a safe water supply.

The ultimate problem of water pollution stems from our using natural resources in greater and greater amounts because of additional industrialization, population growth, a greater dependence on appliances, and a subsequent increase in the need for sewage disposal. The problem of dissolving waste has put a real strain on waste-disposal systems. Even excessive amounts of treated waste now obstruct the waterways. Current engineering research is attempting to solve some of the problems of water pollution by developing different types of waste-disposal systems.

Water is essential to life. When it contains such a variety of pollutants in ever-increasing amounts, it becomes a threat to human health. It poses a threat, first, because of its increasing unavailability for consumption, and second, because of the harmful proportion of dangerous pollutants contained in what does remain.

A timely example of a health problem associated with water pollution is the controversy surrounding the Love Canal of Niagara Falls, New York. Love Canal has been an active and inactive dump site. The EPA assured the residents that all contamination discovered is within acceptable legal limits. Local residents, however, are not so sure and continue to insist on protection from the hazards of pollution. The controversy rages and water safety is again under government and laboratory scrutiny (79, 112, 113).

We can become diseased from drinking contaminated water. The quality of water service for countless people must be improved; many inhabitants of rural areas and small towns obtain their drinking water from polluted sources. Keeping drinking water separate from water for other uses would help conserve water supplies and ensure greater purity, for water used for other purposes could be refiltered with less expense (91).

Pollution of marshes and shorelines has severely impaired breeding habitats for many types of shellfish and deep-water species, thereby subsequently affecting the nation's food supply. Polluted water cannot be used for recreational purposes. The odor of decay and the unsightliness of polluted water destroy the beauty of any natural setting.

Misuse of our water has far-reaching consequences, threatening people all over the world from every age group and culture. Therefore we must take definite personal responsibility for stopping needless pollution of the water by exercising careful personal use of agents that can ultimately destroy it and by using legal procedures to prevent undue dumping of wastes into streams. Some health problems associated with contaminated water would be eliminated via proper legislation, and needless sickness and death could be avoided. Such legislation as the Clean Water Act of 1977, which promotes water quality standards and imposes a system of emission control in all sources of pollution, is effective and worthy of support. More importantly, the health of future generations and their chance to enjoy the beauty, taste, and power of the water depend on those of us who are so carelessly polluting it.

SOIL POLLUTION

As early as 1950 the federal Food and Drug Administration announced that the potential health hazards of compounds containing chlorinated hydrocarbons, such as dichloro-diphenyl-trichloroethane (DDT), had been underestimated (66). The Federal Environmental Pesticide Control Act, passed in 1972 and amended in 1975 and 1978, requires that all pesticide products sold or distributed in this country must be registered with the United States Environmental Protection Agency (139).

Substances used to kill weeds, rats, mice, worms, fungi, and insects are called **pesticides.** Soil pollution can occur as a result of excessive or improper use of pesticides (insecticides, herbicides, fungicides) or crop fertilizers. Many chemicals used in these preparations are highly toxic and can remain in the soil for long periods of time without being degraded, thus setting the stage for pollution of food, water, and, ultimately, people.

Farmers are the largest users of pesticides, but they are also used by industry; federal, state, and local governmental agencies; and individual people in their homes and gardens. Actual toxic effects of the different compounds vary and some effects occur before the chemicals reach the soil. Vertebrates usually will not suffer acute poisoning from these substances except through accidental ingestion, direct skin contact, or inhalation of the dust or spray of the more toxic pesticides. Workers in pesticide manufacturing plants, agricultural workers, and commercial pest-control operators applying the chemicals to crops or soil can all inhale pesticide dust or spray. Inhalation exposure can occur in a subtle manner at times—for example, by inhaling the dust from storage bags during the filling and emptying process or from cultivated soil previously treated with pesticides. Symptoms occurring as a result of such exposure may not be attributed to the pesticides. Therefore many episodes of acute poisoning go undiagnosed. Direct skin contact can occur when solutions are spilled accidentally or when the moist spray touches exposed skin (5, 67, 69). An occupational history aids early diagnosis of such problems.

Effects of Soil Pollution

Reports from epidemiological studies conducted in Iowa and California indicate that various acute illnesses and physiological changes were observed in farmers after handling agricultural chemicals. Such effects on the central nervous system as forgetfulness, decreased attention and interest span, hyperirritability, anxiety, depression, nervousness, and insomnia have been reported. Skin diseases, eye and respiratory conditions, and digestive disorders have also been identified. In some instances, these problems occurred after a single exposure to a toxic chemical (121, 135, 143).

Pesticides have an immediate toxic effect on birds, bees, and rodents, thus curtailing the necessary natural agents of cross-pollination and insect destruction, which, in turn, can affect the food supply. Surface water may be contaminated during spraying or dusting; or rain may wash pesticides or fertilizers into streams and lakes, again affecting food supply.

Edwards shows that earthworms are capable of concentrating toxic chemicals from the soil and storing these chemicals in their fatty tissues. Because earthworms provide food for other animals that are also capable of concentrating these chemicals, they may prove to be an important source of undesirable chemical residues in higher animals and humans (24).

The effects on people of long-term exposure to pesticides by inhalation or by ingestion of food and water containing residual chemicals are unknown. However, lower activity values of serum lactic dehydrogenase (an enzyme present in large amounts in liver tissue); inhibited cholinesterase activity; and altered hemoglobin, hematocrit, and amino acid levels have been shown to exist in people occupationally exposed to pesticides (69). Experimentally, small doses of pesticides have caused such metabolic changes as lowered estrogen levels, altered glucose metabolism, and inhibition of adenosine triphosphatase (ATP) in a wide variety of vertebrates, including humans (93). In addition, potent **herbicides**, *substances used to kill weeds or plants*, such as 2,4,5-T, have produced spontaneous abortions, birth defects, and skeletal and tissue changes *after birth* in animals and humans (102, 143).

The Environmental Protection Agency's pesticide control program has three major components: registration of pesticides, training of pesticide applicators, and monitoring and research. All pesticides must be registered with the Agency before being marketed. The Agency approves labeling and sets maximum safe levels for pesticide residues in human and animal food. The EPA has developed an applicator training program, certifying individuals permitted to apply restricted-use pesticides. In addition, the Agency sponsors research on pesticides and monitors pesticide levels in the environment. Both acute and long-term pesticide effects are considered in the epidemiological studies (140).

In spite of the EPA's efforts, evidence indicates that EPA standards are not being followed and long-term effects are yet unknown. According to a report from the National Research Council of the National Academy of Sciences, industrial wastes are being dumped on or pumped into the earth's crust and few studies are being done to determine whether the sites are safe. It may be possible to contain wastes safely and to lessen toxicity in wastes in the natural systems of the earth if the chemical nature of the waste and the geologic nature of the disposal area are understood. Geologic mapping is needed as a guide to safe disposal sites and for research on reactions between chemicals and rock or soil, fracture patterns in rocks, fluid flow, and hydrodynamics of deep basins (55).

The widespread contamination by dioxin in Missouri in 1983 following massive flooding illustrates the complexity and extent of the problem. Chemicals were used without awareness of harmful effect. Unregulated use of chemicals for dumping various chemicals by industries has occurred for some time and has only become apparent later. Furthermore, chemicals may not remain where originally used or dumped. Flood waters, underground water, and wind transport chemicals or their residues from one soil site to another. People are now learning that their past and present symptoms or diseases are related to or caused by hazardous pollutants in the environment to which they did not know they were being exposed (107).

Dioxin, for example, is considered the most toxic synthetic compound known to science. A complex organic chemical compound, it is insoluble in water but dissolves in organic solvents mixed with water. It is strongly attracted to lipids: fatty tissue in the body, oils, or related lipid substances. It becomes strongly attached to soil particles. The chemical remains in lipids or soil for many years and can move through water with solvents, soil particles, or colloids to which it is attached, such as during a flood or with soil erosion. Dioxin is also part of many other chemical compounds—for example, chlorophenols, herbicides, and the antiseptic hexachlorophene. It can be generated by incineration of industrial, commercial, and municipal wastes that contain chlorinated aromatics, chlorophenols, or PCBs. It produces a wide range of harmful effects in humans and animals, including

1. Fatal liver damage
2. Birth defects
3. Spontaneous abortions and sterility
4. Many types of cancer
5. Nerve and brain damage
6. Disturbed enzyme production
7. Reduced immunity to infections
8. Chloracne, a disfiguring and painful affliction of the skin
9. Damage to the urinary, genital, and gastrointestinal tracts, the thymus, and spleen

Many effects are chronic and longterm (107).

Dioxin is not only a problem for residents along Missouri rivers outside of St. Louis, however, although that was the scene of much publicity in 1983. Dioxin was a contaminant in Agent Orange, the herbicide sprayed in Vietnam, to which many U. S. service personnel were exposed. These servicemen are also suffering a variety of health problems. Where else dioxin contamination may be found is not yet known (107).

FOOD POLLUTION

Some of the same chemicals found in pesticide preparation are used as **food additives**. These purposely used additives are not designed to be toxic but rather *to preserve, improve, and protect nutritional value.* The average person in the United States consumes approximately three pounds of these additives every year. Artificial flavors and colors make up 80 percent of all chemicals used in our food; preservatives, sweeteners, and thickeners, a total of 11 categories of substances, make up the rest of the additives (37, 62). However, determining their potential health hazard over a life span is difficult. Certain food additives interfere with intestinal mucosa absorptive ability and therefore affect availability of nutrients and drugs. Also, some nontoxic substances or chemicals used as food additives are metabolized into toxic substances in the body. Adverse reactions to synthetic flavors and colors include gastrointestinal, respiratory, neurological, skeletal, and skin disorders. Removal of artificial flavors and colors from the diet has been found to reduce hyperkinesis and certain learning disabilities in 50 percent of the children with these disorders (1, 27, 37, 147). Under certain physiological conditions nitrites used to inhibit bacterial growth in processed foods can combine with certain amines to form chemicals that are potentially mutagenic and carcinogenic (37).

Unexpected side effects due to antibiotic and hormone residues from drugs given to animals for growth promotion and disease prevention have resulted. In people these residues have resulted in (1) allergy and increased drug toxicity or resistance to pathogens when the *same* family of antibiotics is later administered therapeutically and (2) change of normal bacterial flora in a body area so that invasion by pathogens is more likely, causing infection or disease (6). Synthetic estrogen diethylstilbestrol (DES) was used in cattle feed to promote rapid weight gain. Studies have linked DES to increases in a rare genital tract tumor in young women whose mothers were given DES when pregnant. As a result of these studies, use of DES has been restricted. An attempt to ban its use and the use of other sex hormones as feed supplements for cattle is underway (37).

Other food pollution hazards are radioactive materials, such as strontium 90, which has been traced in milk; mercury found in swordfish; worms; and mold, which may be present without noticeable change in the food's appearance, taste, or smell. Food handlers may introduce their infectious diseases into food by touching it or the equipment with soiled hands or by coughing onto it. Prolonged storage of highly acidic foods in aluminum cookware or aluminum foil may cause more aluminum than usual to enter the body. Using unlined copper utensils for cooking or storing food may also be harmful (44). Food sources may become contaminated by the chemicals and metals used in fertilizers and pesticides. In the future, diseases from food additives may assume as much significance in humans as do the **zoonoses,** *diseases transmitted between animals and humans*, such as trichinosis, brucellosis, tuberculosis, psittacosis, salmonellosis, typhus, roundworms, and rabies.

Because of the endless contamination possibilities from bacteria, toxins, viruses, parasites, and protozoa, the Food and Drug Administration and the Department of Agriculture enforce laws passed by Congress, impose various regulations of their own, and, in general, monitor the food industry nationwide. Various state and local authorities also attempt to regulate standards within their respective jurisdictions (5, 150). Yet these agencies cannot possibly determine every breach of regulation. Astute observations must be made about standards in the food store. Demanding to know the growing, cleansing, processing, and handling procedures is not out of line. Reporting suspected breaches is your responsibility for health.

NOISE POLLUTION

Sensory stimulation plays a major role in psychological and physiological development and is therefore directly related to physical and mental health. Sound is but one form of sensory stimulation. **Sound overload,** *unwanted sound that produces unwanted effects*, as well as sound deprivation, can be hazards to health (33, 121, 131).

Sound overload can produce temporary or permanent hearing loss by affecting the tympanic membrane and by slowly deteriorating the microscopic cells that send sound waves from the ear to the brain. The effects produced on each person's hearing vary, depending on the sound intensity and pitch, the location of the source in relation to the person, the length of exposure, and the person's age and history of previous ear problems. Surveys have shown that at least 20 million Americans have measurable hearing deficits and still another 16 million are exposed to occupational noise levels capable of producing permanent hearing loss (75, 130, 133).

One means of determining the potential hazard of any sound is to measure its loudness. *The measurement of sound loudness is stated in* **decibels**. The faintest audible sound is designated 1 decibel; ordinary conversation, measured at 40 to 60 decibels, is considered adequately quiet. The Environmental Protection Agency identifies 55 decibels as the level above which harmful effects occur. Studies have shown that moderately loud sounds of 75 to 80 decibels, such as those produced by a clothes washer, tabulating machine, or home garbage-disposal unit, can be discomforting to human ears and can, over a period of time, produce temporary or permanent hearing loss. Here are examples of common sound pollutants and their decibel readings.

	Decibels
Vacuum cleaner	72
Dishwasher	76-96
Minibike	76
Heavy city traffic	90-95
Food blender in home	93
Pneumatic hammer	95
Air compressor	95
Power lawnmower	95
Farm tractor	98
Outboard motor	102
Jet flying over at 1000 feet	103
Riveting gun	110
Motorcycle	115
Live rock music	120
Jet plane at takeoff	150
Rocket engine	180

Sound louder than 130 decibels, such as that produced by a nearby jet plane, gunshot blast, or a rocket at the launching pad, may cause actual pain (34, 121, 128, 129, 130, 133). Persons who work regularly with any of the machines listed should realize the potential long-range effects of such noise levels.

The Noise Control Act was passed in 1972 and amended in 1978 as the Quiet Communities Act. Under this act the Environmental Protection Agency has the authority to set noise emission standards for transportation vehicles and products that are major sources of noise. The act also provides for research into the psychological and physiological effects of noise on people (140).

Effects of Noise Pollution

Sound overload affects everyone at some time by intruding on privacy and shattering serenity. It can produce impaired communication and social relationships, irritability, chronic headache, depression, fatigue, and tension, in addition to hearing loss. Research indicates that less obvious physiological changes can also occur. These changes include involuntary responses in the digestive, cardiovascular, endocrine, and nervous system. They can produce blood vessel constriction, pallor, dilated pupils and visual disturbance, increased and irregular heart rate, hypertension, headache, gastrointestinal spasm with nausea and diarrhea and eventual peptic ulcer, hyperactive reflexes, and muscle tenseness. These responses do not subside immediately but continue up to five times longer than the actual noise. Noise has also been associated with elevated blood cholesterol levels, atherosclerosis, and accident proneness (20, 34, 106, 121, 143).

We do not adapt to excessive sound, as was once thought; we learn to tolerate it. Even when a person is asleep, noise cannot be shut out completely. We are exhausted by our efforts to remain asleep in the midst of this external stimuli. Perhaps being aware of these environmental stress factors can aid in reducing or coping with them (34, 142, 143).

Although not every harmful form of sound can be avoided, certain measures, such as wearing protective ear coverings, shortening exposure time, having regular hearing examinations, and seeking immediate medical attention for any ear injury or infection, will decrease the possibility of permanent damage or hearing loss. Noise can be brought under control without excessive cost. You can educate the public about the hazards of excess noise and ways to reduce noise in the home environment. Some suggestions to reduce noise are: hang heavy drapes over windows closest to outside noise sources, use foam pads under blenders and mixers, use carpeting in areas of heavy foot traffic, use upholstered instead of hard-surfaced furniture, and install sound absorbing ceiling tile in the kitchen.

The hospital, considered a place to recuperate and rest, may actually contribute to symptoms because of the noise levels in certain areas. One study showed that noise levels in infant incubators, the recovery room, and acute care units were high enough to act as a stressor and stimulate the hypophyseal-adrenocortical axis. Peripheral vasoconstriction affecting blood pressure and pulse, threats to hearing loss in patients receiving aminoglycosidic antibiotics, and sleep deprivation were noted. Noise pollution in the operating room, causing vasoconstriction, pupil dilation, fatigue, and impaired speech communication, has also been found (106).

SURFACE POLLUTION

Until the mid-1960s U. S. residents were not concerned with problems of waste disposal or recycling. Raw materials were plentiful and the open-dump method of disposal was convenient and economical. In the early 1970s, however, people became more concerned with the decreasing supply of natural resources and the health problems created by open dumps.

The Solid Waste Disposal Act was passed by Congress in 1965. The primary focus of this act was on the disposal of waste, not collection or street cleaning. In 1970 Congress passed the Resource Recovery Act, which shifted the emphasis of federal involvement from disposal to recycling, resource recovery, and the conversion of waste into energy. Subsequent laws, such as the Resource Conservation and Recovery Act of 1976, have been passed to facilitate further the safe disposal of waste (77, 140).

The total quantity of solid waste is large and increasing. Over 4 billion tons of solid household, municipal, industrial, agricultural, and mineral wastes are produced yearly in the United States (11, 114). The waste-disposal system of an average city must accommodate about 85 kilograms of refuse per week for every family of four (124). Most present disposal methods for this waste pollute land, air, or water. We can see this pollution everywhere: in open air, foul-smelling dumps, smoking incineration centers, junkyards, and poorly covered landfills.

Solid-Waste Disposal Methods

Solid waste is discarded in four basic ways: (1) open dumps, (2) sanitary landfills, (3) incineration, and (4) salvage. Of these methods, the *open dump* (now illegal in most states) is the oldest, most convenient, and most economical. It creates many health problems, however, and is esthetically undesirable. Dumps serve as breeding areas for rodents, flies, and other insects, such as cockroaches; they also attract seagulls, notorious as thieves and litterers. Houseflies carry poliomyelitis, tuberculosis, diarrhea, dysentery, hepatitis, and cholera. Rats carry plague, tapeworm, Rocky Mountain spotted fever, and rat-bite fever. Water running off from these dumps pollutes local streams and lakes. Rain and surface water can seep through the wastes and pollute underground water. Any attempt to burn the surface waste in the dumps emits large quantities of foul-smelling fumes that increase air pollution and thus respiratory problems among local inhabitants. Dumps also invite accidents and fires, in addition to lowering the value of surrounding property (66, 121).

Landfills, when handled properly, can be economical, sanitary, and esthetically acceptable. These areas should be placed far from water sources. Even with this precaution, underground or surface water may become polluted. The waste should be quickly covered to avoid foul smells, spontaneous combustion, breeding of rats and flies, and scavenging by rodents (121, 122, 124).

Approximately 80 percent of household solid wastes are combustible and therefore suitable for *incineration*. Decentralized incineration is usually poorly controlled and it frequently produces gaseous emissions and particulates that pollute the air and damage our health. Central incineration conducted by federal, state, or local governmental bodies is expensive, although necessary for large urban areas. The controlled-combustion process used in these centers prevents the emission of harmful gases and uses the byproduct, heat, for an energy source. Through incineration the volume of waste can be reduced to one-fifth of its original bulk. The remaining material can be removed to landfills or compressed for use in soil conditioners or construction material (5).

The composition of solid waste has changed in past years; today it includes larger amounts of paper, plastics, aluminum cans, and other packaging and wrapping materials. Many such materials will not decompose or rust; therefore they present new problems in disposal. If these products are *salvaged*, they can be **recycled**, *treated by mechanical, thermal, or biological means so that they can be used again*, thus promoting resource recovery and reuse (6, 77, 104).

Hazardous-Waste Disposal

Congress has defined **hazardous waste** as *discarded material that may pose a threat or hazard to human health or the environment*. These wastes can be solids, liquids, sludges, or gases. They are toxic, ignitable, corrosive, infectious, reactive (react with air, water, or other substances, resulting in explosions and toxic fumes), or radioactive (23).

Hospitals, medical research laboratories, mining operations, service stations, retailers, and householders contribute in small amounts to hazardous-waste production. The Armed Forces with their obsolete explosives, herbicides, and nerve gases contribute significantly to the total volume. Most hazardous wastes generated, however, come from manufacturing industries. According to the Environmental Protection Agency, only about 10 percent of the hazardous waste currently generated is disposed of in an environmentally sound manner. The rest threatens our water and air quality and our water and land ecosystems. The EPA estimates that if available recycling and resource recovery technologies were used, the production of hazardous wastes could be reduced by as much as 20 percent (23). The task of tracking hazardous waste to ensure its safe disposal is enormous. Every month 90 million kilograms of hazardous waste are produced. At least 20,000 facilities exist to store, treat, or dispose of chemical refuse, plus 10,000 transporters of waste (118).

An example of the problems associated with hazardous-waste disposal can be found in the small community of Wilsonville, Illinois. In 1977, Wilsonville residents learned that a national disposal firm was burying dirt contaminated with polychlorinated biphenyls, a cancer-causing substance, in a landfill near their town. After a long legal battle, the landfill was closed and the hazardous wastes were to be removed. Removal of the waste did not begin until late 1982. Because the company has no way of disposing of the material completely, it was transferred to a landfill in the Midwest (43). Thus a task that will take several years to complete will decrease the danger at Wilsonville but may pose a threat to another community.

Nuclear Waste

One type of hazardous-waste product that has attracted considerable attention is radioactive waste. Some fission products that must be stored are cesium-137, strontium-90, iodine-131, and plutonium-239. Some decay rapidly in hours or days while others require thousands and millions of years to lose their radioactive potency (136). No satisfactory method of permanent disposal has been developed; the cost and fear of leakage from the storage area have been stumbling blocks.

The use of nuclear energy or power produced by fission reactors has caused much concern and debate among the people of the United States. The concerns center around two major issues: the long-term disposal of radioactive wastes and the safety of the actual reactors.

When a utility shuts down a reactor at the end of its period of usefulness, the utility is faced with the problem of what to do with intensely radioactive materials. At present, only three means of disposal exist: dismantlement of the reactor with the debris shipped to a burial site, entombment of the reactor in a concrete structure, and protective storage that would prevent public access for 30 to 100 years. Even though nuclear power is a quarter-century old, the problem of safe disposal of radioactive waste is not yet critical. At present, only four reactors are potential candidates for shutdown (87).

The seriousness of problems associated with the safety of nuclear reactors for generating electricity is well illustrated by the following highly publicized event. In Pennsylvania, in March 1979, an accident occurred at the nuclear reactor site known as Three Mile Island. In retrospect, the accident was preventable and was less severe than originally reported. Residents near the site, however, were exposed to the radioactive isotope xenon-133, which has a half-life of approximately 5 days. The radiation release has the potential for causing the death, by cancer, of less than one person in the next 30 or 40 years (64). The major health effect of the accident appears to have been on the mental health of the people in the region. The fear, anger, and confusion felt by the Three Mile Island community are shared nationally and internationally. The majority of citizens now have serious second thoughts about the safety and reliability of nuclear power (64, 96). Diminishing resources lead to the need for alternative energy sources. The problems in this area must be explored.

Hospital Waste

The amount of solid waste being produced by hospitals should be a primary concern to health workers. The average citizen accumulates and disposes of 5.5 pounds of solid waste daily whereas the average hospital patient accumulates 24.16 pounds daily. Hospitals add 170,000 tons of pathologic materials yearly to the waste load (124). This increase in hospital wastes can be attributed to the increase in disposable products: syringes, needles, surgical supplies, dishes and utensils, linens, uniforms, and medication containers. Many hospitals use disposable products because they are considered cheaper, easier to store, and less likely to produce cross-infection. Yet hospitals often fail to consider the cost or inconvenience of transporting or discarding large quantities of these contaminated objects. Much of a hospital's solid waste, often contaminated by infectious organisms, is removed to open dumps or sanitary landfills without proper initial sterilization, thus spreading pathogens to land and water (68). Most hospital workers don't consider the implications of casually using disposable items.

One study conducted in an urban area with 16 participating hospitals revealed that the nurse influences decisions regarding the purchase of patient care items more than any other hospital worker. If these decisions are largely your responsibility, know how much trash your hospital creates, where the waste goes, the decontamination procedures used before disposal, the cost of disposal, why your agency uses disposable products, and how much your agency contributes to environmental pollution. Form an interdepartmental committee, perhaps of administrators, nurses, doctors, and patients. Report your findings to them and together consider all the advantages and drawbacks of various products. Consider cost, convenience, infection control, and quality. Give each new product a careful clinical trial and adopt it for use only after careful consideration about contributions to patient care. Avoid using disposable items if nondisposables will do the job as well. Pass this information on to the patients and families. Encourage health workers in homes to demonstrate and teach proper disposal of such items as syringes and dressings. Work to reduce the huge volume of solid waste that is taking space and depleting natural resources (57). And work for disposal of infectious wastes in non-air-polluting incinerators, which many cities and hospitals do not have.

Lead Poisoning

Lead is another surface pollutant. We inhale lead as an air pollutant and ingest traces of lead daily through a normal diet. Because lead wastes have increased during the past century, particularly from industry and automobile use, exposure and intake into the body have multiplied. Consequently, the rate of absorption by soft tissue exceeds the rate of excretion or storage by bone (10, 22, 144). An urgent problem is controlling the lead exposure that occurs from drinking or eating from improperly lead-glazed earthenware, using leaded gasoline, consuming lead-contaminated "moonshine," or working in or living near industries where lead exposure is not controlled (63). Two-thirds of the lead found in canned foods comes from solder. This source of lead constitutes one-third of the lead that the average person ingests from food (12).

Individuals who work in areas with high lead levels show evidence of chronic lead poisoning. Persistent abdominal pain is the cardinal symptom in adults. They also exhibit fatigue, nervousness, and sleep disturbances as well as cognitive deficits and peripheral neuropathy. Kidney damage occurs slowly and may not be detected until two-thirds of the kidney function is destroyed. The male workers have a decrease in the quantity and quality of sperm, and the female workers have an increased risk of fetal damage and/or abortion (42).

Another urgent problem arises when young children, mainly in urban slums, form the *habit of eating nonfood substances, including peeling paint, plaster, or putty containing lead. This behavior is called* **pica.** The precise cause of pica is not completely understood, but it may be related to nutritional, cultural, and emotional factors. Acute or chronic lead poisoning, an insidious disease, results from this eating pattern and is a major source of brain damage, mental deficiency, and behavior problems. The pathological changes that occur affect the nervous, renal, and hematopoietic systems. Kidney damage is usually reversible, but chronic lead poisoning in childhood may lead to gout or kidney disease later in life. Damage to the hematopoietic system is evident by the reduction in the number and quality of red blood cells produced, thus leading to severe anemia. The most serious effects are on the nervous system. The mortality rate from lead encephalopathy (disease of the brain) is 5 percent. Of the children who survive acute lead poisoning, 40 percent have convulsive disorders and another 20 percent have significant neurological deficits (21, 40, 97, 98).

Studies show that

1. Blood lead levels are higher in Blacks than Caucasians among all socioeconomic and urbanization levels.
2. Young children from both Black and Caucasian families with incomes under $6000 have a significantly higher prevalence of elevated blood lead than those from households with incomes of $6000 or more.
3. Almost one-fifth of Black children from low-income families, the group with the highest proportion of elevated blood lead levels, should be referred for medical followup.
4. Mean blood lead level in young children increases with the degree of urbanization where they live (45).

Although there seems to be a trend toward reduced lead screening, child health programs should consider routine screening of all children from 1 to 5 years of age. Reduction of leaded gasoline and establishment of auto-emissions standards set by the EPA have been steps in the right direction, for the mean blood lead level in the United States fell significantly between 1976 and 1980 (45).

OCCUPATIONAL HAZARDS

Increasingly we learn of the health hazards that many workers face daily at their jobs. Monotony, paced work, and performance pressures are major sources of stress in many jobs and can contribute to disease pathology. The muscle strains, backaches, fractures, burns, eye injuries, and other accidental emergencies are taken for granted by the public. But workers may not suffer the consequences of the hidden environmental hazards—the chemicals or radiation they work with directly or indirectly—until years later. Often in the past the etiology of the physical illness remained unsolved. Not only do miners and factory workers become ill because of their work environment, hospital workers also may suffer. Those who work regularly with certain anesthetics, for example, may develop cancer, leukemia, or lymphoma. Those who work with high levels of radiation risk sterility or defective offspring if adequate protection is not maintained. Nurses may suffer infections, back and muscle injuries, varicose veins, and any of the other physical or emotional effects of stress.

The Occupational Safety and Health Act of 1970, the Coal Mine Health and Safety Act of 1969, and the Toxic Substances Control Act of 1976 are some of the laws passed by Congress that have been responsible for making occupational safety and health a public health concern rather than a private matter. Through these laws the federal government works to prevent work-related accidents and disease, to correct hazardous working conditions, to promote good health for working men and women, and to improve compensation. The Occupational Safety and Health Act established the Occupational Safety and Health Administration, which conducts inspections of industries to force compliance and research to establish the hazardous levels of various chemicals. Relatively few of the many chemicals in industry have been researched, but the standards, as well as prevention and treatment measures, are published periodically in *The Federal Register*, which can be obtained from the Department of Labor. The act has forced industries to become more active in seeking health services for employees and has assisted the occupational health nurse to offer additional services related to disease prevention and education of employees (105). Health screening is also being emphasized, for contamination from some substances can be detected early enough to prevent disease. In one community where smelter employees were manifesting symptoms of nerve damage, for instance, high levels of arsenic were found in the urine, fingernails, and hair (83). Earlier screening could have prevented arsenic poisoning.

The Federal Register also publishes updated guidelines on occupational hearing conservation. Basically each hearing program must consist of five parts.

1. Employee education. Each employee must be told the significance of the program.
2. An analysis of the noise in the workplace, now required every two years or as noise levels change.
3. Engineering and administrative controls. The environmental noise must be altered if possible.
4. Audometric texting. All employees exposed to 85 decibels or more (over a period of 8 hours) must be tested yearly as well as on preemployment.
5. Personal protective equipment. A variety of hearing protectors must be available.

Along with these guidelines are specific requirements for those who administer and interpret tests, circumstances under which tests are administered, and the instruments for measuring noise levels and hearing (117).

Hazards of the factory or mine can extend beyond the workplace and endanger workers' families and other residents of the community. Workers carry out dust particles on skin and clothing; wind currents also deposit particles. Even if workers shower before leaving work, the total removal of all dust particles of some chemicals or elements is difficult. As a result, some communities become well known for a high incidence of certain types of cancer or skin or respiratory disease.

Another group of health hazards related to a large industry in the United States is cosmetics, including aerosol preparations, hair dyes, and feminine sprays, which increasingly are related to skin and other diseases, including cancer. As with other occupational chemicals, effects of the use of these products are usually not known until years after their regular usage (143). The World Health Organization estimates that 75 to 85 percent of all cancers are environmentally caused. No one knows how much occupational factors contribute to these causes (149).

Laryngeal cancer has been found among workers exposed to asbestos, cutting oil, wood dust, grease, and oil; among workers in the paper, metal, construction, leather, food, and textile industries; and among barbers, sheet metal workers, electricians, and naphthalene cleaners (29).

Often occupational health hazards are taken for granted. They are seen as part of the job. Employees in laundries and dry cleaning establishments, for example, suffer hazards of excess heat, humidity, and noise; falls and accidents from slipping on wet floors; back injury and muscle strains from lifting; and circulatory problems from standing. Janitorial workers may have contact with dangerous chemicals in cleaning agents. Asthma is an occupational hazard for animal workers, veterinarians, farmers, bakers, carpenters, welders, and many other workers.

Industrial nurses and safety engineers emphasize wearing protective clothing and using protective equipment. Yet there are problems. The employee may not want to be bothered with cumbersome protective clothing. Or the protective clothing and equipment given to the female employee may be too large or too heavy, thus ill-fitting and not protective, for it is designed for the male employee. (However, a few companies do specialize in protective clothing designed for females.) Hard hats, safety shoes and gloves, and ear muffs that fit improperly may actually contribute toward an accidental injury.

To compound the problem of prevention, length of exposure to an industrial substance often determines if it will cause disease. The amount of exposure to the worker often depends on the production phase involved. Additionally, each substance appears likely to produce disease, such as cancer, in a specific body part; such information becomes available after workers become ill. Sex is also a factor, for some substances affect the reproductive organs of the female (or fetus) but do not affect the male. Some substances do not affect the male reproductive organs, but the father's genes may contribute to fetal damage. *

*Information about health hazards for women employees and preventive or corrective measures is available from the Woman's Occupational Health Resource Center, American Health Foundation, 320 East 43rd Street, New York, New York, 10017.

Table 9-1 summarizes common industrial agents (various substances, elements, or chemicals) and their major known effects.

TABLE 9-1 Effects of Some Common Industrial Agents Upon the Worker

AGENT	TYPE OF INDUSTRY OR OCCUPATION	BODY AREA AFFECTED
Acetaldelhyde	Chemical, Paint	All body cells, especially brain and respiratory tract.
Acetic Anhydride	Textile	Exposed tissue damage, especially eye and respiratory tract.
Acetylene	Welding, Plastic, Dry Cleaning	Respiratory tract asphyxiant. Explosive, especially when combined with certain substances.
Acrolein	Chemical	Skin, eye, respiratory tract.
Allyl Chloride	Plastic	Skin, respiratory tract, kidney.
Ammonia	Chemical, Leather, Wool, Farmers, Refrigeration Workers	Eyes, skin, respiratory tract.
Anesthetic Gases	Medical, Dental, and Veterinary Workers	Reproductive (increased rate of spontaneous abortions and congenital anomalies whether male or female exposed).
Aniline	Paint, Rubber	Skin, hematopoietic system.
Arsenic	Mine, Smelter, Leather, Chemical, Oil Refinery, Insecticide Makers and Sprayers.	Skin, lung, liver (cancer). Nervous system damage.
Asbestos	Mine, Textile, Insulation, Shipyard Workers, Construction	Respiratory and gastrointestinal tract (cancer) as well as asbestosis (lung scarring). More harmful to people who smoke.
Benzene	Rubber, Chemical, Explosives, Paint, Shoemakers, Dye Users, Office Workers	Skin, liver, brain, hematopoietic system (cancer, leukemia).
Beryllium	Foundry, Metallurgical, Aerospace, Nuclear, Household Appliance Production	Skin and eye (inflammation, ulcers), respiratory tract (acute inflammation and berylliosis—chronic lung infection), systemic effects on heart, liver, spleen, kidneys.
Butyl Alcohol	Lacquer, Paint	Eye, skin, respiratory tract.
Carbon Disulfide	Rubber, Viscose Rayon	Gastrointestinal, heart, liver, kidney, brain.
Carbon Tetrachloride	Solvent, Dry Cleaning	Skin, gastrointestinal, liver, kidney, brain.

TABLE 9-1 (cont.)

AGENT	TYPE OF INDUSTRY OR OCCUPATION	BODY AREA AFFECTED
Chlorine	Industrial Bleaching, Laundry Workers	Eye, respiratory tract, skin.
Chloroform	Chemical, Plastic	Heart degeneration, liver, kidney.
Chromium	Chrome Plating, Chemical, Industrial Bleaching, Glass and Pottery, Linoleum Makers, Battery Makers	Irritating to all body cells. Skin, eye, respiratory tract, (cancer) liver, kidney.
Coal Combustion Products (Soot, Tar)	Gashouse Workers, Asphalt, Coal Tar, or Pitch Workers, Mine, Coke Oven Workers	Skin, respiratory tract, scrotum, urinary bladder (carcinogenic to all areas).
Cotton, Flax, Hemp, Lint	Textile	Respiratory tract (byssinosis-chest tightness, dyspnea, cough, wheezing; chronic bronchitis). Cigarette smokers especially affected.
Creosal	Chemical, Oil Refining	Denatures and precipitates all cellular protein. Skin, eye, respiratory tract, liver, kidney, brain.
Dichloroethyl Ether	Insecticide, Oil Refining	Respiratory tract.
Dimethyl Sulfate	Chemical, Pharmaceutical	Eye, respiratory tract, liver, kidney, brain.
Ethylene Oxide	Hospital Sterilization	Possible fetal damage.
Formaldehyde	Textile	Liver, lung, skin (infection and cancer).
Fungus, Parasites, Microorganisms	Food, Animal, Outdoor Workers, Clinical Laboratory Workers	Skin, respiratory tract (infection, including hepatitis B).
Germicidal Agents	Health Care Workers, Maintenance/Cleaning Workers	Skin (contact allergy, dermatosis).
Hydrogen Chloride	Meat Wrappers	Respiratory tract (irritation and asthma).
Iron Oxide	Mine, Iron Foundry, Metal Polishers and Finishers	Respiratory tract (cancer).
Lead	Auto, Smelter, Plumbing, Paint, Metallurgical, Battery Making, Exposure in 120 different industries	Hematopoietic, liver, kidney, brain, muscles, bone, gastrointestinal tract. Causes fetal damage during first trimester of pregnancy.
Leather	Leather, Shoe	Nasal cavity and sinuses, urinary bladder (carcinogenic for each).
Manganese	Mine, Metallurgical, Welders	Respiratory tract, liver, brain.
Mercury	Electrical, Laboratory Workers, Exposure in 80 different types of industries	Toxic to all cells. Dermatosis. Respiratory tract, liver, brain damage. Exposure of pregnant

TABLE 9-1 (cont.)

AGENT	TYPE OF INDUSTRY OR OCCUPATION	BODY AREA AFFECTED
		woman causes congenital defects and retardation.
Mica	Rubber, Insulation	Respiratory tract.
Nickel	Metallurgical, Smelter, Electrolysis Workers	Skin, respiratory tract (infection and cancer).
Nitrobenzene	Synthetic dyes	Skin, hematopoietic system, brain.
Nitrogen Dioxide	Chemical, Metal	Eye, respiratory tract, hematopoietic system.
Organophosphates	Agriculture	Brain dysfunction, memory loss, disorientation, ataxia, liver and kidney damage.
Petroleum Products	Rubber, Textile, Aerospace, Workers in contact with fuel oil, coke, paraffin, lubricants	Skin, respiratory tract, scrotum (carcinogenic to each); dermatosis.
Phenol	Plastics	Corrosive to all tissue. Liver, kidney, brain.
Polyurethane	Plastics and most other industries	Respiratory tract (asthma, cancer). Dermatosis.
Rubber Dust	Rubber	Respiratory tract (chronic disease). Dermatosis.
Silica	Mine, Foundry, Ceramic or Glass Production	Respiratory tract (silicosis).
Talc Dust	Mine	Respiratory tract (cancer), calcification of pericardium.
Tetraethyl Lead	Chemical	Hematopoietic system, brain.
Thallium	Pesticide, Fireworks or Explosives	Skin, respiratory and gastrointestinal tract, kidney, brain.
Toluene	Rubber, Paint, Clerical Workers, Printers	Skin, respiratory tract, liver, hematopoietic system, brain (may cause drunken state and accidents).
Trichloroethylene	Chemical, Metal Degreasing	Skin, liver, kidney, brain.
Vinyl Chloride	Plastic, Rubber, Insulation, Organic-Chemical Synthesizers, Polyvinyl Resin Makers	Skin, respiratory tract, (asthma), cancer in the liver, kidney, spleen and brain. Exposure of pregnant woman to polyvinyl chloride causes defective fetus.
Wood Products	Furniture	Respiratory tract (asthma).

Knowing that the worker may come in contact with a variety of harmful substances and that presenting symptoms may often seem unrelated to the occupation should help you be more careful and thorough in assessment. Also, as a citizen you can work for enforcement of preventive measures for known hazards and for continued research.

NURSING RESPONSIBILITY

Personal Responsibility

Consider the environment, the various social institutions, and the population as a complex of interacting, interdependent systems. Environmental problems are a concern to everyone and are of equal consequence to every part of the world. Each of us shares the earth and so we are all responsible for its well-being. Environmental pollution is our collective fault and requires our collective solutions. In the United States alone discarded materials amount to 4 billion tons yearly and the quantity is growing by 8 percent annually.

Linton describes a fourfold environmental protection system for continuously identifying, analyzing, and controlling environmental hazards:

1. Surveillance—maintaining an awareness of what people are doing to the air, water, and land, and of the effect of these actions on health.
2. Development of criteria for the detection of pollution.
3. Research.
4. Compliance—getting local government and industry to accept and implement new standards (66).

An informed public can help establish such a system, but the financial support and legislative and administrative guidance of federal, state, and local governments seem to be the most feasible solution. Chanlett, Rogers, and Hurst speak strongly of the need for environmental health planning on a widespread scale, involving the citizen and the government (8).

The Resource Conservation and Recovery Act of 1976 (PC 94-580) provides for recycling of our natural resources, safe disposal of discarded materials, and management of hazardous wastes, those that contribute to increased mortality or pose a substantial present or potential hazard to human health or environment. But these goals are not possible without individual effort.

As a citizen, you should conserve natural resources to the best of your ability and learn about the environmental pollution in your own area. Remember that metallurgical and chemical companies are the greatest source of hazardous waste. Campaign for minimized waste and for safe disposal of unavoidable waste. Encourage the development of additional burial sites for long-term safety as well as the monitoring of present sites for escape of wastes (114).

Avoid unnecessary use of water, electricity, and fuel. Don't litter. Buy beverages in returnable bottles and save cans and papers for recycling. Most cities have aluminum recycling points for beverage cans, gutters, siding, furniture, or household items for your use.

Use undyed paper products. Avoid high-phosphate detergents and aerosols. Don't carelessly dispose of used batteries, used engine oil, or empty pesticide containers. Walk or bicycle instead of driving a car when feasible. Avoid cigarette smoking in closed, crowded areas. Avoid contact with pesticides by thoroughly scrubbing or peeling foodstuffs and, if possible, maintain your own garden without use of pesticides. Quiet surroundings are a natural resource, too. Make your own quieter through personal habits. Help plan for local recreation sites that offer natural surroundings. Campaign for adequate acoustical standards in homes, apartments, hospitals, and industrial buildings, and for noiseless kitchen equipment. Participate in local governmental planning to decrease town and city noise in relation to transportation routes, zoning, and industrial sites. Don't burn leaves; contribute to a natural resource —soil—by composting plants or organic content in garbage. Plant a rooftop or patio garden to contribute to the oxygen cycle. Limit the number of pet animals. Join citizens' crusades for a clean environment or a conservation organization and attend workshops given by the Cancer Society, Sierra Club, Conservation Foundation, and League of Women Voters to learn more about problems, preventive measures, and means of strengthening legislation. Support antipollution and noise-control laws. Be an involved citizen!

The momentum that surrounded much of the environmental effort in its earliest stages has lead to some degree of apathy. It is a never-ending task to make the environment safe for the public and attitudes must be positive to maintain this serious concern.*

Professional Responsibility

Although nursing responsibilities have been interwoven throughout this chapter, consider that your primary responsibilities are detection through thorough assessment, making suggestions for intervention, and health teaching. You can play a significant role in the early detection of lead poisoning, for example. Assessment of a child's health should include observation for physical signs, such as tremors, abdominal discomfort, decreased appetite, and vomiting, as well as questions related to a pica behavior. Ask the mother about her child's interest in play, ability to get along with playmates, coordination, and level of developmental

*For more information on specific measures for wasting less and practicing ecologically sound living, see Saltonstall, *Your Environment and What You Can Do About It* (102) and the booklets published by the United States Department of Labor and the Environmental Protection Agency that are listed in the references.

skill attainment. Phrase your questions and comments carefully, in a nonjudgmental manner, so that the mother will not feel that her fitness as a parent is being judged. If the persons for whom you are caring live in unsatisfactory, low-income housing, work for improvement through local legislation. Emphasis must be placed on repair and deleading of dwelling places, not just on moving the present dweller to a new house or apartment. You can encourage the formation of screening and case-finding programs, already started in many cities, and you can assist with their activities. Be as thorough in assessment as possible. An example of questions usually not asked on standard health history forms that you could use in assessment of the employed client is presented in Table 9-2.

TABLE 9-2 Occupational History Form

1. Occupational History (start with last job first).

	COMPANY	DATE EMPLOYED	JOB
(a)	______	______	______
(b)	______	______	______
(c)	______	______	______
(d)	______	______	______

2. In these jobs, have you ever been exposed to:
   Excessive radiation or radioactive material? ______
   Excessive noise? ______ Excessive heat or light? ______
3. Have you worked in dusty trades? ______
   With any specific chemicals? ______
   In any vapors or fumes? ______
   If your answer is yes to any questions in (2) or (3), please elaborate. ______
   ______
   ______
4. Has a job ever made you "sick"? ______ If so, which job? ______
   Explain how you were sick. ______
5. Have you ever worn any protective equipment or a specific support? ______
   If so, what? ______
6. Have you ever had a serious work injury? ______ If so, please describe.
   ______
7. Have you had several minor work injuries? ______ If so, please describe.
   ______
8. Have you ever applied for, or received, workers' compensation? ______
9. Have you ever had a pension for disability? ______

Natural or manmade chemical pollution in soil, water, and food products can produce various adverse effects, ranging from slight health impairments to death. Higher-than-normal concentrations of nitrates in water, for example, can cause acute methemoglobinemia (a type of anemia) in infants (75, 84). Although local public health officials are responsible for maintaining safe nitrate levels in the water supply, your responsibilities are to aid in the education of the public concerning the health hazards of such pollutants and to use the epidemiological method in your work. Be aware of such symptoms as fatigue, listlessness, and sleepiness that might indicate an untoward reaction to this particular form of pollution.

Another dangerous problem associated with chemical pollution is its possible carcinogenic effect (as seen on Table 9-1). Incidence of specific forms of cancer can be higher or lower, depending on exposure to specific compounds, a common example being the high incidence of lung cancer in the United States and England because of heavy tobacco use. Be aware and knowledgeable of the incidence of chemically produced cancer in your particular locale. Health teaching can then be directed at trying to eliminate or control the responsible carcinogenic chemical. Radiation is also carcinogenic. Encourage the use of protective clothing and sunscreen lotions to prevent overexposure to the sun. Prevent overexposure to ionizing radiation by making certain that unnecessary x rays are not taken, by keeping a record of the frequency of x rays, and by using a lead shield when x rays are given.

The biochemical response to chemical pollution or radiation can influence the cell in various ways. *Teratogenic* (producing malformations) and *mutagenic* (producing hereditary changes) are two such changes in cells. Be aware that these changes can occur in both the client and the health care worker who are exposed to radiation. Genetic counseling might be indicated for couples who have been exposed to radiation. Citizens should know of the possibility for dealing effectively and therapeutically with biochemical changes, whether prenatally or in any stage of growth and development (38).

In the past 100 years disease and death have been reduced because of preventive public health measures in the form of environmental control, such as water and waste management, rodent and insect control, development of housing codes. Now we are again faced with problems and diseases that have an environmental impact. Prevention can begin with informed consumer groups who have educational and work projects as their goals. It can begin with your responsibility for the patient's environment.

The Patient's Immediate Environment

Besides a feeling of responsibility for the community and physical environment in which the patient lives, you also have a responsibility for that individual's immediate environment while receiving health care.

The patient's *surroundings should constitute a* **therapeutic milieu** *free of hazards and conducive to recovery, physically and emotionally.*

The patient's surroundings should be clean and adequately lighted, ventilated, and heated. Precautions should always be taken during care to prevent injury, such as burns from a hot-water bottle. Falls should be prevented by removing obstacles from walking areas and having the person wear well-fitted shoes and use adequate support while walking. Lock the bed or wheelchair while the patient is moving to and from them. Be sure that electrical cords and scatter rugs are not so placed that the patient could fall. Wipe up spilled liquids immediately. Use sterile technique and proper handwashing methods to ensure that you bring no pathogenic organisms to the patient. Avoid excessive noise from personnel and equipment to the degree possible.

The esthetic environment is also important for rest. Arrange articles on the bedside table in a pleasing manner if the patient is unable to do so. Keep unattractive equipment or supplies out of sight as much as possible. Electrical equipment should be in proper repair and function. Minimize offensive odors and noise. Place the person's bed or chair by a window or door so that the person can watch normal activity rather than stare at the ceiling and walls. As a nurse, involve yourself in making the entire ward as well as the patients' rooms look pleasing. Consider color combinations and the use of drapes, furniture, clocks, calendars, pictures, and various artifacts to create a more homelike atmosphere. The committee in charge of decorating and building should include at least one nurse. You may need to volunteer to ensure that nursing and, indirectly, patients are represented in such programs.

The patient's surroundings should not only be safe and attractive, but the emotional climate of the unit and entire institution affects patients and staff as well. The patient and family are quick to respond and react to the attitudes and manner of the staff. Here are some questions you might ask yourself. How do I treat delivery workers who bring gifts and flowers to patients? Do I participate in the joy such remembrances bring to the patient? Do I help arrange the flowers into a pleasant pattern or just stick them quickly into whatever can be found? Do I treat visitors as welcome guests or as foreign intruders? The emotional climate should radiate security and acceptance. A sense of warmth should prevail that promotes a feeling of trust, confidence, and motivation within the patient as he/she and the staff work together to cope with problems. The emotional relationship between the patient and the health care staff should help the patient reach the goal of maximum health.

In a truly therapeutic milieu the staff also feel a sense of harmony among themselves. There are mutual trust and acceptance between staff and supervisors, and supervisors recognize work well done by the staff.

As a result, staff feel motivated to continue to learn and to improve the quality of patient care. Staff members are not likely to give individualized, comprehensive, compassionate care in an agency where they are not treated like individuals or where their basic needs are not met.

Be aware of environmental pollution in the health care environment. "No Smoking" should be the rule not only when oxygen is in use but also in any health care setting. Often the conference or dining rooms or lounges for health care workers are polluted with cigarette or cigar smoke and ashtrays are full. It is difficult to teach a client the adverse effects of smoking and nicotine when an odor of cigarette smoke hangs on the uniform. Moreover, health care workers will benefit from practicing what they teach others. Health care workers and clients may also come in contact with agents listed in Table 9-1. Constant vigilance is necessary to detect harmful agents and prevent or reduce their usage. Early assessment of harmful effects to reduce the symptoms and proper intervention for dermatoses, allergens, or other symptoms is essential.

There are times when the treatment for the client may also affect the health care worker—for example, radiotherapy. Proper precautions should be taken to protect the worker from excess exposure and to protect any body areas of the client that should not be exposed. Constant monitoring of the dosage and duration of exposure to radiation, whether from a portable x-ray machine or a radium implant, is essential.

Patients who are receiving radiotherapy should be assessed for the following side effects (151):

1. Redness, edema, itching, denuding, and atrophy of skin.
2. Inflammation, dryness, pain, and impaired physiological function of mucous-lined areas of the body, including the oral cavity, esophagus, and vagina.
3. Sloughing of epithelial cells in various body areas, such as the esophagus, stomach, intestine, and genitourinary tract, resulting in ulceration, chronic inflammation, pain, necrosis, and impaired physiological functions of the organ system affected (vomiting, diarrhea, cystitis).
4. Depression of bone marrow, resulting in reduced white and red blood cells and platelets, which, in turn, causes infections, anemia, and hemorrhagic tendencies.
5. Inflammatory and fibrotic damage to the lungs and heart, causing pneumonitis, pericarditis, and occasionally myocarditis.
6. Temporary or permanent loss of hair, depending on dosage and duration of exposure.

Intervention for these side effects includes skin and mouth care; dietary modifications; use of mild analgesics, antiemetics, and antidiarrheal drugs; and reverse isolation technics. Refer to a medical-surgical text for specific interventions for the patient who is suffering side effects from radiotherapy.

If you are caring for a person in the home, you are limited in the amount of change you can make. You can point out such hazards as electrical cords in the walking area, however. You can make suggestions for furniture rearrangement if you think that the person could function more easily with the change. You can put a clock in sight, pull the drapes, or put needed materials within the patient's reach if feasible.

Specific ways of meeting the patient's environmental needs also differ for various developmental stages. The components of a therapeutic milieu are different for the baby than for the middle-aged man. However, a safe, secure environment, physically and psychologically, must be present for both. Accurately determining the factors that make up the environment and making appropriate changes may be the first step in promoting health.

It is past time for all of us to ask ourselves some basic questions. How much energy and natural resources do we need to sustain life, to maintain the high standard of living in the United States? How much are we willing to pay for benefits that will not poison us with side effects? How does population growth affect the use and abuse of natural resources? Will strictly controlled energy allocation be necessary because people refuse to abide by suggested limits? Must people continue to grow up with strontium-90 in their bones, DDT in their fat, and asbestos in their lungs? What more can each of us do personally and professionally to maintain a health-fostering environment?

REFERENCES

1. "Additives at Fault in Hyperactivity," *Science News*, 117, no. 13 (1980), 199, 204.
2. **Althouse, Harold,** "How OSHA Affects Hospitals and Nursing Homes," *American Journal of Nursing*, 75, no. 3 (1975), 450–53.
3. **Beck, Alan,** "The Public Health Implications of Urban Dogs," *American Journal of Public Health*, 65, no. 12 (1975), 1315–18.
4. **Brown, Mary,** *Occupational Health Nursing*. New York: Springer Publishing Company, 1981.
5. **Brubaker, Sterling,** *To Live on Earth*. New York: New American Library, 1972.
6. **Burton, Lloyd,** and **Hugh Smith,** *Public Health and Community Medicine for the Allied Medical Professions* (2nd ed.). Baltimore: The Williams & Wilkins Company, 1975.
7. "Cancer: The Environmental Connection," *Science Challenge*, 5, no. 3 (1982), 3–11.
8. **Chanlett, Emil, D. Rogers,** and **G. Hurst,** "The Necessity for Environmental

Health Planning," *American Journal of Public Health*, 63, no. 4 (1973), 341–44.
9. "Chemical Wastes–Illegal Hazards and Legal Remedies," *American Journal of Public Health*, 71, no. 9 (1981), 985–86.
10. **Chisolm, Julian,** "Lead Poisoning," *Scientific American*, 224, no. 2 (1971), 15–23.
11. **Cimino, J.,** "Health and Safety in the Solid Waste Industry," *American Journal of Public Health*, 65, no. 1 (1975), 38–46.
12. **Corwin, Emil,** "On Getting the Lead Out of Food," *FDA Consumer*, 16, no. 2 (1982), 19–21.
13. **Commoner, Barry,** *Science and Survival*. New York: The Viking Press, 1969.
14. _____, *The Closing Circle*. New York: Alfred A. Knopf, Inc., 1972.
15. **Croft, Harriet,** and **Sallie Frenkel,** "Children and Lead Poisoning," *American Journal of Nursing*, 75, no. 1 (1975), 102–4.
16. **Davies, J., W. Edmundson,** and **A. Raffonelli,** "The Role of House Dust in Human DDT Pollution," *American Journal of Public Health*, 65, no. 1 (1975), 53–57.
17. **Deland, Michael,** "Disposal of Liquid Hazardous Waste," *Environmental Science and Technology*, 16, no. 4 (1982), 225A.
18. _____, "Hazardous Waste: The Controversy Continues," *Environmental Science and Technology*, 16, no. 2 (1982), 193A.
19. **deNevers, Noel,** "Measuring and Managing Pollutants," *Environment*, 23, no. 5 (1981), 25–35.
20. **Dobrzanski, T.,** and **T. Rychta,** "Cattell's 16 Personality Factors and Biochemical Responses to Occupational Noise Exposure," *Poland's Archives of Medicine*, 58, no. 5 (1977), 427–35.
21. **Drummond, A. G.,** "Lead Poisoning in Children," *Journal of School Health*, January 1981, pp. 43–47.
22. **Duffus, John H.,** *Environmental Toxicology*. New York: John Wiley & Sons, Inc., 1980.
23. **Durso-Hughes, Katherine,** and **James Lewis,** "Problems in Recycling Hazardous Waste," *Environment*, 24, no. 2 (1982), 14 ff.
24. **Edwards, Clive,** "Soil Pollutants and Soil Animals," *Scientific American*, 220, no. 4 (1969), 88–99.
25. **Falk, S.,** and **N. Woods,** "Hospital Noise Levels and Potential Health Hazards," *New England Journal of Medicine*, 289 (October 11, 1973), 744–81.
26. **Fears, Thomas, J. Scott,** and **M. Schneiderman,** "Skin Cancer, Melanoma, and Sunlight," *American Journal of Public Health*, 66, no. 5 (1976), 461–64.
27. **Feingold, Ben,** "Hyperkinesis and Learning: Disabilities Linked to Artificial Food Flavors and Colors," *American Journal of Nursing*, 75, no. 5 (1975), 797–803.
28. **Fine, L.,** and **J. Peters,** "Studies of Respiratory Morbidity in Rubber Workers. Part III. Respiratory Morbidity in Processing Workers," *Archives of Environmental Health*, 31 (May–June 1976), 136–40.
29. **Flanders, W.,** and **Kenneth Rothman,** "Occupational Risk for Laryngeal Cancer," *American Journal of Public Health*, 72, no. 4 (1982), 369–72.
30. **Gibbons, Don,** "Acidic Confusion Reigns," *Science Quest*, 55, no. 1 (1982), 10–15.

31. **Glass, Norman R.**, et al., "Effects of Acid Precipitation," *Environmental Science and Technology*, 16, no. 3 (1982), 162A-69A.
32. **Gold, Michael**, "Indoor Air Pollution," *Science '80*, 1, no. 3 (1980), 30-35.
33. **Golden, Jack, Robert Ovellette, Sharon Saari,** and **Paul Cheremisinoff,** *Environmental Impact Data Book*. Ann Arbor, MI: Ann Arbor Science Publishers, Inc., 1979.
34. **Goldsmith, John,** and **Erland Jonnson,** "Health Effects of Community Noise," *American Journal of Public Health*, 63, no. 9 (1973), 782-93.
35. **Graves, C. K.**, "Rain of Troubles," *Science '80*, 1, no. 5 (1980), 75-79.
36. **Guralnik, David,** ed., *Webster's New World Dictionary of the American Language* (2nd college ed.). New York: The World Publishing Company, 1972.
37. **Guthrie, Frank,** and **Jerome Perry,** *Introduction to Environmental Technology*. New York: Elsevier North-Holland, Inc., 1980.
38. **Hamilton, Michael,** ed., *The New Genetics and the Future of Man*. Grand Rapids, MI: William B. Eerdmans Publishing Company, 1972.
39. **Haque, Rizwanul,** ed., *Dynamics, Exposure and Hazard Assessment of Toxic Chemicals*. Ann Arbor, MI: Ann Arbor Science Publishers, Inc., 1980.
40. **Hardy, Harriet, Robert Goyer,** and **Vincent Guince,** eds., *Epidemiology and Detection of Lead Toxicity*. New York: MSS Information Corporation, 1976.
41. **Haslam, P.**, "Noise in Hospitals: Its Effect on the Patient," *Nursing Clinics of North America*, 5, no. 4 (1970), 715-24.
42. **Hattis, Dale, Robert Goble,** and **Nicholas Ashford,** "Airborne Lead: A Clear-cut Case of Differential Protection," *Environment*, 24, no. 6 (1982), 14-20.
43. **Hazelwood, Mary,** "Wilsonville: What Went In, Must Come Out," *Alton Evening Telegraph*, October 9, 1982, Sec. B, p. 8.
44. **Henderson, Doug,** "Cookware as a Source of Additives," *FDA Consumer*, 16, no. 2 (1982), 11-B.
45. **Hickey, Susan,** "Report: Lead Poisoning Worse Than Predicted," *The Nation's Health*, 12, no. 10 (1982), 7.
46. **Hileman, Bette,** "Acid Disposition," *Environmental Science and Technology*, 16, no. 6 (1982), 323A-27A.
47. _____, "Carbon Dioxide Buildup: The Greenhouse Effect," *Environmental Science and Technology*, 16, no. 2 (1982), 90A-93A.
48. _____, "Nuclear Power Plants," *Environmental Science and Technology*, 16, no. 7 (1982), 373A-78A.
49. _____, "Nuclear Waste Disposal," *Environmental Science and Technology*, 16, no. 5 (1982), 271A-75A.
50. _____, "Radiation and Health," *Environmental Science and Technology*, 16, no. 8 (1982), 442A-4A.
51. **Hill, Gladwin,** "Cleansing Our Waters." Washington, D.C.: Public Affairs Pamphlet No. 497, February 1974.
52. **Hinga, K. R.**, et al., "Disposal of High Level Radioactive Wastes by Burial in the Sea Floor," *Environmental Science and Technology*, 16, no. 1 (1982), 28A-37A.
53. **Horne, Amy,** "Groundwater Policy: A Patchwork for Protection," *Environment*, 24, no. 3 (1982), 6-11.

54. "Indoor Air Pollution: An Emerging Hazard," *The Nation's Health*, 10, no. 11 (1980), 12.
55. "Industrial Wastes and the Earth," *The Nation's Health*, 12, no. 10 (1982), 7.
56. **Jamann, Joann,** "Health Is a Function of Ecology," *American Journal of Nursing*, 71, no. 5 (1971), 970–73.
57. **Jennings, Betty,** and **Susie Gudermuth,** "Hospital Solid Waste: A Challenge for Nurses," *Missouri Nurse*, 47, no. 2 (1973), 5–7.
58. **Josephson, Julian,** "Immobilization and Leachability of Hazardous Wastes," *Environmental Science and Technology*, 16, no. 4 (1982), 219A–23A.
59. **Kermode, G. O.,** "Food Additives," *Scientific American*, 226, no. 3 (1972), 15–21.
60. **Kilburn, K., G. Kilburn,** and **J. Merchant,** "Byssinosis: Matter from Lint to Lungs," *American Journal of Nursing*, 73, no. 11 (1973), 1952–56.
61. **Lee, Jean,** *The New Nurse in Industry*. Cincinnati: National Institute for Occupational Safety and Health Division of Technical Services, 1978.
62. **Lehmann, Phyllis,** "What Are Those Additives in Food?" *Consumer's Research Magazine*, 65, no. 3 (1982), 13–17.
63. **Levine, R.,** et al., "Occupational Lead Poisoning, Animal Deaths and Environmental Contamination at a Scrap Smelter," *American Journal of Public Health*, 66, no. 6 (1976), 548–52.
64. **Lewis, Harold,** "The Safety of Fission Reactors," *Scientific American*, 242, no. 3 (1980), 53–65.
65. **Likens, Gene, Richard Wright, James Galloway,** and **Thomas Butler,** "Acid Rain," *Scientific American*, 241, no. 4 (1979), 43–51.
66. **Linton, Ron,** *Terracide*. Boston: Little, Brown & Company, 1970.
67. **Lippman, Morton,** and **Richard Schlesinger,** *Chemical Contamination in the Human Environment*. New York: Oxford University Press, 1979.
68. **Litsky, Warren, Joseph Martin,** and **Bertha Litsky,** "Solid Waste: A Hospital Dilemma," *American Journal of Nursing*, 72, no. 10 (1972), 1841–47.
69. **Long, Keith,** "Pesticides: An Occupational Hazard on Farms," *American Journal of Nursing*, 71, no. 4 (1971), 740–43.
70. "Lung Cancer Rates Rising Rapidly," *The Nation's Health*, 12, no. 4 (1982), 12.
71. **Marshall, Eliot,** "Turnabout on EPA Lead Rules," *Science*, 217, no. 4561 (1982), 711.
72. ———, "EPA May Allow More Lead in Gasoline," *Science*, 215, no. 4538 (1982), 1375–78.
73. ———, "The Senate's Plan for Nuclear Waste," *Science*, 216, no. 4547 (1982), 709–10.
74. **Maugh, Thomas,** "Just How Hazardous Are Dumps?" *Science*, 215, no. 4532 (1982), 490–93.
75. **McKee, William,** ed., *Environmental Problems in Medicine*. Springfield, IL: Charles C Thomas, Publisher, 1974.
76. **Medalia, Nahum Z.,** "Air Pollution as a Socio-Environmental Health Problem: A Survey Report," in *Patients, Physicians, and Illness* (2nd ed.). ed. E. Gartly Jaco. New York: The Free Press, 1972.
77. **Melosi, Martin,** "Waste Management: The Cleaning of America," *Environment*, 23, no. 8 (1981), 6 ff.

78. **Melville, Mary,** "Risks on the Job: The Worker's Right to Know," *Environment*, 23, no. 9 (1981), 12–20, 42–45.
79. **Miller, Stanton,** "Is This the Last Word on Love Canal?" *Environmental Science and Technology*, 16, no. 9 (1982), 500A–01A.
80. ______, "Trends in Air Measurement," *Environmental Science and Technology*, 16, no. 9 (1982), 506A–07A.
81. **Minckley, Barbara,** "Space and Place in Patient Care," *American Journal of Nursing*, 68, no. 3 (1968), 510–16.
82. **Morse, E.,** et al., "Canine Salmonellosis: A Review and Report of Dog to Child Transmission of Salmonella Enteritidis," *American Journal of Public Health*, 66, no. 1 (1976), 82–24.
83. "Nerve Damage Among Workers Proved in Test," *The Nation's Health*, 7, no. 9 (1977), 3.
84. **Newberne, Paul,** ed., *Trace Substances and Health*. New York: Marcel Dekker, Inc., 1976.
85. **Neylan, Margaret,** "The Nurse in a Healing Milieu," *American Journal of Nursing*, 61, no. 4 (1961), 72–74.
86. **Niewoehner, D.,** et al., "Pathologic Changes in the Peripheral Airways of Young Cigarette Smokers," *New England Journal of Medicine*, 291 (October 10, 1974), 755–58.
87. **Norman, Colin,** "A Long-Term Problem for the Nuclear Industry," *Science*, 215, no. 4531 (1982), 376–78.
88. **Norris, Ruth,** "Toxic Waste: EPA's Misleading List of 114 'Worst' Sites," *Audubon*, 84, no. 1 (1982), 106–8.
89. **Norton, Boyd,** "Supercritical: A Nuclear Excursion," *Audubon*, 82, no. 3 (1980), 80–105.
90. "Occupational Cancer." Reprinted from *Job Safety and Health*, 3, no. 7, Washington, D.C.: U.S. Department of Labor, Occupational Safety and Health Administration, July 1975.
91. **Okum, Daniel,** "Drinking Water for the Future," *American Journal of Public Health*, 66, no. 7 (1976), 639–43.
92. **Parrish, Henry,** "Animal-Man Relationships in Today's Environment," *American Journal of Public Health*, 63, no. 3 (1973), 199–200.
93. **Peakall, David,** "Pesticides and the Reproduction of Birds," *Scientific American*, 222, no. 4 (1970), 72–78.
94. "Pesticide Risks to Laborers Called Great," *The Nation's Health*, 9, no. 1 (1979), 1, 4.
95. **Peterson, Ivars,** "Keeping Radwaste Out of Sight," *Science News*, 121, no. 1 (1982), 9–11, 15.
96. **Purcell, Arthur,** "Three Mile Island's Three Fateful Dates . . . And the Fate of Nuclear Energy," *Science Digest*, 87, no. 4 (1980), 44–48.
97. **Raloff, J.,** "Childhood Lead: Worrisome National Levels," *Science News*, 121, no. 5 (1982), 88.
98. **Reed, Jane,** "Lead Poisoning: Silent Epidemic and Social Crime," *American Journal of Nursing*, 72, no. 2 (1972), 2181–84.
99. **Revelle, Roger,** "Carbon Dioxide and World Climate," *Scientific American*, 247, no. 2 (1982), 35–43.
100. **Ritz, W.,** "Investigating the Aerosol Issue," *Today's Education*, September-October 1972, 46–49.

101. **Robinson, J.,** and **W. Forbes,** "The Role of Carbon Monoxide in Cigarette Smoking," *Archives of Environmental Health*, 30 (September 1975), 425–34.
102. **Saltonstall, Richard,** *Your Environment and What You Can Do About It: A Citizens' Guide*. New York: Walker and Company, 1970.
103. "Secondhand Smoke and Lung Cancer," *Newsweek*, January 26, 1981, p. 63.
104. **Seldman, Neil,** and **Jon Huls,** "Waste Management: Beyond the Throwaway Ethic," *Environment*, 23, no. 9 (1981), 23–25.
105. **Serafini, Patricia,** "Nursing Assessment in Industry," *American Journal of Public Health*, 66, no. 8 (1976), 755–60.
106. **Shapiro, R.,** and **T. Berland,** "Noise in the Operating Room," *New England Journal of Medicine*, 287 (December 14, 1972), 1236–37.
107. **Shaeffer, Mark,** "Alert on Dioxin" (a series of articles), *Alert Newsletter—Coalition for the Environment*, 13, no. 1 (1983).
108. **Smith Dorothy,** "Patienthood and Its Threat to Privacy," *American Journal of Nursing*, 69, no. 3 (1969), 509–13.
109. **Smith, Evelyn,** "For Occupational Asthma, The Best Treatment Is Prevention," *American Lung Association Bulletin*, 68, no. 6 (1982), 12–15.
110. ———, "The Work and Asthma Connection," *American Lung Association Bulletin*, 68, no. 5 (1982), 12–16.
111. **Smith, R. Jeffery,** "A Battle Over Pesticide Data," *Science*, 217, no. 4559 (1982), 515, 518.
112. ———, "How Safe Is Niagara Falls?" *Science*, 217, no.. 4562 (1982), 809.
113. ———, "The Risks of Living Near Love Canal," *Science*, 217, no. 4562 (1982), 808–10.
114. "Solid Waste Disposal—A Long Standing Public Health Problem Comes of Age," *American Journal of Public Health*, 67, no. 5 (1977), 419–20.
115. "Some Cancers May Increase Due to Ozone Depletion," *The Nation's Health*, 12, no. 6 (1982), 7.
116. **Stellman, Jeanne,** "The Effects of Toxic Agents on Reproduction," *Occupational Health and Safety*, April 1979, pp. 36–43.
117. **Stewart, Andrew P.** Oral presentation at an Industrial Hearing Conservationist Training Course, November 10–12, 1982, Carrboro, NC.
118. **Sun, Marjorie,** "EPA Relaxes Hazardous Waste Rules," *Science*, 216, no. 4543 (1982), 275–76.
119. **Swanson, R. L.,** and **M. Devine,** "Ocean Dumping Policy," *Environment*, 24 no. 5 (1982), 14–20.
120. **Trainer, Daniel,** "Wildlife as Monitors of Disease," *American Journal of Public Health*, 63, no. 3 (1973), 201–3.
121. **Turk, Amos, Janet Wittes, Jonathan Turk,** and **Robert Wittes,** *Environmental Science* (2nd ed.). Philadelphia: W. B. Saunders Company, 1978.
122. United States Department of Labor, Occupational Safety and Health Administration, *Handling Hazardous Materials*, Washington, D.C.: U.S. Government Printing Office, 1975.
123. United States Environmental Protection Agency, *Cleaning the Air*. Washington, D.C.: Office of Public Affairs, 1975.
124. ———, *Hazardous Wastes*. Washington, D.C.: U.S. Government Printing Office, 1975.
125. ———, *Is Your Drinking Water Safe?* Washington, D.C.: Office of Public Affairs, March 1977.

126. _____, *Measuring Air Quality*, Washington, D.C.: Office of Public Affairs, July 1978.
127. _____, *Mission 5000*. Washington, D.C.: U.S. Government Printing Office, 1972.
128. _____, *Noise and Its Measurement*. Washington, D.C.: Office of Public Affairs, February 1977.
129. _____, *Noise and Recreational Vehicles*. Washington, D.C.: Office of Public Affairs, December 1976.
130. _____, *Noise Around Our Homes*, Washington, D.C.: Office of Public Affairs, February 1977.
131. _____, *Noise at Work*. Washington, D.C.: Office of Public Affairs, February 1977.
132. _____, *Noise Control Programs of the Federal Government*. Washington, D.C.: Office of Public Affairs, June 1976.
133. _____, *Noise on Wheels*. Washington, D.C.: Office of Public Affairs, February 1977.
134. _____, *Ozone, Its Effects and Control*. Washington, D.C.: Office of Public Awareness, April 1979.
135. _____, *Pollution and Your Health*. Washington, D.C.: Office of Public Affairs, May 1976.
136. _____, *Radioactive Wastes*. Washington, D.C.: Office of Public Affairs, 1976.
137. _____, *Toxics Information Series: Asbestos*. Washington, D.C.: Office of Pesticides and Toxic Substances, April 1980.
138. _____, *Trends in the Quality of the Nation's Air—A Report to the People*. Washington, D.C.: Office of Public Awareness, October 1980.
139. _____, *What You Should Know about the Pesticide Law*. Washington, D.C.: Office of Public Affairs, December 1976.
140. _____, *Your Guide to the Environmental Protection Agency*. Washington, D.C.: Office of Public Awareness, December 1980.
141. **Upton, Arthur**, "The Biological Effects of Low-Level Ionizing Radiation," *Scientific American*, 246, no. 2 (1982), 41–49.
142. **Van Sickle, Derek**, *The Ecological Citizen*. New York: Harper & Row, Publishers, Inc., 1971.
143. **Waldbott, George**, *Health Effects of Environmental Pollutants* (2nd ed.). St. Louis: The C. V. Mosby Company, 1978.
144. **Waldron, Harry**, and **D. Stofen**, *Sub-Clinical Lead Poisoning*. New York: Academic Press, Inc., 1974.
145. "Warning Issued Again on Carbon Dioxide Use," *The Nation's Health*, 11, no. 2 (1981), 1, 14.
146. **Weber, A., C. Jermini**, and **E. Grandjean**, "Irritating Effects on Man of Air Pollution Due to Cigarette Smoke," *American Journal of Public Health*, 66, no. 7 (1976), 672–76.
147. **Weiss, Bernard**, et al., "Behavioral Responses to Artificial Food Colors," *Science*, 207, no. 4438 (1980), 1487–88.
148. **West, Susan**, "Acid from Heaven," *Science News*, 117, no. 5 (1980), 76–78.
149. "WHO: Most Cancers Are in the Developing World," *The Nation's Health*, 11, no. 12 (1981), 18.

150. World Health Organization, *Health Hazards of the Human Environment.* Geneva: Office of Publications and Translation, World Health Organization, 1972.
151. **Yasko, J.**, *Care of the Client Receiving Radiation Therapy: A Self-Learning Module for the Nurse Caring for the Client with Cancer.* Reston, VA: Reston Publishing Company, 1982.

10

Sociocultural Influences on the Person

Study of this chapter will help you to

1. Define *culture* and *subculture* and describe various types of subcultures.
2. Discuss the general features of any culture and how they affect the persons under your care.
3. Identify the dominant cultural and social class values in the United States and how they influence you as a health care worker as well as the client and family.
4. Compare the cultural values of the traditional Greek, the Mexican-American living in the southwestern United States, and the Japanese in relation to the family unit, male and female relationships, childrearing patterns, the group versus privacy, time orientation, work, and use of leisure, education, and change.
5. Contrast the attitudes toward health and illness of persons living in the main cultures of the United States, Greece, Spanish-American neighborhoods in the southwestern United States, and Japan.
6. Interview a person from another culture and contrast his/her values with those described in this chapter.
7. Discuss influences of culture and social class on the health status of the person and group.
8. Describe how knowledge of cultural and social class values and

attitudes toward daily living practices, health, and illness can influence the effectiveness of your health care.

9. Discuss ways to meet the needs of another with cultural and social class values different from your own.
10. Apply knowledge about the teaching-learning process to a health education program for a person or family from another culture or social class.
11. Assess and care for a person or family from another culture and social class and identify your own ethnocentric tendencies.

When someone talks or acts differently from you, consider that to him you may also seem to talk or act differently. Many such differences are cultural and should be understood rather than laughed at.

The great divide between humans and animals is culture. Culture includes using language, art forms, and games to communicate with others; cooperating in problem solving; deliberately training children; developing unique interpretations; forming organizations; and making, saving, using, and changing tools. Humans are heir to the accumulation of wisdom and folly of preceding generations and, in turn, they teach others their beliefs, feelings, and practices. The patient, family, and you are deeply affected by the culture learned during the early years, often more so than by that learned later. An understanding of the cultural and social class systems and their influence on behavior is essential to understanding yourself and the person under your care.

DEFINITIONS

Culture *is the sum total of the learned ways of doing, feeling, and thinking, past and present, of a social group within a given period of time. These ways are transmitted from one generation to the next or to immigrants who become members of the society.* Culture is a group's design for living, a shared set of socially transmitted assumptions about the nature of the physical and social world, goals in life, attitudes, roles, and values. *Culture is a complex integrated system that includes knowledge, beliefs, skills, art, morals, law, customs, and any other acquired habits and capabilities of the human being. All provide a pattern for living together.*

A **subculture** *is a group of persons, within a culture, of the same age, socioeconomic status, ethnic origin, education, or occupation, or with the same goals, who have an identity of their own but are related to the total culture in certain ways* (82). Mexican-Americans, Latin-

Americans, American Indians, and Afro-Americans (American Blacks) represent subcultures within the overall culture of the United States. Regional, social-class, religious, and family subcultures also exist. A description of each follows.

Regional culture *refers to the local or regional manifestations of the larger culture.* Thus the child learns the sectional variant of the national culture—for example, rural or urban, Yankee, Southern, Midwestern. Regional culture is influenced by geography, trade, and economics; variations may be shown in values, beliefs, housing, food, occupational skills, and language.

A social class also has its own culture. A **social class** *is a cultural grouping of persons who, through group consensus and similarity of occupation, wealth, and education, have come to have a similar status, lifestyle, interests, feelings, attitudes, language usage, and overt forms of behavior.* The people belonging to this group meet each other on equal terms and have a consciousness of cohesion (82, 159). Social class is not only economic in origin; other factors also contribute to superior status, such as age, sex, and personal endowment.

The more a class as a group becomes fixed, the more predictable is its patterns of attitudes and behavior. The child learns the patterns of his/her own class and the class attitude toward another class. The attitude patterns make up a culture's **value system,** *its concept of how people should behave in various situations as well as which goals they should pursue and how.* The value systems of the general culture and of the subculture or social class may conflict at times.

Religious culture also influences the person, for a *religion constitutes a way of living and thinking and therefore is a kind of culture.* Religious influences on values, attitudes, and behavior are discussed in Chapter 11.

Family culture *refers to the family life, which is part of the cultural system.* The family is the medium through which the large cultural heritage is transmitted to the child. *Family culture consists of ways of living and thinking that constitute the family and sexual aspects of group life.* These ways include courtship and marriage patterns, sexual mores, husband-wife relationships, status of men and women, parent-child relationships, childrearing, responsibilities to parents, and attitudes toward unmarried women, illegitimate children, and divorce (19).

The family gives the child status. The family name gives the child a social position as well as an identity; the child is assigned the status of the family and the reputation that goes with it. Family status has a great deal to do with health and behavior throughout life because of its effect on self-concept (19).

Family rituals are the collective way of working out household routines and using time within the family culture. **Ritual** *is a system of* *definitely prescribed behaviors and procedures and it provides exactness in daily tasks of living and has a sense of rightness about it.* The more often the behavior is repeated, the more it comes to be approved and therefore habitual. Thus rituals inevitably develop in family life as a result of the intimacy of relationships and the repetition and continuity of certain interactions. Rituals change from one life cycle to another—for example, at marriage, after childbirth, when children go to school, and when children leave home. Rituals are important in child development because

1. They are group habits that communicate ways of doing things and attitudes related to events, including family etiquette, affectionate responses between family members, organization of leisure time, and education for group adjustment.
2. They promote solidarity and continuity by promoting habitual behavior, unconsciously performed, which brings harmony to family life. Many rituals will continue to the next generation, increasing the person's sense of worth, security, and family continuity or identity.
3. They aid in maintaining self-control through disciplinary measures.
4. They promote feelings of euphoria, sentimentality, or well-being—for example, through holiday celebrations.
5. They dictate reactions to threat, such as at times of loss, illness, or death (19).

You must consider the person's standard rituals as you plan care. Family influences are dealt with more extensively in Chapter 12.

CHARACTERISTICS OF CULTURE

Culture as Learned

Culture has three basic characteristics. First, *culture is learned.* People function physiologically in much the same way throughout the world, but their behavior is learned and therefore relatively diverse. Because of his/her culture, a child is ascribed or acquires a certain **status** *or position of prestige.* The child also learns or assumes certain **roles,** *patterns or related behaviors expected by others, and later by him/herself, that define behavior and adjustment to a given group.* The behavior, values, attitudes, and beliefs, learned within his/her culture become a matter of tradition, even though the culture allows choices within limits and may even encourage certain kinds of deviancy. The way in which a person experiences the culture and society and what he/she learns during development are of great significance. Culture determines the kinds of experiences the person encounters and the extent to which responses to life situations will be either unhealthy, maladaptive, and self-defeating, or healthy, adaptive, constructive, and creative (27, 140). What the person has learned from the culture determines how and what you will be able to teach him/her, as well as your approach during care.

Culture as Stable but Changing

The second characteristic of culture is that *it is subject to and capable of change in order to remain viable and adaptive, although it is basically a stable entity*. The culture of a society, like a human body, is dynamic but maintained at a steady state by self-regulating devices. *Stabilizing features are traditions and the ready-made solutions to life's problems* that are provided for the group, enabling the person to anticipate the behavior of others, predict future events, and regulate his/her life within the culture. Behavior, carefully defined by the culture, is difficult to change because of group pressure. Norms and customs that persist may have a negative influence on the group. Food taboos during pregnancy, a high-animal-fat diet, or crowding of people into a common dwelling that provides an apt incubator for spread of contagious disease are examples (131).

Another stabilizing, limiting aspect of culture is the use of language. Although language forms vary from culture to culture, the terms for *mother* and *father* sound very much alike across cultural lines, perhaps because certain vocalizations are easy for a child to articulate and learn.

Learning cultural and family language is primarily by ear and can affect the child who learns better by sight. In addition, use of language is determined considerably by age and sex—for example, baby talk, child talk, adult talk, girl talk, and boy talk. Subcultural groups, particularly the family, differ in conversational mores—that is, permitted topics of conversation; proper situations for discussing certain topics, such as during mealtime or before bedtime; level of vocabulary used; reaction to new words used; number of interruptions permitted; who can be interrupted; and who talks most (19).

The meeting ground between cultures is in language and **dialect**, *a variety of a language spoken by a distinct group of people in a definite place*. All immigrants to the United States brought their own ethnic and cultural heritage and language. No doubt all had problems being acculturated to mainstream America, but generally their different lifestyles and accents were considered interesting and eventually accepted. Until recently Blacks were the least accepted and understood group of "immigrants," brought to America by force and separated from their culture and awareness of their past in Africa. They were expected to express their cultural and racial identity through the White man's culture and image of what it meant to be Black. Thus English was superimposed on the many African languages that were forced together. An artificial subculture characterized by Aunt Jemima and Uncle Remus was created.

With the movement of the Black American minority to express its identity, dialect, as well as other components of its subculture, has received attention (51, 52, 133, 206, 207). Understanding of the Black subculture and dialect can help you to talk with, understand, and care for the Black person, just as an understanding of the subculture and dialect of any ethnic group enhances acceptance and care of that person. NonBlacks often do not understand Black dialect. Although it often coincides with "standard American English," it has its own grammatical rules (and errors), slang, cadence, and intonation. Black dialect will vary from region to region and with the age, sex, and economic status of the user. Some Blacks avoid using Black dialect, especially those more highly educated and in the higher social classes. And keep in mind that dialect usage changes, as all language usage changes, with time. A word that is first specific to a minority ethnic group can later be adopted by members of the mainstream culture.

Black dialect has words for which there are no analogies in "standard American English," such as the *hawk*: a severe, bone-chilling wind (originally blowing off the Great Lakes). The verbs *am, is*, and *are* are often omitted in dialect, being unnecessary for a complete sentence. The verb form *be* can indicate extended or repeated action, and *been*, completed or past action: "He be hurtin' " means "He has been in pain for some time." "He been hurtin' " means "He was in pain." A sentence without an auxiliary verb indicates an activity going on now that does not usually occur—for example, "She workin'." "She *be* workin' " indicates the person is doing the work she usually does. Possession can be expressed without the use of *'s*—for example, as in "my baby clothes," instead of "my baby's clothes." The letter *g* is commonly dropped as an end sound; two syllables may be shortened into one, and *th* pronounced like *v* or *d*. To avoid grammatical redundancy, the *s* is omitted in plural noun forms if some other word in the sentence indicates plural—for example. "She have three brother." *Man* may be used instead of the name of the person addressed or to convey emphasis. The word *ain't* can be used to negate verbs in the past tense: "Dey ain't like dat" can mean "They *didn't* like that" rather than "They *aren't* like that."

An undifferentiated form of the possessive pronoun occurs—as in "He a nice girl."

You will find a variety of regional dialects in the United States—for example, "Brooklynese"; southern mountain; "Tex-Mex" along the Texas–Mexico border; Texas cotton country; Missouri Ozarkian, and Pennsylvania Dutch. Language differences may give a false impression about the intelligence of the person, for some people have difficulty switching from dialect to "standard American English." Listen carefully to the language spoken, be accepting of the dialect, and validate meanings of words when necessary.

Von Bertalanffy discusses how language emphasizes the values of a culture. For example, neither the language of the Nootka Indians on Vancover Island nor that of the Hopi has a separate subject and predicate or parts of speech, as does English. These languages instead describe an event as a whole with a single term. He points out that Americans are complex, abstract, and fragmentary in their descriptions of the world around them. The Indo-European languages, of which English is one, emphasize time. Cultures using these languages keep records, use mathematics, do accounting, use clocks and calendars, and study archeology to learn of their historical past. In contrast, past, present, and future tenses do not exist in the Hopi language; the validity of a statement is not based on time or history but on "fact," memory, expectations, or customs. The Navaho language has little mention of clock time and instead emphasizes type of activity, duration, or aspects of movement. Moreover, von Bertalanffy shows how Indo-European languages, like English, describe nonspatial relationships with spatial metaphors—for example, *long* and *short* for duration; *heavy* and *light* or *long* and *short* for intensity; *rise* and *fall* for tendency. In the Hopi language psychological metaphors are used to name mental processes; for example, *heart* can be used for *think* or *remember*. Thus various cultures have different conceptualizations with which to perceive the same matter or reality. The kinds of conceptualizations influence the values, behavior, stability, and progress of a culture (217). Assessment of the person's intellectual ability must consider culture as well as age. People from non-Western cultures may learn differently and at a different rate because of different language and perceptual skills and value orientations (77). Most cultures are less technical and verbal than ours.

Analyses of the habits and practices of various peoples show that traditional language and behavior patterns practiced between parent and child within a culture are related to the interactions within that culture between employer and employee, among peers, and between nurse and patient, making for predictability and stability. Stability of culture promotes adaptability and economy of energy (140).

Cultures also change, sometimes imperceptibly, so that norms, the usual rules for living, are modified to meet the group's needs as new life challenges arise. Cultures change primarily in response to technological innovation or by borrowing from another culture. For example, the harnessing of electrical power and the subsequent invention and use of electrical appliances and tools changed the way of life in the United States: in work, recreation, food preservation, communication, education, vocabulary, women's roles, health care, and the entire value system.

Cultures also change for other reasons:

1. Competition among groups for geographical regions in order to meet the members' sustenance and safety needs.
2. Use of deferred gains for members to induce them to work for the good of the culture, such as in communist countries.
3. Change in political leadership, such as in China.
4. Increased scientific and industrial complexity.
5. Increased population.
6. Change in economic practices and standards, such as the change from feudalism to industrialism seen in Africa and Asian countries.
7. Use of behavior modification techniques by groups in power.
8. Promotion of values, lifestyle, and products through mass media programming and advertisements (159).

You need to realize that our culture is continually shaped by forces and people outside our awareness; some are discussed in *The People Shapers* by Vance Packard. He discusses how we could use our growing knowledge of science and technology to enslave and depersonalize people and thus radically change our culture (161).

Toffler describes how the United States is moving into a postindustrial society. He identifies some of the problem areas of such a society as

1. The need for more professional knowledge.
2. Greater expectations by the public.
3. More goods considered to be public goods.
4. Lack of measurements to show what is actually needed and thus where money and resources should be directed.
5. A changing demography with more urban concentration.
6. Increased life expectancy.
7. Changing values.

Resulting problems in health care will include: rising costs, maldistribution of health personnel and specialized services, and greater demand by the consumer for professional competence and accountability and more procedures for ensuring it (212).

Each culture is a whole, but not every culture is integrated in the same way to the same extent. Some cultures are so tightly integrated that any change threatens the whole. Other cultures are characterized by traditional patterns that are easy to manipulate and change.

When significant numbers of people begin to respond other than usual to one or more facets of a culture, this factor may cause others in the society to realize that a particular custom or norm is no longer useful. Such customs might pertain to marriage, burial, childrearing, or moral codes. If a group of people (or isolated persons) can consistently adapt while at the same time following the norm imperfectly, they may establish a new norm, which may be gradually adopted by others until it becomes the generally established pattern. Thus the culture and the people in it can be changed in spite of initial resistance. Such changes can have a positive or negative influence on health (140).

Cultural Components and Patterns

The third characteristic of culture is that *certain components or patterns are present in every culture*, regardless of how "primitive" or "advanced" it may be (159, 234). Understanding them can help you understand yourself, your patient, and the health care system in which you work.

A Communication System, which may include only the language itself or the complexities of mass media, computers, and satellites, is the basis for interaction and cohesion between persons and a vehicle for the transmission and preservation of culture (19). In addition to vocabulary and word taboos, gestures, facial expressions, and voice qualities—intonation, rhythm, speed, pronunciation—vary among families or groups within a culture and carry specific meanings. Because millions of U. S. residents nightly watch television, it has become the most powerful cultural communication force in the United States today. Television could be used more effectively for mass health teaching, just as it is used now for mass advertising (104).

Methods and Objects Are Used by a Culture to Provide for Physical Welfare. Methods include getting food; establishing personal care habits; making, using, saving, and improving tools; and manufacturing. Objects include instruments and machines used to change land terrain for farming, home building, or industrialization, and equipment used to diagnose and test disease.

Means or Techniques of Travel and Transportation of Goods and Services are particularized to a culture. Whether walking, use of dog or horse, or a complex system of cars, trucks, railways, and airplanes, they will affect the person's ability to obtain health care, among other services and goods.

Exchange of Goods and Services may occur through barter, trade, commerce, involve occupational roles, and affect work and payment in a health care system.

Forms of Property, real estate and personal, are defined by the culture in terms of their necessity and worth. Respecting the person's property in the hospital or home shows that you respect him/her personally.

Sexual and Family Patterns, which may vary considerably from culture to culture, affect how you care for and teach the person. Such patterns include wedding ceremonies, divorce proceedings, forms of kinships, guardianship roles, inheritance rights, the family's division of labor, and roles assigned men, women, and children.

Societal Controls and the Institution of Government include **mores,** *morally binding attitudes, and* **customs,** *long-established practices having the force of unwritten law.* Other controls include public or group opinion, laws, political offices and the organization of government, the regulation of time, and institutionalized forms of conflict within the society or between tribes, states, or nations, such as war. These factors all influence the health care system in which you work. Increasingly, the nurse must become familiar with the political system and skilled in using it for improving health care.

Artistic Expression through architecture, painting, sculpture, music, literature, and dance is universal, although what is considered art by one culture may not be so considered by another. Knowledge of these factors can be useful in therapy and rehabilitation.

Recreational and Leisure-Time Interests and Activities, as defined by each cultural group, are essential for health and must be considered in the nursing history and in medical diagnosis.

Religious and Magical Ideas and Practices exist in the form of various beliefs, taboos, ethical codes, rituals, mythology, philosophy, or the organized institution of the church and serve to guide the behavior of a cultural group during health and illness.

Knowledge Basic to Survival and Expansion of the Group is always present. In developed countries **science,** *systematized knowledge based* *on observation, study, and experimentation*, is basic to technological innovation and improving material living standards. Education has traditionally been considered a bridge that enables the person to move up in socioeconomic status in the United States. In modern Western cultures science is highly valued as a basis for health care. Medical science influences people biologically and socially.

Cultural Structuring of Basic Human Patterns includes rules for competition, conflict, cooperation, collaboration, and games. Also, the intimate habits of daily life, both personally and in groups, the manner in which one's house and body are perceived, and the many "taken-for-granted" activities between people are basically structured.

All the foregoing components and patterns influence and are influenced by climate, natural resources, geography, sanitation facilities, diet, group biological and genetic factors, and disease conditions and health practices.

COMPARISON OF CULTURES

Cultural Values in the United States

Several orientations and value systems may be simultaneously present in a given society or culture, but only one orientation dominates over a given period of time. The following middle-class orientation and values are dominant in the United States at present:

1. Speed, change, progress, activity, punctuality, and efficiency.
2. Personal achievement, occupational and financial success, and status consciousness.
3. Youth, beauty, health, self-reliance.
4. Science and the use of machines and various social institutions.
5. Materialism, consumerism, and use of disposable items.
6. Conformity to the group simultaneously with emphasis on rugged individualism and personal pleasure.
7. Competitive and aggressive behavior and exploitation of others rather than cooperation and contemplation.
8. Social and geographical mobility.
9. Pursuit of recreational activities.
10. Equality of people, but recognition of social differentiation and inequality based on personal abilities, education, and opportunity.
11. Future orientation; interest in long-term goals and willingness to defer immediate satisfaction.

In the past (and to some degree still now), the Protestant ethic described by sociologist Max Weber was the prime influence on American culture, even for those Americans who were not Protestants. An **ethic** *is defined as an outlook or view made up of assumptions that are not often noticed and still less often questioned or tested.* These assumptions are blindly and passively accepted because they have been handed down from generation to generation and had their origins in an unimpeachable, but long forgotten, authority. With new knowledge, the assumptions are often found invalid, but assumptions about living undergo a slow process of change. The Protestant ethic encompasses a harsh, pessimistic view of the human race. It upholds the five following assumptions.

1. Man is basically imperfect and must struggle against imperfection.
2. Man was placed on earth to struggle and so struggle must be valued. Any sign of surrender or softness denotes weakness in the person and is bad.
3. Self-sacrifice and aspiring to good conduct are essential to overcome evil and gain personal salvation.
4. Emotions cannot be overtly expressed. Displaying anger is basically un-Christian. One should love one's neighbor, but expressing love openly is suspect, especially if related to sexuality, for sex is considered an animal pleasure and therefore a taboo topic. Even too intense an expression of nonsexual love can be a sign of weakness and one must be strong and self-controlled in order to struggle. Anxiety must be avoided or denied, for it shows that the struggle is not going well.
5. The world is seen as useful to man and should provide for material satisfaction. Thus the exploitation of land, even ruthlessly, is acceptable. Mastery of the environment is emphasized. Conservation of natural resources is secondary, for the resources of the world (which are supposedly inexhaustible) were put there to be used (223).

Earlier in this century Puritanical values and rigid Christian morality upheld the tenet of fear of God's judgment. A strong conscience was developed in fear of punishment and social disfavor. Society was stable because traditions were adhered to and proverbs were taken seriously. Hard work, plain living, thrift, self-control, responsibility, willpower, honesty, and initiative were emphasized. Family and community roles were clearly defined: father was the patriarch; mother was subservient to him; and children were obedient to all. Education also emphasized discipline, order, and obedience to authority. People were tradition-bound and hard-working, and they provided stability in society. Your understanding that many elderly and middle-aged persons still live by these values can help you better accept them and plan their care.

You need only look around at what Toffler calls our superindustrial society to realize that the Protestant ethic has lost its hold (212). Yet parts of this ethic are being revived by some of the growing fundamentalist religious groups.

The value system of the United States is worldly, in spite of its religious roots, for the most highly valued activities involve competitive, practical, secular pursuits rather than contemplation, devotion, cooperation, or esthetic satisfaction. Thus the ideal society, originally the Kingdom of God on earth, has for many people been secularized into a good society with ideals of liberty, justice, general prosperity, and equality of opportunity (19).

Various cultural groups may have values and behaviors or a lifestyle that are in conflict with the dominant values of society. A persistent sense of family responsibility is traditional to American Indians, for example. Although family members leave the reservation to find work, they are expected to return to visit relatives or for emergencies and life-cycle, or tribal, events. When the cultural values of sharing, cooperation, and mutual dependence conflict with the demands of a job, American Indians face a difficult choice. If the call to attend a funeral or help a sick relative comes when a worker cannot take time off, the decision may be to give up the job. Employers are not always understanding of the values underlying the behavior (98).

For many second- and third-generation Latin Americans, educational and socioeconomic advances have paralleled a reduction in the sizes of their households and the development of individual and family rather than community orientation. But for the majority, loyalty to the family and a preference for large kin groups that act as support networks are very strong. Thus the competitiveness against others that is part of the educational system is avoided; the children may not make the high grades in school that are likely to ensure continued educational and employment success.

Many non-Jewish Caucasian U. S. ethnic cultures inherited work and family values from European Catholic peasant societies—values that seem to set family interests against individual achievement. Generations of underemployment, fear of losing what little wealth the family had managed to accumulate, and the contrast struggle to feed ever-growing families encouraged European immigrants to favor economic security over risk taking (96).

The southern Appalachian person may have a value system that is almost on the opposite end of the continuum from the upper-middle-class professional as shown by Table 10-8.

Keniston describes how the issue of violence is to this generation in the United States what the issue of sex was to the Victorian world.

Today's young adults have grown up with the ever-present possibility of instantaneous death or permanent maiming by thermonuclear, chemical, or biological warfare agents. The threat and fear of violence are therefore constant facts of life. Fear of violence has led to a fascination with violence that further surrounds people with its symptoms. U. S. society is preoccupied with, almost mesmerized by, the violence of organized crime, urban rioting, and political assassinations. Violence on television and in the movies shows the potential for brutality and aggression in all (104).

People react differently to constant exposure to violence: they may tolerate it, develop disease symptoms, project their own aggression onto others, develop a neurotic preoccupation with it, or act violently themselves in order to discharge rage. We see examples of each reaction in our society in the form of physical, emotional, and social illness.

Persad discusses how concepts of aggression and dependency vary from culture to culture. In U. S. culture aggression is regarded as an innate force that has survival value and that requires appropriate channels for its expression; it is considered an integral part of social success. If aggression is not dealt with appropriately, however the person becomes psychopathic. In some cultures aggression is considered the result rather than the cause of psychopathy. Americans teach their children to be independent and emphasize the importance of the adolescent or young adult leaving home. Psychiatric therapy in the United States is often directed toward these goals. In traditional Oriental cultures, however, indirect communication, modesty, cooperation with the team, and conformity to the group are valued rather than assertiveness of the individual. Touch or physical contact between business colleagues is avoided. The young adults may be castigated for abruptly leaving home or striving for independence. Consideration for family elders is more important than one's desires to pursue personal goals. In our culture a well-developed ego is considered necessary for maturity. In Oriental cultures personal preoccupation with the ego is considered absurd (168). In the Saudia Arabian culture, behavior that is normal for the United States businessperson is considered offensive, such as abrupt or interrupting speech, asking about the man's wife, or emphasizing a time schedule (141).

Three Cultures: Greek, Spanish-American, and Japanese

Tables 10-1 through 10-7 contrast Greek culture, American culture in the southwestern United States, and Japanese culture. Although many nationality groups fit under Spanish-American and each nationality group has its unique values and customs, the values, norms, customs, and behaviors described in the following tables are applicable to people who have a Spanish background whether they are from Spain, Mexico,

TABLE 10-1 A Comparison of Cultures: The Family Unit

COMPONENT	GREEK	SPANISH-AMERICAN	JAPANESE
Basis for Marriage	Social and family welfare. All of society patterned on family.	Family welfare central.	Value family and household lineage.
Type of Family System	Paternalistic. Extended family. Monogamy. Marriage bond strong.	Paternalistic. Extended. Monogamy. Marriage bond strong.	Traditional value on authority of father and elderly. Family strongly identified with father. Subordinate position of women and arranged marriage still accepted by older generation.
Family Size	Want many children.	Large so parents not alone in old age.	Family planning, including use of abortion to control size in modern family.
Pattern of Interaction	Authoritarian; man dominant in conversation and decision making. Man head of house and disciplinarian. Sex roles traditional male and female. Mother powerful in own way; credited with sustaining child with moral strength. Children subordinate. Oldest son responsible for family if husband not present. Child not focus of family activity. No special activities for child, even birthday a time to wish family long happiness with child rather than focus on child. Family together most of time with child learning to enjoy adult behavior and anticipate adulthood. Peer contacts through family.	Authoritarian. Man head of house; woman subordinate socially. Sex roles traditional male and female. Child seldom center of activity or attention. Avoid admiration of child for fear of "evil eye." Child proud of home responsibilities. Age and authority figures highly respected. Family loyalty strong. Obedience emphasized. Family ties may extend beyond biological relatives, including godparents, the boss.	Family revered as an institution, but interrelationships lacking companionship and warmth. Major decisions made by family. Subordination of individual to family interest. Traditional autocratic family system stronger in rural areas, with eldest son inheriting family property and hesitant to rebel against father. Young generation choosing own marriage partner, establishing own household, and daughter-in-law gaining freedom from mother-in-law's dominance. Increasing premarital and extramarital sexual affairs.

TABLE 10-2 A Comparison of Cultures: Childrearing Patterns

COMPONENT	GREEK	SPANISH-AMERICAN	JAPANESE
Process of Childbirth	Considered normal process, not to be feared.	Considered normal process. Husband little involved. Special practices surrounding process.	Considered normal process.
Philosophy of Childrearing	Effectiveness sought as parent, not as a pal. Child raised to be strong, hard, firm, straight, for that is ideal personality. Wishes of elders put before child's wishes.	Effectiveness sought as parent, not as a pal. Child taught to do as parents do, to listen to parents' advice, learn from their experience, and not advance further than their parents.	Traditionally child to be dutiful and responsible. Young urban generations not bound as firmly by traditions.
Practices of Childrearing	Mother firm, not overprotective. Baby kept in straight position when carried or in bed. Follow rigid schedule, consistent.	Consistent, traditional, faith in own judgment.	Mother enveloping child in warmth during early years, but when child older, relationship more distant. Oldest son reared differently from other brothers, and brothers from sisters, so every child aware of his/her place.
Responsibility for Child Care	Primarily mother, but older children involved in daily activities, including care of younger siblings. Attitude of love and responsibility among siblings; new baby not seen as competition.	Husband ultimately responsible as head of household. Any family member, including siblings and cousins, responsible at times.	Mother primarily, but all of family involved.

TABLE 10-2 (cont.)

COMPONENT	GREEK	SPANISH-AMERICAN	JAPANESE
Discipline	Consistent. Obedience very important and taught to child at early age. Child praised when good and told when bad. Taught that it is important to be good and not shame family. Use group pressure to set limits on behavior.	Consistently correct child because his/her behavior is bothersome and warned not to act in a way to provoke father. Instill fear of consequences. Pride in self-control and fear of being shamed instilled in child. Seldom told he/she is "good" or "bad."	Firm, consistent, lack strong emotions. Emphasis on responsibility, duty, loyalty. Promote feeling of insecurity when do wrong.
Training of Child	Taught to value interdependence, cooperation. Sibling rivalry when new baby arrives but does not last long. Mother delighted with new baby but shares self equally with older child, including offer of free breast during feeding. Older child invited to share excitement about baby. Parents never clowning for child's amusement or giving many material things.	Taught to value interdependence, companionship. Little sibling jealousy. Freely show affection and attention.	Taught to value interdependence but responsible for own behavior. Taught to carry out obligation regardless of personal cost and to control behavior to avoid personal shame and disgrace of group. Develop strong sense of responsibility. Poor communication between generations because of differences in experiences, education, language comprehension, and values fostering problems in modern society.

TABLE 10-3 A Comparison of Cultures: Interaction with Others Versus Privacy

COMPONENT	GREEK	SPANISH-AMERICAN	JAPANESE
Basic Values of Person and Behavior	Strong sense of self-esteem. Inner core of personality not to be exposed or shamed. Value equality, individuality. Aloneness not sought, but borne with fortitude. Pride in glorious past of Greece.	Anxiety about being alone and concern for people who are alone. Not considered proper to compete, push self forward in group through achievements. Better to submit than provoke anger in another. Self-restraint emphasized. Violence atypical.	Strong sense of self-respect and important to be treated respectfully by others. Privacy not valued, apparently unwanted, and seen as loneliness.
Personal Possessions	Value in shared living and sharing possessions, especially with family and friends.	Sharing of possessions. One's own house nebulous; frequent unannounced visiting among family and friends.	Possessions not highly valued. Shared living space and possessions in family.
Status of Person	Valued for what he/she is rather than position or achievement. Family unit valued, not individual.	Valued for what he/she is, depends on family.	Belonging to right clique or faction important to status and future success. Try to join influential group at early age.
Interaction among Persons	Resented when treated impersonally, mechanically, or like a number on a chart. No word for "group," but born into group of family and friends. Extended family working together for benefit of each other. Units of cooperation retained from past, not created. Work to achieve common goal with those to whom he/she feels loyalty. Speech of much importance because it establishes interactions; expressive of feelings	Much neighborhood socializing, especially among women to borrow, help, consult, discuss, or exchange gifts. Interchange of gifts and services frequent. Accepting as gracious as giving, and person not satisfied until he/she has returned a gift to show appreciation; return gift not necessarily same kind or form. Strangers not completely accepted unless related to established family by marriage. Interdependence between family and close friends does not extend to broader community. Few formalized social groups.	Suppression of emotion in many situations. Most docile with strong urge to conform. Pleasant, polite, correct but aloof behavior to others in all classes. Restrained, formal, hierarchal relationships in family, company, and political party rather than horizontal, comradely behavior. Ceremonious, at ease, and apologetic to acquaintances and friends but less so with strangers. Man unappreciative of domineering woman.
Social Activities	Family basic social group. Circle of friends important. Enjoy social affiliations, great loyalty to all groups to which belong. Food important with social activities.	Family basic social group. Women thought of as one social group, men another. Remain close to own social group for job or marriage partner.	Fondness for crowds and physical proximity of people. Participation and spectator roles in social activities and sports enjoyed.

TABLE 10-4 A Comparison of Cultures: Time Orientation

COMPONENT	GREEK	SPANISH-AMERICAN	JAPANESE
Concept of Time	Present important but prepare for something in future that is sure part of life. No automatic faith in future. Distasteful to organize activities according to clock. Life regulated by body needs and rhythms, daily pattern of light and dark, and seasons.	Present important but validated by past. Expect future to be like present. Perform with distinction in present rather than emphasize efficiency, quantity. Life not regulated by clock but by body needs and rhythms, light and dark, seasons, religious holidays.	Time neither an absolute nor objective category but a process—the changing of nature with man as part of it. Planning for future valued. Present considered important, and past priceless.
Use of Time	Time used spontaneously. Elastic attitude toward time; governed by cycles of nature. "Tomorrow" thought of as tomorrow, next week, or never. Activities and appointments usually not starting on time, but person not hurried.	Time used spontaneously. Little value in planning ahead. **"Right now" means now or later.**	Appreciation of time. Calmness and time for daily ceremony highly valued. Ceremony carried out in spite of rush of work.

TABLE 10-5 A Comparison of Cultures: Work and Use of Leisure Time

COMPONENT	GREEK	SPANISH-AMERICAN	JAPANESE
Concept of Work	Work thought of as life, a joy and dignity, not drudgery. Work interrupted primarily for religious reasons, not as claim to idleness or leisure. Women as hard workers as men. Tenacious and resourceful at making the best of what they have and coping with difficulty. Person not to be hurried but works efficiently at own pace.	Work considered inevitable part of daily life. Not done just to keep busy or earn more money if present needs met. No moral corruption in being idle. Work at own pace and no specially defined working hours if possible. Everyone expected to cooperate and do his/her part. Work shared to decrease loneliness. Work roles of sexes and age groups distinct but each aware of tasks performed by the other. Able to take over work roles of other family members. Child a part in work of home and family and feels important. No special rewards.	Enjoyment of work more important than money earned. Strong ties between person, the job, and the company. Job mobility frowned on. Independence in work traditionally valued but younger workers adjusting to Western concept of employment.
Concept of Leisure	Leisure an attitude, a dimension of all life and work. Not confined to certain time but a continual expression of internal freedom, at work or rest.	Leisure synonymous with free time. No emphasis on leisure for own sake. Intersperse work with rest, socialize during work. Free time spent visiting.	Some leisure time used in solitude. Much leisure time spent in traveling with peers. Freer expression of emotion in recreational pursuits.

TABLE 10-6 A Comparison of Cultures: Education

COMPONENT	GREEK	SPANISH-AMERICAN	JAPANESE
Value on Education	Highly prized, especially professional education. Curiosity and creativity valued. Educated person accorded much respect. Use of creative intellect and being cultured citizen valued, but can be achieved through life's experiences and work as well as by education.	Learns that which interests him/her. Absent from school if learning little or if something more interesting going on elsewhere. Not seen as only way to achieve.	Education highly valued, with emphasis on scientific information. Eager to learn. Believe in value of practical experience as well. Choice of college influences status in life. Much competition in education.
Educational Methods	Emphasize quickness, curiosity, cleverness, realism, reason. Education applied to matters of life.	No emphasis on excelling or competing against other family members for high grades or honors. Use of native language may interfere with success in school.	Educational reform by U.S. occupation after World War II counter to traditional methods: replaced rote memorization with progressive methods, deemphasized moral training and unquestioning acceptance of authority, granted equal status to women, broadened opportunity for women.

TABLE 10-7 A Comparison of Cultures: Attitudes Regarding Change

COMPONENT	GREEK	SPANISH-AMERICAN	JAPANESE
Value of Change	Not valued for itself. Progress hoped for but not taken for granted. Change not necessarily bringing progress or improvement.	Change condemned simply because it is change. Patience and postponing personal desires emphasized. Little faith in progress or control over own destiny.	Physical world considered transient. Person appreciative but does not cling to things; thus change accepted.
Pace of Change	Deliberate.	Slow. Deliberate.	Able to adjust lifestyle to rapid economic, industrial, and urban changes.
Effect of Change	No value on unlimited progress. Wants what is better than present but what is known and can be achieved. A plan to an American synonymous with a dream to a Greek. Adaptive to change. Use material goods. Do not discard useful articles. Repair to maintain usefulness of object. Traditional Greek culture changing, becoming Westernized, affecting behavior of young.	Value system seen as constant. Feel many individuals not amenable to change by human endeavor. Adjust to environment. Use material goods to capacity. Generally remain near traditional home, maintaining stable relationships with people. Change in main culture affecting behavior of young, causing insecurity in elders.	Urgency of Western-like activity a new phenomenon. Breaking traditional patterns and solidarity, increased individualism, competition, and individual insecurity. Youth seeking new values to replace old dogmas. Parent generation generally revere authority of family and state—now rejected by younger generation.

the Caribbean Islands, or South America. Furthermore, values may be lived differently, outwardly, if the person resides in Greece, Mexico, or Japan rather than the United States.

Yet much of the behavior of the third- or fourth-generation family or person from a country reflects the original cultural-ethnic values. That fact explains the differences among groups of people and should not be considered abnormal. Discussion centers on the family unit, male and female relationships, childrearing, the group versus privacy, time orientation, work and use of leisure time, education, and attitudes regarding change. The following discussion then compares the attitudes of U. S. residents toward health and illness with the corresponding attitudes in each of these cultures (9, 12, 27, 53, 59, 84, 125, 140, 165, 198, 212).

Table 10-8 summarizes Kluckhorn's presentation of five basic value questions, the range of beliefs derived from these questions, and examples of some (sub)cultural groups adhering to these beliefs (109). You may wish to assess your clients and their families according to these values as well as the characteristics presented in Tables 10-1 through 10-7. Although neither a comprehensive study nor a stereotype of everyone in these cultures, these comparisons indicate that subtle as well as obvious differences, along with some similarities, exist among different groups' values and behavior. Understand that these cultural patterns will be followed by different persons in each culture to varying degrees, denied by some, and not identified, yet taken for granted by others. Chapter 12 will discuss some of these values in relation to the culture of the United States.

Attitudes Toward Health and Illness

How health is identified, physically and emotionally, varies from culture to culture, as do ideas about the factors related to health and disease. American definitions are emphasized in Chapter 1.

Attitudes in the United States toward health are influenced considerably by society's emphasis on mastery of the environment as opposed to adjustment to it. Illness is seen as a challenge to be met by mobilizing resources: research, science, funds, institutions, and people. Americans tax themselves to finance health and welfare organizations and persons giving time and effort to these organizations are given special status by the community. Because independence is highly valued, the weak are expected to help themselves as much as possible. The strong help the weak as long as their problems are caused by events beyond their control; otherwise the physically, socially, or emotionally weak, deformed, or unsightly are devalued.

A person is evaluated on productivity or "doing good." Because the ability to be productive depends in part on health, individual health is highly valued. Health in the broadest sense is considered necessary

TABLE 10-8 Basic Values of Cultures with Selected Cultural Examples

VALUE	RANGE OF BELIEFS	EXAMPLE OF CULTURAL/ SUBCULTURAL GROUP ADHERING TO VALUE
Human nature (What is innate nature of man?)	A. The person is basically *evil but capable of achieving goodness* with self-control and effort.	Puritan ancestors. Protestants of Pentecostal or Fundamentalist background. Appalachian subculture.
	B. The person is a *combination of good and evil,* with self-control necessary but lapses in behavior understood.	Most people in the United States.
	C. The person is basically *good.*	Some religious groups, such as Society of Friends; some philosophical groups, such as humanistic psychologists or members of Ethical Society.
Man-Nature (What is relation of man to nature or supernatural?)	A. The person is *subjugated to nature* and cannot change whatever is destined to happen.	Spanish-American culture. Appalachian subculture.
	B. The person lives in *harmony with nature;* man-nature-supernatural exist as a whole entity.	Oriental cultures. Navaho Indian culture.
	C. The person is to gain *mastery over nature;* all natural forces can be overcome.	Middle- and upper-class and highly educated people in the United States.
Time (What is temporal focus on human life?)	A. *Past time* is given preference; most important events to guide life have happened in the past.	Historic China.
	B. *Present time* is the main focus; people pay little attention to the past and regard the future as vague.	Spanish-American cultures. Appalachian subculture.
	C. *Future* is the main emphasis, seen as bigger and better; people are not content with the present.	Educated, professional, and middle-class people in the United States

TABLE 10-8 (cont.)

VALUE	RANGE OF BELIEFS	EXAMPLE OF CULTURAL/ SUBCULTURAL GROUP ADHERING TO VALUE
Activity (What is the main purpose in life?)	A. *Being orientation.* The person is important just because he/she is and may spontaneously express impulses and desires.	Appalachian subculture. While no culture allows complete expression of impulses and all cultures must have some work done, the Mexican fiesta and Mardi Gras in New Orleans are manifestations of this value.
	B. *Becoming-in-being orientation.* The person is important for what he/she is, but must continue to develop.	Most religious cultures. Native American subcultures.
	C. *Doing orientation.* The person is important when he/she is active or accomplishing something.	Most people in the United States.
Relational (What is one's relation to other people?)	A. *Individualistic relations* emphasize autonomy of the person; he/she does not have to fully submit to authority. Individual goals have primacy over group goal.	Most Gemeinschaft societies, such as folk or rural cultures. Yankee and Appalachian subcultures. Middle-class America, with emphasis on nuclear family.
	B. *Collateral relations* emphasize that the person is part of a social and family order and does not live just for him/herself. Group or family goals have primacy.	Most European-American ethnic groups, especially Italian-American. Spanish-American culture. Native American tribal subcultures. Most cultures adhere to somewhat through sibling relations in family.
	C. *Lineal relations* emphasize the extended family and biological and cultural relationships through time. Group goals have primacy.	Cultures that emphasize hereditary lines. Upper-class America. Oriental cultures. Middle-East cultures.
	D. Relations are impersonal, focused on role behavior.	Business interactions, upper middle class, and those moving up the social ladder.

for successful interaction with others, educational accomplishment, ability to work, leadership, childrearing, and capacity to use opportunities. Thus development of medical, nursing, and other health sciences and technology is considered important. The physical cause of illness is generally accepted. Only recently have the sociocultural causes of disease also been emphasized.

The importance of health has been accentuated by industrialization, high-level technology, greater social controls, and mass communications, as well as by a high level of responsibility and stress placed on the person. Americans at times react to the complexities of society by retreating into ill health, physically, emotionally, or socially. Levels of pathology that could be tolerated in pre-industrial societies cannot be tolerated in complex modern life. Americans are more likely to interpret a person's difficulty in fulfilling social-role expectations as illness than would some other societies. Thus the person who is ill is less likely to be tolerated or kept in the family. When ill, the person is supposed to leave home, isolate self from the family, and be cared for in a strange place, the hospital, by strange people who are authorities on illness. One's capacity for meeting social-role expectations is developed primarily through family socialization and education, but it is protected and restored through the health care system. The ill person is expected to want to return to normal roles and to leave behind the feelings of alienation, regression, and passivity that are part of the deviance of illness. The impersonal agency of the hospital exerts pressures that discourage staying dependent and ill.

In Greece health is important and desired, but it is not a preoccupation. One should not pamper the self. Straight living gives a healthy body and so fortitude, hardness, and a simple standard of living are pursued. Excesses in living–in eating, drinking, or smoking–are avoided, and, in general, the level of public health is high. Because children are prized, their health needs take precedence over adults' needs.

Going to bed is a sign of weakness except for recognized disease. People do not go to a doctor unless there is something seriously wrong; but then they expect the doctor, who is a father figure, to have the answers for their problems. Home remedies and the services of an herbalist are tried first as treatment. Prayers are said and vows are made. Illness is thought to arise from evil or magical sources that can be counteracted through magical practices. Entering the hospital is a last resort. The whole family is involved when the person is sick; each person has a specific role and a role gap exists during illness.

The organs of highest significance are the eyes, for they reflect the real person. Next in importance are the lips because of the words that come out of them. A girl's hair and a man's mustache are important symbols of sexual identity and attractiveness. The genital organs are not freely talked about but are respected for their reproductive functions. The body is meant to be covered and exposed only when necessary. Dress and ornamentation are essential to complete one's body image.

Childlessness is unfortunate and in the past the woman was held responsible. The woman dislikes any examination or treatment of the reproductive organs and will accept gynecological problems rather than seek medical care for fear fertility will be affected. Special care is given to the woman during pregnancy, when special regulations about hygiene, rest, activity, and a happy environment are followed.

The handicapped are not easily accepted because of the emphasis on a whole, strong, firm body. To be crippled, blind, or lame means that one is not a whole person, is dependent, and is unable to do anything for oneself.

Attitudes among Spanish-Americans in the U. S. Southwest are very unlike attitudes in mainstream America. The Spanish-American considers the self to be a whole person; thus "better health" has no meaning. Good health is associated with the ability to work and fulfill normal roles, for one gains and maintains respect by meeting one's responsibilities. Criteria of health are a sturdy body, ability to maintain normal physical activity, and absence of pain. The person does not have to perfect his/her health; as long as the family is around, he/she is all right. Thus preventive measures are not highly valued. The person does seek to care for self, however, through moderation in eating, drinking, work, recreation, and sleep, and by leading a good life.

The Spanish-American believes that hardship and suffering are part of destiny and that reward for being submissive to God's will and for doing good will come in the next life. Ill health is accepted as part of life and is thought to be caused by an unknown external event or object, such as natural forces of cold, heat, storms, water, or as the result of sinning—acting against God's will. The Spanish-American, for example, thinks that one cause of illness is bad air, especially night air, which enters through a cavity or opening in the body. Thus a raisin may be placed on the cord stump of the newborn and surgery is avoided if possible; both practices help prevent air from entering the body. Avoiding drafts, keeping windows closed at night, keeping the head covered, and following certain postpartum practices have the same basis. Other causes of disease (according to Spanish-American beliefs) include overwork, poor food, excess worry or emotional strain, undue exposure to weather, uneven wetting of the body, taking a drink when overheated, and giving blood for transfusion. Underlying this thinking is the hot-cold theory of disease that stems from the Hippocratic humoral theory and was carried to the Western Hemisphere by the Spanish and Portuguese in the sixteenth and seventeenth centuries. Basically all diseases are classified as hot or cold. Arthritis is a cold disease and an ulcer is a hot disease, for instance. All foods, herbs, medicines are classified as hot or cold. Avocado is a cold food and aspirin and corn meal are considered hot. A goal is to balance the body: a hot disease is cured with a cold food and a cold disease is cured with a hot food, herb, or medication. Thus aspirin could be taken for arthritis—which also fits into the Western medical system (87).

Evil eye, *mal ojo, is a cause of disease that results when a person looks admiringly at the child of another.* Usually children are not openly admired, but precautions against illness include patting the child on the head or a light slap. (Do you know people in other subcultures with similar beliefs? Such causes are commonly stated when illness occurs.) A common illness, in this culture, *susto*, with symptoms of agitation and depression, results from traumatic, frightening experiences and may result in death. Psychosocial forces causing disease are also seen in *empacho*, a gastrointestinal disease that results from eating food that is disliked, or from overeating, or from eating hot bread. Disease may also result from organs or parts of the body moving from the normal position. Little attention is paid to colds, minor aches, or common gastrointestinal disorders.

The role of the family is important in time of illness. The head of the house, the man, determines whether illness exists and what treatment is to be given. The person goes to bed when too ill to work or to move. Treatment from a lay healer is sought if family care does not help. The medical doctor is called only when the Spanish-American is gravely ill; this is combined with visiting so the patient does not get the rest and isolation advised by health workers in the majority culture. The sick person does not withdraw from the group; doing so would only make him/her feel worse. Acceptance of present fate amounts to saying "If the Lord intends for me to die, I'll die." The discomfort of the present is considered, but not in terms of future complications. Being ill brings no secondary advantage of care or coddling. Communicable diseases are hard to control, for resistance to isolation is based on the idea that family members, relatives, and familiar objects cannot contaminate or cause illness. Taking home remedies, wearing special articles, and performing special ceremonies are accepted ways of getting and staying well. The person feels he/she will keep well by observing the ritual calendar, being brotherly, being a good Catholic and member of the community. If the health worker uses any procedure, such as an x ray, it is considered to be the treatment and hence the person should be cured.

Accidents are feared because they disrupt the wholeness of the person. In addition, the Spanish-American fears surgery, the impersonality of the hospital and nurses, and any infringement on modesty. The hospital represents death and isolation from family or friends. The "professional" (Anglo) approach of the majority culture is regarded as showing indifference to needs and as causing anxiety and discomfort.

Attitudes in Japan toward health strongly reflect the belief in a body-mind-spirit interrelationship. Spiritual and temporal affairs in life are closely integrated; thus health practices and religion are closely intertwined, influenced considerably by the magicoreligious practices of Shinto, Japan's ancient religion. Bathing customs stem from Shinto purification rites, for example, and baths are taken in the evening before eating not only for cleanliness but for ceremony and relaxation as well.

There is a strong emphasis on physical fitness, an intact body, physical strength, determination, and long life. Self-discipline in daily habits is highly valued, as are the mental, spiritual, and esthetic aspects of the person. These traits remain equally important to the sick person.

As a child, the person is taught to minimize reactions to injury and illness. Hence to the Westerner the sick person may appear stoic. Part of the reserve in expressing emotion and pain is also influenced by childrearing and interaction practices, which emphasize correct behavior and suppression of emotion. Yet the sick person, as much as the well, expects to be treated with respect and resents being addressed abruptly or informally by first name. The person also resents people entering the hospital room without knocking. The Japanese male resents being dominated by women and he may feel uncomfortable with an American female nurse because he interprets her behavior as overbearing. The person is eager to cooperate with the medical care program but wishes to be included in planning and decisions regarding care. The so-called professional approach of the average U. S. health worker is likely to insult the average Japanese, although he/she may be too polite to say so.

By studying the life patterns of people in various cultures (especially those of patients for whom you care) and by taking into account the factors discussed in the following chapters on religion and family, you can better understand and handle varying levels of health, health problems, and attitudes toward care of different groups.

You may obtain additional information about people from the following (sub)cultures and their specific nursing needs from references at the end of the chapter:

1. American Indian (22, 27, 78, 95, 98, 103, 110, 118, 124, 172, 173, 194, 197, 220, 222, 224, 235).
2. Appalachian (154, 157, 178, 192, 204, 215).
3. Black American (15, 16, 30, 41, 42, 91, 94, 97, 118, 169, 175, 227, 228, 231).
4. Eskimo (17, 23, 40, 48, 56, 69, 144, 213, 226).
5. German-American (13, 180, 191, 232).
6. Greek-American (13, 27, 89, 125, 187, 232).
7. Gypsy (6).
8. Irish-American (13, 232, 236, 237).
9. Italian-American (13, 28, 43, 118, 232, 236, 237).
10. Jewish (73, 151, 175, 196, 236).

11. Migrant farmer (11, 21, 34, 35, 68, 162, 219).
12. Oriental American (22, 24, 33, 47, 54, 86, 108, 112, 128, 148, 175, 202, 205, 221).
13. Polish-American (13, 27, 123, 189, 232).
14. Puerto Rican (24, 47, 65, 119).
15. Southeast Asian refugees (36, 67, 74).
16. Spanish-American of the southwestern United States (4, 7, 8, 9, 22, 27, 32, 57, 63, 71, 105, 118, 138, 142, 145, 149, 152, 171, 175, 230, 233).
17. Vietnamese (50, 118, 218).

SOCIAL CLASS SUBCULTURE

Research about social stratification indicates that the person's class position is influenced by economic and social status and political power of the family and affects formation of values, attitudes, and lifestyle. Each class tends to have a more or less well-specified set of values and role expectations regarding practically every area of human activity: sex, marriage, male–female and parent–child responsibilities and behavior, birth, death, education, dress, housing, home furnishings, leisure, reading habits, occupational status, politics, religion, and status symbols. Social class includes a group consciousness (132). Most persons can be objectively placed within a certain class, but they are sometimes accorded a status by others around them that might be different. Furthermore, they may see themselves at yet a different status level, based on race, sex, religion, ancestry, ethnic origin, or wealth in material goods. What seems natural and logical in determining status to some people may be rejected by others.

Profile of Socioeconomic Levels

The Upper-Upper or Corporate Class consists of a relatively small number of people who own a disproportionate share of personal wealth and whose income is largely derived from ownership. This group has both money and power and it can control how its assets are used as well as various other economic and political aspects of society. The decisions made by this group affect everyone else. Coleman refers to the upper-upper class as the *Successful Elite* (100). Coles (39) refers to them as the *affluent*. These are the people who have had lineage, inherited wealth, and power for several generations. They are acknowledged by the general public and themselves as leaders nationally and internationally. They feel obliged to tend their own financial and material resources well, to obtain the best possible education, and to take care of their health so that they can meet their obligation of giving of themselves personally and philanthropically to society (39, 100).

This person or family lives in an exclusive residential area in a house whose atmosphere is spatial and formal and that affords privacy from the masses. This person or family may own several estates in different areas of the country (or world) that are used in different seasons or for different purposes. The family may have a number of people to help it maintain its lifestyle, such as a maid, butler, gardener, and other staff members (39).

The children are reared by a governess or maid as well as by the parents. The mother usually is selective in her teaching, guiding, and care. Certain aspects of rearing are done only by the mother, others only by the maid. The children, like the parents, live with choices, for they have more animate and inanimate objects and possessions than others and many opportunities to follow the arts; to learn certain sports, such as horseback riding, tennis, swimming, or skiing; and to travel. But even the children know the importance and value of the objects and opportunities that surround them. They recognize the importance of self-control, behaviorally and in their various activities and sports. They seek reverie and disciplined activity even though in the public view. They are able to move smoothly from one activity to another without being *driven* to excel. Yet they expect to be competent at their chosen academic, recreational, and social pursuits (39).

Although the upper class is adult oriented, children know at an early age that they are special and parents try to instill a feeling that the child must do well because he/she has special responsibilities to society on reaching adulthood. The child, like the parent, associates with others from the same class, observing the average person from the sidelines, never really understanding what life is like for the average citizen or why middle- or lower-class people live as they do. Although both adults and children take a lot for granted and feel entitled to the fine things in life, they feel a sense of responsibility and try to live up to their ideals. Destiny is abundance and limitless possibility. They are confident that life will be rewarding. Even crisis, such as illness or surgery, can be made into something basically pleasant, for the best of specialized health care professionals and comprehensive facilities can be obtained, and convalescence frequently involves a trip to and rest at a secluded place (39, 90).

The Lower-Upper Class consists of people whose wealth is more recently acquired and who have become well known (actors, famous doctors or lawyers, athletes) or they may be less famous but have large incomes, homes, and lifestyles that show off their money. They have social position and prestige because of what they *do*. The upper-upper-class person has position and prestige because of *who* he/she is; the person doesn't lose them even if encountering financial setbacks. The lower-upper-class person may slide down into middle-class anonymity if wealth is lost. The lower-upper-class person or family also has an abundance of possessions and opportunity, however, but may be less humble about or more self-conscious of it than the upper-upper-class person. Although this person or family may attend the same activities, travel to the same areas, or send the children to the same schools as the upper-upper-class family, this person or family is seen as different by the upper-upper class (39, 111). Often a fine line separates the upper-upper and lower-upper classes in a community; such intangibles as social charm or likeability, family background, religion, value of residence, and schooling often make the difference. Money is only loosely related to social standing in many communities (93, 100). Increasingly, the wives of the lower-upper class are working—starting a business or doing consultant work—for fun, for a sense of identity, to be worthwhile, to provide structure to the day or to life, to avoid the image of being dumb (they are usually college educated), to avoid being important only through the husband. Often the women enjoy having their own money to spend as well (174).

The Upper-Middle Class is described by Coleman as *Those Who Are Doing Well*. Income is above $40,000 to $60,000, depending on geographical area. Each spouse is college educated and at least one is a professional—the average doctor, dentist, engineer, business manager, or lawyer. The main work of these people is intellectual instead of manual, requires professional training, and offers upward mobility. They live in a large house in the better part of town or suburb, may have a maid and often a gardener, have more than one car, travel abroad, usually belong to a semi-elite country club, and send the children to private schools and college (5, 83, 100). Both family stability and community leadership are valued. The children have a number of opportunities educationally and culturally; in return, they are expected to be successful academically and socially. The children are often involved in a number of prestigious out-of-home activities and organizations, as are parents, and the children may actually have fewer home responsibilities than the upper-class child. Childrearing is permissive; children are given explanations instead of punishment. The parents will exert more direct influence on the child's schooling than will the middle or working class (39, 83, 111).

The Middle Class, according to Coleman, is divided in two categories: Middle American Dream and the Average-Man Comfortable Existence (100). Members of the *Middle-American Dream* group have education above the high school level in a professional or specialized school and include business people with small or medium-sized enterprises who employ a few or many workers; self-employed business people, artists; skilled workers; office and sales workers; and public or private school teachers. Nurses and other professional health workers typically are in this class. These people have a special status because of education and occupation (many *work with* people), although they do not have much wealth. Typically they work in occupations that involve thinking rather than hard physical labor. They live in a pleasant residential section or suburb, in a nicely furnished house, have two cars, usually including a station wagon or camper (one car may be older). The family eats out weekly and vacations annually (100). The middle-class family is usually a nuclear family, but it has linkages through kin for social and family goals. The family is active in community activities and organizations and pursues some sports or other leisure activities as a family unit, but the family members frequently go to separate activities several evenings a week. Members of the *Average-Man Comfortable Existence* group tend to have less education and less material goods than the first group, but they live comfortably. They have more than the necessities and are somewhat active in the community.

The middle class is child oriented; family life often revolves around children and their interests. Parents have high aspirations for children and take pride in their accomplishments. Parents emphasize education and value and encourage verbal and problem-solving skills (111). The middle (and upper) class(es) uses an elaborate code in speech, which is characterized by precision, differentiation of ideas, and extensive use of modifiers and clauses. Its verbosity may bury the meaning, and the abstractness of such speech causes lack of understanding among the working and lower classes (37). Parents teach the importance of hard work, self-reliance, thrift, patience, planning ahead, and postponing immediate rewards for later rewards. Parents are responsive to research results about childrearing and advice of experts and change childrearing practices accordingly. Parents try to understand the dynamics of the child's behavior and mix discipline with permissiveness. Discipline is often in the form of withdrawal of privileges or of disapproval, threats, or appeals to reason. The child is expected to be expressive verbally and emotionally, happy and cooperative, to confide in them, to want to learn, and to have self-control. Fathers are frequently as involved in childrearing as mothers; parental roles are not sharply differentiated (93, 109, 111).

Overall the middle class uses the internist, family practice physician, and pediatrician for routine health care, but the services of specialists are wanted when indicated. The middle class respects health professionals and wants thorough and scientific diagnosis and treatment.

Middle-class people see themselves as knowledgeable about health, but they appreciate and will try to use additional information. They tolerate, although they don't like, the high medical costs (93).

The Lower-Middle or Working Class is described by Coleman as *The World of Just Getting By* (100). Generally both spouses have graduated from high school and both work as industrial or blue-collar workers, clerical or service workers, agricultural wage earners, technicians, skilled or semiskilled workers, as telephone operators or waitresses. Many working-class people work with things. The family rents either a small home with two or three bedrooms or an apartment and takes good care of its home and belongings, including an older car. It has some conveniences but does not own many luxuries, such as a dishwasher or expensive household gadgets. The family depends on the extended family instead of on social agencies for economic and emotional support and may be active in church but not active in other community organizations. The husband is typically head of the house and the woman is considered responsible for the home. The family enjoys recreational activities as a family unit, such as bowling or drive-in movies, and eating at fast-service or local "home-style" restaurants (100, 111, 175).

Members of the working class value patriotism, religion, authority, the work ethic, honesty, respectability, self-reliance, conformity, consumerism, competition, achievement, education, the home, saving for the future, and law and order. They believe people with money aren't happy. They accept their position and are basically proud of their hard work and accomplishment, even with less education. They believe that on-the-job, collective action is important. They believe that the poor are lazy, deserve their poverty, and should not be given welfare (93, 100, 111, 115). (A natural economic depression and forced unemployment are the only two causes for poverty without moral blame.) Being higher in the social scale than the poor and minorities gives them a social identity and a measure of social worth. They feel that equality of all people, including the poor, minorities, and women, is threatening and would pose problems of social adjustment. Another danger of equality is that friends or neighbors might surpass them. The present inequality allows the upper class or supervisors to be an elite group, to take care of people, to be friendly, helpful leaders. Equality of income would deprive people of their incentive to work. Working-class people are stable breadwinners, churchgoers, voters, and family men/women. They may have two jobs and little leisure. Leisure is usually focused on activities that help the person forget the life situation and work temporarily. Many do not like their jobs but fear not finding another; therefore they keep the job because of family responsibilities and the hold on respectability that the job brings. What they want most is a decent standard of living (111, 115, 175).

Because they are less educated and read less, they are less responsive to research results and expert advice about childrearing. They don't view childrearing as something to discuss or do with a plan. They expect their children to be obedient, neat and clean, honest, to conform to adult expectations, to respect the rights of others. Discipline includes more physical punishment and less emphasis on reasoning than in the preceding classes. Mother is seen by father as the main childrearer, although sometimes he is the main disciplinarian and she is the supportive parent. As in childrearing, the work and social roles of man–woman, mother–father, and parent–child are sharply differentiated (111). Health care is sought when they are too sick to work; prevention is less emphasized than for the foregoing classes. They may try home or folk remedies first and then go to a general practitioner. The neighborhood health center will be used if one exists. Dental care is more likely to be neglected than other medical care. They respond well to an approach that is respectful, personable, prompt, and thorough. They do not understand why health care should be so costly and they may omit very expensive treatments or drugs whenever possible (93, 153).

The Upper-Lower Class is identified by Coleman as *Having a Real Hard Time*. The family is often only one step away from poverty and welfare. The person has fewer chances of acquiring education. Thus upper-lower-class people work at menial tasks, usually nonunion, but are proud to be working. These people may work as domestics, gardeners, hospital or school maintenance or cafeteria workers, junk collectors, garbage collectors, or street cleaners. Neither husband nor wife has completed high school and sometimes one may not have completed junior high. The family lives in a substandard flat in an older building, usually with an absentee landlord. The family enjoys picnics in the park and other free diversions. The family's only long trips are for funerals of relatives (100). Often the upper-lower-class family had its beginning in lack of motivation for education, resulting in high school dropout for pregnancy or lack of academic success, an early parenthood, a poor first job, a rapid succession of children, or an early separation or divorce. As life progresses, the chance to advance becomes even less likely (111).

The Poor may be classified into those in acute poverty and those in chronic poverty. The person or family in **acute poverty** *has reduced economic means because of given circumstances for a limited time* but anticipates being able to return to work and a better lifestyle. The person or family in **chronic poverty** *has a long family history of being un-*

employed and without adequate economic means and is unlikely to see much chance for improvement (37, 163). The lines are not always so clearly drawn, however. Because of the unemployment problems of the late 1970s and the 1980s, more traditionally middle-class people are economically classified as poor. The single parent raising several children, although middle class by birth, may become acutely poor when a job is not available or a prolonged illness or other crisis occur. The elderly person who considered him/herself middle class or even affluent may now barely be able to pay for the essentials of life or may be living in poverty conditions.

Although the poor or lower-class person has traditionally not finished high school, perhaps not even elementary school, and is an unskilled or semiskilled worker, often employed in temporary or seasonal jobs, the person with a doctorate degree may also be unemployed and living in poverty. Often the woman is better able to get a job than the man, but neither may have the necessary job skills for our competitive and technologically changing society. The poor person lives primarily on welfare in the rural area or in an inner city or ghetto tenement, often infested by rats and roaches and without hot water. Recreation for the man consists of talking with peers on the street corner or at a cheap bar, sitting alone in a park, or watching television. The women's chief leisure activity may be attending church and visiting relatives. The family unit may be nuclear or extended and frequently there are a number of offspring (37, 111).

Much of the results of the research of the 1960s on people in the lower socioeconomic class and "the culture of poverty" reflected the bias or race of the researchers or focused on institutionalized populations or people in trouble, perhaps without reflecting on the many variables that influence people. Typically only negative traits were assigned to the poor person or family—traits at the opposite end of the continuum from the desired middle-class characteristics. The victim of social oppression and racism was blamed for his/her problems. Fortunately, later research findings give a more balanced view, which should help health workers to offer the same quality of care to the poor as to the middle and upper classes (37, 163).

Characteristics describing the lower class—reliance on the extended family, response to authoritarian leadership as well as using authoritarian childrearing practices, inability to delay gratification, fatalism, and concrete thinking—may be seen as adaptive practices or subcultural values (37, 139, 163).

Most minority and ethnic cultures value kinship ties and the emotional, social, and economic support that the extended family provides in contrast to dominant middle-class America, which values individualism and independence. Much visiting goes on between relatives in the lower and working classes; assistance is sought and appreciated. All get along better by sharing meager resources or by working together to gain resources. The grandmother (and grandfather if living) is valued as caretaker for the child if the mother works. But the grandmother is also valued because she is the carrier of the culture; she is wise and can teach the young a great deal. The grandparent also benefits from being valued as a person (31, 37, 111).

Authoritarian childrearing practices, which may be an euphemism for discipline, has as the explicit objective to develop toughness and self-sufficiency for survival. Yet in spite of the authoritarian, direct approach, the parent is warm and expressive. An attachment exists between parent and child. In his/her own home the child is also likely to be expressive, although the child may seem restrained with strangers (37). The child is often given adult responsibilities early; he/she is not the focus of the family in the way that the middle-class child is. Everyone must fend more for self (31, 111).

Ability to delay gratification appears related to the situation. If the minority person is being tested by a White person or has experienced broken promises—either by the researcher or others—he/she does not delay gratification. That is, the person requests an immediate reward in the experiment instead of being willing to wait. Moreover, ability to wait is related to **internal locus of control**, *a feeling that the self has some control over events.* Frequently the poor person learns early that he/she is at the mercy of the system, whether the system is White, economic, educational, or health (31, 37). Then, too, if hungry, cold, or without necessities, small wonder that the person takes whatever possible to appease hunger or feel more comfortable. The child learns to delay gratification if he/she can trust that what is needed will be there when needed. The poor child may seldom have this opportunity because of economic problems in the family. If meager resources are used to meet today's needs, it is difficult or impossible to plan ahead, to save, or to anticipate that planning and saving have merit. The lower class is present-oriented, in contrast to the future perspective of middle and upper classes, because of necessity, cultural values, or inability to trust what is not tangible (37, 163).

Often the poor person appears to need an authoritarian, directive approach. The poor person (or the parents) may work in a situation in which he/she takes orders; the poor person's expectancy is to be *told* rather than *invited to talk with* someone about his/her ideas, problems, tentative solutions, or insight. Or the person may not understand the health care worker's professional jargon but is too polite or fearful to ask for an explanation. Also, if previous attempts to share ideas were met with rejection or ridicule by parent, teacher, or health care worker, the person learned that it was safer not to respond. Finally, the poor person values action—getting something accomplished—more than words or promises (25, 37).

Impaired verbal communication and problem-solving ability may be present, not because the poor person is cognitively deficient but for other reasons. Many ethnic or minority groups speak a dialect in the home; the child then has difficulty understanding standard English or being understood. Essentially the child must become bilingual to be successful in school (41). The poor person uses a restricted code that is characterized by short sentences, lack of specificity, and lack of subordinate clauses for elaboration of meaning. The poor person speaks directly to the point. Such language is said to be concrete and to indicate lack of abstract thinking. In contrast to the middle-class elaborate and sometimes vague speech, the speech of the poor class is logical and expressive. Thought is not buried in verbosity and vagueness. The blunt speech may be uncomfortable to listen to, both in words and ideas (37).

Linguists have found that dialects do have grammatical structure (51, 52). Use of a dialect does not necessarily inhibit abstract thinking. The child must be taught problem-solving and abstract thinking, however. If parents are seldom at home because of work, if the subculture values action more than words, if parents talk little with the child or brush aside questions, and if the child associates more with peers than with adults, he/she is not likely to be stimulated to try new speech forms or new thought patterns. School teachers try, but unfortunately they often have classes too large to give the needed individual instruction, to form a motivating relationship, or to assess fully what the child doesn't know. Parents often wish to help the child learn more; in fact, most poor parents repeatedly emphasize that their children must get an education so that they can achieve more than their parents did. Unfortunately, good intentions and admonitions are not enough. Poor parents often lack the education, energy, time, or resources to help the child advance educationally or even keep up minimally. The farther behind the child gets, the less the likelihood of ever catching up with cognitive skills. The cycle is repeated each generation. Yet most poor parents are receptive to suggestions on how to make the best possible use of their limited resources or what specific measures to follow to enhance the child's development (37, 41, 42, 99, 111).

There is a clear relationship between poverty and ill health. Long-term ill health may contribute to poverty. Poverty predisposes to certain illnesses or causes the person to suffer adverse consequences of illness. The ill child who is poor is less likely to attend school. The poor have a higher infant and maternal mortality rate from accidents, preventive measures are less likely to be carried out in the family (203).

The lower-class person defines self as ill when unable to work for days or weeks. The lower-class person first uses folk or home remedies when ill or may go to a cultural healer. Reluctantly, and only when absolutely necessary, does he/she enter the scientific health care system. The person in abject poverty may not go for professional, scientific care at all because of the lack of knowledge, money, transportation, or an inadequate sense of self-worth. The lower-class person is suspicious of the health worker or feels that there is a distance between the health worker and him/herself. These feelings can be overcome only by a gentle, respectful, courteous, prompt approach and straightforward speech. Although many people feel that much financial assistance is available for the poor and sick, such assistance is limited. Moreover, the poor person is unfamiliar with or unlikely to use community agencies wisely without your assistance. Because the poor person often does not have the resources to practice preventive physical or dental care, he/she may be very ill—even irreversibly—on entry to the health care system (10, 31, 37, 45, 62, 93).

Living in poverty takes its toll physically, emotionally, and mentally. The person who lives in chronic poverty is more likely to have behavioral characteristics opposite to the dominant culture because of not being involved with or learning from the dominant culture. Such behaviors, however, should not be viewed as innately bad, predetermined, irreversible, or the fault of the victims (37).

INFLUENCES OF CULTURE ON HEALTH

Because every culture is complex, it can be difficult to determine whether health and illness are the result of cultural or other factors, such as physiological or psychological factors. Yet there are numerous accounts of the presence or absence of certain diseases in certain cultural groups and reactions to illness that are culturally determined.* Cultural influences may include food availability, dietary taboos, methods of hygiene, and effects of climate—all factors related to culture. Several examples of the influences of culture on health and illness follow. The examples are necessarily limited.

Leaf studied three cultures in which many people live to be very old. These people live in Vilcabamba, Ecuador; in Hunza, located in Pakistani-controlled Kashmir; and in Abkhazia in the Caucasus Mountain region of the Soviet Union. In each of these cultures the old people share in a great deal of the hard labor. Exercise appears to be a major factor in their longevity. In each culture the aged are accorded high social status and occupy a central and privileged position in the ex-

*For further information, see references 9, 103, 130, 136, 150, 166, 184, 195, 209, 236.

tended family. They live with close relatives, are given useful roles, continue daily to perform useful tasks, contribute to the economy of the community, and are sought for counsel and for their wisdom. Sense of family continuity is strong. The elderly are not shunted aside as in Western industrial societies, nor are they forced to retire; instead they remain independent and expect great longevity. Once they lose their useful roles in the community, however, they die quickly (117).

The influence of other cultural folkways on health has been studied. Race, social class, ethnic group, and religion influence distribution of disease and death (22, 75, 85, 92, 118, 127, 143, 188). Epidemiological findings suggest that Jewish women have less cancer of the cervix than non-Jewish women and that these results can be related to circumcision of the Jewish male or to abstinence from intercourse as prescribed by Jewish law for a certain period after the menses. Nuns also have low risk for cancer of the cervix. Generally lower-class and Black women in the United States, with earlier sexual intercourse and early and more frequent childbirth, run a higher risk than the rest of the population—than Jews, in particular. Prostitutes also have a higher incidence of cancer of the cervix, possibly because of multiple sex partners (75). Graham was influenced by the etiological theory proposed by Martin that the uncircumcised non-Jewish male is more likely to harbor a carcinogenic virus, although only certain men carry it. Therefore a woman who has sexual intercourse with a greater number of men during her life has a greater chance of being exposed to the virus and hence runs a greater risk of cervical cancer (137).

To determine the effect of ethnic group on respiratory disease occurrence, average annual sex, ethnic, and disease specific mortality rates for the period of 1969 to 1977 were calculated for New Mexico's American Indian, Hispanic, and Anglo populations. Incidence data were available for respiratory tract cancer. This study corroborates previous findings of reduced mortality from lung cancer in American Indians of both sexes and in Hispanic males. American Indian mortality from tuberculosis and from influenza and pneumonia was high. Hispanic males and American Indians of both sexes showed low mortality rates for chronic obstructive pulmonary disease (COPD). Differing cigarette usage is the most obvious explanation for the variations in COPD and lung cancer occurrence with ethnic groups (188).

Culturally induced belief in magic can cause illness and death. The profound physiological consequences of intense fear, including inability to eat or drink, may be responsible. Yet there may be no physiological changes except in the terminal moments. If the behavior of friends and relatives—what they say or do—strongly reinforces the person's conviction of imminent death, the victim becomes resigned to fate and soon meets it (130).

A culture's favored drink may have implications for health. Health workers in a remote Mexican village found that the only available beverage was an alcoholic drink made from the juice of a local plant. A safe water supply was brought in, but the people did not fare well on it. The local drink was a rich source of essential vitamins and minerals not otherwise present in the local diet. Thus although it may have appeared desirable to change a cultural pattern for certain health reasons, the unanticipated consequences proved detrimental to health in another way.

NURSING IMPLICATIONS

Importance of Cultural Concepts for Nursing

If you live or work in a culture different from your own, you may suffer **cultural shock**, *the feelings of bewilderment, confusion, disorganization, frustration, and stupidity and the inability to adapt to the differences in language and word meanings, activities, time, and customs that are part of the new culture.* An antidote for cultural shock is to look for similarities between your native and new cultures. In order to adapt to a new culture, be interested in the culture and be prepared to ask questions tactfully and to give up some of your own habits. Leininger and Weis give a number of specific suggestions for adapting to another culture (118, 225).

In the United States, you are working in a **pluralistic society** *in which members of diverse ethnic, racial, religious, and social groups maintain independent lifestyles and adhere to certain values within the confines of a common civilization.* Knowledge of other cultures helps you examine your own cultural foundations, values, and beliefs, which, in turn, promotes increased self-understanding. But avoid **ethnocentricity**, *believing that your own ways of behavior are best for everyone.* For example, emphasizing daily bathing to a group who has a severely limited water supply is useless, for the water will be needed for survival. Recognize that your patterns of life and language are peculiar to your culture.

Learning about another's cultural background can promote feelings of respect and humility as well as enhance understanding of the person and the family—his/her needs, likes and dislikes, behavior, attitudes, care and treatment approaches, and sociocultural causes of disease. Cultural differences should be anticipated not only in foreigners and first-generation immigrants but also in persons even further reremoved in time from their native country and in persons from other regions within your country. The person's behavior during illness is influenced by cultural definitions of how he/she should act and the meaning of illness. Understanding this situation and seeking reasons for behavior help to avoid stereotyping and labeling the person as uncooperative and resistant just because the behavior is different. As you consider alternate reasons for behavior, care can be individualized. People from different cultural backgrounds classify health problems differently and have certain expectations about how they should be helped. If cultural differences are ignored, your ability to help the patient and his/her ability to progress toward a personally and culturally defined health status may be hampered. You should be able to translate your knowledge of the health care system into terms that match the concepts of your patients/clients.

All people have some prejudice; it emerges in such expressions as "Those upper-crust people always . . . " or "Those welfare people never. . . ." Examine your thinking for unconscious prejudice, understand your own class background, and distinguish your values from those held by people under your care. Try to withhold value judgments that interfere with your relationship with the patient and with objective care. There are too many unknown factors in people's lives to set up stereotyped categories. A family may be in the middle class or upper class in terms of income, education, and goals, for example, and yet live in an upper-lower-class neighborhood because they refuse to emphasize material wealth. A farmer, according to our criteria, may be labeled upper-lower-class and yet regard him/herself very much a part of the middle class. A person who lives in an economically depressed section of the United States and is poor may have an adequate public education, a middle-class value system, and upper-class graciousness.

If you feel you are stooping by helping lower-class people, you may be labelled a "do-gooder" and be ineffective. Recognize the behavior of the lower class not as pathological but as adaptive for their needs. Realize, too, that not only the poor need your help. The upper-class person may need a great deal of help with care, health teaching, or counseling. Having money does not necessarily mean one is knowledgeable about preventive health measures, nutrition, and disease processes. Persons of all classes deserve competent care, clear explanations, and a helpful attitude.

Knowledge about social classes and cultural groups may help explain late or broken agency appointments that result from fear or inferiority feelings, lack of transportation, or someone to care for the children at home rather than from lack of interest in health. The reservation American Indian or poor Black, for instance, may not be accustomed to keeping a strict time schedule or appointments if unemployed, for a strict clock time orientation is not valued as highly as in the industrialized work force. Take time to talk with the person and you will learn of his/her fears, problems, aspirations, and concern for health and family, and his/her human warmth.

To illustrate, a woman in labor who is a product of a parochial background with reliance on lay medical help and suspicious of the impersonal hospital and professional-looking nurses asks to have a knife placed under the bed to help "cut labor pains." While implementing scientific health care, you can be more prepared to act on this belief that psychologically helps the patient. Herbs used by various cultural groups are increasingly found to have medicinal value; they are chemically similar to drugs used by scientific practitioners.

The misinterpretation of behavior typical of a social class does not always go in one direction, from upper to lower. Suppose that you are a nurse with a working-class background whose patient is a 50-year-old corporation president, admitted for coronary disease, a member of the newly rich class. He seems obsessed with learning when he can resume his professional duties, exactly how many hours he can work daily, and his chances for a recurrence. An understanding of his class position, along with his possible motives, values, and status (which he feels must be maintained), will enable you to work with his seeming obession rather than simply label him an "impossible patient."

Try to accept people as they are regardless of culture or social class. Picture the world from the eyes of others—those you care for. In this way, you can maintain your own personal standards without being shocked by theirs.

Your knowledge of cultures will enable you to practice holistic nursing care, including cultural values and norms in the nursing process. Holistic healing practices combine the best of two worlds: the wisdom and sensitivity of the East and the technology and precision of the West. Although holistic practitioners use conventional therapies in many cases, the emphasis remains on the whole person: physical, emotional, intellectual, spiritual, and sociocultural background. The focus is on prevention and overall fitness and on the individual taking responsibility for his/her own health and well-being. Multiple techniques are used to restore and maintain balance of body energy—the life force. These techniques include exercise, acupuncture, massage, herbal medicine, nutritional changes, manipulation of joints and spine, medications, stress management, and counseling. The nurse-client relationship is the key to holistic nursing care, for the person has come to expect a caring interaction from the healer. The curandera (herb healer) of the Spanish Southwest makes a tea from herbs, for example, and the patient slowly sips the tea. The pain is gone. The client's faith is a major factor in herbal cures—faith in God, the plants, and the curandera. The curandera also has faith in recovery as she shows caring, looks, listens, and heals.

As you assess the person, remember that people differ biologically, physically, and culturally. (See Table 10-9.) Studies on biological baselines for growth and development or normal characteristics have usually been done on White populations. These norms may not be applicable to nonwhites. Biological features, such as skin color, body size and shape, and presence of enzymes, are the result of biological adjustments made by ancestors to the environment in which they lived (18, 160, 181).

Various physical differences are known to exist. **Mongolian spots,** *the hyperpigmented, bluish discoloration* occasionally seen in Caucasian neonates, are normal for many Asians, American Indians, and Blacks. Type of ear wax varies and may determine the presence of ear disease in preschoolers. Dry ear wax is recessive and is found primarily

TABLE 10-9 Assessment of Skin Color

CHARACTERISTIC	WHITE OR LIGHT-SKINNED PERSON	DARK-SKINNED PERSON
Pallor: Vasoconstriction present	Skin takes on white hue, which is color of collagen fibers in subcutaneous connective tissue.	Skin loses underlying red tones. Brown-skinned person appears yellow-brown. Black-skinned person appears ashen-gray. Mucous membranes, lips, nail beds pale or gray.
Erythema, Inflammation: Cutaneous vasodilation	Skin is red.	Palpate for increased warmth of skin, edema, tightness, or induration of skin.
Cyanosis: Hypoxia of tissues	Bluish tinges of skin, especially in earlobes, as well as in lips, oral mucosa, and nailbeds.	Lips, tongue, conjunctiva, palms, soles of feet are pale or ashen gray. Apply light pressure to create pallor; in cyanosis tissue color returns slowly by spreading from periphery to the center.
Ecchymosis: Deoxygenated blood seeps from broken blood vessel into subcutaneous tissue	Skin changes color from purple-blue to yellow-green to yellow.	Obtain history of trauma and discomfort. Note swelling and induration. Oral mucous membrane or conjunctiva will show color changes from purple-blue to yellow-green to yellow.
Petechiae: Intradermal or submucosal bleeding	Round, pinpoint purplish red spots on skin.	Oral mucosa or conjunctiva show purplish-red spots if person has black skin.
Jaundice: Accumulated bilirubin in tissues	Yellow color in skin, mucous membranes, and sclera of eyes. Light-colored stools and dark urine often occur.	Sclera of eyes, oral mucous membranes, palms of hand and soles of feet have yellow discoloration.

in American Indians and Asians. Wet ear wax is found in most Blacks and Caucasians. Also, people with dry ear wax have fewer apocrine glands and perspire less; they usually do not have as much body odor. Thus presence of body odor may be indicative of disease. Pelvic shape of the woman, shape of teeth and tongue, fingerprint pattern, blood type, keloid formation, and presence of the enzyme lactase vary among groups. Persons with certain blood types are more prone to certain illnesses. The adult who has lactose intolerance is missing lactase, the enzyme for digestion and metabolism of lactose in milk and milk products. The person becomes ill on ingestion of these foods. Symptoms include flatulence, distention, abdominal cramping, diarrhea, and colitis. Milk intolerance because of enzyme deficiency occurs in over 80 percent of Chinese, Japanese, and Eskimo adults and in 60 to 80 percent of Native American, Black, Jewish, and Mexican-American adults. Only people of northern European Caucasian extraction and members of two African tribes tolerate lactose indefinitely and even some aged Whites will have lactose deficiency. Do not automatically teach everyone to drink milk. Calcium can be obtained in other ways: seafoods (cook fish to yield edible bones); leafy vegetables; yogurt, buttermilk, or aged cheese (lactose has been changed to lactic acid during aging); or homemade soup (add vinegar to the water when cooking a soupbone to decalcify the bone). Most ethnic groups have adapted ways of cooking to ensure calcium intake from nondairy sources; listen carefully to their dietary descriptions. If the lactase-deficient person wishes to ingest considerable milk foods, an enzyme product to add to milk, called Lact-Aid, may be purchased from drug or health food stores (94, 169, 183). An acidophilus milk, which contains a controlled culture of lactobacillus acidophilus bacteria, is also easily digested.

Other biological variations exist. Susceptibility to disease varies with blood type. Rh-negative blood type is common in Caucasians, rarer in other groups, and absent in Eskimos. Myopia is more common in Chinese; color blindness is more common in Europeans and East Indians. Nose size and shape correlate with ancestral homeland. Small noses (seen in Asians or Eskimos) were produced in cold regions, high-bridged noses (common to Iranians and American Indians) were common in dry areas; and the flat, broad noses characteristic of some Blacks were adaptive in moist, warm climates.

Branch and Paxton, Brink, and Leininger present much specific information in their books that will help you assess and intervene with people from various cultures and subcultures (22, 24, 118).

If the person does not speak English as a first language, learn key words of his/her language. Use language dictionaries or a card file of key words. Breach the language barrier so that your assessment is more accurate and care measures will be understood by the person. Muecke offers practical suggestions to overcome language differences (147).

Learn about the significant religious practices and the everyday patterns of hygiene, eating, types of foods eaten, sleeping, elimination, use of space, and various rituals that are a part of the person's culture. Interference with normal living patterns or practices adds to the stress of being ill. You will encounter and need to adapt patient care to the following customs: drinking tea instead of coffee with meals, eating the main meal at midday instead of in the evening, refusing to undress before a strange person, doing special hair care as described by Grier (80), avoiding use of the bedpan because someone else must handle its contents, maintaining special religious or ethnic customs, refusing to bathe daily, refusing a pelvic exam by a male doctor, moaning loudly when in pain, and showing unreserved demonstrations of grief when a loved one dies.

Respecting the person's need for privacy or need to have others continually around is essential. Understand that some patients or families will not be expressive emotionally or verbally. Respect this pattern, recognizing that nonverbal behavior is also significant. Be aware, too, that word meanings may vary considerably from culture to culture so that the person may have difficulty understanding you and vice versa. Be sure the gesture or touch you use conveys the message you intend. If you are unsure, avoid nonverbal behavior to the extent that you can.

A patient with a strict time orientation must take medicines and receive treatments on time or feel neglected. You are expected to give prompt and efficient, but compassionate, service to the patient and family. Time orientation also affects making appointments for the clinic and plans for medication routine or return to work after discharge and influences the person's ideas about how quickly he/she should get well. The person with little future-time orientation has difficulty planning a future clinic appointment or a long-range medication schedule. This person cannot predict now how he will feel at a later date and thinks that clinic visits or medicines are unnecessary if he/she feels all right at the moment.

For some patients, the hurrying behavior of the nurse is distressing; it conveys a lack of concern and lack of time to give adequate care. In turn, the patient expresses guilt feelings when it is necessary to ask for help. Although you may look very efficient when scurrying, you are likely to miss many observations, cues, and hidden meanings in what the patient says.

Examine your own attitude about busyness and leisure in order to help others consider leisure as part of life. The disabled patient, whose inability to work carries a stigma, must develop a positive attitude about leisure and may seek your help.

Relations between the patient and the family may at times seem offensive or disharmonious to you. Differentiate carefully between patterns of behavior that are culturally induced and expected and those that are unhealthy for the persons involved.

The changing society may cause families to have a variety of problems. Be a supportive listener, validate realistic ideas, prepare the family to adapt to a new or changing environment, and be aware of community agencies or resources that can provide additional help. When a patient has no family nearby and seems alone and friendless, you may provide significant support.

Develop a personal philosophy that promotes a feeling of stability in your life so that you, in turn, can assist the patient and family to explore feelings and to formulate a philosophy for coping with change. Toffler speaks about ways in which the person can learn to cope with rapid change. One important way is to develop some ritual or pattern in your personal life that you can practice regardless of where you are and thus maintain some sense of continuity and stability (212).

Several authors have written of their successful experiences in adapting care to certain cultural or social class groups. Success has resulted from an accurate assessment and understanding of the person or group, acceptance of differences, and practical suggestions to promote compliance with prescribed health practices while the person or group also maintained culturally preferred treatments.*

You may also talk with members of the National Association of Hispanic Nurses, the American Indian/Alaskan Indian Nurses Association, and the Black Nurses Association in order to gain information about how to give care that includes cultural values and customs.

Promoting Health in Other Cultures through Education

One way to have a lasting effect on the health practices of a different cultural group is through health teaching that includes a philosophy of prevention. Present-day China compared with China during the 1940s is an example of how public health standards can be effectively raised through an emphasis on prevention (201). Increasingly your role includes health education, as discussed in Chapter 5. Outsiders cannot make decidions for others, but people should be given sufficient knowledge concerning alternate behavior so that they can make intelligent choices themselves.

Various pressures interfere with attempts at health teaching. Behind poor health habits lie more than ignorance, economic pressure, or

*See references 3, 14, 22, 23, 44, 50, 102, 110, 117, 119, 124, 126, 127, 150, 185, 193, 201, 204, 205, 228, and 235.

selfish desires. Motivation plays a great part in continuing certain practices even though the person has been taught differently by you. Motivation, moreover, is influenced by the person's culture, status, and role in that culture and by social pressures for conformity. Starting programs of prevention can be difficult when people place a low value on health, cannot recognize cause-and-effect relationships in disease, lack future-time orientation, or are confused about the existence of preventive measures in their culture. Thus preventive programs or innovations in health care must be shaped to fit the cultural and health profiles of the population. Long-range prevention goals stand a better chance of implementation if combined with measures to meet immediate needs. A mother is more likely to heed your advice about how to prevent further illness in her sick child if you give the child immediate attention.

Be mindful of how people view you. If they cannot understand you, if you threaten their values, or if they view you as an untouchable professional, you will not cross the cultural barrier.

REFERENCES

1. **Abercombie, Thomas,** "Japan's Historic Heartland," *National Geographic*, 137, no. 3 (1970) 295–339.
2. **Aeschleman, Dorothy,** "Guidelines for Cross-Cultural Health Programs," *Nursing Outlook*, 21, no. 10 (1973), 660–63.
3. **Aichlmayr, Rita,** "Cultural Understanding: A Key to Acceptance," *Nursing Outlook*, 17, no. 7 (1969), 20–23.
4. **Ailinger, Rita,** "A Study of Illness Referral in a Spanish Speaking Community," *Nursing Research*, 26, no. 1 (1977), 53-56.
5. **Anderson, Charles,** *White Protestant Americans: From National Origins to Religious Groups*. Englewood Cliffs, NJ: Prentice-Hall, Inc., 1970.
6. **Anderson, Gwen,** and **Bridget Tighs,** "Gypsy Culture and Health Care," *American Journal of Nursing*, 73, no. 2 (1973), 282–85.
7. **Anthony-Tkach, Catherine,** "Care of the Mexican-American Patient," *Nursing and Health Care*, 2, no. 8 (1981), 424-32.
8. **Aramoni, Aniceto,** "Maschismo," *Psychology Today*, 5, no. 8 (1972), 69–72.
9. **Baca, Josephine,** "Some Health Beliefs of the Spanish Speaking," *American Journal of Nursing*, 69, no. 10 (1969), 2172–76.
10. **Becher, Marshall,** et al., "A New Approach to Explaining Sick-Role Behavior in Low-Income Populations," *American Journal of Public Health*, 64, no. 3 (1974), 205–15.
11. **Beck, R. H.,** *Migrant Health Problems*. Washington, D.C.: Inter-America Research Associates, 1975.
12. **Beland, Irene,** and **Joyce Passos,** *Clinical Nursing: Pathophysiological and Psychosocial Approaches* (3rd ed.). London: Collier-MacMillan, Ltd., The Macmillan Publishing Company, 1975.
13. **Bernadino, Stephanie,** *The Ethnic Almanac*. Garden City, NY: Doubleday & Co., Inc., 1981.

14. **Berry, E.**, "HOPE Docks in Guinea," *American Journal of Nursing*, 66, no. 10 (1966), 2238–42.
15. **Billingsley, A.**, *Black Families in White America*. Englewood Cliffs, NJ: Prentice-Hall, Inc., 1968.
16. ——, *Black Families and the Struggle for Survival: Teaching Our Children to Walk Tall*. New York: Friendship Press, 1974.
17. **Birkert-Smith, K.**, *Eskimos*. New York: Crown Publishers, Inc., 1971.
18. **Block, Bobbie**, and **Mary Hunter**, "Teaching Physiological Assessment of Black Persons," *Nurse Educator*, 6, no. 1 (1981), 24–27.
19. **Bossard, J.**, and **E. Boll**, *The Sociology of Child Development* (4th ed.). New York: Harper & Row, Publishers, Inc., 1966.
20. **Bouws, Beth**, "Working with Albanian Families," *American Journal of Nursing*, 74, no. 5 (1974), 902–5.
21. **Bragdon, Ida**, "How to Help Migrant Children," *Today's Education*, January–February 1976, pp. 57–58.
22. **Branch, Marie**, and **Phyllis Paxton**, *Providing Safe Nursing Care for Ethnic People of Color*. New York: Appleton-Century-Crofts, 1976.
23. **Briggs, J. L.**, *Never in Anger, Portrait of an Eskimo Family*. Cambridge, MA: Harvard University Press, 1970.
24. **Brink, Pamela**, ed., *Transcultural Nursing*. Englewood Cliffs, NJ: Prentice-Hall, Inc., 1976.
25. **Brinton, D.**, "Health Center Milieu: Interaction of Nurses and Low Income Families," *Nursing Research*, 21, no. 1 (1972), 46–52.
26. **Brockington, Fraser**, "Health Education as a Cultural Philosophy," *International Journal of Nursing Studies*, 1, no. 1 (1941), 17–25.
27. **Brown, Esther**, *Newer Dimensions of Patient Care, Part III; Patients As People*. New York: Russell Sage Foundation, 1964.
28. **Bruhn, John G.**, "An Epidemiological Study of Myocardial Infarctions in an Italian-American Community," *Journal of Chronic Diseases*, 18 (April 1965), 353–65.
29. ——, et al., "Social Aspects of Coronary Heart Disease in a Pennsylvania German Community," *Social Science and Medicine*, 2 (June 1968), 201–13.
30. **Bucker, Kathleen**, et al., "Racial Differences in Incidence of ABO Hemolytic Disease," *American Journal of Public Health*, 66, no. 9 (1976), 854–58.
31. **Bullough, Bonnie**, and **Vern Bullough**, *Poverty, Ethnic Identity and Health Care*. New York: Appleton-Century-Crofts, 1972.
32. **Cadena, Maxine**, "The Mexican-American Family and the Mexican-American Nurse," in *Family Health Care*, eds., Debra Hymovich and Martha Barnard. New York: McGraw-Hill Book Company, 1979.
33. **Campbell, Teresa**, and **Betty Chung**, "Health Care of the Chinese in America," *Nursing Outlook*, 21, no. 4 (1973), 245–49.
34. **Campbell, W. D.**, "Delivering Health Care to Domestic Farmworkers," *Texas Medicine*, 70 (1974), 113–17.
35. **Chase, L.**, and **F. Kumar**, "Nutritional Status of Preschool Mexican American Migrant Farm Children," *American Journal of Disease of Children*, 122 (1971), 7.
36. **Coakley, T. Anne**, **Paul Ehrlich**, and **Elaine Hurd**, "Southeast Asian Refugees:

Health Screening in a Family Clinic," *American Journal of Nursing*, 80, no. 11 (1980), 2032–36.

37. **Cohen, Susan,** et al., *Culture of Poverty Revisited*. New York: Mental Health Committee Against Racism, n.d.
38. **Cole, Joan,** and **Marc Pilisuk,** "Difference in the Provision of Mental Health Services by Race," *American Journal of Orthopsychiatry*, 46, no. 3 (1976), 510–25.
39. **Coles, Robert,** "The Children of Affluence," *The Atlantic Monthly*, September 1977, pp. 53–66.
40. _____, *Eskimos, Chicanos, Indians*. Boston: Little, Brown & Company, 1978.
41. **Comer, James,** *Beyond Black and White*. New York: Quadrangle Books, 1972.
42. _____, and **Alvin Poussaint,** *Black Child Care*. New York: Simon & Schuster, Inc., 1975.
43. **Cordasco, Francesco, ed.,** *Studies in Italian American Social History*. Totowa, NJ: Rowman and Littlefield, 1975.
44. **Cunningham, M., H. Sanders,** and **P. Weatherly,** "We Went to Mississippi," *American Journal of Nursing*, 67, no. 4 (1967), 801–4.
45. **Davis, Anne,** "The Poor Can Least Afford It: Poverty and Health in the United States," *International Nursing Review*, 18, no. 4 (1971), 360–66.
46. **Davis, Mardell,** "Getting to the Root of the Problem," *Nursing '77*, 7, no. 4 (1977), 60–65.
47. **Davitz, Lois, Y. Sameshima,** and **J. Davitz,** "Suffering as Viewed in Six Different Cultures," *American Journal of Nursing*, 76, no. 8 (1976), 1296–97.
48. **DeLaguna, Frederica,** *Voyage to Greenland*. New York: W. W. Norton & Co., Inc., 1977.
49. **Deutsch, Elizabeth,** "A Stereotype—or an Individual?" *Nursing Outlook*, 19, no. 2 (1971), 106–8.
50. **Devitt, H.,** "Nursing in a Vietnam Village," *Nursing Outlook*, 14, no. 12 (1966), 46–49.
51. **Dilliard, J.,** "Negro Children's Dialect in the Inner City," *Florida FL Reporter*, Fall 1967.
52. _____, "Non-Standard Negro Dialects: Convergence or Divergence?" *Florida FL Reporter*, Fall 1968, pp. 9–12.
53. **Dimancescu, Dan,** "Kayak Odyssey from the Inland Sea to Tokyo," *National Geographic*, 132, no. 3 (1967), 295–336.
54. **Dimond, E., Grey,** *More Than Herbs and Acupuncture*. New York: W. W. Norton & Co., Inc., 1975.
55. "Down and Out in America," *Newsweek*, March 15, 1982, pp. 28–29.
56. **Dumond, Don E.,** *The Eskimos and the Aluets*. London: Thames and Hudson, Ltd., 1977.
57. **Ehling, M. B.,** The Mexican American (el chicano), in *Culture and Childrearing*, ed. A. L. Clark. Philadelphia: F. A. Davis Company, 1981.
58. **Ehrenreich, Barbara,** and **Karin Stallard,** "The Nouveau Poor," *The New Day*, 14, no. 4 (1982), 1.
59. **Eliot, Alexander,** *Greece*, Life World Library. New York: Time, Inc., 1963.
60. **Erkel, E. A.,** "The Implications of Cultural Conflict for Health Care, *Health Values: Achieving High Level Wellness*, 4 (1981), 51–57.

61. *Ethnicity and Health Care*. New York: National League for Nursing, 1976.
62. **Fabrega, Horacio, R. Moore,** and **J. Strawn,** "Low Income Medical Problem Patients: Some Medical and Behavioral Features," *Journal of Health and Social Behavior*, 10 (December 1969), 334–43.
63. **Farge, E. J.,** "Medical Orientation Among a Mexican American Population: An Old and New Model Reviewed," *Social Science Quarterly*, 33 (1977), 46–55.
64. **Feinman, Saul,** "Trends in Racial Self-Image of Black Children: Psychological Consequences of a Social Movement," *Journal of Negro Education*, 48, no. 4 (1979), 488–99.
65. **Fitzpatrick, Joseph,** *Puerto Rican Americans: The Meaning of Migration to the Mainland*. Englewood Cliffs, NJ: Prentice-Hall, Inc., 1971.
66. **Flaskerud, Jacquelyn,** "Perceptions of Problematic Behavior by Appalachians, Mental Health Professionals, and Lay Non-Appalachians," *Nursing Research*, 29, no. 3 (1980), 140–49.
67. **Floriani, Carol,** "Southeast Asian Refugees: Life in a Camp," *American Journal of Nursing*, 80, no. 11 (1980), 2028–30.
68. **Fuentes, J. A.,** "The Need for Effective and Comprehensive Planning for Migrant Workers," *American Journal of Public Health*, 64 (1974), 2–10.
69. **Gadey, Jon,** *Alaska, the Sophisticated Wilderness*. New York: Stein and Day, Publishers, 1976.
70. **Galston, Arthur,** *Daily Life in People's China*. New York: Thomas Y. Crowell Co., Inc., 1973.
71. **Gibson, G.,** "An Approach to Identification and Prevention of Developmental Difficulties Among Mexican American Children," *American Journal of Orthopsychiatry*, 48 (1978), 96–112.
72. **Glenn, Max,** *Appalachia in Transition*. St. Louis: Bethany Press Co., 1970.
73. **Goldstein, Sidney,** *Jewish Americans: Three Generations in a Jewish Community*. Englewood Cliffs, NJ: Prentice-Hall, Inc., 1968.
74. **Gordon, Verona, Irene Matonsek,** and **Theresa Lang,** "Southeast Asian Refugees: Life in America," *American Journal of Nursing*, 80, no. 11 (1980), 2031–36.
75. **Graham, Saxon,** "Cancer, Culture, and Social Structure," in *Patients, Physicians, and Illness* (2nd ed.), ed. E. Gartly Jaco. New York: The Free Press, 1972, pp. 31–39.
76. **Greely, Andrew,** *Ethnicity in the United States: A Preliminary Reconnaissance*. New York: Wiley-Interscience, 1974.
77. **Greenfield, Patricia,** and **Jerome Bruner,** "Work with the Wolof," *Psychology Today*, 5, no. 2 (1971), 40 ff.
78. **Gregg, Elinor,** *The Indians and the Nurse*. Norman: University of Oklahoma Press, 1965.
79. **Gresser, Linda,** "Healing Hands: A New Mexico Herbalist," *The Herbalist*, 5, nos. 4–5 (1980), 7.
80. **Grier, Margaret,** "Hair Care for the Black Patient," *American Journal of Nursing*, 76, no. 11 (1976), 1781.
81. **Grossberg, Kenneth A.,** ed., *Japan Today*. Philadelphia: Ishi Institute for Study of Human Issues, Inc., 1981.

82. **Guralnik, David,** ed., *Webster's New World Dictionary of the American Language* (2nd college ed.). New York: World Publishing Company, 1972.
83. **Handel, George,** "Sociological Aspects of Parenthood," in *Family Health Care*, eds. Debra Hymovich and Martha Barnard. New York: McGraw-Hill Book Company, 1973, pp. 71–92.
84. **Hanson, Robert,** and **Lyle Saunders,** *Nurse-Patient Communication: A Manual for Public Health Nurses in Northern New Mexico*. Washington, D.C.: United States Department of Health, Education, and Welfare, 1964.
85. **Harris, Ralph,** et al., "The Child-Adolescent Blood Pressure Study: Distribution of Blood Pressure Levels in Seventh Day Adventist (SDA) and Non-SDA Children," *American Journal of Public Health*, 71, no. 12 (1981), 1342–48.
86. **Hartley, William,** "The Old Ways Linger: Chinese Herb Doctors Still Treat Taiwanese," *The Wall Street Journal*, October 10, 1969, p. 9.
87. **Harwood, Alan,** "The Hot-Cold Theory of Disease: Implications for Treatment of Puerto Rican Patients," *Journal of American Medical Association*, 216, no. 7 (May 17, 1971), 1153–58.
88. **Hauser, Philip,** "Urban U.S.A.—A Chaotic Society," *Nursing Outlook*, 18, no. 3 (1970), 48–49.
89. **Hecker, Melvin,** and **Heike, Fenton,** eds., *The Greeks in America, 1528–1977*. Dobbs Ferry, NY: Oceana Publishers, Inc., 1978.
90. **Henry, Beverly,** and **Elizabeth Di Giacomo-Geffers,** "The Hospitalized Rich and Famous," *American Journal of Nursing*, 80, no. 8 (1980), 1426–29.
91. **Hill, R.** *The Strengths of Black Families*. New York: Emerson Hall Publishers, Inc., 1972.
92. **Holck, Susan,** et al., "Lung Cancer Mortality and Smoking Habits: Mexican-American Women," *American Journal of Public Health*, 72, no. 1 (1982), 38–42.
93. **Hollingshead, August,** and **Frederick C. Redlich,** *Social Class and Mental Illness: A Community Study*. New York: John Wiley & Sons, Inc., 1958.
94. **Hongladarom, Gail,** and **Millie Russell,** "An Ethnic Difference—Lactose Intolerance," *Nursing Outlook*, 24, no. 12 (1976), 764–65.
95. **Horner, Mary, C. Olson,** and **D. Pringle,** "Nutritional Status and Chippewa Head Start Children in Wisconsin," *American Journal of Public Health*, 67, no. 2 (1977), 185–86.
96. "How Are Things in Your Neighborhood?" *Graduate Woman*, March–April 1980, 17 ff.
97. **Hunt, D.,** "Reflections on Racial Perspectives," *Journal of Afro-American Issues*, 2, no. 4 (1974), 361–69.
98. **Hutchinson, Sarah,** "The American Indian Senior Citizens View of Women," *Bulletin of American Association of Social Psychiatry* ,1, no 3 (1980), 13–15.
99. **Hutto, Ruth,** "Poverty's Children," *American Journal of Nursing*, 69, no. 10 (1969), 2166–69.
100. "Income and Status in the '70's," *St. Louis Post-Dispatch*, January 23, 1976, Sec. A, pp. 3 ff.
101. "Issues on Poverty and Health Care," *Nursing Outlook*, 17, no. 9 (1969), 33–75.

102. **Jacobson, Phyllis,** "The Y. Family," *American Journal of Nursing*, 69, no. 9 (1969), 1951–52.
103. **Jewell, D.,** "A Case of a 'Psychotic' Navajo Indian Male," in *Social Interaction and Patient Care*, eds. J. Skipper and R. Leonard. Philadelphia: J. B. Lippincott Company, 1965, pp. 184–95.
104. **Johnson, Nichols,** "The Careening of America," in *Moral Values in Contemporary Society*. St. Louis, MO: Webster College, 1975, pp. 71–121.
105. **Kagan, Spencer,** and **Philip Ender,** "Maternal Response to Success and Failure of Anglo-American, Mexican-American and Mexican Children," *Child Development*, 46 (1975), 452–58.
106. **Kahl, Joseph A.,** *The American Class Structure*. New York: Holt, Rinehart & Winston, 1967.
107. **Kegeles, S. Stephen,** "A Field Experimental Attempt to Change Beliefs and Behavior of Women in an Urban Ghetto," *Journal of Health and Social Behavior*, 10 (June 1969), 115–24.
108. **Kitano, Harry,** *Japanese-Americans: Evolution of a Subculture*. Englewood Cliffs, NJ: Prentice-Hall, Inc., 1966.
109. **Kluckhorn, Florence,** "Family Diagnosis: Variations in Basic Values of Family Systems," *Social Casework*, 32 (February–March 1958), 63–72.
110. **Kniep-Hardy, Mary,** and **Margaret Burkhardt,** "Nursing the Navaho," *American Journal of Nursing*, 77, no. 1 (1977), 95–96.
111. **Kohn, Melvin,** "Social Class and Parent-Child Relationships," in *Human Life Cycle*, ed. Wm. Sze. New York: Jason Aronson, Inc., 1975, pp. 541–53.
112. **Kuhn, Delia,** and **Ferdinand Kuhn,** *The Philippines—Yesterday and Today*. New York: Holt, Rinehart & Winston, 1966.
113. **LaFargue, J.,** "Role of Prejudice in Rejection of Health Care," *Nursing Research*, 21, no. 1 (1972), 53–58.
114. ——, "A Survival Strategy: Kinship Networks," *American Journal of Nursing*, 80, no. 9 (1980), 1636–39.
115. **Lane, Robert,** and **Michael Lerner,** "Why Hard Hats Hate Hairs," *Psychology Today*, 4, no. 6 (1970), 45 ff.
116. **Lauman, Edward O.,** *Bonds of Pluralism: The Form and Substance of Urban Social Networks*. New York: Wiley-Interscience, 1973.
117. **Leaf, Alexander, M.D.,** "Every Day Is a Gift When You Are over 100," *National Geographic*, 143, no. 1 (1973), 93–119.
118. **Leininger, Madeline,** *Nursing and Anthropology: Two Worlds to Blend*. New York: John Wiley & Sons, Inc., 1970.
119. **Leonard, Sister Margaret Ann,** and **Sister Carol Ann Joyce,** "Two Worlds United," *American Journal of Nursing*, 71, no. 6 (1971), 1152–55.
120. **Lieberman, Harry M.,** and **Rodney M. Powell,** "Health Services for the Poor," *Public Health Reports*, 85, no. 4 (1970), 284–94.
121. "Life Below the Poverty Line," *Newsweek*, April 5, 1982, pp. 20–28.
122. **Lipset, Seymour,** and **Everett Ladd,** "And What Professors Think," *Psychology Today*, 4, no. 6 (1970), 44 ff.
123. **Lopata, H.,** *Polish Americans*. Englewood Cliffs, NJ: Prentice-Hall, Inc., 1976.
124. **Loughlin, B.,** "Pregnancy in the Navajo Culture," *Nursing Outlook*, 13, no. 3 (1965), 55–58.

125. **Lynn, F.**, "An American Nurse Visits Two Mental Hospitals in Greece," *Nursing Outlook*, 14, no. 12 (1966), 50-53.
126. **McCabe, Gracia**, "Cultural Influences on Patient Behavior," *American Journal of Nursing*, 60, no. 8 (1960), 1101-4.
127. **McEvoy, Larry**, and **Garland Land**, "Life Style and Death Patterns of the Missouri RLD's Church Members," *American Journal of Public Health*, 71, no. 12 (1981), 1350-56.
128. **McGregor, Frances**, "Uncooperative Patients: Some Cultural Interpretations," *American Journal of Nursing*, 67, no. 1 (1967), 88-91.
129. **McKenzie, Joan**, and **Noel Chrisman**, "Healing Herbs, Gods, and Magic: Folk Health Beliefs Among Filipino-Americans," *Nursing Outlook*, 26, no. 5 (1977), 326-29.
130. **MacDonald, Anne**, "Folk Health Practices Among North Coastal Peruvians: Implications for Nursing," *Image*, 13, no. 6 (1981), 51-56.
131. **MacLachlan, J.**, "Cultural Factors in Health and Disease," in *Patients, Physicians, and Illness: Behavioral Science and Medicine*, ed. E. Gartly Jaco. Glencoe, IL: Free Press, 1958, pp. 95-105.
132. **Maher, Father Trafford**, *Self—A Measureless Sea*. St. Louis: The Catholic Hospital Association, 1966.
133. **Malmstrom, Jean**, "Dialects—Updated," *Florida FL Reporter*, Spring-Summer 1969.
134. **Mandel, Marjorie**, "Hard Times Displace the New Homeless," *St. Louis Post-Dispatch*, May 2, 1982, Sec. A., p. 7.
135. **Mandell, Arnold**, and **Mary Mandell**, "What Can Nursing Learn from the Behavioral Sciences?" *American Journal of Nursing*, 63, no. 6 (1963), 104-7.
136. **Mangin, William**, "Mental Health and Migration to Cities: A Peruvian Case," *Annals of the New York Academy of Science*, 84 (1960), 911-17.
137. **Martin, C.**, "Marital and Coital Factors in Cervical Cancer," *American Journal of Public Health*, 57, no. 5 (1967), 803-14.
138. **Martines, Edward**, *The Mexican American*. Boston: Houghton Mifflin Company, 1973.
139. **Mason, Diana**, "Perspectives on Poverty," *Image*, 13, no. 3 (1981), 82-88.
140. **Mead, Margaret**, *Cultural Patterns and Technical Change*. New York: The New American Library, Mentor Books, 1955.
141. **Melees, Afaf**, "The Arab American in the Health Care System," *American Journal of Nursing*, 81, no. 6 (1981), 1880-83.
142. **Moore, John**, *Mexican-Americans*. Englewood Cliffs, NJ: Prentice-Hall, Inc., 1976.
143. **Moore, L. G.**, **P. W. VanArsdale**, **J. E. Glittenberg**, and **R. A. Aldrich**, *The Biocultural Basis of Health Care*. St. Louis: The C. V. Mosby Company, 1980.
144. **Morgan, Lael**, *And the Land Provides: Alaskan Natives in a Year of Transition*. Garden City, NY: Anchor Press/Doubleday & Co., Inc., 1974.
145. **Moses, Marion**, "Viva in Causa," *American Journal of Nursing*, 73, no. 5 (1973), 843-48.
146. **Mott, Paul E.** *The Organization of Society*. Englewood Cliffs, NJ: Prentice-Hall, Inc., 1976.

147. **Muecke, Marjorie,** "Overcoming the Language Barrier," *Nursing Outlook*, 22, no. 4 (1970), 53–54.
148. **Mummah, R.,** "Sakaguchi San and I Had a Contract: A Nurse Helps a Patient Surmount Seemingly Insurmountable Setbacks, *Nursing '78*, 8, no. 12 (1978), 36, 38.
149. **Murillo, N.,** "The Mexican American Family," in *Chicanos: Social and Psychological Perspectives*, eds. C. A. Hernandez, M. J. Haug, and N. W. Wagner. St. Louis: The C. V. Mosby Company, 1976.
150. **Murphy, Patricia,** "Tuberculosis Control in San Francisco's Chinatown," *American Journal of Nursing*, 70, no. 5 (1970), 1044–46.
151. **Naimann, H.,** "Nursing in Jewish Law," *American Journal of Nursing*, 70, no. 11 (1970), 2378–79.
152. **Nail, Frank,** and **Joseph Spellberg,** "Social and Cultural Factors in the Responses of Mexican-Americans to Medical Treatment," *Journal of Health and Social Behavior*, 8 (December 1967), 299–308.
153. **Navarro, Vicente,** "The Underdevelopment of Health of Working America: Causes, Consequences, and Possible Solutions," *American Journal of Public Health*, 66, no. 6 (1976), 538–47.
154. **Newman, Monroe,** *The Political Economy of Appalachia*. Lexington, MA: D. C. Heath & Company, 1972.
155. **Newman, William M.,** *American Pluralism: A Study of Minority Groups and Social Theory*. New York: Harper & Row, Publishers, Inc., 1973.
156. **Newton, Jules,** "Childbirth and Culture," *Psychology Today*, 4, no. 6 (1970), 75 ff.
157. **Niekerson, Gifford,** and **Donald Hochstrasser,** "Factors Affecting Non-Participation in a County-wide Tuberculin Testing Program in Southern Appalachia," *Social Science and Medicine*, 3 (April 1970), 575–96.
158. **Norbury, Paul,** ed. *Introducing Japan*. New York: St. Martin's Press, Inc., 1977.
159. **Ogburn, William,** and **M. Nimkoff,** *Sociology* (2nd ed.). Boston: Houghton Mifflin Company, 1950.
160. **Overfield, Theresa,** "Biological Variations: Concepts from Physical Anthropology," *Nursing Clinics of North America*, 12, no. 1 (1977), 19–26.
161. **Packard, Vance,** *The People Shapers*. Boston: Little, Brown & Company, 1977.
162. **Park, Jeanne,** "Children Who Follow the Sun," *Today's Education*, January–February 1976, pp. 53–56.
163. **Parker, S.,** and **R. J. Kleiner,** "The Culture of Poverty: An Adjustive Dimension," *American Anthropologist*, 72 (1970), 516–27.
164. **Parson, Talcott,** *Essays in Sociological Theory* (rev. ed.). London: Collier-Macmillan, Ltd., 1964, pp. 275–97.
165. ———, "Definitions of Health and Illness in the Light of American Values and Social Structure," in *Patients, Physicians and Illness* (2nd ed.), ed. E. Gartly Jaco. New York: The Free Press, 1972, pp. 118–27.
166. **Paul, Benjamin,** "Anthropological Perspectives on Medicine and Public Health," *Annals of the American Academy of Political and Social Science*, 346, no. 3 (1963), 34–43.

167. **Paynich, M.,** "Cultural Barriers to Nurse Communication," *American Journal of Nursing*, 64, no. 2 (1964), 87–90.
168. **Persad, Emmanuel,** "Some Cultural Factors in Psychiatric Training," *Canadian Mental Health*, 19, nos. 3–4 (1971), 11–15.
169. **Pinkney, Alphonse,** *Black Americans*. Englewood Cliffs, NJ: Prentice-Hall, Inc., 1975.
170. **Prather, Jeffrey L.,** *A Mere Reflection: The Psychodynamics of Black and Hispanic Psychology*. Ardmore, PA: Dorrance, 1977.
171. **Prattes, Ora,** "Beliefs of the Mexican-American Family," in *Family Health Care*, eds. Debra Hymovich and Martha Barnard. New York: McGraw-Hill Book Company, 1973, pp. 128–37.
172. **Primeaux, Martha,** "Caring for the American Indian Patient," *American Journal of Nursing*, 77, no. 1 (1977), 91–94.
173. _____, "American Indian Health Care Practices," *Nursing Clinics of North America*, 12, no. 1 (1977), 55–65.
174. **Proctor, Pamela,** "Rich Women Who Work for Fun and Profit," *Parade*, January 23, 1977, pp. 12–14.
175. **Queen, Stuart,** and **Robert Habenstein,** *The Family in Various Cultures* (4th ed.). Philadelphia: J. B. Lippincott Company, 1974.
176. **Rainwater, Lee,** "Crucible of Identity: The Negro Lower Class Family," in *Human Life Cycle*, ed. Wm. Sze. New York: Jason Aronson, Inc. 1975, pp. 109–42.
177. **Ramey, Craig,** and **Frances Campbell,** "Parental Attitudes and Poverty," *Journal of Genetic Psychology*, 128 (1976), 3–6.
178. **Rasmussen, David,** "Black Lung in Southern Appalachia," *American Journal of Nursing*, 70, no. 3 (1970), 509–11.
179. **Richardson, Stephens, N. Goodman, A. Hostorf,** and **S. Dornbusch,** "Cultural Uniformity in Reaction to Physical Disabilities," *American Sociological Review*, 26, no. 2 (1961), 241–47.
180. **Rippley, La Vern J.,** *The German-Americans*. Boston: Twayne Publishers, Division of G. K. Hall and Company, 1976.
181. **Roach, Lora,** "Assessment: Color Changes in Dark Skin," *Nursing '77*, 7, no. 1 (1977), 48–51.
182. **Rose, Peter I.,** ed., *Nation of Nations: The Ethnic Experience and the Racial Crisis*. New York: Random House, 1972.
183. **Rosenberg, Frances,** "Lactose Intolerance," *American Journal of Nursing*, 77, no. 5 (1977), 823–24.
184. **Rubel, Arthur,** "Concepts of Disease in Mexican-American Culture," *American Anthropologist*, 62 (1960), 795–814.
185. **Russell, B.,** and **L. Lofstrom,** "Health Clinic for the Alienated," *American Journal of Nursing*, 71, no. 1 (1971), 80–83.
186. **Sachman, E. A.,** "Sociomedical Variations Among Ethnic Groups," *American Journal of Sociology*, November 1970, pp. 319–31.
187. **Saloutos, Theodore,** *The Greeks in the United States*. Cambridge, MA: Harvard University Press, 1964.
188. **Samet, Jonathan,** et al., "Respiratory Disease Mortality in New Mexico's American Indians and Hispanics," *American Journal of Public Health*, 70, no. 5 (1980), 492–97.

189. **Sanders, I., and E. Morawska,** *Polish American Community Life: A Survey of Research*. Boston: Boston University Press, 1975.
190. **Saunders, Lyle,** *Cultural Differences and Medical Care*. New York: Russell Sage Foundation, 1954.
191. **Schalk, Adolph,** *The Germans*. Englewood Cliffs, NJ: Prentice-Hall, Inc., 1971.
192. **Schmidt, Cheryl,** "Five Become a Team in Appalachia," *American Journal of Nursing*, 75, no. 8 (1975), 1314–15.
193. **Schneider, V.,** "Letter from Lambarene," *American Journal of Nursing*, 65, no. 10 (1965), 128–30.
194. **Schroeder, Albert, ed.,** *The Changing Ways of Southwestern Indians: A Historic Prospective*. Glorietta, NM: The Rio Grande Press, Inc., 1973.
195. **Scotch, Norman,** "A Preliminary Report on the Relation of Sociocultural Factors to Hypertension Among the Zulu," *Annals of the New York Academy of Science*, 84 (1960), 1000–9.
196. **Shiloh, Ailon, and Ida Selavan, eds.,** *Ethnic Groups of America: Their Morbidity, Mortality, and Behavior Disorders, Volume I—The Jews*. Springfield, IL: Charles C Thomas, Publisher, 1973.
197. **Shinkle, Florence,** "An Indian Way of Life, 1975: Insight on the Omaha Indians," *St. Louis Post-Dispatch* (Sunday Pictures), November 23, 1975, pp. 4–14.
198. **Shor, Franc,** "Japan: The Exquisite Enigma," *National Geographic*, 118, no. 6 (1969), 733–77.
199. **Sowell, Thomas,** *Ethnic America: A History*. New York: Basic Books, Inc., 1981.
200. **Sparber, Jean,** "Working with Low-Income Families," in *Family Health Care*, eds. Debra Hymovich and Martha Barnard. New York: McGraw-Hill Book Company, 1973, pp. 149–66.
201. **Stallsmith, J.,** "Treat or Tribulation?" *American Journal of Nursing*, 66, no. 8 (1966), 1782–83.
202. **Stanley, Margaret,** "China: Then and Now," *American Journal of Nursing*, 72, no. 12 (1972), 2213–18.
203. **Starfield, Barbara,** "Child Health and Socioeconomic Status," *American Journal of Public Health*, 72, no. 6 (1982), 532–33.
204. **Steinman, David,** "Health in Rural Poverty," *American Journal of Public Health*, 60, no. 9 (1970), 1813–22.
205. **Stern, Phyllis,** "Solving Problems of Cross-Cultural Health Teaching: The Filopino Childbearing Family," *Image*, 13, no. 6 (1981), 47–50.
206. **Stewart, W.,** "Sociolinguistic Factors in the History of American Negro Dialects," *Florida FL Reporter*, Spring 1967.
207. ——, "Continuity and Change in American Negro Dialects," *Florida FL Reporter*, Spring 1968.
208. **Suchman, Edward,** "Social Patterns of Illness and Medical Care," in *Patients, Physicians, and Illness* (2nd ed.), ed. E. Gartly Jaco. New York: The Free Press, 1972, pp. 262–79.
209. **Tao-Kim-Hai, A.,** "Orientals Are Stoic," in *Social Interaction and Patient Care,* eds. J. Skipper and R. Leonard. Philadelphia: J. B. Lippincott Company, 1965, pp. 142–55.

210. **Tarshis, Barry,** *The Average American Book.* Saddle Brook, NJ: American Book-Stratford Press, 1979.
211. "The Evolution of a Culture," *Psychology Today,* 5, no. 3 (1971), 63–75.
212. **Toffler, Alvin,** *Future Shock.* New York: Bantam Books, 1970.
213. **Torrey, E. F.,** "Mental Health Services for American Indians & Eskimos," *Community Mental Health Journal,* 6, no. 12 (1970), 455–63.
214. **Traeger, T. R.,** *The Chinese: How They Live and Work.* New York: Praeger Publishers, Inc., 1973.
215. **Tripp-Reimer, Toni,** and **Mary Friedl,** "Appalachians: A Neglected Minority," *Nursing Clinics of North America,* 12, no. 1 (1977), 41–54.
216. **Tumin, M.,** *Patterns of Society.* Boston: Little Brown & Company, 1973.
217. **von Bertalanffy, Ludwig,** *General System Theory.* New York: George Braziller, Inc., 1968.
218. **Vuong, G. Thuy,** *Getting to Know the Vietnamese.* New York: Frederick Unger Publishing Co., Inc. 1976.
219. **Walker, G. M.,** "Utilization of Heath Care: The Laredo Migrant Experience," *American Journal of Public Health,* 69 (1979), 667–72.
220. **Wallace, Louella Thornton,** "Patient Is an American Indian," *Supervisor Nurse,* May 1977, pp. 22–23.
221. **Wang, Rosalind,** and **Lona Moore,** "Students Discover Chinatown," *American Journal of Nursing,* 74, no 6 (1974), 113–14.
222. **Wax, Murray,** *Indian American: Unity and Diversity.* Englewood Cliffs, NJ: Prentice-Hall, Inc., 1971.
223. **Weber, Max,** *The Protestant Ethic and the Spirit of Capitalism,* trans. Talcott Parsons. New York: Charles Scribner's Sons, 1930; students' edition, 1958.
224. **Weddle, D.,** "Indian Pow-Wow," *Globe Democrat Sunday Magazine,* October 12, 1975, pp. 6–11.
225. **Weiss, M. Olga,** "Cultural Shock," *Nursing Outlook,* 19, no. 1 (1971), 40–43.
226. **Weyer, E. M.,** *The Eskimos, Their Environment and Folkways.* Boston: Archon Books, 1969.
227. **White, Earnestine,** "Health and The Black Person: An Annotated Bibliography," *American Journal of Nursing,* 74, no. 10 (1974), 1839–41.
228. ———, "Giving Health Care to Minority Patients," *Nursing Clinics of North America,* 12, no. 1 (1977), 27–40.
229. **Whiting, B.,** ed., *Six Cultures: Studies of Child Rearing.* New York: Jurley and Sons, 1968.
230. **Williams, Margaret,** "Easier Convalescence From Hysterectomy," *American Journal of Nursing,* 76, no. 3 (1976), 438–40.
231. **Winsberg, B.,** and **M. Greenlick,** "Pain Responses in Negro and White Obstetrical Patients," *Journal of Health and Social Behavior,* 8 (September 1967), 222–27.
232. **Woods, Sister Frances Jerome,** *Cultural Values of American Ethnic Groups.* New York: Harper and Brothers, 1956.
233. **Yanochik-Owen, Anita,** and **M. White,** "Nutrition Surveillance in Arizona: Selected Anthropometric and Laboratory Observations Among Mexican American Children," *American Journal of Public Health,* 67, no. 2 (1977), 151–54.

234. **Young, Kimball,** *Social Psychology* (2nd ed.). New York: F. S. Crofts and Company, 1944.
235. **Yuki, Trudy,** "Caring for the Urban American Indian Patient," *Journal of Emergency Nursing*, 7, no. 3 (1981), 110–13.
236. **Zborowski, Mark,** "Cultural Components in Response to Pain," in *Sociological Studies of Health and Sickness*, ed. Dorrian Apple. New York: McGraw-Hill Book Company, 1960, pp. 118–33.
237. **Zola, Irving Kenneth,** "Culture and Symptoms: An Analysis of Patients Presenting Complaints," *American Sociological Review*, 31, (October 1966), 615–31.

11

Religious Influences on the Person

Study of this chapter will enable you to

1. Define the terms *religious* and *spiritual* and the connotations of each.
2. Contrast the major tenets of Hinduism, Buddhism, Shintoism, Confucianism, Taoism, Islam, Judaism, and Christianity.
3. Compare the major tenets of the various branches of Christianity: Roman Catholicism, Eastern Orthodoxy, various Protestant denominations, other Christian sects.
4. Gain an overview of the variety of religions in the United States.
5. Discuss how religious beliefs influence lifestyle and health status in the various religious groups and subgroups.
6. Identify your religious beliefs, or lack of them, and explore how they will influence your nursing practice.
7. Discuss your role in meeting the spiritual needs of client and family.
8. Describe specific nursing measures that can be used to meet the needs of persons with different religious backgrounds.
9. Work with a patient who has religious beliefs different from your own or refer the client to an appropriate resource.

Until an illness occurs, the person may give no thought to the meaning of his/her life or spiritual beliefs. But when he/she feels vulnerable and fearful of the future, solace is sought. Religion can provide that solace.

A patient sneezes. You say "God bless you." Why? Perhaps unconsciously you are coordinating the medical-physical with the religious-spiritual. But you may feel afraid to work professionally with the combination. This fear comes in part from the long-lived schism between science and religion.

The attitude that medical science is superior to religion has affected us all. Yet religion is there as it always has been. Each culture has had some organization or priesthood to sustain the important rituals and myths of its people. Primitive man combined the roles of physician, psychiatrist, and priest. The Indian medicine man and the African witch doctor combine magic with religion; with their herbs, psychosuggestion, and appeals to the gods, they realize that man is a biopsychospiritual being (79).

I had the cancer patient visualize an army of white blood cells attacking and overcoming the cancer cells. Within two weeks the cancer had diminished and he was rapidly gaining weight. He is alive and well today (13).

Is this a priest or a faith healer talking? No, this is a prominent tumor specialist talking in the late 1970s. An internationally known neurosurgeon says, "In a very real sense, medicine is now—as it has always been—faith healing" (13). Dr. Elisabeth Kübler-Ross, internationally known for studies of dying, states that there is definitely life after death (36). Thus some health workers are trying to reunite the biopsychospiritual being.

The 1980s are showing an increased awareness of the link between health and religion and the subject is being discussed more openly.

DEFINITIONS

Religion is defined on various levels: *a belief in a supernatural or divine force that has power over the universe and commands worship and obedience; a system of beliefs; a comprehensive code of ethics or philosophy; a set of practices that are followed; a church affiliation; the conscious pursuit of any object the person holds as supreme* (23).

This definition, however, does not portray the constancy and at times the fervency that can underlie religious belief. In every human there seems to be a **spiritual dimension,** *a quality that goes beyond religious affiliation, that strives for inspiration, reverence, awe, meaning,* *and purpose, even in those who do not believe in any god. The spiritual dimension tries to be in harmony with the universe, strives for answers about the infinite,* and comes into focus when the person faces emotional stress, physical illness, or death.

In the midst of our specialized health care you have an opportunity to go beyond the dogma to bring together the biopsychospiritual being through the study of the religions and religious symbols of your patients/clients. And those are world religions, not your personal or country's basic religion. Mass media, rapid transportation, and cultural exchanges have nullified the provincial approach.

WORLD RELIGIONS

Studying world religions poses a semantic difficulty in that an expression in the Chinese-based religion of Confucianism may have no equivalent in the English language. Thus language has dictated what people think, how they act, and how their religious beliefs are carried out (49).

Concepts, however, are often basically the same but are rephrased in each religion's own linguistic style. The saying "Love one another as I have loved you" will appear to the Hindu as "This is the sum of religion, do not unto others what causes pain to you"; to the Taoist as "Return goodness for hatred"; and to the Muslim as "No one is a believer unless he desires for his brother what he desires for himself."

Each religion also has other characteristics in common:

1. Basis of authority or source(s) of power.
2. A portion of scripture or sacred word.
3. An ethical code that defines right and wrong.
4. A psychology and identity so that its adherents fit into a group and the world is defined by the religion.
5. Aspirations or expectations.
6. Some ideas about what follows death.

The major world religions can be divided into categories in an attempt to group characteristics even further (49). The *alpha* group includes Christianity, Judaism, and Islam. All adhere to a Biblical revelation of a supernatural, monotheistic God. People in these religions are "doers." They obey because God commands; they make covenants with God for protection; they have a historical fixed scripture that is canonized for public use; and they often proselytize. Into the *gamma* group go Taoism,* Confucianism, and Shintoism. In these religions people be-

*Pronounced "dowism."

lieve either that everything is in the being of God or that there is no Godhead (still a definite belief). These people try to be in harmony with the world around them. Their most immediate concern is in relationships with others. Scripture is a family affair. They can be characterized as simple in faith, spontaneous, and straightforward in feelings of affection for people, flowers, and birds. The final grouping is the *beta* group, which includes Buddhism and Hinduism. These religions have their roots in Indian soil and teach that everything is in the being of God. Adherents are interested in "being" rather than "doing." They have a collective literature for private devotion. Control of mind and body is desired, as some of the yoga practices show. The beta and gamma groups do not define God as clearly as the alpha group. The beta and gamma groups look inside themselves for answers: common sense rather than commands from God determines good.

The following discussion presents a more detailed insight into each major world religion through personality sketches. Each person has a fictitious name and represents not a single person but a composite of knowledge gained from the authors' interviewing, reading, and personal experience. Although these personalities are presented as acting and thinking in a certain way, remember that the person's culture, family background, and personality affect how that person lives out a religious experience. Thus a particular Hindu and a given Roman Catholic may be more in agreement religiously than two Lutherans. You cannot make generalizations about a religion from knowing a single follower.

HINDUISM

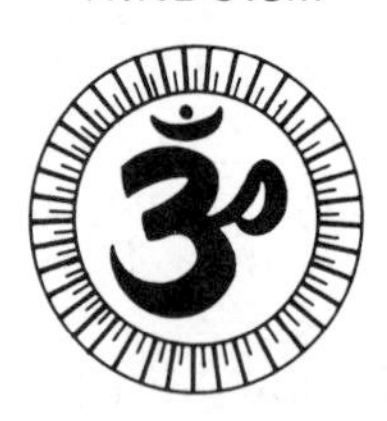

Rama tells us that nothing is typically Hindu and that anyone who puts religion in neat packages will have difficulty comprehending his outlook. Rama is named after Ramakrishna, the greatest Hindu saint of the nineteenth century. The history of Rama's religion goes back to approximately 1500 B.C., when the **Vedas**—*divine revelations*—were written. His main religious texts are the **Upanishads,** *or scriptures*, and the **Bhagavad-Gita,** *a summary of the former with additions. The most expressive*

and universal word of God is **Om,** *or* **Aum**—providing the most important auditory and visual symbol in Rama's religion.*

Rama speaks of some of the worship popular in India today: of the family and local deities; of the trinity—**Brahma,** *the creator;* **Vishnu,** *the preserver and god of love*; and **Shiva,** *the destroyer.*

Rama tells of his own shrine in his home where, in the presence of various pictures of **incarnations** *(human forms of God)* and with incense burning, he meditates. He also thinks of Buddha, Muhammed, and Jesus as incarnations and sometimes reads from the scriptures inspired by their teachings, although they represent other major religions.

In spite of this vast array of deities and the recognition that all religions are valid, Rama believes in one universal concept—**Brahman,** *the Divine Intelligence, the Supreme Reality*. Rama believes all paths lead to the understanding that this "reality" exists as part of all physical beings, especially humans. Rama's entire spiritual quest is directed toward uniting his *inner and real self*, the **atman,** with the concept of Brahman. So although Rama has gone through several stages of desire—for pleasure, power, wealth, fame, and humanitarianism—the last stage, his desire for freedom, for touching the infinite, is his main goal.

Rama is interested in health and illness only as a guide to this goal. He feels that the human love for the body is a cause for illness. He says, for example, that we overeat and get a stomachache. He views the pain as a warning—in this case, to stop overeating. He does not oppose medical treatment if absolutely necessary, but he feels that medicine can sometimes dull the pain and then the person overeats again, thus perpetuating the cause of the problem. Medical or psychiatric help, Rama says, is at best transitory. The cause of the pain must be rooted out.

In order not to dwell on physical concerns, Rama strives for moderation in eating as well as in other bodily functions. He considers only the atman as real and eternal, the body as unreal and finite. The body is a temple, a vehicle, no more. He tries to take care of it so that it will not scream at him because of overindulgence or underindulgence. Rama is a vegetarian. He feels that meat and intoxicants would excite his senses too much. Yet the Hindu diet pattern is flexible; definite rules are not set. If Rama is sick, he tries to bear his illness with resignation, knowing its temporary nature. He believes that the prayer of supplication for bodily cure is the lowest form of prayer whereas the highest form is devotion to God. To him, death and rebirth are nearly synony-

*See the symbol at the beginning of this section. A transliteration of the script is *a, u, m*. It is written in English as *Om*, or *Aum. Om, God*, and *Brahman* are synonymous and mean a *consciousness* or *awareness* rather than a personified being.

mous, for the atman never changes and always remains pure. He compares the atman to the ocean: as ocean water can be put into various containers without changing its nature, so can the atman be put into various physical and human containers without changing its nature.

Thus if death is imminent, Rama believes that the body, mind, and senses weaken and become lifeless but that the never-changing atman is ready to enter into a new form of life, depending on the person's knowledge, deeds, and past experiences. Full acceptance of death is encouraged. Death is a friend to be faced bravely, calmly, and confidently.

Rama says that as a devotee of God he is following a *training course* called **yoga**. As a preliminary, however, he must establish certain moral qualifications. He must strive for self-control, self-discipline, cleanliness, and contentment. He must avoid injury, deceitfulness, and stealing. His overwhelming desire to reach God can be implemented through one or a combination of the four yoga paths: (1) **inana yoga** through *reading and absorbing knowledge,* (2) **bhakti yoga** through the *devotion of emotion and love,* (3) **karma yoga** through *work dedicated to God,* and (4) **raja yoga** through *psychological experiments on oneself.* Rama combines the first three by reading and memorizing portions of the ancient scriptures, by meditating daily at his shrine, and by dedicating the results of his professional work to God.

Rama mentions that various forms of yoga have spread around the world to form hybrid groups with varied purposes. One branch that has appeared in medical centers is **hatha yoga**, meaning *sun and moon*, symbolizing an inner balance that is achieved through *muscle and breathing exercises.* Ultimately the body is prepared for meditation through these exercises.

From another branch, **bhakti yoga,** has come the Hare Krishna movement in the United States, starting in 1965 when A. C. Bhaktivedanta came to New York City. The first Krishna temple was established on the Lower East Side (14). Rama reports that there are now reportedly 150,000 Krishnas in the United States, almost all of them converts from Catholicism, Judaism, or Protestantism. At New Vrindaban Krishna community in Moundsville, West Virginia, a palace has been built solely by community members. It contains $500,000 worth of gold, silver, onyx, marble, stained glass, teak, and crystal chandeliers. In contrast, the lifestyle is austere: work, study, and praise beginning about 3:30 A.M., no meat eating, no stimulants, no intoxicants, and no sex except for procreation (40).

For Rama, religion is not something to be picked up and put down according to a schedule or one's mood. It is a constant and all-pervading part of his life and the life of his country. India's literature and art are witness to this fact.

If you give nursing care to someone with Rama's background, consider how his religious beliefs will influence your approach. Be accepting if the person seems to minimize bodily ills. Keep in mind the view of the body as only a vehicle to carry the atman and the belief that the desire for bodily cure is a low form of prayer. Yoga training, emphasizing self-control and devotion to God through reading and meditation, may cause the person to seek help from inner resources and the literature of Hinduism rather than from medication or consultation with staff. Providing an atmosphere conducive to this practice will be appreciated. Should death seem imminent, remember that death is perceived as a rebirth. The person will want rebirth to have as much dignity as possible.

BUDDHISM AND SHINTOISM

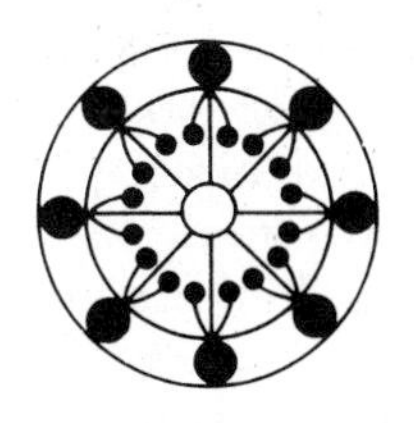

Umeko Sato is a member of the *Buddhist sect* **Soka Gakkai.** This sect is now a powerful religion in Japan, with a government party, a university, and a grand temple representing it. Based on the **Lotus Sutra,** *part of the Buddhist scriptures,* its doctrine advocates the three values of happiness: profit, goodness, and beauty. Sato is attracted by the practicality of the teaching, the mottoes that she can live by, the emphasis on small group study, and present world benefits, especially healing.

Although Sato's beliefs at some points seem in direct contrast to the original Buddhist teachings, she is happy to explain the rich multireligious tradition that her family has had for generations. She emphasizes that she is affected by the Confucian emphasis on the family unit, by Christianity's healing emphasis, by Shintoism, the state religion of Japan until 1945, and by Buddhism, which originated about 600 B.C. in India with a Hindu named *Siddhartha Gautama.*

Gautama, shortly after a historic enlightenment experience during which he became the Buddha, preached a sermon to his followers and drew on the earth a wheel representing the continuous round of life and death and rebirth. Later eight spokes were added to illustrate the sermon and to provide the most explicit visual symbol of Buddhism*

*See the symbol at the beginning of this section.

today. Sato repeats Buddha's four noble truths: (1) life is disjointed or out of balance, especially in birth, old age, illness, and death; (2) the cause of this imbalance is ignorance of one's own true nature; (3) removal of this ignorance is attained by reaching **Nirvana,** *the divine state of release, the ultimate reality, the perfect knowledge* via (4) the eightfold path.

The eight spokes of the wheel represent the eightfold path used to reach Nirvana. Sato says that followers subscribe to right knowledge, right intentions, right speech, right conduct, right means of livelihood, right effort, right mindfulness, and concentration. From these concepts has arisen a moral code that, among other things, prohibits intoxicants, lying, and killing of any kind (which explains why Buddhists are often vegetarians). She further explains that the Mahayana branch of Buddhism took hold in Japan as opposed to the Theravada branch. The **Theravada branch** *emphasizes an intellectual approach through wisdom, man working by himself through meditation and without ritual.* The **Mahayana branch** *emphasizes involvement with mankind, ritual, petitionary prayer, and concern for one's sibling.* Sato feels that the Mahayana branch provides the happier philosophy of the two and she tells of the ritual of celebration on Gautama's birthday. But most Japanese believe in **Amitabha Buddha,** *a god rather than a historical figure*, who in replacing the austere image of Gautama is a glorious redeemer, one of infinite light. Also, the people worship **Kwannon,** *a goddess of compassion.*

Sato explains that she cannot omit mention of the one austere movement within the Mahayana branch, the *Zen* sect. Taking their example from Gautama's extended contemplation of a flower, Zen followers care little for discourse, books, or other symbolic interpretations and explanations of reality. Hours and years are devoted to meditation, contemplation of word puzzles, and consultation with a Zen master. In seeking absolute honesty and truthfulness through such simple acts as drinking tea or gardening, the Zen student hopes to experience enlightenment.

Sato next turns to her former state religion, *Shintoism*. While Buddhism produced a solemnizing effect on her country, Shintoism had an affirmative and joyous effect. Emperor, ancestor, ancient hero, and nature worship form its core. Those who follow Shintoism, she says, feel an intense loyalty and devotion to every lake, tree, and blossom in Japan as well as to the ancestral spirits abiding there. They also have a great concern for cleanliness, a carryover from early ideas surrounding dread of pollution in the dead.

Sato says that her parents have two god shelves in their home. One contains wooden tablets inscribed with the name of the household's patron deity and a symbolic form of the goddess of rice, as well as other texts and objects of family significance. Here her family performs simple rites, such as offering a prayer or a food gift each day. In a family crisis, perhaps an illness, the family conducts more elaborate rites, such as lighting tapers or offering rice brandy. The other god shelf, in another room, is the Buddha shelf; and if a family member dies, a Buddhist priest, the spiritual leader, performs specified rituals there.

Sato strongly emphasizes that if illness or impending death causes a family member to be hospitalized, another well family member will stay at the hospital to bathe, cook for, and give emotional support to the patient. Sato feels that recovery largely depends on this family tie. If death occurs, Sato will be reminded of the Buddhist doctrine teaching that death is a total nonfunction of the physical body and mind and that the life force is displaced and transformed to continue to function in another form. Every birth is a rebirth, much as in the Hindu teaching, and rebirth happens immediately after death, according to some Buddhists. Others believe that rebirth occurs 49 days after death, during which time the person is in an intermediary state. The difference in quality of death, birth, and existence depends on whether the person lived a disciplined or undisciplined life.

Buddhist teachings teach the living how to die well. The elderly, or feeble, are to prepare themselves mentally for a state that would be conducive for a good rebirth. The person is to remain watchful and alert in the face of death, to resist distraction and confusion, to be lucid and calm. Distinct instructions are given in what to expect as life leaves the body, as the person enters an intermediary state, and as Nirvana is about to occur.

So although Sato has grasped a new religious path for herself, her respect for tradition remains.

In giving care to a person with Umeko Sato's background, be aware of the varied religious influences on life. The sect's emphasis on the here and now rather than on the long road to Nirvana may place a high value on physical health so that the person can benefit from the joys and beauty of this life. The person may readily voice impatience with the body's dysfunction. You can also respond to the great concern for cleanliness, the desire to have family nearby, and the need for family rites that are offered for the sick member. Should a family member be dying, you may see some ambivalence. The family member may want to prepare himself or herself in the traditional way while someone with Sato's background, with emphasis on present world benefits and healing, may deny that there is a valid preparation for death.

CONFUCIANISM AND TAOISM

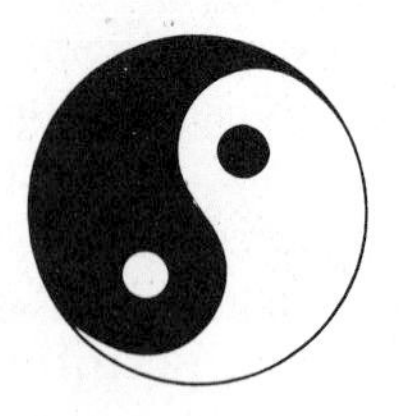

Wong Huieng is a young teacher in Taiwan simultaneously influenced by **Taoism,** *the romantic and mystical,* and **Confucianism,** *the practical and pragmatic.* To provide insights into these Chinese modes of thinking, although it is more representative of Taoism, Wong Huieng uses the *yin-yang symbol.** The symbol is a circle, representing **Tao** or *the absolute,* in which two tear shapes fit perfectly into one another, each containing a small dot from the other. Generally yang is light or red, and yin is dark. Ancient Chinese tradition says that everything exists in these two interacting forces. Each represents a group of qualities. Yang is positive or masculine—dry, hot, active, moving, and light. Yin is feminine or negative—wet, cold, passive, restful, and empty. For example, fire is almost pure yang and water almost pure yin—but not quite. The combination of yin and yang constitutes all the dualisms a person can imagine: day-night, summer-winter, beauty-ugliness, illness-health, life-death. Both qualities are necessary for life in the universe; they are complementary and, if in harmony, good. Yang and yin energy forces are embodied in the body parts and affect food preferences and eating habits.

Huieng translates this symbol into a relaxed philosophy of life: "If I am sick, I will get better. Life is like going up and down a mountain; sometimes I feel good and sometimes I feel bad. That's the way it is." Though educated, she is not interested in climbing up the job ladder, accumulating wealth, or conquering nature. Her goal is to help provide money to build an orphanage in a natural wooded setting.

Huieng thinks of death as a natural part of life, as the peace that comes when the body is worn out. She admits, however, that when her father died, human grief took hold of her. Before his death, her mother went to the Taoist temple priest and got some incense that was to help cast the sickness from his body. After death, they kept his body in the house for the required time, 49 days. The priest executed a special

*See the symbol at the beginning of this section.

ceremony every seven days. Her mother could cry only one hour daily, 2:00 until 3:00 in the morning. Now her mother talks through the priest to her father's ghost. Although Huieng regards this practice as superstitious and thinks that painting a picture of a lake and mountain is a more fitting way to erase her grief, she looks at the little yellow bag, containing a blessing from the priest, hanging around her neck, and finds it comforting if not intellectually acceptable.

Now Huieng turns to her practical side and talks about **Confucius,** *the first saint of the nation.* Although **Lao-tzu,** *the founder of Taoism,* is a semilegendary figure said to have vanished after he wrote the *bible of Taoism,* **Tao-te-ching,** Confucius has a well-documented existence.

Confucius, born in 551 B.C., wrote little. His disciples wrote the **Analects,** *short proverbs embodying his teachings.* He is revered as a teacher, not as a god. Huieng does not ask him to bless her but tries to emulate him and his teachings, which she has heard since birth. The temple in his memory is a place for studying, not for praying. And on his birthday, a national holiday, people pay respect to their teachers in his memory.

Five important terms in Confucius' teaching are **Jen,** *a striving for goodness within;* **Chun-sui,** *establishing a gentlemanly/womanly approach with others;* **Li,** *knowing how relationships should be conducted and having respect for age;* **Te,** *leading by virtuous character rather than by force*; and **Wen,** *pursuing the arts as an adjunct to moral character.* Huieng stresses that in *Li* are the directives for family relationships. So strongly did Confucius feel about the family that he gave directives on proper attitudes between father and son, elder brother and junior brother, husband and wife. Also, Huieng feels she can't harm her body because it was given to her by her parents. Her concept of immediate family includes grandparents, uncles, aunts, and cousins. Her language has more words for relationships between relatives than the English language does.

Huieng feels that in caring for her body, she cares for her family, the country, and the universe. Essentially, to her, all people are family.

Important in your understanding of a person with Wong Huieng's background is the dualism that exists in such thinking. Acceptance of the particular version of mysticism and practicality, and of the yin and yang forces that are seen as operating within self, will help in building a foundation of personalized care.

The person may have more respect for older than younger staff members and may respond well to teaching. There may be a strong desire to attain and maintain wellness. These factors are directly related to the religious teaching; you can use them to enhance care.

ISLAM

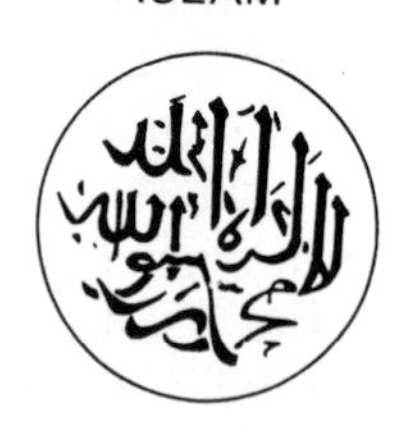

Omar Ali is **Muslim,** *a member of Islam, the youngest of the major world religions.* This faith, with its Arabic coloring and tenacious monotheistic tradition, serves as a bridge between Eastern and Western religions. "There is no God but Allah; Muhammed is His Prophet"* provides the key to Omar's beliefs. He must say this but once in his life as a requirement, but he will repeat it many times as an affirmation.

Omar is an Egyptian physician whose religious tradition was revealed through Muhammed, born approximately A.D. 571 in Mecca, then a trading point between India and Syria on the Arabian peninsula. Hating polytheism and influenced by Judaism and Christianity, Muhammed wrote *God's revelation to him* in the **Quran,**† *scriptures* that to Omar confirm the truths of the Jewish-Christian Bible. Omar believes in the biblical prophets, but he calls Muhammed the greatest—the Seal of Prophets.

Through the *Quran* and the **Hadith,** *the traditions*, Omar has guidelines for his thinking, devotional life, and social obligations. He believes he is a unique individual with an eternal soul. He believes in a heaven and hell and while on earth he wants to walk the straight path.

To keep on this path, Omar prays five times a day: generally on rising, at midday, in the afternoon, in the early evening, and before retiring. Articles needed are water and a prayer rug. Because the *Quran* emphasizes cleanliness of body, Omar performs a ritual washing before each prayer. Then, facing Mecca, he goes through a series of prescribed bodily motions and repeats various passages in praise and supplication.

Omar also observes **Ramadan,** *a fast month,*‡ during which time he eats or drinks nothing from sunrise to sunset; after sunset he takes nourishment only in moderation. He explains **fasting** *(abstinence from eating)* as a *discipline aiding him to understand those with little food.* At the end of Ramadan, he enters a festive period with feelings of goodwill and gift exchanges.

Omar has made one pilgrimage to Mecca, another requirement for all healthy and financially able Muslims. He feels the experience created

*These words are a translation of the sacred calligraphy in the symbol shown at the beginning of this section. The prophet's name is sometimes spelled *Muhammad.*

†Sometimes spelled *Koran.*

‡Coming during the ninth month of the Muslim year, always at a different time each year by the Western calendar, and sometimes spelled *Ramazan.*

a great sense of brotherhood, for all the pilgrims wore similar modest clothing, exchanged news of followers in various lands, and renewed their mutual faith. The *twelfth day of the Pilgrimage month is the* **Feast of Sacrifice**, when all Muslim families kill a lamb in honor of Abraham's offereing of his son to God.

In line with the *Quran's* teaching, Omar does not eat pork (including such items as bologna, which might contain partial pork products), gamble, drink intoxicants. He worships no images or pictures of Muhammed, for the prophet is not deified. He gives a portion of his money to the poor, for Islam advocates a responsibility to society.

Omar mentions that parts of the basic Islam faith are used by a United States-based group called the Black Muslims (Nation of Islam). Known to have stringent, seclusionist rules, the Black Muslims have taken some new positions since 1976 and seem to be moving toward more orthodox Islam. Members may now get politically involved; membership is open to Whites; dress codes have changed; and some of the myths about the American founder, W. D. Fard, have been erased.

Omar outlines the ideas of his religion as it applies to his profession. He feels that he can make a significant contribution to health care, but that essentially what happens is God's will. Submission to God is the very meaning of Islam.

Muslim patients are excused from religious rules, but many will still want to follow them as closely as possible. Even though in a body cast and unable to get out of bed, a patient may want to go through prayers symbolically. The person might also recite the first chapters of the *Quran*, centered on praise to Allah, which are often used in times of crises. Family is a great comfort in illness and praying with a group is strengthening, but the Muslim has no priest. The relationship is directly with God. Some patients may seem completely resigned to death, whereas others, hoping it is God's will that they live, cooperate vigorously with the medical program. After death, a body must be washed and the hands folded in prayer. Knowledge of these attitudes and traditions can greatly enhance your care.

JUDAISM

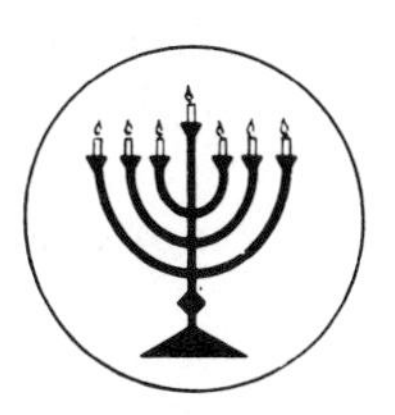

Seth Lieberman, strongly influenced by the social-concern emphasis in Judaism, is a psychiatrist. In the Jewish community each member is expected to contribute to others' needs according to his/her ability.

Jews have traditionally considered their community as a whole responsible for feeding the hungry, helping the widowed and orphaned, rescuing the captured, and even burying the dead. Jewish retirement homes, senior citizens' centers, and medical centers are witness to this philosophy.

Seth can't remember when his religious instruction began—it was always there. He went through the motions and felt the emotion of the Sabbath eve with its candles and cup of sanctification long before he could comprehend his father's explanations. Book learning followed, however, and he came to understand the fervency with which his people study and live the law as given in the **Torah,** *the first five books of the Bible*; and in the **Talmud,** *a commentary and enlargement of the Torah.* His *spiritual leader is the* **rabbi.** His spiritual symbol is the *menorah.**

His own *entrance into a responsible religious life and manhood* was through the **Bar Mitzvah,** a ceremony which took place in the synagogue when he was 13. (Girls are also educated to live responsible religious lives, and a few congregations now have a similar ceremony, the **Bas Mitzvah,** for girls.)

Although raised in an *Orthodox* home, Seth and his family are now *Reform.* And he mentions another group, the *Conservatives. The* **Orthodox** *believe God gave the law*; it was written exactly as He gave it; it should be followed precisely. **Reform** *Jews believe the law was written by inspired men* at various times and therefore is subject to reinterpretation. Seth says he follows the traditions because they are traditions rather than because God demands it. **Conservatives** *are in the middle*, taking some practices from both groups. Overriding any differences in interpretation of ritual and tradition is the fundamental concept expressed in the prayer "Hear, O Israel, the Lord our God, the Lord is One." Not only is He one, He loves His creation, wants His people to live justly, and wants to bless their food, drink, and celebration. Judaism's double theme might be expressed as "Enjoy life now, and share it with God." Understandably, then, Seth's religious emphasis isn't on an afterlife, although some Jewish people believe in one. And although Jews have had a history of suffering, the inherent value of suffering or illness isn't stressed. Through their observance of the law, the belief of their historical role as God's chosen people, and their hope for better days, Jews have survived seemingly insurmountable persecution.

Seth works with physically, emotionally, and spiritually depressed

*See the symbol at beginning of this section, page 485. The seven-branched candelabrum stands for the creation of the universe in seven days; the center light symbolizes the Sabbath; and the candlelight symbolizes the presence of God in the Temple.

persons. He feels that often the spiritual depression is unnoticed, misunderstood, or ignored by professional workers. He cites instances in which mental attitudes have brightened as he shared a common bond of Judaism with a client. He offers guidelines for working with a Jewish person in a hospital or nursing home. Although Jewish law can be suspended when a person is ill, the patient will be most comfortable following as many practices as possible.

Every Jew observes the **Sabbath,** *a time for spiritual refreshment, from sundown on Friday to shortly after sundown on Saturday*. During this period Orthodox Jews may refuse freshly cooked food, medicine, treatment, surgery, and use of radio, television, and writing equipment lest the direction of their thinking be diverted on this special day. An Orthodox male may want to wear a **yarmulke** *or skullcap* continuously; use a *prayerbook called* **Siddur**, and use **phylacteries,** *leather strips with boxes containing scriptures*, at weekday morning prayer. Also, the ultra-Orthodox male may refuse to use a razor because of the Levitical ban on shaving.

Some Orthodox Jewish women observe the rite of **Mikvah,** an *ancient ritual of family purity*. From marriage to menopause (except when pregnant) these women observe no physical-sexual relations with their husbands from 24 hours before menstruation until 12 days later when a ritual immersion in water renders them ready to meet their husbands again.

Jewish dietary laws have been considered by some scholars as health measures: to enjoy life is to eat properly and in moderation. The Orthodox, however, obey them because God so commanded. Food is called **treyfe** (or treyfah) if it is *unfit* and **kosher** if it is *ritually correct.* Foods forbidden are pig, horse, shrimp, lobster, crab, oyster, and fowl that are birds of prey. Meats approved are from those animals that are ruminants and have divided hooves. Fish approved must have both fins and scales. Also, the kosher animals must be healthy and slaughtered in a prescribed manner. Because of the Biblical passage stating not to soak a young goat in its mother's milk, Jews do not eat meat products and milk products together. Neither are the utensils used to cook these products ever intermixed, nor the dishes from which to eat these products.

Guidelines for a satisfactory diet for the Orthodox are as follows:

1. Serve milk products first, meat second. Meat can be eaten a few minutes after milk, but milk cannot be taken for 6 hours after meat.
2. If a person completely refuses meat because of incorrect slaughter, encourage a vegetarian diet with protein supplements, such as fish

and eggs, considered neutral unless prepared with milk or meat shortening.

3. Get frozen kosher products marked Ⓤ, K, or *pareve*.
4. Heat and serve food in the original container and use plastic utensils.

Two important holy days are *Rosh Hashanah* and *Yom Kippur*. **Rosh Hashanah,** *the Jewish New Year*, is a time to meet with the family, give thanks to God for good health, and renew traditions. **Yom Kippur,** *the day of atonement*, a time for asking forgiveness of family members for wrongs done, occurs 10 days later. On Yom Kippur Jews fast for 24 hours, a symbolic act of self-denial, mourning, and petition. **Tisha Bab,** *the day of lamentation*, recalling the destruction of both Temples of Jerusalem, is another 24-hour fast period. **Pesach** or **Passover** (eight days for Orthodox and Conservative, seven days for Reform) *celebrates the ancient Jews' deliverance from Egyptian bondage*. **Matzo,** *an unleavened bread*, replaces leavened bread during this period.

The Jewish person is preoccupied with health. Jews are future-oriented and want to know diagnosis, how a disease will affect business, family life, and social life. The Jewish people as a whole are highly educated, and although they respect the doctor, they may get several medical opinions before carrying out a treatment plan.

While family, friends, and rabbi may visit the ill, especially on or near holidays, they will also come at other times. Visiting the sick is a religious duty. And although death is final to many Jews except for living on in the memories of others, guidelines exist for this time. When a Jewish person has suffered irreversible brain damage and can no longer say a **bracha,** *a blessing to praise God*, or perform a **mitzvah,** *an act to help a fellow,* he/she is considered a "vegetable" with nothing to save. Prolonging the life by artificial means would not be recommended. But until then the dying patient must be treated as the complete person he/she always was, capable of conducting his/her own affairs and entering into relationships.

Jewish tradition says never to leave the bedside of the dying person, which is of value to the dying and the mourners. The dying soul should leave in the presence of people and the mourner is shielded from guilt of thinking that the patient was alone at death or that more could be done. The bedside vigil also serves as a time to encourage a personal confession by the dying, which is a *rite de passage* to another phase of existence (even though unknown). This type of confessional is said throughout the Jewish life cycle whenever one stage has been completed. Confessional on the deathbed is a recognition that one cycle is ending and that another cycle is beginning. Recitation of the *Shema* in the last moments before death helps the dying to affirm faith in God and focus on the most familiar rituals of life.

Death, being witnessed at the bedside, helps to reinforce the reality of the situation. Immediate burial and specified mourning also move the remaining loved ones through the crisis period. (Note, however, that if a Jew dies on the Sabbath, he cannot be moved, except by a non-Jew, until sundown.) After the burial, the mourners are fed in a meal of replenishment called *se'udat havra'ah*. This step symbolizes the rallying of the community and the sustenance of life for the remaining. Also, Jews follow the custom of sitting *shiva* or visiting with remaining relatives for one week after the death (33).

Judaism identifies a year of mourning. The first three days are of deep grief; clothes may be torn to symbolize the tearing of a life from others. Seven days of lesser mourning follow, leading to 30 days of gradual readjustment. The remainder of the year calls for remembrance and healing. During that year a prayer called the mourner's *Kaddish* is recited in religious services. It helps convey the feeling of support for the mourner (33). At the annual anniversary of death, a candle is burned and special prayers said.

So from circumcision of the male infant on the eighth day after birth to his deathbed, and from the days of the original menorah in the sanctuary in the wilderness until the present day, the followers of Judaism re-enact their traditions. Because many of these traditions remain an intrinsic part of the Jew while striving to maintain or regain wellness, the preceding guidelines offer a foundation for knowledgeable care.

CHRISTIANITY

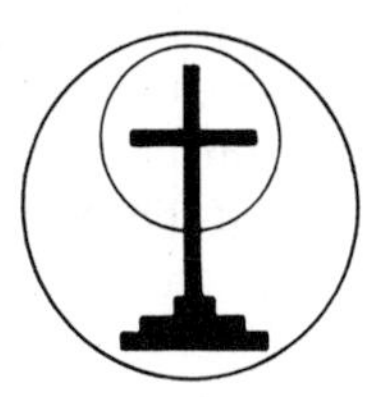

Beth Meyer, a *Roman Catholic*, Demetrius Callas, an *Eastern Orthodox*, and Jean Taylor, a *Protestant*, are Christian American nurses representing the three major branches of Christianity. Although Christianity divided into Eastern Orthodox and Roman Catholic in A.D. 1054, and the Protestant Reformation provided a third division in the sixteenth century, these nurses share some basic beliefs, most importantly that Jesus Christ as described in the Bible is God's son. Jesus, born in Palestine, changed "B.C." to "A.D." The details of His 33 years are few, but His deeds and words recorded in the Bible's New Testament show quiet authority, loving humility, and an ability to perform miracles and to visit easily with people in varied social positions.

The main symbol of Christianity is the cross,* but it signifies more than a wooden structure on which Jesus was crucified. It also symbolizes the finished redemption—Christ rising from the dead and ascending to the Father in order to rule with Him and continuously pervade the personal lives of His followers.

Christians observe **Christmas** *as Christ's birthday*; **Lent** *as a season of penitence and self-examination preceding* **Good Friday,** *Christ's crucifixion day*; and **Easter,** *His Resurrection day*.

Beth, Demetrius, and Jean rely on the New Testament as a guideline for their lives. They believe that Jesus was fully God and fully man at the same time, that their original sin (which they accept as a basic part of themselves) can be forgiven, and that they are acceptable to God because of Jesus Christ's life and death. They believe God is three persons—the Father, the Son, and the Holy Spirit (Holy Ghost), the last providing a spirit of love and truth.

Beth, Demetrius, and Jean differ in some worship practices and theology, but all highly regard their individuality as children of God and hope for life with God after death. They feel responsible for their own **souls,** *the spiritual dimension of themselves*, and for aiding the spiritual needs of their patients.

Roman Catholicism, according to Beth, is a religion based on the dignity of man as a social, intellectual, and spiritual being, made in the image of God. She traces the teaching authority of the church through the scriptures: God sent His Son to provide salvation and redemption from sin. He established the Church to continue His work after ascension into heaven. Jesus chose apostles to preach, teach, and guide. He appointed Saint Peter as the Church's head to preserve unity and to have authority over the apostles. The mission given by Jesus to Saint Peter and the apostles is the same that continues to the present through the Pope and his bishops.

Beth believes that the seven Sacraments are grace-giving rites that give her a share in Christ's own life and help sustain her in her efforts to follow His example. The Sacraments that are received once in life are Baptism, Confirmation, Holy Orders, and usually Matrimony.

Through **Baptism** *the soul is incorporated into the life of Christ and shares His divinity*. Any infant in danger of death should be baptized, even an aborted fetus. If a priest is not available, you can perform the sacrament by pouring water on the forehead and saying, "I

*See the symbol at the beginning of this section.

baptize thee in the name of the Father, of the Son, and of the Holy Spirit." The healthy baby is baptized some time during the first weeks of life. Adults are also baptized when they convert to Catholicism and join the church.

Confirmation *is the sacrament in which the Holy Spirit is imparted in a fuller measure to help strengthen the individual in his/her spiritual life.* **Matrimony** *acknowledges the love and lifelong commitment between a man and a woman.* **Holy Orders** *ordains deacons and priests.*

The Sacraments that may be received more than once are Penance (Confession), the Eucharist (Holy Communion), and the Anointing of the Sick (Sacrament of the Sick). Beth feels that **Penance,** *an acknowledgment and forgiveness of her sins in the presence of a priest,* should be received according to individual need even though it is required only once a year by church law. The Mass, often called the **Eucharist,** is the *liturgical celebration* whose core is the sacrament of the Holy Eucharist. Bread and wine are consecrated and become the body and blood of Christ. The body and blood are then received in Holy Communion. The Eucharist is celebrated daily and all Roman Catholics are encouraged to participate as often as possible; they are required by church law to attend on Sundays (or late Saturdays) and specified holy days throughout the year unless prevented by illness or some other serious reason.

Beth is glad that the Anointing of the Sick has been modified and broadened and explains the rite to patient and family to allay anxiety. Formerly known as Extreme Unction or the last rites, this sacrament was reserved for those near death. Now **Anointing of the Sick,** *symbolic of Christ's healing love and the concern of the Christian community,* can provide spiritual strength to those less gravely ill. Following anointing with oil, the priest offers prayers for forgiveness of sin and restoration of health. Whenever possible, the family should be present to join in the prayers.

If the patient is dying, extraordinary artificial measures to maintain life are unnecessary. At the hour of death the priest offers communion to the dying person by means of a special formula. This final communion is called *Viaticum.* In sudden deaths the priest should be called and the anointing and *Viaticum* should be administered if possible. If the person is dead when the priest arrives, there is no anointing, but the priest leads the family in prayers for the person who just died.

Beth divides the Roman Catholic funeral into three phases: the **wake,** *a period of waiting* or vigil during which the body is viewed and the family is sustained through visiting; the **funeral mass,** *a prayer service* incorporated into the celebration of the Mass; and the **burial,** *the final act* of placing the person in the ground. (This procedure may vary somewhat, for some Catholics are now choosing cremation.) The mourners retain the memory of the dead through a Month's Mind Mass, celebrated a month after death, and anniversary masses. Finally, the priest integrates the liturgy for the dead with the whole parish liturgical life.

Beth is convinced that her religious practice contributes to her health. She feels that the body, mind, and spirit work together and that a spirit rid of guilt and grievances, and fortified with the strength of Christ's life, has positive effects on the body. She believes that suffering and illness are allowed by God because of our disobedience (original sin), but that they are not necessarily willed by God or given as punishment for personal sin.

While in the hospital, a Roman Catholic may want to attend Mass, have the priest visit, or receive the Eucharist at bedside. (Fasting an hour before the sacrament is traditional, but in the case of physical illness, fasting is not necessary). Other symbols that might be comforting are a Bible, prayer book, holy water, a lighted candle, crucifix, rosary, and various relics and medals.

The Greek Orthodox Faith is discussed by Demetrius. The Eastern Orthodox Church, the main denomination, is divided into groups by nationality. Each group has the **Divine Liturgy**, *the Eucharistic service,* in the native language and sometimes in English also. Although similar in many respects to the Roman Catholic, the Eastern Orthodox have no pope. The seven sacraments are followed with slight variations. Baptism is by triple immersion: the priest places the infant in a basin of water and pours water on the forehead three times. He then immediately confirms the infant by anointing with holy oil. If death is imminent for a hospitalized infant and the parents or priest cannot be reached, you can baptize the infant by placing a small amount of water on the forehead three times. Even a symbolic baptism is acceptable, but only a living being should receive the sacrament. Adults who join the church are also baptized and confirmed.

The **unction of the sick** has never been practiced as a last rite by the Eastern Orthodox; *it is a blessing for the sick.* Confession at least once a year is a prerequisite to participation in the Eucharist, which is taken at least four times a year: at Christmas, at Easter, on the Feast Day of Saint Peter and Saint Paul (June 30), and on the day celebrating the Sleeping of the Virgin Mary (August 15).

Fasting from the last meal in the evening until after **Communion,** *another term for the Eucharist*, is the general rule. Other fast periods include each Wednesday, representing the seizure of Jesus; each Friday, representing His death; and two 40-day periods, the first before Christmas and the second before Easter. Fasting to Demetrius means avoiding meat, dairy products, and olive oil. Its purpose is spiritual betterment, to avoid producing extra energy in the body and instead think of the spirit. Fasting is not necessary when ill. Religion should not harm one's health.

Demetrius retains the Eastern influence in his thinking. He envisions his soul as blending in with the spiritual cosmos and his actions as affecting the rest of creation. He is mystically inclined and feels insights can be gained directly from God. He tells of sharing such an experience with a patient, Mrs. A., also Greek Orthodox.

Mrs. A. had experienced nine surgeries to build up deteriorating bones caused by rheumatoid arthritis. She faced another surgery. On the positive side, the surgery promised hope for walking; on the negative, it was a new and risky procedure. Possibly she would not walk; possibly she would not live. Demetrius saw Mrs. A. when he started working at 3:30 P.M. She was depressed, fearful, and crying. Later, at 6:30 P.M., he saw a changed person—fearless and calm, ready for surgery. She explained that she had seen Jesus in a vision, and that He said, "Go ahead with the surgery. You'll have positive results. But call your priest and take Communion first." Demetrius called the priest, who gave her Communion. She went into surgery the next day with supreme confidence. She now walks.

In addition to Communion, other helpful symbols are prayer books, lighted candles, and holy water. Especially helpful to the Orthodox are **icons,** *pictures of Jesus, Mary, or a revered saint.* Saints can intercede between God and the person. One of the most loved is **Saint Nicholas,** *a third-century teacher and father figure* who gave his wealth to the poor and became an archbishop. He is honored on Saint Nicholas Day, December 6, and prayed to continuously for guidance and protection.

Every Sunday morning Demetrius participates in an hour-long liturgy. Sitting in an ornate sanctuary with figures and symbols on the windows, walls, and ceiling, facing the tabernacle containing the holy gifts and scripture, Demetrius finds renewal. He recites "I believe in one God, the Father Almighty, Maker of Heaven and Earth, and of all things visible and invisible. And in one Lord Jesus Christ, the only begotten Son of God."

Protestantism is divided into many denominations and sects. Jean Taylor is a member of the *Church of God* (Anderson, Indiana). She identifies the church by its headquarters because there are some 200 independent church groups in the United States using the phrase "Church of God" in their title. Her group evolved late in the nineteenth century because members of various churches felt that organization and ritual were taking precedence over direction from God. They banded together in a drive toward Christian unity, toward a recognition that any people who followed Christ's teachings were members of a universal Church of God and could worship freely together.

This example speaks of one of the chief characteristics of Protestantism: the insistence that God has not given any one person or group of persons sole authority to interpret His truth to others. Protestants use a freedom of spiritual searching and reinterpretation. Thus new groups form as certain persons and their followers come to believe that they see God's teaching in a new and better light. Jean feels that reading the Bible for historical knowledge and guidance, having a minister to teach and counsel her, and relying on certain worship forms are all important aids. But discerning God's will for her life individually and following that will are her ultimate religious goals.

Jean explains that she "accepted Christ into her life" when she was 8 years old. This identified her as personally following the church's teaching rather than just adhering to family religious tradition. A later experience, in which the Holy Spirit gives the person more spiritual power and discernment, is called *sanctification*.

Jean defines her corporate worship as free liturgical, with an emphasis on congregational singing, verbal prayer, and scripture reading. A sermon by the **minister,** *the spiritual leader*, may take half the worship period. As with many Protestant groups, two sacraments or ordinances are observed: (1) baptism (in this case, **believer's** or **mature baptism** *by total immersion into water*) and (2) Communion. To Protestants, the bread and wine used in Communion are symbolic of Christ's body and blood rather than the actual elements. One additional ordinance practiced in Jean's church and among some other groups is **footwashing,** *symbolic of Jesus washing His disciples' feet*. These ordinances are practiced with varied frequencies.

Because of the spectrum of beliefs and practices, defining Protestants, even within a single denomination or sect, is almost impossible. Some Protestant groups, retaining their initial emphasis on individual freedom, have allowed no written creed but expect members to follow an unwritten code of behavior. Jean does suggest some guidelines, however. She lists some of the main Protestant bodies in the United States, beginning with the most formal liturgically and sacramentally, the *Protestant Episcopal* and *Lutheran* churches. The in-betweens are the *Presbyterians, United Church of Christ, United Methodists,* and *Disciples of Christ* (*Christian Church*). The liturgically freest and the least sacramental are the *Baptists* and *Pentecostals*.

Among these groups, some of the opposing doctrines and practices are as follows: living in sin versus living above sin; predestination versus free will; infant versus believer's baptism; and loose organization versus tightly knit organization. Some uphold **fundamental precepts,** *holding to the Scriptures as infallible* whereas others uphold **liberal precepts,** *using the Scriptures as a guide, with various interpretations for current living.*

With this infinite variety, Jean feels that learning the individual beliefs of her Protestant patients is essential. When and if a patient wants Communion; if an infant should be baptized; and what will be most helpful spiritually to the patient—these factors are learned by careful listening. Generally Jean feels that prayer, a scriptural motto such as "I can do all things through Christ who gives me strength," or a line from a hymn can give strength to a Protestant. Some patients will also want anointing with oil as a symbolic aid to healing.

Jean has discovered that there are wide differences in Prostestantism, sometimes even within the same denomination, about the theology and rituals of death. Some Protestant theologies have come to grips with the realities and meaning of death; others block authentic expression of grief by denying death and focusing on "If you are a Christian, you won't be sad."

Some Protestants view death as penalty and punishment for sins; others see death as a transition when the soul leaves the body for eternal reward; and still others view death as an absolute end. All agree that death is a biological and spiritual event, a mystery not fully comprehended.

Rituals surrounding death vary widely. Some churches believe that the funeral service with a closed casket or memorial service with no casket present is more of a testimony to the joy and victory of Christian life than the open-casket service. Others believe that death is a reality to be faced instead of denied and that viewing the dead person promotes the grief process and confrontation with death in a Christian context.

Jean believes that, for most Protestants, the minister represents friendship, love, acceptance, forgiveness, and understanding. His presence seems to help the dying face death with more ease. She also feels that Protestants are becoming more active in ministering to the bereaved through regularly scheduled visits during the 12 to 18 months after the funeral, although there are no formal rituals.

OTHER GROUPS OF INTEREST

Practices or beliefs unique to certain groups should be part of every health worker's knowledge.*

Seventh-Day Adventists rely on Old Testament law more than do other Christian churches. As in Jewish tradition, the Sabbath is from

*See *Nursing* '77, December 1977, pp. 64–70, for more detailed study.

sundown Friday to sundown Saturday. And like the Orthodox Jew, the Seventh-Day Adventist may refuse medical treatment and the use of secular items, such as television, during this period and prefer to read spiritual literature. Diet is also restricted. Pork, fish without both scales and fins, tea, and coffee are prohibited. Some Seventh-Day Adventists are **lacto-ovo-vegetarians:** *they eat milk and eggs but no meat*. Tobacco, alcoholic beverages, and narcotics are also avoided. Because Adventists view the body as the "temple of God," health reform is high on their list of priorities and they sponsor health institutes, cooking schools, and food-producing organizations. They have pioneered in making foods for vegetarians, including meatlike foods from vegetable sources. Worldwide they operate an extensive system of over 4000 schools and 400 medical institutions and are active medical missionaries (55, 78). Much of their inspiration comes from Ellen G. White, a nineteenth-century prophetess who gave advice on diet and food and who stressed Christ's return to earth.

The Church of Jesus Christ of Latter-Day Saints (Mormons) takes much of its inspiration from the **Book of Mormon,** *translated from golden tablets found by the prophet Joseph Smith*. The Mormons believe that this book and two others supplement the Bible. Every Mormon is an official missionary. There is no official congregational leader, but a **seventy** and a **high priest** *represent successive steps upward in commitment and authority*.

The Articles of Faith of the Church of Jesus Christ of Latter-day Saints, as given by Joseph Smith, include statements of belief:

1. God and His Son, Jesus Christ, and the Holy Ghost.
2. The same organization that existed in the Primitive Church.
3. Worship of God according to personel conscience while obeying the law of the land.
4. People being punished for their own sins and not for Adam's transgression.
5. All people being saved, repentance, and obedience to the laws and ordinances of the Gospel.
6. Being honest, true, chaste, benevolent, virtuous, hopeful, persistent, and doing good to all people.

Specific Mormon beliefs are that the dead can hear the Gospel and can be baptized by proxy. Marriage in the temple seals the relationship for time and eternity. After a special ceremony in the temple, worthy members receive a white garment. This garment, worn under the clothes, has priesthood marks at the navel and at the right knee and is considered a safeguard against danger. The church believes in a whole-being approach and provides education, recreation, and financial aid for its members. A health and conduct code called "Word of Wisdom" prohibits tobacco, alcohol, and hot drinks (interpreted as tea and coffee) and recommends eating, though sparingly and with thankfulness, herbs, fruit, meat, fowl, and grain, especially wheat.

The Mormon believes that disease comes both from failure to obey the laws of health and from failure to keep the other commandments of God. However, righteous persons sometimes become ill simply because they have been exposed to microorganisms that cause disease. They also believe that by faith the righteous sometimes escape plagues that are sweeping the land and often, having become sick, the gift of faith restores the obedient to full physical well-being.

Statistics indicate that the Mormon population succumbs to cancer and diseases of the major body systems at a much lower rate than the general population in this country. The death rate for patients suffering from cancer is less than 50 percent that of the general population; 50 percent less for those with diseases of the nervous, circulatory, and digestive systems; 33 percent less for kidney diseases, and 10 percent less for those with respiratory diseases. Mental illness occurs only half as often among Mormons as among the general population (57). An explanation for these differences from the norm might be that the Mormons literally believe that the body is the "temple of God." And they have programs of diet, exercise, family life, and work to help that "temple" function at optimum level.

Although the two groups just discussed—the Seventh-Day Adventists and the Mormons—generally accept and promote modern medical practices, the next two groups hold views that conflict with the medical field. The first group, *Jehovah's Witnesses*, refuses to accept blood transfusions. Their refusal is based on the Levitical commandment, given by God to Moses, declaring that no one in the House of David should eat blood or he would be cut off from his people, and on a New Testament reference (in Acts) prohibiting the tasting of blood. Jehovah's Witnesses in need of surgery, if they are fortunate to be near New York City, can take advantage of the rapid skills of surgeon Termo Hirose. He uses no blood transfusions because he has reduced operating time to one-sixth the usual required time. Thus far he has saved the lives of over 4000 Jehovah's Witnesses (20). Several other surgeons around the country are beginning to be willing to do surgery without using blood, using intravenous fluids like the body's fluid composition instead. The new plasma expanders can also be used.

Every Jehovah's Witness is a minister. Members meet in halls rather than in traditional churches and they produce massive amounts of literature explaining their faith.

The second group, *Church of Christ, Scientist (Christian Scientists),* turn wholly to spiritual means for healing. Occasionally they allow an orthopedist to set a bone if no medication is used. Parents do not allow their children to get a physical examination for school; to have eye, ear, or blood pressure screening; or to receive immunizations. In addition to the Bible, Christian Scientists use as their guide Mary Baker Eddy's *Science and Health with Key to the Scriptures*, originally published in 1875. The title of this work indicates an approach to wholeness and those who follow its precepts think of God as Divine Mind, of spirit as real and eternal, of matter as unreal illusion. Sin, sickness, and death are unrealities or erring belief. Christian Scientists do not ignore their erring belief, however, for they have established nursing homes and sanitoriums, the latter recognized in the United States under the federal Medicare program and in insurance regulations. These facilities are operated by trained Christian Science nurses who give first-aid measures and spiritual assistance.

A Christian Science graduate nurse must complete a 3-year course of training at one of a number of accredited sanitoriums. The training includes, among other subjects, classes in basic nursing arts, care of the elderly, cooking, bandaging, nursing ethics, care of reportable diseases, and theory of obstetrical nursing. The training is nonmedical and in the work of a Christian Science nurse no medication is administered. The nurse supports the work of the **practitioner**, *who devotes full time to the public practice of Christian Science healing*. Healing is not thought of as miraculous but as the application of natural spiritual law.

The practitioner helps people apply natural spiritual law. Such a person is not a clergyman and does not necessarily hold special church office. Becoming a practitioner is largely attained through self-conducted study and a short course of intensive study from an authorized teacher of Christian Science, but daily study, prayer, application, and spiritual growth are the foundation of practice. The practitioner will treat anyone who comes for help and is supported, like other general practitioners, by patients' payments. A Christian Scientist who is in a medical hospital has undoubtedly tried Christian Science healing first, may have been put there by a non-Scientist relative, or may be at variance with sacred beliefs. If brought in while unconscious, the person would want to be given the minimum emergency care and treatment consistent with hospital policy. The person may also appreciate having a Christian Science practitioner called for treatment through prayer.

Two more groups of special interest because of their positive personal and health emphasis are the *Unity School of Christianity* and the *Society of Friends (Quakers)*. While most Roman Catholics acknowledge the earthly spiritual authority of the Pope and most Protestants regard the Bible as their ultimate authority, the Friend's authority resides in direct experience of God within the self. A Friend obeys the **light with-**

in, *the* **inner light** *or the* **divine principle;** *this spiritual quality causes the Friend to esteem self and listen to inner direction.* All Friends are spiritual equals. Without a minister and without any symbols or religious decor, unprogrammed corporate worship consists of silent meditation with each person seeking divine guidance. Toward the end of the meeting, people are free to share their inspiration. The meeting closes with handshaking. Always interested in world peace, Friends have been instrumental in establishing organizations that work toward human brotherhood and economic and social improvements resulting in better health. Friends have staffed hospitals, driven ambulances, and served in medical corps, among numerous other volunteer services.

The *Unity School of Christianity* believes that health is natural and that sickness is unnatural. Followers think illness is real but they believe it can be overcome by concentrating on spiritual goals. Late in the nineteenth century Charles and Myrtle Fillmore started this group after studying, among other religions, Christian Science, Quakerism, and Hinduism. Thus it blends several established concepts in a new direction. Today Unity Village in Missouri has a publication center that publishes several inspirational periodicals, is beautifully landscaped and open for guests to share in the beauty, and houses its real force, Silent Unity. **Silent Unity** *consists of staff who are available on a 24-hour basis to answer telephone calls, telegrams, and letters from people seeking spiritual help.* They offer prayer and counseling to all faiths with no charge.

Some religious groups have retained lifestyle and geographical solidarity as well as theological unity. These groups originated in other countries and immigrated to America.

The Mennonites, for example, some of whom settled in Pennsylvania, are part of a group called the Pennsylvania Dutch, who are of German, rather than Dutch or Holland descent. The Mennonites generally emphasize plain ways of dressing, living, and worshipping. They do not believe in going to war, swearing oaths, or holding offices that require the use of force. Many of them farm the land or are inclined toward service professions. They are well known for their missionary efforts. Another group, the Amish, is a split from the Mennonite family.

A group with northern headquarters in Bethlehem, Pennsylvania, and southern headquarters in Winston-Salem, North Carolina, are the Moravians. These people have also been noted for their missionary work. A restored Moravian village is open for touring in Winston-Salem and during Christmas and Easter special services are shared with non-Moravian friends.

The Waldenses, a Presbyterian group, have their headquarters in Rome but largely populate the town of Valdese, North Carolina. Each summer an outdoor drama portrays their pilgrimage to freedom.

Neo-Pentecostalism

Another facet of Christianity in the United States is *Neo-Pentecostalism*. This is not a group but a trend or phenomenon that has gained support from small groups in all major denominations—some Roman Catholics, Presbyterians, and Lutherans—as well as from those churches traditionally closer to the Pentecostal spirit.

The heart of the Pentecostal spirit is an enthusiastic personal relationship with Christ. Those who are a part of this trend tell about getting out of dead, organized religion or of getting out of a religious tradition that no longer has meaning. They are anxious to share their insights. The hallmark of this experience is "speaking in tongues" or "glossolalia." Christians trace this experience back to the first century A.D. In 1914, however, the phenomenon became institutionalized with the organization of the Pentecostal Assembly of God Church. This group placed its emphasis of a right relationship with God on glossolalia. Three other Pentecostal denominations have come into being: Church of God (Cleveland, Tennessee), Foursquare, and United Evangelical Brethren (11).

Neo-Pentecostalism is thought of as the *renewed interest in glossolalia; it is sometimes called the Charismatic Movement.*

Just what is **glossolalia**? Oral Roberts describes it as the *prayer language of the spirit*; he feels that it is a release of thoughts so deep within the person that ordinary words do not suffice. Sounds made by the person are not in any known language and the conscious mind, through prayer, should interpret the glossolalia after the experience so that the person can use the gained insight in everyday living (58).

Agnosticism and Atheism

This chapter has concentrated so far on worship of God, the divine spirit, with an emphasis on traditional teaching. Some people live by ethical standards, considering themselves either **agnostic**, *incapable of knowing whether God exists*, or **atheistic**, *believing that God does not exist.*

Cults

In the 1970s various *cults* gained publicity. Some older cults are based on fundamental religions, but they are unique in their own way. The Snake People, for example, incorporate the holding of snakes into their services. Newer cults have arisen from communal groups whose goals are stated as religious. Some cults spring from the philosophy and schedule of a self-chosen leader who entices youth in search of identity from their parents and formalized church. The youth involved may evolve into robots; parents have had to "kidnap" their children in order to get them home and "deprogram" them in order to recognize their original personalities (17). You may be involved in the long-term therapy of such a youth.* Lately attention has focused on cults that are attracting not only the young but also the elderly. There are thought to be 2000 cults throughout the world with a membership of 3 million (56).

Devil worship is also practiced as a cult. One young man spoke of how he became a precocious student of Satan. He read dozens of books on Satan as "Light-Bearer, the strongest and wisest angel in heaven, robbed of his rightful worship by a jealous God." He spoke of putting a hex on others, drinking ghoulish concoctions, and being obsessed with certain rites as he moved through the hierarchy to priesthood (80). Counselors and psychiatrists, as well as some ministers and priests, have had to deal with devil possession in treating clients. Although we do not often speak in these terms in our scientific age, devil possession is a recurring theme in patients' self-diagnosis and one that you should listen for.

Summary of American Religions

The Encyclopedia of American Religions (1978, two volumes) by J. Gordan Meltan would be a good addition to the reference shelf in any health care facility in the United States. It is the first reference work to gather detailed information on all 1200 American religions from the well-known to the lesser cults. This work encompasses all religionists from mystical Hassidic Jews, metaphysicians, psychics, and witches to believers in the imminent end of the world, magic, and UFOs, as well as traditional Catholics, Lutherans, and Methodists. The author places all 1200 groups into 18 families (45) with common heritages and lifestyles and identifies these families as

Liturgical	Lutheran
Reformed-Presbyterian	Liberal
Pietist Methodist	Holiness
Pentecostal	European Free Church
Baptist	Independent Fundamentalists
Adventist	Latter Day Saints
Communal	Metaphysical
Psychic and New Age	Magick
Eastern	Middle Eastern

*See *Christian Life*, April 1978, pp. 22-25, 62-65, for more information on cults.

NURSING IMPLICATIONS

You can use the foregoing—basic beliefs, dietary laws, and ideas of illness, health, body, spirit, mysticism, pragmatism, pain, death, cleanliness, and family ties—as a *beginning*. Even more basic than understanding these concepts is respecting your patient as a person with spiritual needs who has a right to have these needs met, whether he/she has formal religious beliefs. No one will respect your spiritual aid if you do not appear competent and thoughtful in your work. You are not expected to be a professional spiritual leader, for which lengthy training and experience would be required. You can, however, aid patients. You are the transition, the key person between the patient and spiritual help.

If you feel inadequate, you may want to imitate several nurses who also felt the same. They decided that they could not meet the spiritual needs of others because they had not met—or even identified—their own. They had a series of discussions focusing on their own needs and used the book *Spiritual Care: The Nurses Role* (18), along with the accompanying workbook (64). When they had a clear vision of their own value system and made plans to meet their own needs, they could begin to focus on others. They also discussed appropriate and inappropriate spiritual intervention and learned to be comfortable making appropriate referrals when they felt that their lack of time or expertise did not allow them to intervene (7).

Case Study

Consider the following case of a man with spiritual needs.

> Jason Smith is a 40-year-old, middle-class, Caucasian bank president. He lives in a small town with his wife and four children. He also deals in real estate, works with civic and Roman Catholic church groups, and is developing an advertising company. He seems constantly busy. He discusses business over lunch and competes with friends when playing golf or tennis.
>
> One evening he started vomiting and defecating blood and learned, after being hospitalized locally, that he had a bleeding duodenal ulcer. He was then taken in an ambulance to a metropolitan hospital 200 miles away, where a specialist successfully performed a partial gastrectomy, surgical removal of part of the stomach.
>
> For the first time in his life, Jason was stopped. He was away from family and friends and was confined. Good and bad memories flooded his mind. He began to evaluate his activities, his emphasis on material gain and competition, how his children were growing so fast, how his religious activities were superficial, and how, without skilled surgery, he might have died.
>
> At first he tried being jovial with the staff in order to strike out these

new and troubling thoughts. But he couldn't sleep well. He was dreaming about death in wild combinations with his past life. He began to mention these dreams, along with questions about how the surgery would affect his life span, diet, and activities. He mentioned a friend who seemed severely limited from a similar surgery. He also said he was worried about the problems his teenagers were beginning to face and about his own ability to guide them properly.

The staff members never forced Jason to express more than he wished but answered the questions that were medically based and asked him if he would like to see the chaplain, since his own priest was not available. Jason agreed. An appointed nurse then informed the chaplain of Jason's physical, emotional, and spiritual history to date. In the course of several sessions the chaplain helped Jason work through a revised philosophy of life that put more emphasis on spiritual values, family life, and healthy use of leisure.

Assessment

Although you can learn a great deal by picking out points in case studies, remember that they provide only a basis. You will have to accept each patient's individual spiritual development. For example, the sacraments have a very different meaning to Jason than to a child. To a 10-year-old, the meaning of baptism might be carrying an ugly little baby on a pillow to the front of the church, pouring water on its head, and trying to believe that the baby emerges as a beautiful child of God. An adolescent or young adult caught up in sorting out various facets of learned idealism and trying to fit them into more realistic daily patterns may temporarily discard religious teaching. He/she may reject the guidance of a spiritual leader because the latter is associated with the parents' beliefs; yet the adolescent is nevertheless searching and needs guidance. An elderly person suffering the grief of a recently lost mate may repeatedly question how a God of love could allow this loss. Some physiologically mature people are not religiously mature; they may expect magic from God. The spiritually maturing individual experiences the fruits of faith in God in behavioral terms of love, trust, and security. The external spiritual stimuli of God's word, sacraments, and relationships with other believers create an inner peace and love through which the person experiences God within and then reaches out to others in supporting relationships.

Furthermore, realize that people can use the same religious terms differently: *saved, sanctified, fell out, slain by the spirit*, and *deathbed conversion* all connote religious experiences. You should listen carefully and you may have to ask questions to determine accurately the individual person's meaning.

For too long there has been no communication between the nurse and the chaplain. You can fill that gap. Nurse and chaplain rapport can mean that the *whole* person is served rather than segmented parts. Chaplains are especially helpful to clients, as well as to nurses, when they assist with the expression of anger, death, and the expression of grief (15). Nurse and chaplain, however, need to know what to expect from each other; there is no substitute for talking about these expectations and agreeing on strategies.

When determining medical background, such as drug or food allergies, you could also ask about religious dietary laws, special rituals, or restrictions that might be an important part of the patient's history. Recording and helping the patient follow beliefs could speed recovery.

The spiritual needs of the patient have become a part of the evolving nursing diagnosis system of classification. Three areas have been pinpointed: spiritual distress related to the need for (1) love and relatedness, (2) forgiveness, and (3) meaning and purpose. As nurses become more attuned to this situation, perhaps meeting the patient's spiritual needs will not be unattached from other care. Perhaps you could share with the chaplain the responsibility for asking some of the following questions as you give patient care. No specific set of questions will be right for every patient, but the following questions might draw helpful responses as you make a nursing assessment-diagnosis in the spiritual realm.

1. Who is your God? What is He like? (Or, what is your religion? Tell me about it.)
2. Do you believe that God or someone is concerned for you?
3. Who is the most important person to you? Is that person available?
4. Has being sick (what's been happening to you) made any difference in your feelings about God? In the practice of your faith? If it has, could you explain how it has changed?
5. Do you feel that your faith is helpful to you? If it is, how? If it is not, why not?
6. Are there any religious beliefs, practices, or rituals that are important to you now? If there are, could you tell me about them? Can I help you carry them out by showing you where the chapel is? By telling the dietary department about your vegetarian preference? By allowing you specific times for prayer or meditation?
7. Is there anything that would make your situation easier? (Such as a visit from the minister, priest, rabbi, or chaplain? Someone who would read to you? Time for reading your religious book or praying? Someone to pray with you?)
8. Is prayer important to you? (If so, has being sick made a difference in your practice of praying?) What happens when you pray?
9. Do you have available religious books or articles, such as the Bible,

prayer books, phylacteries, or crucifix, that mean something to you?
10. What are your ideas about illness? About life after death?
11. Is there anything especially frightening or meaningful to you right now?
12. If these questions have not uncovered your source of spiritual support, can you tell me where you do find support (69, 70)?

Be sure to look for the patient's strengths, not weaknesses. And remember that you must not preach or reconstruct. Allow the patient to assume his/her own spiritual stance.

Because your relationship with the patient may be of short duration, be sure to document well the results of this interview. And later, when you or others care for the patient, you should watch for religious needs that may be expressed through nonreligious language. You must again let the patient know what options are open for spiritual help. If you hide behind busyness and procedures, you may lose a valuable opportunity to aid in health restoration.

Your greater understanding of social-class and cultural differences gleaned from Chapter 10 should help you comprehend some of the religious differences. For instance, a poor Protestant American who has grown up with the barest survival materials, who has no economic power, no money for recreation, no hope for significant gain, and no positive attitude about this life may center his/her whole being in the church. It provides as best it can for his/her emotional, recreational, and spiritual needs. When the person sings about heaven in terms of having beautiful clothes, a crown, and a mansion, he/she is singing with a much different meaning than the wealthy Protestant American who is really more concerned about mansions *here* than *over there*.

In a wider sense, an Egyptian Christian and an American Christian, although voicing the same basic beliefs, will differ in their approaches to religion. The Egyptian, influenced by the Islamic attitudes of his/her country, might say, "No matter what happens, it's God's will. I can do no more about it." The American Christian may be more influenced by the individual drive to guide his/her life, a philosophy so prevalent in this culture. Another cultural difference centers on the influence of the family with an ill member. The Egyptian, accustomed to having family and friends around nearly constantly, will expect a continuation of such activity during illness. Their presence provides spiritual and emotional support. The American, more mobile and used to the American hospital system of limiting visitors in number and time, may be better able to detach self from the emotional and religious support given by the presence of family.

Religion influences behavior and attitudes toward:

1. Work–whether you work to expiate sin, because it's there to do, or because of a conviction that it is a God-given right and responsibility.
2. Money–whether you save money to deny yourself something, do installment buying, buy health insurance, consider money the root of all evil, or believe that it is to be used for the betterment and development of persons and society.
3. Political behavior–ideas about the sanctity of the Constitution, effects of Communism, importance of world problems, spending abroad versus spending for national defense, school or residential desegregation, welfare aid, and union membership.
4. Family–kinds of interaction within the family, honoring of parents or spouse, children, or siblings.
5. Childrearing–interest in the child's present and future, attitudes toward punishment or rewards for behavior, values of strict obedience as contrasted with independent thinking, or how many children should be born.
6. Right and wrong–what is sin, how wrong is gambling, drinking, birth control, divorce, smoking, and abortion (4).

Consider how essentially the same situation can be diversely interpreted by two teenagers of different faiths. One, a fundamentalist Protestant, may spend an evening dancing and playing cards and suffer crushing guilt because she participated in supposed sinful acts. The other, a Jewish teenager, may participate in the same activities and consider it a religiously based function. Your knowledge of and sensitivity to such differences are important, for essentially similar kinds of decisions–right and wrong as religiously defined–will be made about autopsy, cremation, and organ transplants. (See reference 30 for additional information.) Furthermore, although religious bodies may hand down statements on these issues, often the individual person will alter the group's stand while incorporating individual circumstances into the decision.

Ideally, religion provides strength, an inner calm and faith with which to work through life's problems. But you must be prepared to see the negative aspect. To some, religion seems to add guilt, depression, and confusion. Some may blame God for making them ill, for letting them suffer, or for not healing them in a prescribed manner. One Protestant felt she had made a contract with God: if she lived the best Christian life she could, God would keep her relatively well and free from tragedy. When an incurable disease was diagnosed, she said, "What did I do to deserve this?" Another Protestant, during her illness, took the opposite view of her contract with God. She said "I wasn't living as well as I should and God knocked me down to let me know I was backsliding."

Healing, too, has varied meanings. Some will demand that God provide a quick and miraculous recovery whereas others will expect the process to occur through the work of the health team. Still others combine God's touch, the health workers' skill, and their own emotional and physical cooperation. Some will even consider death as the final form of healing.

Sometimes you must deal with your own negative reactions. Your medical background and knowledge may cause you to be dismayed at some religious practices. For instance, how will you react as you watch a postoperative Jehovah's Witness patient die because she has refused blood? How will you react to a Christian Scientist patient who, in your opinion, should have sought medical help a month ago to avoid present complications? Here is one response given by a Christian Science nurse: "People can be ruined psychologically by going against a long held belief. They may live and get better physically, but will suffer depression, guilt, and failure in not holding to their standard." Basically they prefer to die. Should you dictate otherwise? You may need to think through and discuss such situations with a spiritual leader.

Intervention

With all these aspects to consider, a team approach that includes the patient, family, health workers, and chaplain or other spiritual leader is imperative. Because Americans want weekends away from the job, the weekend hospital staff often has double responsibility. Furthermore, weekends are when most people attend corporate worship. Preparing the patient for chapel service, or seeing that the Sabbath ritual is carried out, puts a special responsibility on you, the nurse.

If a patient is confined to a room, you can simply prepare a worship center or shrine by arranging flowers, prayer book, relics, or whatever other objects have spiritual meaning.

You should keep one or more calendars of various religious holidays. The Eastern Orthodox Easter usually does not coincide with the Roman Catholic and Protestant Easter. Jewish holidays usually do not fall on the same dates of the Western calendar in successive years. Remember, also, that holidays are family days and that ill people separated from the family at such times may be especially depressed.

Maintaining a list of available spiritual leaders, knowing when to call them, and knowing how to prepare for their arrival are other important responsibilities. If a patient can't make the request, consult with the family. One woman said, "If my sister sees a priest, she will be sure she is dying." Once a health worker took the initiative to call an Eastern Orthodox priest who, unfortunately, represented the wrong nationality; the patient's main source of comfort was to have come from discussion and prayers in the native language. Sometimes the family needs reassurance and guidance from the chaplain. You can suggest this option.

As you prepare the patient and the setting for a spiritual leader, help create an atmosphere that reflects more than sterile procedure. Privacy has previously been emphasized by drawing curtains and shutting doors. Although acceptable to some, this approach may produce a negative response in others. Perhaps more emphasis should be given to cheerful surroundings: sunshine, flowers, lighted candles, openness, and participation by family and staff in at least an introductory way. Perhaps the patient and spiritual leader could meet outdoors in an adjoining garden. The Shintoist and Taoist would especially benefit from the esthetic exposure. If the patient is a child on a prolonged hospitalization, a special area might be designated for religious instruction.

Brief the spiritual leader on any points that might provide special insight and be sure that the patient is ready to receive him/her. Prepare any special arrangements, such as having a clean, cloth-covered tray for Communion. Guard against interruption by health workers from other departments who may be unaware of the visit. Finally, incorporate the results of the visit into the patient's record.

Many will benefit from the sacraments, the prayers, Scripture reading, and counseling given by the spiritual leader, but others will want to rely on their own direct communication with God. The Zen Buddhist, Hindu, Muslim, and Friend might be in the latter category. All may wish reading material, however. Most will bring their sacred book with them, but if they express a desire for more literature, offer to get it. Some hospitals furnish daily and weekly meditations as well as copies of the King James Version of the Bible (which recently has been updated). Or you might suggest the Bible paraphrased in modern language by Kenneth Taylor, called *The Living Bible* (Tyndale House, 1971). The same edition is available as *The Children's Living Bible* (Tyndale House, 1972) with appropriate illustrations. *The Way* (Tyndale House, 1972) has the same wording as *The Living Bible* with guidelines and illustrations for youth. The *Amplified Bible* (Zondervan Publishing House, 1965) is especially good for translating the original Greek into comparable English meaning. A positive interfaith magazine is *Guideposts* (Guideposts Associates, Inc.). A novel with religious insights is *Christy* (Avon Books, 1968) by Catherine Marshall. A spiritually based autobiography is *Joni* (World Wide Publication, 1976) by Joni Eareckson. A delightful biography about a spiritually mature preschool-school-age child is *Mister God, This Is Anna* (Ballantine

Books, 1974) by Fynn, *In Search of God: The Story of Religion* by Marietta Maskin is written for youth but is also recommended for adults who work with youth. Don't overlook the opportunity to share the ministry of books.

If you feel comfortable doing so, you can at times say a prayer, read a Scripture, or provide a statement of faith helpful to the patient. If you do not feel comfortable in providing this kind of spiritual care, you can still meet the patient's spiritual needs through respectful conversation, listening to the patient talk about beliefs, referral to another staff member, or calling one of the patient's friends who can bolster his/her faith. If spiritual leaders aren't available, you could organize a group of health workers willing to counsel with or make referrals for patients of their own faiths.

The atheist is not to be neglected because he/she does not profess a belief in God. He/she has the same need for respect as anyone else and may need you to listen to fears and doubts. The person doesn't need your judgment.

Moreover, just as health teaching is often omitted for health workers who are patients, so is spiritual guidance often omitted for spiritual leaders who are patients. You must recognize that each person, regardless of religious stand or leadership capacity, may need spiritual help.

Although a hospital setting has been used as a point of reference throughout this chapter, you can improvise in your setting—nursing home, school, industry, clinic, home, or other health center—in order to provide adequate spiritual assistance.

Exactly what constitutes spiritual intervention needs further research. In an attempt to identify which practices are used by individuals to establish or maintain a relationship with God, three groups within the Judeo-Christian religion completed a 23-item questionnaire. The questionnaire listed 16 practices that individuals in the Judeo-Christian religion might do to establish or maintain a relationship with God; study participants were asked to check if the practice was "helpful" or "not helpful" to them. The questionnaire focused on religious practices that do not require the clergy. The three groups, one Protestant, one Catholic, and one Jewish, were randomly selected from churches and synagogues listed in the Yellow Pages of a Midwestern city. The Protestant church so selected was Pentecostal and the Jewish synagogue was Orthodox. At least 25 individuals from each group completed the questionnaire.

Table 11-1 lists the practices from the questionnaire and the number and percentage of subjects that identified the practice "helpful" from each of the three groups.

Subjects who had had contact with nurses were also asked if they

TABLE 11-1 Practices Rated Helpful by Individuals in the Judeo-Christian Religion to Establish and/or Maintain a Relationship with God

USING RELIGIOUS LITERATURE	CATHOLICS	N	PROTESTANTS	N	JEWS	N
Reading from the Bible by yourself.	21 (68%)	31	48 (98%)	49	23 (92%)	25
Reading from the Bible with others.	18 (56%)	32	48 (96%)	50	20 (83%)	24
Discussing Bible passages with others.	21 (66%)	32	50 (100%)	50	23 (96%)	24
Reading from religious writings of people of your religious group or denomination.	22 (71%)	31	45 (92%)	49	20 (87%)	24
Reading religious books, magazines, and/or religious newspapers	29 (83%)	35	45 (92%)	49	21 (88%)	24
USING PRAYER						
Praying silently, using your own words.	37 (100%)	37	48 (96%)	50	25 (100%)	25
Praying silently, using written or memorized prayers.	36 (95%)	38	7 (14%)	49	11 (69%)	16
Praying aloud with your religious leader.	31 (91%)	34	44 (90%)	49	23 (85%)	27
Praying aloud when a group of your faith is listening and praying with you.	29 (85%)	34	46 (94%)	49	21 (84%)	25
Praying aloud when you are alone.	31 (84%)	37	48 (98%)	49	16 (64%)	25
Praying aloud with one or two others.	22 (65%)	34	46 (94%)	49	12 (48%)	25
Praying aloud when people not of your faith are in the vicinity and may overhear you.	10 (33%)	30	35 (73%)	48	8 (33%)	24

USING RELIGIOUS LITERATURE	CATHOLICS	N	PROTESTANTS	N	JEWS	N
ATTAINING SPIRITUAL SUPPORT THROUGH THE ASSISTANCE OF OTHERS						
Listening to me talk through my problems.	33 (97%)	34	47 (94%)	50	19 (76%)	25
Reading Bible passages to me.	13 (41%)	32	44 (88%)	50	4 (20%)	20
Praying with me.	28 (78%)	36	47 (98%)	48	12 (52%)	23
Saying prayers for me (when I was not with the person).	36 (95%)	38	47 (94%)	50	12 (48%)	25

believed a nurse could be helpful to them in establishing or maintaining a relationship with God. Only 5 of 24 Jewish subjects responded "yes." One subject added the comment, "No one, nurse or otherwise, can help in my relationship with God." However, 42 (91%) of the Protestant respondents and 26 (72%) of 36 Catholic respondents checked "yes." The subjects indicating a nurse could be helpful were asked to rate "helpful" or "not helpful" to five possible nursing interventions. The Catholic and Protestant responses are in Table 11-2.

This study is limited by the small number of subjects in each of the three groups. The responses, however, can give direction for more investigation to other Catholic, Protestant, and Jewish groups. Additional studies also need to determine which practices are helpful to individuals in hospitals, hospices, and nursing homes.

TABLE 11-2 Nursing Interventions Rated Helpful

HAVING A NURSE:	CATHOLIC	N	PROTESTANT	N
Read to me Bible passages I have chosen.	15 (75%)	20	36 (88%)	41
Read or recite Bible passages of the nurse's choice.	12 (55%)	22	31 (78%)	40
Listen to me talk through my problems.	22 (92%)	24	32 (80%)	40
Pray with me at my bedside.	20 (83%)	24	37 (93%)	40
Tell me that the nurse is praying for me (when not with me).	23 (96%)	24	36 (92%)	39

REFERENCES

1. **Abbott, Walter M.**, and **Joseph Galleger**, eds., *The Documents of Vatican II.* New York: The America Press, 1966. pp. 37-39. 158, 363.
2. **Allport, Gordon,** *The Individual and His Religion.* New York: The Macmillan Company, 1961, pp. 24-27.
3. **Berkowitz, Philip,** and **Nancy Berkowitz,** "The Jewish Patient in the Hospital," *American Journal of Nursing,* 67, no. 11 (1967), 2335-37.
4. **Bossard, J.,** and **E. Boll,** *The Sociology of Child Development* (4th ed.). New York: Harper & Row, Publishers, Inc., 1966.
5. **Brown, Robert,** *The Spirit of Protestantism.* New York: Oxford University Press, 1961.
6. **Butler, Richard,** "The Roman Catholic Way in Death and Mourning," in *Concerning Death: A Practical Guide for the Living,* ed. Earl Grollman. Boston: Beacon Press, 1974, pp. 101-18.
7. **Buys, Ann,** "Discussion Series Sensitizes Nurses to Patient's Spiritual Needs," *Hospital Progress,* 62 (October 1981), 44-45.

8. **Campbell, Teresa,** and **Betty Chang,** "Health Care of the Chinese in America," *Nursing Outlook*, 21, no. 4 (1973), 245–49.
9. **Carson, Verna,** "Meeting the Spiritual Needs of Hospitalized Psychiatric Patients," *Perspectives in Psychiatric Care*, 18, no. 1 (1980), 17–20.
10. **Coles, Robert,** "God & the Rural Poor," *Psychology Today*, 6, no. 1 (1972), 33–40.
11. **DeVol, Thomas,** "Ecstatic Pentecostal Prayer and Meditation," *Journal of Religion and Health*, 13, no. 4 (1974), 285–88.
12. **Dixon, Dorothy,** *World Religions for the Classroom*. West Mystic, CT.: Twenty-Third Publications, 1975.
13. "Doctors Use Psychic Tools for Healing," *St. Louis Globe-Democrat*, September 30, 1975, Sec. A, p. 12.
14. **Eck, Diana,** "Roots" in *Who Are They?* Los Angeles: The Bhaktivedanta Book Trust, 1982.
15. **Eickhoff, Alice,** "The Chaplain–Nurse Relationship," *Nursing Management*, 13, no. 3 (1982), 25–26.
16. **Ellis, Donelda,** "Whatever Happened to the Spiritual Dimension?" *The Canadian Nurse*, September 1980, pp. 42–43.
17. **Enroth, Ronald,** *Youth, Brainwashing, and the Extremist Cults*. Grand Rapids, MI.: Zondervan Publishing House, 1977.
18. **Fish, Sharon,** and **Judith Allen Sheely,** *Spiritual Care: The Nurses Role*. Downers Grove, IL: Inter-Varsity Press, 1978.
19. **Fleeger, Rebekah,** and **Judy Van Heukelein,** "The Patient's Spiritual Needs—A Part of Nursing Diagnosis," *The Nurses Lamp*, 28, no. 4 (1977).
20. **Galton, Lawrence,** "Surgeon of the Impossible," *Parade*, March 6, 1977, 17–19.
21. **Glustrom, Simon,** *When Your Child Asks: A Handbook for Jewish Parents*. New York: Block Publishing Company, 1959.
22. **Gordon, Audrey,** "The Jewish View of Death: Guidelines for Mourning," in *Death, the Final Stage of Growth*, ed. Elizabeth Kubler-Ross. Englewood Cliffs, NJ: Prentice-Hall, Inc., 1975, pp. 44–51.
23. **Guralnik, David,** ed., *Webster's New World Dictionary of the American Language* (2nd college ed.). New York: World Publishing Company, 1972.
24. **Hackney, E. J.,** personal letter on Zen Buddhism, January 19, 1973.
25. **Hostetler, John,** *The World Book Encyclopedia*. Chicago: World Book-Childcraft International, Inc., 1979, pp. 325–26.
26. "How to Stop a Doctor from Prolonging Life," *St. Louis Globe-Democrat*, February 26, 1976, Sec. A, p. 15.
27. **Hudson, Virginia,** *O Ye Jigs and Juleps*. New York: MacFadden-Bartell Corporation, 1964.
28. **Jordan, Merle,** "The Protestant Way in Death and Mourning," in *Concerning Death: A Practical Guide for Living*, ed. Earl Grollman. Boston: Beacon Press, 1974, pp. 81–100.
29. **Kepler, Milton,** "The Religious Factor in Pediatric Care," *Clinical Pediatrics*, 9, no. 3 (1970), 128–30.
30. ——, "Human Values in Medicine: Some Helping Organizations," *Journal of the American Medical Association*, 15, no. 3 (1973), 305–7.
31. **Kertzer, Morris N.,** *Today's American Jew*. New York: McGraw-Hill Book Company, 1967.

32. ——, *What Is a Jew?* (rev. ed.). New York: The Macmillan Company 1969.
33. **Kushner, Harold,** *When Bad Things Happen to Good People.* New York: Schocken Books, Inc., 1981.
34. **Lamna, Maurice,** *The Jewish Way in Death and Mourning.* New York: Jonathan David Publishing Company, 1969.
35. **Lang, Bruce,** "The Death that Ends Death in Hinduism and Buddhism," in *Death, The Final Stage of Growth,* ed. Elizabeth Kubler-Ross. Englewood Cliffs, NJ: Prentice-Hall, Inc., 1975, pp. 52–57.
36. "Life After Death? 'Beyond Shadow of Doubt,' Psychiatrist Says," *St. Louis Globe-Democrat,* November 15–16, 1975, Sec. A, p. 15.
37. **Long, Luman,** ed., *The World Almanac and Book of Facts, 1971.* New York: Newspaper Enterprise Association, 1971, pp. 327–28.
38. **Luce, Henry R.,** ed., *The World's Great Religions.* New York: Time, Inc., 1957.
39. *Manual on Hospital Chaplaincy.* Chicago: American Hospital Association, 1970, pp. 55–66.
40. **Marshall, Gary,** "Growing up in Krishna," *Parade: St. Louis Post-Dispatch,* February 24, 1980, pp. 4–10.
41. **Marty, Martin,** "Religion in America, 1972," *P.T.A.,* December 1972, pp. 15–19.
42. **Mastrantonis, George,** ed., "St. Nicholas: The Popular Wonder Worker," *Ologos.* St. Louis: Ologos, n.d.
43. **McConkie, Bruce R.,** *Mormon Doctrine.* Salt Lake City: Bookcraft, 1966.
44. **Mead, Frank,** *Handbook of Denominations in the United States* (4th ed.). Nashville: Abingdon Press, 1965.
45. **Melton, J. Gordon,** *The Encyclopedia of American Religions,* I & II. Wilmington, NC: McGrath Publishing Co., 1978.
46. **Morris, Karen,** and **J. Foerster,** "Team Work: Nurse and Chaplain," *American Journal of Nursing,* 72, no. 12 (1972), 2197–99.
47. **Naimann, H.,** "Nursing in Jewish Law," *American Journal of Nursing,* 70, no. 11 (1970), 2378–79.
48. **Noss, John,** *Man's Religions* (rev. ed.). New York: The Macmillan Company, 1956, pp. 399–427.
49. **Okamoto, Abraham,** "Religious Barriers to World Peace," *Journal of Religion and Health,* 15, no. 1 (1976), 26–33.
50. **Petersen, Mark,** *A Word of Wisdom.* Salt Lake City: Church of Jesus Christ of Latter-Day Saints, n.d.
51. **Piepgras, Ruth,** "The Other Dimension: Spiritual Help," *American Journal of Nursing,* 68, no. 12 (1968), 2610–13.
52. **Pill, Robert,** "The Christian Science Practitioner," *Journal of Pastoral Counseling,* 4, no. 1 (1969), 39–42.
53. "Pope Paul Eases the Rules for Anointing the Sick," *St. Louis Globe-Democrat,* January 19, 1973, Sec. A, p. 8.
54. **Porath, Thomas,** "Humanizing the Sacrament of the Sick," *Hospital Progress,* 53, no. 7 (1972), 45–47.
55. "Prophet or Plagarist? E.G. White," *Time,* August 2, 1976, p. 43.
56. "Religious Cults and the Elderly," *Information on Aging.* Institute of Gerontology at Wayne State University, Michigan, July 1982, p. 2.

57. **Richards, LeGrande,** *A Marvelous Work and a Wonder*. Salt Lake City: Deseret Book Company, 1975.
58. **Roberts, Oral,** *A Daily Guide to Miracles*. Tulsa: Pinoak Publications, 1975.
59. **Rosten, Leo,** ed., *Religions in America* (rev. ed.). New York: Simon & Schuster, 1963.
60. **Russell, Douglas L.,** personal letter on Christian Science beliefs and practices, December 1, 1975.
61. **Satprakashananda, Swami,** ed., *The Use of Symbols in Religion*. St. Louis: The Vedanta Society, 1970.
62. **Saunders, E. Dale,** *Buddhism in Japan*. Philadelphia: University of Philadelphia Press, 1964, pp. 265–86.
63. "Second Thoughts About Man: Searching Again for the Sacred," *Time*, April 9, 1973, pp. 90–93.
64. **Shelly, Judith Allen,** *Spiritual Care Workbook*. Downers Grove, IL: Inter-Varsity Press, 1978.
65. **Shibata, Chizuo,** "The New Religions and the Christian Church," *Japan Christian Quarterly*, Summer 1971, pp. 173–80.
66. **Slimmer, Lynda,** "Helping Students to Resolve Conflicts Between Their Religious Beliefs and Psychiatric-Mental Health Treatment Approaches," *Journal of Psychiatric Nursing and Mental Health Services*, 18 (July 1980), 37–39.
67. **Smith, Huston,** *The Religions of Man*. New York: Harper & Row, Publishers, Inc., 1965.
68. **Smith, Wilfred,** *The Faith of Other Men*. New York: The American Library of World Literature, Inc., 1963.
69. **Stoll, Ruth,** and material presented at the workshop for the "Whole Person: Spiritual Dimensions of Patient Care," St. Louis University School of Nursing and Allied Health Professions, February 11–12, 1976.
70. ——, "Guidelines for Spiritual Assessment," *American Journal of Nursing* 79, No. 9 (1979), 1574–77.
71. **Suzuki, D. T., E. Fromm, and R. DeMartino,** *Zen Buddhism and Psychoanalysis*. New York: Grove Press, 1960, p. 5.
72. **Thomas, David M.,** "Religion as a Family Life-Style," *Marriage and Family Living Magazine*, 1979, pp. 1–4.
73. "Those Who Preserve the Ritual Bath," *St. Louis Post-Dispatch*, January 9, 1977, Sec. H, p. 3.
74. **Tinney, James, S.,** "Black Muslims," *Christianity Today*, 20 (March 12, 1976), 51–52.
75. ——, "State of the Nation," *Christianity Today*, 20 (March 26, 1976), 42–43.
76. **Ujhely, Gertrud,** "On Being Possessed by the Devil," *Perspectives in Psychiatric Care*, 10, no. 5 (1972), 202–9.
77. *Unity School of Christianity*. Unity Village, MO: Unity School of Christianity, n.d.
78. **Utt, Richard,** *The Builders: A Photo Story of Seventh-Day Adventists at Work Around the World*. Mountain View, CA: Pacific Press Publishing Association, 1970.
79. **Walker, H. B.,** "Why Medicine Needs Religion," *International Surgery*, 56, no. 8 (1971), 37B–40B.

80. **Warnke, Michael,** "When Evil Fights Back," *Guideposts*, November 1972, pp. 22-25.
81. **Wasson, Elgin,** personal letter and paper from Christian Science Committee on Publication for Missouri, January 8, 1973.
82. **Westerhoff, John, III,** *Will Our Children Have Faith?* New York: Seabury Press, 1976.
83. **Williams, Dennis A.,** and **Elaine Sciolino,** "Rebirth of the Nation," *Newsweek*, 87 (March 15, 1976), 33.
84. **Wilson, John,** *Religion in American Society*. Englewood Cliffs, NJ: Prentice-Hall, Inc., 1981.
85. **Wood, Verna,** personal letter on Religious Society of Friends, January 29, 1973.
86. **Zborowski, Mark,** *People in Pain*. San Francisco: Jossey-Bass, Inc., 1969, pp. 110--28.

Personal Interviews

87. **Andrews, Constantine,** pastor, St. Nicholas Greek Orthodox Church, St. Louis, January 26, 1973.
88. **Bregman, Alan,** rabbi, Temple Israel, St. Louis, January 27, 1973.
89. **Crump, Ronald,** pastor, Rock Hill Church of God, St. Louis, January 30, 1973.
90. **Danker, William,** professor of world mission, Concordia Seminary, St. Louis, January 26, 1973.
91. **Dickes, Hans,** a seventy in the Church of Jesus Christ of Latter-Day Saints, St. Louis, January 20, 1973.
92. **Gowing, Peter,** regional professor, Southeast Asia, Graduate School of Theology, Singapore, January 10, 1973.
93. **Griswell, John,** pastor, Seventh-Day Adventist Central Church, St. Louis, January 31, 1973.
94. **Guirguis, Youssef,** and **Laila Guirguis,** Egyptian Christians, January 13, 1973.
95. **Katsarus, Georgia,** Greek Orthodox, January 19, 1973.
96. **Khalifa, Saeed, Soheir Eltòumi, E. Z. Eltoumi, Mohamed Ahmed,** and **Fatma Ahmed,** Egyptian Muslims, January 13, 1973.
97. **Kimelman, Dr. Nathan, Mrs. Nathan Kimelman, Dr. Harry G. Mellman,** and **Jane Tarlow,** American Jews, January 29 and February 2, 1973.

12

The Family— Basic Unit for the Developing Person

Study of this chapter will enable you to

1. Define *family* and discuss the family as a system and the implications for the developing person.
2. Describe the purposes, tasks, roles, and functions of the family and their relationship to the development and health of its members.
3. List the stages of family life and the developmental tasks for the establishment, expectancy, and parenthood phases.
4. Discuss your role in helping the family achieve its developmental tasks.
5. Relate the impact of feelings about the self and childhood experiences on later family interaction patterns.
6. List and describe the variables affecting the relationship between parent and child and general family lifestyle, including single-parent, step-parent, and adoptive families.
7. Identify ways in which your family life has influenced your present attitudes about family.
8. Discuss the influence of twentieth-century changes on family life and childrearing practices.
9. Predict how a changing culture may affect the development and health of the family system.

10. Explore your role in promoting physical and emotional health of a family and assess community services that might assist you.
11. Assess and work with a family to enhance its welfare while simultaneously giving health care to one of its members.

It's an uncanny feeling—to suddenly know that I am answering my son's question with the same words—even the same tone—as my father used with me 30 years ago.

Even though I have a happy, successful marriage, two loving children, a nice home, and a profession in which I feel competent, I constantly fight a feeling of inferiority. A contributing factor must be that my parents never encouraged or complimented me. When I took a test, they emphasized the 2 wrong, not the 98 right.

I always admired my aunt. If my cousin, her son, had told her he wanted to build a bridge to the moon, she would have furnished the nails.

These three men are speaking of aspects of a social and biological phenomenon that is often taken for granted: the family. So strongly can this basic unit affect our development that we may live successfully or unsuccessfully because of its influence. Much that the person learns about loving, coping, and the various aspects of life is first learned in the family unit.

Between society and the individual person, the family exists as a primary system and social group, for most people share many of life's experiences with the family. Thus the family has a major role in shaping the person; it is a basic unit of growth, experience, adaptation, health, or illness.

This chapter is not an exhaustive study of families or family life. Rather, it is an overview of the various forms, stages, and functions of contemporary American families and of how nursing can use this knowledge. Although various aspects of the family are discussed separately, keep in mind that family purposes, stages of development, developmental tasks, and patterns of interaction are all closely interrelated, all influenced by historical foundations, and all continually evolving into new forms. Thus the family should be viewed as a system.

DEFINITIONS

The **family** *is a social system and primary reference group made up of two or more persons living together who are related by blood, marriage, or adoption or who are living together by agreement over a period of time*. The family unit is *characterized by face-to-face contact, bonds of* *affection, love, harmony, simultaneous competition and mutual concern, a continuity of past, present, and future, shared goals and identity, and behaviors and rituals common only to the specific unit* (78, 87). With the family, the person can usually let down his/her guard and be more himself/herself than with other people.

The family may be **nuclear** *(mother, father, child)*, **extended** *(nuclear plus other relatives of either or both spouses live together)*, **patriarchal** *(the man has the main authority and decision-making power)*, **matriarchal** *(the woman has the main authority)*, or **reconstituted** *(one divorced or widowed adult with all or some of his/her children and a new spouse with all or some of his/her children, so that parents, stepparents, children, and stepchildren live together.)* Or the family may be made up of siblings, especially in middle or late life, homosexuals, friends in a commune, or a male and female living together without being married. The family may be symbolically duplicated in the work setting: a woman may be perceived as a grandmother, mother, or sister, or a man may be perceived as a grandfather, father, or brother to an employee. The family member who is dead or missing may remain clearly in the other members' memory; they may refer to the person on special occasions. Or the deviant of the family—the alcoholic or runaway—may influence other family members to act in an opposite manner.

The family may also be a series of separate but interrelated families. The middle-aged parents are helping the adolescent and young adult offspring to be emancipated from the home while simultaneously caring for increasingly dependent parents and sometimes up to four pairs of grandparents and older aunts and uncles as well. All related family members may not live under the same roof (in fact, they never did in America), but the extended family exists psychologically—in spirit. Often the responsibility is nearly overwhelming to the middle-agers, who have no time or resources to spend on themselves. The conflict inherent in having to care for a number of relatives and in-laws can contribute to marital disharmony as well as poor relationships between the generations (13).

The elderly person is sometimes aware of such a situation and will try to make minimal demands. Often he/she feels that more attention is deserved and may make extra demands or chastise the middle-aged offspring for not doing more for elder family members.

The mass media present a picture of family life dissolving in the United States. Although the divorce rate is approximately 40 to 50 percent, most divorced people remarry. Because of greater life expectancy and the young age at which people marry, the young couple of today enter and remain in marriage longer than did their grandparents.

PURPOSES, TASKS, ROLES, AND FUNCTIONS OF THE FAMILY

Although the institution of the family is being scrutinized and predictions are made that it is about to pass into oblivion, the family has demonstrated throughout history that it is a virtually indestructible institution. Family structure, roles, and responsibilities have always been influenced by technology and the resulting social changes. But technological advances alone do not determine family structure and function. Family systems are a force in themselves endlessly adaptive, and very resistant to outside pressure. In a society where objects are often disposable and people feel uneasy and dispensable, they seek secure relationships.

The U.S. family has passed through major transitions. The family was once a relatively self-contained, cohesive domestic work unit; it has become a group of persons dispersed among various educational and work settings. Various agencies have absorbed many purposes once handled solely by the family group. Schools educate; hospitals care for the sick; mortuaries prepare the dead for burial; churches give religious training; government and private organizations erect recreational facilities; nursing homes care for the aged; and various manufacturing firms bake, can, or bottle food and make clothes.

When the family changed from a production unit to a consumption unit, it also lost some degree of authority to regulate its members' behavior. The emphasis is now on democratic sharing, togetherness, the child's potential as an individual, and the fun aspects of parenthood. Enjoyment and relaxation in every human relationship are considered important. Technology is seen as the reason for this view, and the way to attain the happy state, but the person who believes too strongly in what technology can accomplish may have unrealistic expectations about living and thus undergo considerable stress in marriage and childrearing.

Yet the family is still considered responsible for the child's growth and development and behavioral outcomes; indeed, the family is a cornerstone for the child's competency development. Because the family is strongly influenced by its surrounding environment as well as by the child itself, the family should not bear full blame for what the child is or becomes. Few parents deliberately set out to rear a disturbed, handicapped, or delinquent offspring, although many such failures occur (30).

The family is expected to perform the following tasks:

1. Provide for physical safety and economic needs of its members and obtain enough goods, services, and resources to survive.

2. Create a sense of family loyalty and a mentally healthy environment for the family's well-being.
3. Help members to develop physically, emotionally, intellectually, and spiritually, as well as to develop a personal and family identity.
4. Foster a value system built on spiritual and philosophical beliefs and the cultural and social system that is part of the identity.
5. Teach members to communicate effectively their needs, ideas, feelings, as well as respect for each other.
6. Provide social togetherness simultaneously with division of labor, patterning of sexual roles, and performance of family roles with flexibility and cooperation.
7. Reproduce and socialize the child(ren), inculcating values and appropriate behavior, providing adult role models, and fostering a positive self-concept and self-esteem in the child(ren).
8. Provide relationships and experience within and without the family that foster security, support, encouragement, motivation, morale, and creativity.
9. Help the members to cope with crises and societal demands.
10. Maintain authority and decision making, with the parents representing society to the family as a whole and the family unit to society.
11. Promote integration into society and the ability to use social organizations for special needs when necessary.
12. Release family members into the larger society—school, church, organizations, work, and politics.
13. Maintain constructive and responsible ties with the neighborhood, school, and local and state government (1, 20, 40, 97, 128).

The family's ability to meet its tasks depends on the maturity of the adult members, the support given by the social system—educational, work, religious, social, welfare, governmental, and leisure institutions. The family that is most successful as a unit has a working philosophy and value system that is understood and lived, uses healthy adaptive patterns most of the time, can ask for help and use the community services available, and develops linkages with nonfamily units and organizations (128). Refer to Chapter 7 for additional information about family adaptive mechanisms and patterns that maintain internal equilibrium so that it can fulfill its purposes, roles, deal with stress and crises, and promote growth and maturity of individual family members.

To remain adaptive, families maneuver to secure compliance of all members with the family rules through verbal and nonverbal communication to each other. Usually one member is designated as the one who must maintain a specific pattern of dependent behavior, sometimes negative or unhealthy, in order to keep all other family members comfortable. If the designated member tries to change behavior and become more independent, he/she receives no support. The feedback received is that he/she is disrupting the status quo and the other family members are uncomfortable. Thus sick behavior will be maintained at the expense of the development of the designated person and of the family.

Signs of strained or destructive family relationships include

1. Lack of understanding and communication between spouses.
2. Each family member alternately acting as if the other didn't exist or harassing through arguments.
3. Lack of family decision making.
4. Parents' possessiveness of the children or the mate.
5. Children's derogatory remarks to parents or vice versa.
6. Extreme closeness between husband and his mother or family or the wife and her mother or family.
7. Parent being domineering about performance of household tasks.
8. Few outside friends for parents or children.
9. Scapegoating or blaming each other for difficulties.
10. High level of anxiety or insecurity present in the home.
11. Lack of creativity.
12. Pattern of immature or regressive behavior in parents or children. (59).

Roles of the Family

The family apportions **roles,** *prescribed behaviors in a situation*, in a way similar to society at large (87). In society there are specialists who enforce laws, teach, practice medicine, and fight fires. In the family there are also such performance roles: breadwinner, homemaker, handyman (or handywoman), the expert, political advisor, chauffeur, and gardener. There are also emotional roles: leader, nurturer, sustainer, protector, healer, arbitrator, scapegoat, jester, rebel, dependent, "sex-pot," and "black sheep." Members may fill more than one role. The fewer people there are to fulfill these roles, as in the nuclear family, the greater the number of demands placed on one person. If a member leaves home, someone else takes up his/her role. Any member of the family can satisfactorily fulfill any role in either category unless he or she is uncomfortable in that role. The man who is sure of his masculinity will have no emotional problems diapering a baby or cooking a meal. The woman who is sure of her femininity will have no trouble gardening or taking the car for repair.

The emotional response of a person to the role he/she fulfills should be considered. Someone may perform the job competently and yet dread doing it. The man may be a carpenter because his father taught him the trade, although he wants to be a music teacher. Changes in performance roles also necessitate emotional changes—for example, in the man who takes over household duties when his wife becomes incapacitated.

The child learns about emotional response to roles in the family while imitating adults. The child experiments with various roles in play and eventually finds one that is emotionally comfortable. The more pressure put on the child by the parents to respond in a particular way, the more likely that child is to learn only one role and be uncomfortable in others, as evidenced by the athletic champion who may be a social misfit. The child becomes less adaptive socially and even within the family as a result.

Exercising a capacity for a variety of roles, either in actuality or in fantasy, is healthy. The healthy family is the one in which there is opportunity to shift roles intermittently with ease (87). Through these roles family functions are fulfilled.

Functions of the Family as a Social System

The family is a system. It functions as a unit to fulfill its purposes, roles, tasks. It provides shelter, stability, security, and a setting for nurturance and growth. It is a safe place to experiment with the dynamics and role behaviors required in a system. It has an energy that provides a support system for individual members. As the social system changes, the family system must also adapt if it is to meet individual needs and prepare its members to participate in the social system.

The organization of a family system is hierarchal, although it may not be directly observable. The usual family hierarchies are built on kinship, power, status, and privilege relationships that may be related to individual characteristics of age, sex, education, personality, health, strength, or vigor. We can infer a hierarchy by observing each person's behavior and communication. For instance, who talks first? Last? Longest? Who talks to whom? When? Where? About what? If one family member consistently approaches the staff about the client's health care, he/she probably holds an upper position in the family and has the task of being "expert" on the client's status. Your attempt to communicate with family members may meet with resistance if the communication inadvertently violates the family communication hierarchy (105).

Hierarchal relations in the family system determine the role behavior of family members. These hierarchal role relationships typically have great stability and ordinarily family members can be counted on to behave congruently with their roles. When there are differences in behavior from situation to situation, they are almost inevitably in response to the family's expectations for that particular situation or circumstance (105). Families develop a system of balanced relationships. When one member leaves the family or experiences a change, such as illness, other family members must adapt as well. Roles and relationships are based on reciprocal interaction, each member of the family contributing to the total unit in a unique and functional way. If a member should fail to meet the expectations of the roles established by his or her position in the hierarchy for the moment, the remaining members of the family generally react by using pressure (for example, persuasion, punishment, argument, being ignored) on the "deviant" person (105). Ackerman states that all family functions can be reduced to two basic ones: (1) ensuring the physical survival of the species and (2) transmitting the culture, thereby ensuring essential humanness. The union of mother and father, of parent and child, forms the bonds of identity that are the matrix for the development of this humanness (1).

Physical Functions of the family are met by the parents providing food, clothing, and shelter, protection against danger, provision for bodily repairs after fatigue or illness, and by reproduction. In "primitive" societies these physical needs are the dominant concern. In Western societies many families take them for granted (87).

Affectional Functions are equally important. Although many traditional family functions, such as education, job training, and medical care, are being absorbed by other agencies, meeting emotional needs and promoting adaptation and adjustment are still two of the family's major functions. The family is the primary unit in which the child tests emotional reactions. Learning how to reach and maintain emotional equilibrium within the family enables him/her to repeat the pattern in later life situations. The child who feels loved is likely to contract fewer physical illnesses, learn more quickly, and generally have an easier time growing up and adapting to society (87).

Satir believes a healthy family has five dominant attitudes

1. No distinctions are made about worth of people; all members are perceived as equal.
2. All persons are seen as unique and developing.
3. When a disturbing situation arises, members understand that many factors were involved—people were not simply trying to be difficult.
4. Members accept that change is continuous.
5. Members freely share their thoughts and feelings with a minimum of blame and feel good about each other and themselves (113).

Other important attitudes are

1. The feeling of unity between man and woman and a separateness from their families of origins so that interfamily interference with the marriage is avoided.
2. An ability to invest in the marriage to a greater degree than in other relationships.
3. A feeling of balance or complementarity, for perfect equality is probably impossible.
4. A movement from a romantic "falling in love" to a warm, loving, companionable, accepting relationship.
5. An ability to maintain variety and frequent interactions with each other (113).

Social Functions of the modern family include providing social togetherness, fostering self-esteem and a personal identity tied to family identity, providing opportunities for observing and learning social and sexual roles, accepting responsibility for behavior, and supporting individual creativity and initiative. The family actually begins the indoctrination of the infant into society when it bestows a name and hence a social position or status in relation to the immediate and kinship-group families. Simultaneously, each family begins to transmit its own version of the cultural heritage and its own family culture to the child. Because the culture is too vast and comprehensive to be transmitted to the child in its entirety and all at once, the family selects what is to be transmitted. In addition, the family interprets and evaluates what is transmitted. Through this process, the child learns to share family's values (1, 87, 118).

Thus socialization is a primary task of the parents, for they teach the child about the body, peers, family, community, and age-appropriate roles as well as language, perceptions, social values, and ethics. The family also teaches about the different standards of responsibility society demands from various social groups. For example, the professional person, such as a physician, nurse, or lawyer, those in whom people confide and to whom they entrust their lives and fortunes, are held more accountable than the farmer or day laborer. There is also a difference in the type of contact that society has with a particular group: for example, the mail or milk deliverer does not enter the home, but the exterminator is free to enter a home and look into every corner.

The parent generation educates by literal instruction and by serving as models (87). Thus the child's **personality**, *a product of all the influences that have and are impinging on him/her*, is greatly influenced by the parents. The types and importance of family interactions in carrying out these functions in each life era are further discussed by Murray and Zentner (90).

STAGES OF FAMILY DEVELOPMENT

Like an individual, the family has a developmental history marked by predictable crises. The developmental crises are normal, but they are also disturbing or frightening because each life stage is a new experience. The natural history of the family is on a continuum: from marriage or cohabitation; choosing whether to have children; rearing biological or adoptive offspring, if any; and releasing children into society to establish homes of their own. In later life the aging parents or grandparents are a couple once again, barring divorce or death. The nurturing of spouse or children goes on simultaneously with a multitude of other activities: work at a job or profession, managing a household, participation in church and community groups, pursuit of leisure and hobbies, maintaining friendships and family ties. Or the person may decide to remain single but live with a person of the same or opposite sex; then the purposes, tasks, and roles of family life must also be worked out.

Initial or Establishment Stage

When the couple establish a home of their own, their main psychological tie is no longer with family of orientation (parental family). They commit themselves to living together, usually through marriage. [Readiness for marriage in U. S. society is discussed in relation to young adulthood by Murray and Zentner (90).] They must work out patterns of communication, daily living, sexual relations, a budget, and a philosophy of life. Often this work begins during courtship. Relationships with family and friends are also different after marriage and must be worked out (40).

Today families may choose to have no children, one child and adopt, or one, two, or three children instead of a larger family. Some women feel that motherhood is not necessary for fulfillment. Certainly the man's chief fulfillment is not necessarily from fatherhood. Some people are wise enough to know that children do not automatically bring happiness to a marriage. Children bring happiness to parents who want them and who are selfless enough to become involved in the adventure of rearing them. Children bring trauma to a troubled marriage.

Limitation of family size and birth spacing yield substantial family health benefits. Certain associations in death, disease, and disability are apparent. Maternal deaths increase when maternal age is below 20 or above 40 years and after the third pregnancy for women of all age groups except those over 40. Increased maternal disease, obstetric complications, maternal deaths, and postnatal mortality occur with six or more pregnancies. Unwanted pregnancy increases maternal disease and death, especially if the pregnancy is terminated by illegal abortion that results in infection or hemorrhage. Other effects of unwanted pregnancy include excessive nausea and vomiting, spontaneous abortion, toxemias, complications of labor and delivery, emotional illness prenatally or postnatally, marital friction, and divorce. Infant mortality rate increases for birth order above three in the lower social class and rises among women under 17 years of age. The safest years for a normal delivery are between ages 20 and 29. Infants of youngest mothers of highest parity are at greatest risk for disease and death regardless of social class. Mothers are less likely to have premature or low-birth-weight, and therefore healthier, infants when spacing is greater than 2 years but less than 6 years (121).

The number of children in a family is related to the quality of care provided by the mother. A long-term follow-up study of 13,000 British infants revealed that the smaller the family size, the better the quality of infant care and management, use of medical services, interest in the child's school progress, and the less the tendency for child abuse. Additionally, the child of the smaller family does better in school and finishes more schooling than does the child from a large family. Incidence of infectious diseases, such as gastroenteritis and respiratory infections, are greater in larger-sized families. Children in large families are smaller in physical size, and first-born children with one or more siblings do not reach the height and weight obtained by those who remain only children. Intellectual development in children is affected negatively by large family size (121).

The establishment phase ends when the woman becomes pregnant or when the couple work out their living patterns and philosophy of life (which may include a decision not to have children).

The Expectant Stage

During pregnancy, which is a development crisis, many domestic and social adjustments must be made. The couple are learning new roles and gaining new status in the community. Attitudes toward pregnancy and the physical and emotional status of both partners will affect parenting abilities. Now the couple think in terms of family instead of a pair. They explore beliefs about childrearing and plan for the expanded family in terms of space, budget, and necessary supplies.

The woman may initially dislike being pregnant because it interferes with her personal plans or she may feel proud and fulfilled. Sexual desire may either increase or decrease. She may be more or less interested in her surroundings. Usually she is more preoccupied with herself, her new feelings, and changing body image, and she experiences fantasies and fears regarding the baby and the childbirth experiences.

The man experiences a variety of feelings on learning of the pregnancy, feelings that change during the pregnancy. The reality of the pregnancy increases with time. One study showed that 70 percent of the men experienced ambivalent feelings initially, but fatherly feelings developed. The men also felt guilty about the wife's pregnancy and her physical symptoms, anxious and depressed about their own adequacy, proud of their virility, and fearful of approaching the wife sexually. Concerns identified by fathers were as follows: caring for the infant (80 percent), adequacy as a father (68 percent), financial security (35 percent), and concern related to the baby's effect on the marital dyad (30 percent) (61, 96).

Early and thorough prenatal care for the woman is essential. Both the woman and the man may experience similar physical and emotional symptoms, such as nausea, indigestion, backache, distention, irritability, and depression. Symptoms may result from hormonal changes or feelings about the pregnancy in the woman. In the man they are part of the **couvade syndrome**, *which may be a reaction based on identification with or sympathy for the woman, ambivalence or hostility toward the pregnancy, or envy of the woman's childbearing ability*. The physical symptoms, complex feelings, and changes in body image that accompany pregnancy are described by several authors (31, 33, 65, 101, 109, 110).

Major decisions for the couple are whether to attend childbirth preparation classes and whether the man should be present in the labor and delivery rooms. The woman may feel eager to have the man with her or she may fear that he will think of her as sexually unattractive or be repulsed. The man may be curious about what is happening and want to attend his child's birth, or he may feel guilty about not wanting to when he feels others expect him to be there. He may be embarrassed about his wife's behavior and appearance during labor and delivery, or he may fear that he cannot cope with the childbirth event if present. Sexual fantasies triggered by labor and delivery may threaten the man who has tenuous emotional equilibrium. If the man has considerable unconscious conflicts or a weak self-image as a man, he may wish not to be involved in childbirth preparation, labor, or delivery. Some men and women cannot participate in childbirth preparation classes and should not be made to feel guilty about their decision. Participation may not enhance the couple's self-esteem and may create additional emotional crisis. Participation in Lamaze classes and childbirth does not change the woman's perception of her partner as ideal man, husband, or father, but it does improve her self-image as ideal woman, wife, and mother (61). In addition, the woman is more likely to be in good physical condition for labor if she has had preparation.

Although the woman needs extra "mothering" from the partner during pregnancy, the man also needs extra attention and nurturing or he may be unable to continue to support the mother-to-be emotionally (61). You can listen to the woman's and man's concerns and help them understand that what they are experiencing is normal. Various teaching aids explaining pregnancy and what to expect during the birth experience are also useful. Your care should be family centered, directed toward both parents-to-be. You can help the woman to gain maternal feelings and the man to see the importance of his role as provider as well as nurturer.

The man must be prepared for fathering just as the woman is for mothering. Fathers also go through the five operations (mimicry, role play, fantasy, introjection-projection-rejection, and grief work) identified by Rubin as necessary to attain the maternal role (109).

For additional information about prenatal influences on the mother and baby, see *Nursing Assessment and Health Promotion Through the Life Span* (90). Several authors give further information on the fathers' reactions and responsibilities (44, 52, 66, 69, 81, 98).

Parenthood Phase

With the birth of a child, the couple assume a status that they will never lose as long as each has memory and life—that of parent. The stages of parenthood are

1. Anticipatory stage. The woman is pregnant and the couple are learning the new roles and perceptions associated with pregnancy discussed earlier.
2. Honeymoon stage. The time following birth when the parents feel excited about the new relationship but also uncertain about the meaning of parental love. A parent-child attachment is being formed. During this time difficult adjustments need to be made. Because the parents lose sleep, husband-wife intimacy diminishes and there is less freedom for the couple to follow their own interests.
3. Plateau stage. The years during the child' development when the parents are active in the role of mother and father. During this time the parents deal with problems in the family, community, church, school, and immediate social sphere. They are concerned

with family planning, socialization and education of the child, and participating in community organizations.

4. Disengagement stage. The termination of the parent-child family unit that occurs when the last child marries or leaves home permanently and the parents let go of their major childrearing responsibilities to allow the offspring to be autonomous (107, 108).

Americans value creativity and individuality; thus no set patterns of parenthood exist. Parents rely on their own uniqueness, wisdom, and skills, how their parents raised them, or on books. Youth are poorly prepared to make the transition to parenthood. Yet how parents treat a child is the single most important influence on the child's physical, emotional, and cognitive development and health.

The couple may accept the idea of parenthood but reject a particular child because of the child's sex, appearance, time of the birth in their life cycle, or the child's threatening helplessness. Or the couple may reject the idea of parenthood but genuinely love the baby who was unplanned. Often parents have difficulty because pregnancy, childbirth, and parenting are romanticized in our society, and the romantic ideal differs considerably from the reality of 24-hour responsibility and submersion of their personal desires for many years to come.

How the parents care for and discipline the child are influenced considerably by the parents' own maturity; how they were cared for us children (as shown by studies on child abuse); their feelings about self; culture, social class, and religion (see Chapters 10 and 11); their relationship with each other; their perceptions of and experiences with children and other adults; their values and philosophy of life; and life stresses that arise. Moreover, the historical eras in which the parents were reared and are now living in and the prominent social values of each era subtly influence parental behavior.

Each critical period in the child's development reactivates a critical period in the parent. Demands made on the parent vary with the age of the child. The infant needs almost total and constant nurturance. Some parents thrive during this period and depend on each other for support. Other parents feel overwhelmed by the infant's dependency because their own dependent needs are stimulated but unmet. The baby's cry and behavior evoke feelings of helplessness, dependency, and anger associated with their unacceptable dependency needs and feelings, and then guilt and fatigue. The toddler struggles with individuality and autonomy, exploring and vacillating between dependency and independency. At this stage the child is intense and often unreasonable in demands and refusal to obey commands. The parents may enjoy this explorative, independent behavior of the child, even though the toddler leaves the parent feeling tired and frustrated. Or the primitive behavior of the child may stimulate primitive impulses in the parent, who may feel threatened by the will of the toddler. The parent who has difficulty controlling angry impulses may find the toddler's temper outbursts totally unacceptable. Parents who have difficulty caring for the dependent infant may do very well with the independent preschooler or adolescent or the reverse may be true. The parent may be able to resolve personal conflicts and move to a more advanced level of integration as he/she works with the developing child or the parent may be unable to cope with the aroused feelings (14).

Some parents feel that they must possess a child and will try to fit that child into a mold—their image. Other parents see their task of parenthood as stewards—to be a guide, helping friend, standard setter for the child. They invest themselves in the creative potentialities of their young—nurturing, educating, and protecting the child. They love but do not smother; guide but do not control; discipline but do not punish; offer freedom but do not abandon. They see the child as a lamp to be lit rather than a vessel to be filled (93).

Parents who possess their children feel that they have the right to dictate the terms of their child's life. Then the child has only half a life; parental need to control is greater than real love for child. Too much pressure is placed on the growing child, disturbing his/her emotional development (93).

Just as detrimental are the parents who abandon the child to rear itself, parents who spend too little time with and give too little affection to the child. Such children spend considerable time with television and peers; they learn that the adult world doesn't want them. In one study children who spent most of their time with peers were more influenced by the lack of the parents' presence, attention, and concern than by the attractiveness of the peer group. The peer-oriented child held negative views of self and peer group and expressed dim views of the future. The peer-oriented children rated parents lower in both expression of affection and support and in exercise of discipline control than did children who spent more time with adults. Peer-oriented children reported engaging in more antisocial behavior, such as doing something illegal, playing hooky from school, or lying (24).

Parents should rethink their priorities when they have children. Parents need to invest time in such a way that it brings quality to their relationship with the child. Children need the encouragement of doing things and talking through things with adults (24, 93).

Developmental tasks for the couple, which are reworked with the birth to each child, include to

1. Provide for the physical and emotional needs of the child, conveying love and security freely regardless of the child's appearance or temperament.
2. Reconcile conflicting roles—wife-mother, husband-father, worker-homemaker or family man, and parent-citizen.
3. Accept and adjust to the demands and stresses of parenthood,

learning or relearning basics of child care, adjusting personal routines and needs to meet the child's needs, and trying to meet the spouse's needs as well.
4. Provide opportunities for the child to master competencies expected for each developmental stage, to allow the child to make mistakes and learn from them, to restrict the child reasonably and consistently for safety, and to attain the emotional developmental tasks described by Erikson (43).
5. Share responsibilities of parenthood and together make necessary adjustments in space, finances, housing, lifestyle, and daily routines that are healthy for the family (meals, sleep).
6. Maintain a satisfying relationship with spouse—emotionally, sexually, intellectually, spiritually, and recreationally—while maintaining a personal sense of autonomy and identity.
7. Feel satisfaction from being competent parents and the parenting experience but maintain contacts with relatives and the community.
8. Provide socialization experiences to help the child make the emotional shift from family to peers and society so that the child can become a functioning citizen.
9. Refine the communication system and relationships with spouse, children, and others and permit offspring to be autonomous after leaving home (30, 40, 43).

Other authors also describe the reactions, roles, and responsibilities involved in parenting (7, 10, 13, 16, 24, 39, 51, 60, 62, 72, 90, 91, 93, 94, 103, 105, 120, 122).

As the children mature and leave home, the parents must rework their self-concepts as parents and people in order to take on new roles, responsibilities, and leisure activities so that the last stage of parenthood, disengagement, can be accomplished.

Disengagement Stage of Parenthood

Sometimes the last stage, disengagement, does not last too long. The young adult who is unemployed, a college dropout, or divorced may return home to live. The aged parents or other relatives may be unable to continue to live independently and then are included in the household of middle-aged offspring. Consequently, the tasks, functions, roles, and hierarchical relationships of the family must be reworked. Space and other resources must be reallocated. Time schedules for daily activities may be reworked. Privacy in communication, use of possessions, and emotional space must be ensured. Old parent–child conflicts, ideas about who is boss and how rules are set and discipline accomplished may resurface and should be discussed and worked through. These families can benefit from counseling; your guidance may be crucial.

Fox offers the following suggestions to adult children and their parents to make living together more harmonious.

1. Remember what it was like when a new baby came home. No matter how beloved the child, disruptions are bound to occur. Realize that another relative's homecoming will be the same.
2. Everyone involved should remember whose house it is.
3. Realize that no matter how many years sons or daughters have been away, family procedures don't change. Mom may still be critical. Dad may be the constant advice-giver. Expect it.
4. Talk about resentments. Discuss problems if you think it will help.
5. Parents may say offspring are grown up. But that doesn't mean they believe it. Still, they can't exert the same authority with a 30- or 40-year-old as with a youngster.
6. Offspring and elderly parents need to be flexible. It's unfair to expect the middleagers who are the "hosts" to change their household and life routines too much.
7. Even if parents refuse money, adult offspring should insist on paying something, no matter how minimal. Otherwise the offspring are reinforcing the idea that parents are taking care of them. Elderly parents can also contribute financially most of the time.
8. When grandchildren are involved, set rules about who's in charge. To decrease dependency, babysitters should be hired when possible. Then family members don't feel obligated or constrained.
9. Determine length of the adult offspring's stay. It need not be a precise date, but future plans about leaving the home should be explicitly stated.
10. Both adult offspring and older relatives should share responsibilities if possible. But don't upstage mom or dad; for example, if mom loves cooking, don't make her feel useless by taking over in the kitchen.
11. Space permitting, privacy is important. The relative who has lived on his or her own is probably used to time and space alone.
12. Middleagers should resist meddling in the affairs of either offspring or parents. They can advise. But grown offspring need to think for themselves and older relatives expect to make their own decisions.
13. Realize that the living situation may be temporary. Living together may not be ideal for anyone. But some parents and offspring or middleagers and their parents become closer during such periods (46).

FAMILY INTERACTION

Family interaction *is a unique form of social interaction based on a set of intimate and continuing relationships. It is the sum total of all the family roles being played within a family at a given time* (40). Families function and carry out their tasks and lifestyles through this process.

Family therapists, psychiatrists, and nurses are giving increased attention to the emotional balance in family **dyads** *or paired role positions,* such as husband and wife or mother and child. They have noted that a shift in the balance of one member of the pair (or of one pair) alters the balance of the other member (or pair). The birth of a child is the classic example (77). Dyads and emotional balance also shift in single-parent and step-parent families.

Interaction of the husband and wife, or of the adult members living under one roof, is basic to the mental, and sometimes physical, health of the adults as well as to the eventual health of the children. Two factors strongly influence this interaction: (1) the sense of self-esteem or self-love of each family member and (2) the different socialization processes for boys and girls (134).

Importance of Self-Esteem

The most important life task for each person—to feel a sense of self-esteem, to love and have a positive self-image—evolves through interaction with the parents from the time of birth onward and, in turn, affects how the person interacts in later life with others, including spouse and offspring.

The adult in the family who lacks self-acceptance and self-respect is not likely to be a loving spouse or parent. Behavior will betray feelings about self and others because he/she will perceive no automatic acceptance and little love from others in the family. Because perception of an event is the person's reality, such a person, in turn reacts in ways designed to defend self from the rejection that he/she *thinks* will be received: he/she may criticize, get angry, brag, demand perfection from others, or withdraw. In this way, he/she builds up self, the emotional reasoning being: "I may not be much, but others are worse." Such behavior is corrosive to any relationship but particularly one as intimate as the family's. Because of overt behavior, those intimate with him/her are not likely to appreciate or respond to the basic needs for love, acceptance, and respect. Indeed, the common responses to such behavior are counterattack or withdrawal, which, in turn, perpetuate the other's negative behavior. To remain open and giving in such situations is difficult for the mate but may be the only way to elevate the other's self-esteem. Perhaps only then can he/she reciprocate loving behavior. You can help family members realize the importance of respecting and loving one another and help them work through problems stemming from the low self-esteem of a family member (134).

Influence of Childhood Socialization

The second crucial influence on interaction between adults in the family is the difference in socialization processes for boys and girls. These differences are so embedded in the U. S. social matrix that until recently they had gone nearly unnoticed. There is a different social source for self-love in boys and girls. The girl is loved simply because she exists and can attract, as shown by the admiration pretty little girls receive. The girl is also taught to be subtle, for such behavior is part of her attraction. The boy is loved for what he can do and become; he must prove himself. Boys, especially from school age on, are given less recognition than girls for good looks and much recognition for what they can do. A boy learns to be direct, to brush aside distractions (sometimes including a woman's voice, for most disciplining will come from the mother and female schoolteachers and can be perceived as nagging after a while), and to get to the essence of things (134).

These concepts of what is appropriate boy and girl behavior are taught early and continue to affect heterosexual interactions throughout life. In traditional courtship, for example, the boy is expected to be in charge, to be dominant, to prove himself; the girl is expected to attract, to be passive. In marriage, however, these expectations cause problems, for the man is proving himself largely through his work, and this aspect of his earlier courtship behavior is now less visible to his wife. If the woman does not understand the dynamics of his behavior, she is likely to feel rejected and unloved, thinking she can no longer attract him. If the wife is also working, the husband may think of her as a competitor and work harder to keep his self-esteem. His physical self, including his involvement in lovemaking, is very much intertwined with his social, professional, and financial self, and failure in one is likely to cause feelings of failure in the total self, affecting his sense of masculinity, sexuality, and personhood (134).

All these facts are compounded by the shift in balance between the man and woman found in modern marriage, especially with the advent of the women's liberation movement. The husband often labors under the illusion that he enjoys the rights and responsibilities inherent in a patriarchal family system. Yet he must recognize the qualifications and drive for independence, the basic humanness, of his wife. You can help the couple to recognize the effect of their early socialization on their behavior and expectations and to work through misunderstandings. Help parents to overcome sexual stereotypes so that they do not inflict them on their children. Carmichael's book, *Nonsexist Childrearing*, may be helpful (27).

Variables Affecting Interaction Between the Child and Adult

Long before the child learns to speak, sensory, emotional, and intellectual exchanges are made between the child and other family members. Through such exchanges, and later with words, the child receives and tests instructions on how to consider the rights of others and how to respond to authority. The child also learns how to use language as a symbol, how to carry out certain routines necessary for health, how to compete, and what goals to seek. The games and toys purchased for and played with the child, the books selected and read, and the television programs allowed can provide key learning techniques.

The child's spontaneity can evoke in the adult fresh ways of looking at life long buried under habit and routine. The child says "It's too loud, but my earlids won't stay down" or "I want one of those little red olives with the green around" or "Give me that eraser with the handle." The child can also recreate for the adult the difficulty of the learning process: "Is it today, tomorrow, or yesterday? You said when I woke up it would be tomorrow, but now you call it 'today.' "

Family interaction for the child and adult is also affected by the ordinal position and sex of the children, as well as by the presence of an only child or of multiple births, such as twins.

Parents tend to identify with their children and to treat them according to how they were treated as siblings. A parent can identify best with the child who matches his/her own sibling position. A man from a family of boys may not know how to interact with a daughter and may not empathize with her. In the process of identifying with the parent, the child picks up many of the parent's characteristics, especially if the child is the oldest or lone child. For example, the oldest boy may be dependent instead of independent if his father was the youngest sibling and retained his dependent behavior into adulthood. Using family constellation theory, Toman describes features of each child in a family, based on sex and ordinal position, how the child feels about and interacts with people, and which ordinal position spouse he/she will most happily marry (131, 132).

The Ordinal Position of the Child is important to development (78, 87). Siblings have an important influence on each other. The firstborn, who is an only child until the second one comes along, may enjoy some advantages in achievement of intellectual superiority and perspective about life, including a greater sense of responsibility. He/she has more contact with adults and is the sole recipient of attention for a time. He/she becomes dominant over younger siblings. Secondborn boys with an older sister are more feminine than those with an older brother. The younger children benefit from the parents' experience with childraising and from having older siblings to imitate. Lastborns are also more sociable, possibly to ensure acceptance by older siblings or to gain parental attention. The lastborn may be more dependent. The middle child is likely to become caught between the jealousy of the older child and the envy of the younger, who may form a coalition against him/her. But he/she learns double or triple roles and is prepared for more kinds of relationships in adulthood. If two siblings are more than 6 years apart, they tend to grow up like only children (131, 132).

The Only Child may feel more loneliness but develops more rapidly and may seem older and more serious than peers who have siblings. He/she lacks the opportunities siblings could provide. Thus he/she usually does not share feelings and experiences with someone close, or cope with jealousy and envy from rivals in the home, or learn intimately about ways of the opposite- or same-sexed peers. He/she learns less about compromising with peers, sharing adult attention, and erecting strong defenses against the feelings displaced on him/her by adults and peers (74).

Children are the logical targets for fulfilling many of the parents' frustrated ambitions and needs. In a large family these yearnings and aspirations can be parceled out among a number of children, but when there is only one child, this child can sense the parents' manipulation and expectations. Thus the only child tends to be a peacemaker if he/she and the parents are the only household members. He/she is inadvertently brought into the parents' conflicts and is forced to help maintain harmony and preserve equilibrium in the household (87, 131, 132).

In a family with only one child, there are few people to fulfill the many roles of a family; thus more is demanded of each member. The only child may be forced prematurely to assume roles for which he/she is ill equipped. The child may become deft at performing adult tasks and roles, but self-confidence in the capacity to do so may be uncertain (87, 131, 132).

The only child sometimes has special problems on becoming a parent, seeing in the child a longed-for brother or sister. The danger in the situation is that the child is also a rival for the spouse's attention. On reaching adolescence, the offspring may then pose a threat to the parent's own adult roles, and the parent may unconsciously become overly competitive (87, 131, 132). Yet the only child is now regarded as an answer for the parents who want the parenting experience but who also want time to fulfill their own careers.

Certainly the only child can develop into a wholesome, well-adjusted person. The qualities of being more serious, assertive, responsible, independent, curious, and able to entertain self, and find satisfaction in personal pursuits frequently develop because of parental and home demands. These demands can enhance abilities to be a mature, capable adult. The greater opportunities available for adult contact, beginning at home, develop the only child's creativity, language skills, planning abilities, and intellectual potential. He/she has a high need to achieve and prefers the novel or complex. Firstborn and only children, such as Isaac Newton, Franklin Roosevelt, Emile Zola, Herbert Spencer, Rainer Maria Rilke, and some of the American astronauts, rank high on the roster of outstanding leaders, artists, and scientists. As you counsel parents who plan for or have only one child, emphasize the need for peer activity and the danger of too much early responsibility and pressure.

Multiple Births, such as twins, have considerable impact on family interaction. If ovulation has been inhibited with contraceptive pills, multiple births are more likely once this method stops being used (50). The needs and tasks of these parents will differ from the parents who have a single birth. Your suggestions and support can influence how well the parents cope with their responsibility.

Because multiple births are often premature, the first four or five months are very demanding on the parents in terms of the amount of energy and time spent in child care; this means that the parents have less energy and time for each other or other children. The mother should have help for several months if possible—from the husband, a relative, friend, or neighbor. Financial worries and concern about space and material needs may also intrude on normal husband-wife relationships or on relationships with other children.

Although books discourage the mother of twins from breast-feeding or using alternate breast-and-bottle-feeding, the mother may be able to breast-feed both twins successfully, by alternating breast- with bottle-feedings. The babies will not necessarily be poor breast-feeders with this arrangement.

You can suggest shortcuts in, or realities about, care that will not be detrimental to twin babies and that will give the parents more time to enjoy them. A diaper service, for example, is well worth the investment, for 1000 diapers may be used in a month's time. The parents should not be made to feel guilty if they are not as conscientious with two babies as they would be with one. Each can be given a total bath every other day instead of daily. Heating bottles before feeding is not necessary. The parents should try to avoid getting so wrapped up in meeting the babies' physical needs that resentment, anger, or excessive fatigue creep in. Multiple offspring should be fun as well as work.

Encourage the parents of twins (or multiple offspring) to perceive the babies as individuals and to consider the long-term consequences of giving them similar-sounding names, dressing them alike, having doubles of everything, and expecting them to behave alike. Tell parents about the national organization, Mothers of Twins, whose local branch can be a place to share feelings and ideas and gain practical suggestions.

Multiple-birth children are likely to be closer than ordinary siblings. They soon learn about the extra attention resulting from their birth status and may take advantage of the situation. Interaction between them is often complementary; for example, one twin may be dominant and the other submissive. Each learns from reinforcement of his/her experiences about the advantages of the particular role chosen. Twins may each receive less parental affection and communication because parents have less time to devote to each child. Thus twins are often slower to talk and many have a slower intellectual growth unless parents work to prevent it (74).

The Gender of the Child also influences development within the family (78). In most cultures a higher value is placed on male than on female children. Actually, in some cultures only a boy's birth is welcomed or celebrated and the family's status is partially measured by the number of sons. Or a family with several girls and no boys may perceive another baby girl as a disappointment. The girl may discover this attitude in later years from overhearing adult conversations and she may try to compensate for her sex and gain parental affection and esteem by engaging in tomboy behavior and later assuming masculine roles.

If a boy arrives in a family that hoped for a girl, he may receive pressure to be feminine. He may even be dressed and socialized in a feminine manner. If the boy arrives after a family has two or three girls, he will receive much attention but also the jealousy of his sisters. He will grow up with three or four "mothering" figures (some may be unkind) and in a family more attuned to feminine than to masculine behavior. Developing a masculine identity may be more difficult for him, especially if there is no male nearby with whom to relate. In spite of being pampered, he will be expected by his family to be manly. The boy may feel envious of his sisters' position and their freedom from such great expectations.

The girl who arrives in a family with a number of boys may also receive considerable attention, but she may have to become tomboyish in order to compete with her brothers and receive their esteem. Feminine identity may be difficult for her. You can help parents understand how their attitude toward their own sexuality and their evaluation of boys and girls influence their relationship with their children. Emphasize the importance of encouraging the child's unique identity to develop.

The Adopted Child may suffer some problems of the only child. In addition, the adopted child may have to work through feelings about rejection and abandonment by the biological parents versus being wanted and loved by the adoptive parents. The child should be told that he/she is adopted as early as the idea can be comprehended. Usually by the preschool years he/she can incorporate the idea of being a wanted child.

Social and legal changes have affected the kinds of children in need of adoption. Earlier adoption agencies served mainly White unmarried mothers who saw adoption as the only alternative for their babies. Today fewer infants are available because there is greater social acceptance of out-of-wedlock births; more unmarried mothers keep their babies. Contraceptives and abortions have also reduced the number of unwanted infants. A different category of adoptable children has grown in size, however. These children with "special needs" have at least one of the following characteristics: over age 5; Black, biracial; or physically, emotionally, or cognitively handicapped. Increasingly, state legislatures terminate parental rights in the case of children in long-term foster care who have remained unvisited and ignored by their biological parents and when the likelihood of the child's returning to his/her own home is minimal. New legislation has allowed abused children to become eligible for adoption.

Definition of "suitable" adoptive parents has been liberalized. Adoption agency requirements of age, marital status, race, and mother's employment status are more flexible.

Additionally, today's couples consider adoption even if they have their own children. Some believe they have a responsibility and enough love to provide a home for an existing child rather than add to the total population. Others are single persons who want to offer love and security to a child.

In spite of more liberal definitions of adoptability, the number of people applying to adopt a child, homes approved, placements made, and adoptions completed declined compared to the number of available children. Thus an increasing number of older children need permanent placement. You may have an opportunity to educate adults about the opportunity for adopting an older child with special needs or to work with adoptive parents, who also have needs.

Adoption of a child with special needs involves four phases: (1)

commitment of adults and child, (2) honeymoon or placement period, (3) storm period, and (4) adaptation and adjustment. The phases do not abruptly begin and end; each phase builds on the preceding phase and sometimes reversals occur. The phases, along with thoughts, emotions, and activities accompanying each phase, are summarized in Table 12-1. The adoptive process can terminate at any point. If termination is necessary, both sides—the family and child—need help to understand what happened and to understand that no *one person* is responsible. Future adoption procedures are enhanced if proper guidance is given with the first failure (23).

TABLE 12-1 The Adoptive Process

PHASES	THOUGHTS AND EMOTIONS	ACTIVITIES
1. Commitment of Adult(s) and Child(ren) "Courting Stage"	*Adult(s)* make general decision to adopt (stage 1), leading to decision to adopt specific child(ren) (stage 2).	*Adult(s)* prepare for adoption through dialogue with helpful people/agencies, and sometimes attend sessions on adoption given by adoption agency.
	Child(ren) express desire for adoption (stage 1), leading to decision on specific family (stage 2).	*Child(ren)* are counseled for potential adjustment by adoption agency staff. Visits are arranged and made between potential family—child(ren). All members involved (including existing children in family) get to know each other.
2. Placement "Honeymoon Period" (Child(ren) come to live with parent(s).)	*Parent(s)* are on an "emotional high"; excitement.	Household routines are altered to accommodate child(ren). Limit-setting is minimal. Parent(s) meet child(ren)'s whims.
	Child(ren) are excited but somewhat scared. "Can I trust these people?" "Will they send me away when I don't act my best?"	*Child(ren)* put on best behavior. Sometimes *parent(s)'* show of affection for child(ren) is not accepted because of child(ren)s' past negative parenting.
3. "Storm Period"	*Parent(s)* are tired of permanent house guest(s), feel anger, disappointment, guilt, and displace these feelings on each other and the child. They may wish the child would leave.	*Parent(s)* treat child(ren) or other family members with decreasing tolerance for behavior not in family norm.
	Child(ren) can no longer keep up good behavior but want to be loved and accepted.	*Child(ren)* may have tantrums, run away, try to reject parents before they reject him/her.

TABLE 12-1 (cont.)

PHASES	THOUGHTS AND EMOTIONS	ACTIVITIES
	Parent(s) may feel sense of failure. They may have expected too much of themselves and child(ren), and now may strike out at each other and other family members. Spouse may be jealous of time and energy mate gives to child(ren). *Child(ren)* may think, "They don't want me. What's going to happen to me?" and may live with anticipatory grief, fears of rejection, and insecurity based on past hurts. Parent(s) and child(ren) test each other.	If the outcome is positive, the *parent(s)* will use problem solving, limit-setting with flexibility, sense of humor, ongoing empathy and caring, supportive others, and community resources.
4. Adaptation and Adjustment Phase (Equilibrium occurs.)	*All* feel they can live and work together; mutual trust is growing; family feels fused as a unit and able to handle frustrations and crises. Child(ren) feel good about self, feel love and acceptance.	Parent(s) are consistent with child(ren). *Parent(s)* and *child(ren)* can attend to outside interests without threatening family status.

The Stepchild grieves and mourns the loss of a biological parent from death or divorce and must also deal with problems associated with integration into a new family unit. The stepchild may have conflicting feelings of loyalty to the natural parent and to the stepparent, thinking that acceptance of the stepparent is rejection of the natural parent. The stepchild may also feel rejected by his/her remarried natural parent, seeing the stepparent as a rival for the parent's attention. More on the stepparent family follows in the next section.

FAMILY LIFESTYLES AND CHILDREARING PRACTICES

There is no single type of contemporary U. S. family, but the lifestyles of many correspond to the factors discussed in this section, including family structure, family cultural pattern, and the impact of the twentieth century. These factors, in addition to those already discussed, influence family interaction and so understanding them will assist you in family care.

Family Structure

Childrearing and family relationships are influenced primarily by family structure. The biological and reproductive unit most commonly found in the United States is the mother–father–child group. Ordinarily the parents are married, have established a residence of their own, are viewed (along with their children) as an integral social unit, and live in an intimate, monogamous relationship. Emphasis in U. S. marriage is on pursuit of love in a romanticized way and on individual happiness rather than on family bonds, as in many other cultures. Yet kinship ties are usually recognized on both sides of the family.

In many situations, however, a child may grow up in a family that differs from the typical one. An aunt, uncle, or grandparent may be a continuing member of the household unit; one or the other parent may be absent because of death, divorce, illegitimacy, military service, or occupation involving travel.

Families in which only one parent is living full time with offspring are called **single-parent families**. Although death and illegitimacy may cause the family to have only one parent, divorce of the natural parents is the more common reason. In most cases, these families have undergone a major change in lifestyle. A parent may have died either suddenly or after a long illness. If the parents are divorced, the family may have experienced considerable disruption prior to the breakup. These families—and society—may ignore the changed family structure, for they do not fit the traditional social norm, thereby putting even more stress on people attempting to deal with the situation.

In the single-parent family the children may experience grief for the absent parent, guilt for their real or imagined part in the loss, shame for the change in their family structure, and fear about what changes the future may bring. Roles are changed. Each person may need to assume additional responsibilities and tasks. Parents may change their lifestyles. Mother may go to work or school, for instance; father may move into an apartment; or both parents may begin dating. An adolescent may serve as a parent substitute to younger siblings, or other children may assume new household tasks. The initial task of this family is to accept its family structure as a workable option for family living. Often an open discussion of the changed lifestyle along with support from relatives, friends, and other single-parent families, enhances the problem-solving abilities of these persons. Occasionally some family members may need professional help if they exhibit symptoms of more extreme dysfunction, grieving, or prolonged "acting-out" behaviors.

The *remarriage of a divorced or widowed parent with children may form a composite family unit known as the* **"reconstituted," "blended,"** or **stepparent family**. The "wicked stepmother" myth pervades our culture; in addition, the common usage of the word "stepchild" denotes inferior status. These families may be formed in a variety of ways: a mother with children may remarry; a father whose children visit may remarry; either of the new partners may have an ex-spouse or children from a previous marriage (children add stepsiblings) and, to complicate this family even more, the remarried couple may decide to have children of their own. In-laws and several sets of grandparents complete the picture. This family is now a far cry from the typical nuclear family and the interaction becomes increasingly complex.

When a couple marries for the second time and either or both have children from a previous marriage, the new husband and/or wife becomes an instant stepparent. This addition of children to a couple's life differs from the situation of first-marriage couples, whose children are added at a slower pace. Additionally, the myth that familial love occurs via the marriage ceremony is common.

Adjustment to a new, unique family unit is the major task of the stepfamily. New members cannot be assimilated with an existing family; instead a new family unit is formed. New rules, customs, and activities must be developed.

All members of this new family bring a history of life experiences, relationships, and expectations to the stepfamily. Conflict often occurs when the values and rules of individuals or the former single-parent family differ from those of the second.

In time family members develop agreement about what is "right." Such agreement may include the "correct" church to attend, the "right" time for dinner, and how birthdays are to be celebrated. Open communication between members is essential if decisions that are livable for all members are to be made.

In addition to adjusting in the family, stepfamilies must adjust to expectations of the outside world. Often differences in the reconstituted family are ignored because the family appears to be intact. Feelings of frustration, inadequacy, and isolation in family members stem from expectations that they feel as close to one another as blood relatives are expected to. The absent parent may still be an active influence in the original family. For instance, a divorced father may still contribute to his children's support and spend time with them on a regular basis, but they may be living with a stepfather. Even a deceased parent is remembered, not always accurately, and sometimes the stepparent is compared to the memory.

The child's ability to work through these feelings is influenced by age, sex, level of development, adaptive capabilities, and the understanding and support received from significant adults. He/she may need professional help to work through the difficulties of integration into a new family structure.

The stepfamily, like the single-parent family, needs to accept and be accepted as a combination of persons living together in a unique family unit. It is a potentially stressful situation that requires flexibility and adaptability of its members. Yet this family offers many opportunities for growth and friendship through the differing experiences of its members.

In early 1983 there were about 25 million stepparents in the United States. One out of every five children in America had at least one stepparent. In response to the growing number of these families, support groups, such as the National Stepfamily Association, operate to help these families face their unique situations (127). In spite of the old adage that children are flexible and can "bounce back," one child psychologist says that the trauma of divorce is second only to death. Often the problems that arise in the second marriage are more devastating than earlier ones. The children now know that the original parent will not return and they are faced with a new parent whom they often initially neither want nor accept emotionally. Counseling groups have started in schools, courts, and private practice to help these children (47).

Yet the stepfamily, like the single-parent family, needs to accept itself and be accepted as a combination of persons living together in a unique family unit. It is predicted that by 1990 these two groups will constitute more than 50 percent of U. S. families (127). Even though frequently the complexity of the stepfamily or single-parent unit is initially a stressful situation, the members, through flexibility and adaptability, can offer many opportunities for growth and friendship.

Another type of family structure has been termed *Apartners*. Instead of getting married, a couple, who may have children by a previous marriage, choose to maintain separate residences, take care of their own children, professional lives, and everyday affairs but share special times with each other on a regularly scheduled basis. Personal time and freedom, coupled with intimacy, are what the participants say they seek. Homosexual couples may also have this arrangement, often because of social constraints rather than choice.

Family Size

Family size is related to distinctive patterns of family life and child development. Most children in the United States are members of a small family system—that is, one with three children or less.

Common features observable in the small family system are that (1) emphasis is on planning (the number and the frequency of births, the objectives of childrearing, and educational possibilities); (2) parenthood is intensive rather than extensive (great concern is evidenced from pregnancy through every phase of childrearing for each child); (3) group actions are usually more democratic; and (4) greater freedom is allowed individual members. The child or children in the small family usually enjoy advantages beyond those available to children in large families of corresponding economic and social level, including more individual attention. On the other hand, these children may retain emotional dependence on their parents, grow up with extreme pressure for performance, and retain an exaggerated notion of self-importance.

The large family, generally thought of as one with six or more children, is not a planned family as a rule. Parenthood is commonly extensive rather than intensive, not because of less love or concern but simply because parents must divide their attention more ways. In the large family emphasis is on the group rather than on the individual member. Conformity and cooperation are valued above self-expression. Discipline in the form of numerous and stringent rules is frequently stressed and there is a high degree of organization in the activities of daily living (12). Or if parents lack initiative and use their resources unwisely, disorganization may exist.

A family may be small in size either because the parents wanted a small family or because they failed to achieve a large family. In either case, there is a low probability of unwanted children and they may take great interest in their children. In contrast, a large family is large either because the parents achieved the size they desired or because they have more children than they wanted. Large families therefore have a higher probability than small families of including unwanted and unloved children. Adolescents in small families, for example, have better relations with their parents than adolescents in large families, and mothers of large families are more restrictive toward their children than mothers of small families. Thus, lastborn children may be less wanted than the firstborn or middleborn children, especially in large families. This is consistent with what is known of abortion patterns among married women who typically resort to abortion only when they have achieved the number of children they want or feel they can afford to have. Yet only a small percentage of women faced with such unwanted pregnancies actually resorts to abortion, although these women may not be happy with the child later. Most parents are aware of greater parental skills and confidence with lastborn than with firstborn children. But it does not mean that the attitude of the parent is more positive toward the last child than the first. There is no necessary correlation between skills in and enjoyment of a role. Older homemakers are more skillful in domestic tasks, but they may experience less enjoyment than younger homemakers. Older people rate their marriages as "very happy" less often than younger people. Women may find less enjoyment in the maternal role with the passage of time, although women know the difference between the romantic expectation concerning the first baby and the more realistic expectation and sharper assessment of their own ability to do an adequate job of mothering as they face a second or third pregnancy (108).

Family Cultural Pattern

The ways of living and thinking that constitute the intimate aspects of family group life are the **family cultural pattern** (20). The family transmits the cultural pattern of its own ethnic background and class to the child, together with the parents' attitudes toward other classes.

Within the national cultural pattern of the United States, significant variations have been found in family cultural patterns and social systems (20). In Millstadt, Illinois, for instance, the German farm family provides a distinctive social system with cultural features distinct from its Italian neighbors across the river in St. Louis. The Maine Yankee and the North Carolina rebel may speak the same language, but the meanings of the words used may be quite different because of regional variables. Thus how families rear their children will depend on ethnic group and class, region, nation, and historical period.

Influence of Twentieth-Century Changes

The shift in this century from an agrarian to a complex technological society has produced dramatic changes for the U. S. family (82). A greater percentage of children now survives childhood than in 1900 and a higher percentage of mothers survives childbirth. Marriage, on the average, occurs at an earlier age than in former generations. Fewer children are born to most parents and they are spaced closer together. Middle-aged couples now have more time together after their children are grown and leave home. And because of an increased life expectancy, families now have more living relatives than formerly, especially elderly relatives (40).

There are other trends related to living in a complex industrial society. Families live primarily in urban areas. More women work outside the home. The U. S. woman who formerly stayed home and was the "homemaker" has also gone through several changes. Once homemaking took a good deal of time. Now modern conveniences make tasks easier. The woman who stays home today concentrates more on "mothering." Her outside activities may include volunteer work, so she can control her hours, feel she has prime time at home but yet is contributing outside the family unit. Family members are becoming better educated. Family incomes are increasing and acquisition of personal housing and equipment comes earlier in the marriage. Greater individual freedom exists. Sexual mores are changing, with trial and serial marriages.

The emphasis on the family-kinship group has been replaced by acceptance of the nuclear family. Because Americans are so mobile and are increasingly living in smaller homes or in apartments, many ties with kin other than the immediate family are loosened or at least geographically extended. Sometimes close friends become "the family." Yet many Americans strengthen kinship ties through letters, telephone calls, and holiday and vacation visits. Religious influences affect family ties. Jews, with their many family traditions, are generally more embedded in a network of relatives than White Protestants are.

Rapid change is a fact that families must acknowledge. Medical, pharmacological, and scientific advances in birth technology and all areas of health, the increased number of single-parent families, the growing emphasis on the civil and economic rights of minority groups, and the women's liberation movement are only a part of the cultural expansion of this century. As people live longer, more older people will divorce, remarry, or cohabitate. Those who lack healthy emotional roots within their nuclear families, who have few or no kinship ties, who cannot adjust to rapid change, and who have little identity except as defined by job and income are more likely to become depressed, alcoholic, unfaithful to mate, or divorced (87). Today's changing social environment makes it increasingly difficult for a parent to be certain of his identity. How, then, is he to provide emotional roots for the child?

U. S. Childrearing Practices have no one traditional national pattern, only the general concern that children develop "normally." Parents are encouraged through culture, education, and the mass media to use whatever the dominant childrearing theory is at the time. At the turn of the century the dominant theory reflected the prevailing scientific belief in the primacy of heredity in determining behavior. In the early 1900s child care emphasized the importance of environment, and by the midthirties Freudian Psychoanalytic theory had gained ascendency. Today NeoBehavioristic theories are prominent. With each new wave of "knowledge," parents are bombarded by conflicting reports and condemnation of previous practices. Often the change in theory application occurs during the same parental generation so that parents do not trust their own judgment and considerable inconsistency results. The inconsistency, rather than the theory, probably creates the main problems in childrearing. Sometimes parents strive to avoid rearing their children as they were reared, but nevertheless do so unwittingly because of the permanency of enculturation. Children are often given approval and disapproval for their behavior and told they are "good" or "bad." This practice, along with inconsistency and other factors, contributes to competition and sibling rivalry.

The importance of the father's role is being reconsidered and he is more active in child care. Still, the mother is primarily responsible for the crying baby and young child care. The infant is often unconsciously trained in privacy, individualism, and independence by being left alone in the crib or playpen much of the time. There is still, unfortunately, the fear of "spoiling" the infant if he/she is held too much or responded to spontaneously. Thus the infant may develop behavioral extremes in order to get needs met. He/she is being given the foundation to later stand out, push forward, to compete and achieve.

Then when the children are old enough to be out of the home, parents often strive to do things for their children and center their activities around their children's activities. Work responsibilities are not necessarily demanded, but there is subtle pressure for the children to repay by pleasing the parents through use of talents, organizational achievements, or honors won. Because of the small size of the nuclear family, the school-age child or adolescent may spend more time with peers than with family members. And because of the youth idealization of our culture, seniority does not invoke special respect for the older person (parent). The childrearing parent must offer more than age if he/she wants to maintain control.

A growing trend is for children to be cared for by day-care centers or babysitters who are usually not relatives. What happens if the mother and parent-surrogate differ greatly about childrearing practices? The child generally acknowledges the authority of parents, or at least the mother, but parent-surrogates affect him/her nevertheless. Any adult who is with the child reinforces behavior in the child that conforms to the adult's own standard of behavior. The child conforms to the adult's desires in order to gain approval. If the parent-surrogate acts in a way contrary to the values of the parents, both parents and child are likely to be distressed (87).

NURSING IMPLICATIONS

The family as the basic unit for the developing person cannot be taken for granted. Although family forms have changed and will continue to change, each person, in order to develop healthfully, needs some intimate surroundings of human concern. "No man is an island."

You will frequently encounter the entire family as your client in the health care system, regardless of the setting. You may be asked to do family-centered care, to nurse the patient and the family, or to do "family thereapy." Yet you will not be able to carry out the nursing process with the family even minimally unless you understand the dynamics of family living presented in this chapter.

Rapid change, increasing demands on the person, technological progress, and other trends mentioned seem to isolate people. A glance at one vanishing symbol of American family life—the front porch—can illustrate this point. What happened to the porch where the family used to gather? Where mother sat when the evening dishes were done? Where father rested after a day's work? Where toddlers rode their kiddie cars? Where Susie got her first kiss? Where neighbors stopped to chat? The porch has been converted into a private patio in the back of the house and is used briefly when the family can force themselves to leave the air-conditioned comfort of indoors. Susie and her boyfriend are gone in his car. Father is absorbed in his TV programs. Mother can't hear the toddler calling because the dishwasher, clothes washer, dryer, and garbage disposal block out all human sounds. The older children are carpooled to separate activities.

You cannot call back the front-porch era. Nor do all families live with the foregoing luxuries and isolated from each other. But you should understand that many families are not even aware of the forces that are pulling them apart. More than ever, they need one place in their living where they can act without self-consciousness, where the pretenses and roles demanded in jobs, school, or social situations can be put aside. The living center should be a place where communication takes place with ease; where each knows what to expect from the other; where a cohesiveness exists that is based on nonverbal messages more than verbal; and where a person is accepted for what he/she is. The family may need your help in becoming aware of disruptive forces, of their maladaptive patterns (such as those described in Chapter 8), and of ways to promote an accepting home atmosphere.

In doing a family assessment, ask questions related to achieving the developmental tasks that were described earlier. Also, determine communication patterns and relationships, family health, access to health care, occupational demands and hazards, religious beliefs and practices, childrearing practices, participation in the community, and support systems.

You can help families understand some processes and dynamics underlying interaction so that they, in turn, learn to respect the uniqueness of the self and of each other. Certainly members in the family need not always agree with each other. Instead they can learn to listen to the other person, about how he/she feels and why, accepting each person's impression as real for self. This attitude becomes the basis for mutual respect, honest communication, encouragement of individual fulfillment, and freedom to be. There is then no need to prove or defend the self.

Once the attitude "We are all important people in this family" is established, conflicts can be dealt with openly and constructively.

Name calling and belittling are out of place. Families need to structure time together; otherwise individual schedules will allow them less and less time to meet. Parents need to send consistent messages to their children. To say "Don't smoke" while immediately lighting a cigarette is hardly effective (137).

Times of communication are especially necessary when children are feeling peer pressure; children, moreover, should be praised for what they do right rather than reprimanded for what they do wrong. Children need structure but should be told the reason for the structure if old enough to comprehend (137). As you help the family achieve positive feelings toward and interaction with one another, you are also helping them to fulfill their tasks, roles, and functions (134). Review the adaptive mechanisms of families described in Chapter 7.

The person's health problems, especially emotional ones, may well be the result of the interaction patterns in childhood or present family. Knowledge of the variables influencing family interaction—parents' self-esteem and upbringing, number of siblings, the person's ordinal position in the family, cultural norms, family rituals—all will help you assist the person in talking through feelings related to past and present conflicts. Sometimes helping the person understand these variables in relation to the spouse's upbringing and behavior can be the first step in overcoming current marital problems.

You are a nurse, not a specialized family counselor, although with advanced preparation you could do family therapy. But you can often sense lack of communication in a family. Through use of an empathic relationship and effective communication, teaching, and crisis therapy, you can encourage family members to talk about their feelings with one another and assist in the resolution of their conflicts. Help them become aware of the need to work for family cohesiveness just as they would work at a job or important project. Refer them to a family counseling service if the problems are beyond your scope. Your work with them should also help them better use other community resources, such as private family or psychiatric counseling or family and children's services.

One family self-help resource that does not use the traditional "medical model" (wait until problems surface and then intervene) but rather the "educational model" (learn new information and skills while basically well) is called Family Clusters. Devised by Margaret Sawin and first used in 1970, the Family Cluster is a group of four or five complete family units (including blended, single-parent, cohabitation, or the traditional unit) who contract to meet together over an extended period of time for shared educational experiences that concern relationships within their families. Where available, it provides a positive approach and affirms family members because a commitment is made for all persons—no matter what their age—to have both power and input into the cluster. Training to lead family clusters is available. For more information, write to Family Clustering, Inc., PO Box 18074, Rochester, NY 14618 (115).

Your knowledge of the family life cycle, with developmental tasks to be performed at each stage, provides a foundation for learning the specifics of sequential development discussed in the companion text (90). This combined knowledge will help you in assessing the status of the family and the individual person in planning care, in intervention, and in objectively evaluating your effectiveness.

One liability in working with families of various social classes and cultures may be *you*. For example, if you come from a middle-class U. S. background, that fact will affect your opinions about what constitutes family life. Your attitude toward nonconforming families or unconventional living arrangements may interfere with your objectivity and thus with your ability to assist some families. You will need to go through your own maturation process of learning that your way is not always the best or only way. The process is difficult.

Role of the Nurse in Well-Baby Care

You may care for well babies and mothers in a variety of settings—the clinic, hospital, home, or doctor's office. Your actions contribute significantly to their health.

Prenatal care to the mother and her partner may include physical assessment, teaching healthful practices for mother and baby, listening to mother vent frustrations or share fears, counseling her during periods of depression or uncertainty, and sharing her happy feelings about becoming a mother. You may conduct childbirth classes for mother and father so that they can better understand changes occurring in the mother as well as the nutrition and hygiene necessary during pregnancy; know what to expect during labor, delivery, and postpartum; and prepare for an active role during birth. An obstetric nursing book will give adequate detail to help you do prenatal assessment and care as well as intrapartal and postpartal assessment and intervention.

If the mother-to-be is unwed, you may also try to work with the father-to-be if both are willing. The father-to-be needs help in talking about his feelings and needs to support her, if they are compatible. He may also seek sex education.

To help the unwed parents, as well as break the cycle for future generations, we must gain a better understanding of the unwed father. Do not perceive him as irresponsible or having taken advantage of an innocent girl. The relationship between the unwed mother and the father is not necessarily a hit-and-miss affair but often meaningful to both. If the parents-to-be are adolescents, they realize that a new life has been created as a result of their actions. They want to act in a responsible way. They are concerned about the child's well-being (98).

The unwed father can be encouraged to stand by the unmarried mother. Often he feels proud of fathering; he has proven his masculinity. The long-term consequences of having a child are such, however, that alternate solutions regarding the future of the child should be thoroughly explored with and by both partners. Alternatives include marriage, placing the child for adoption, or assumption by either parent or the grandparents of the responsibility for caring for and rearing the child. The man needs help in understanding how and why he became a father and the serious implications for the mother, the child, and himself (98).

Adolescents may admit that their sexual experiences were unsatisfactory, leaving them depressed, guilty, and scared. The good relationship with the girlfriend may have begun to deteriorate when sexual relations were started. Pregnancy comes as a shock to both. They know about contraceptives, but their use may have been sporadic, if at all, for some people believe that the spontaneity and sincerity of the sexual act are lessened when prepared for (98).

Sex education must relate to the values of interpersonal relations and concern for others if it is to be successful. The implications and responsibilities of sexual behavior need to be discussed with the teenagers. The difference between teenage love and a more mature relationship between people who are ready to meet the problems and responsibilities of adulthood should be discussed (98).

Parents of the unwed father must be involved in helping their son; communication between the boy and parents should be reestablished. In addition, parents should assert themselves in helping the boy take responsibility for his actions and assist the boy in the case of marriage (98).

Efforts to prevent unwed pregnancies must be directed to improving and strengthening family life and developing a better respect for the father's role in the family. Many unwed fathers come from female-dominated homes or from homes in which the father is absent or inadequate in his role (98).

Fathers can help adolescent sons by talking with and listening to them, by being slow to judge, by taking them to the job so the youth can see how the father earns a living, by being a role model in relating maturely to the spouse and other women. Fathers can create an atmosphere in which the sons will want to talk about emerging sexual feelings and experiences (98). If the adolescent son comes from a home where no father is present, the mother can work at listening to and discussing problems and feelings with the son. She may also be able to foster a bond between the son and another male member of the family.

If you conduct childbirth education classes, try to interview each couple in their home early in the pregnancy, by the fourth month if possible, to observe their relationship and determine their response to pregnancy. Their response may be different and more honest in their own home than in class. During the classes include opportunities for men, as well as women, to talk about the problems they feel are uniquely theirs, their feelings, or the commonality of the couvade syndrome. Provide anticipatory guidance about the couvade syndrome. Avoid pushing the father into participation and provide support for him. Focus childbirth education on the known benefits to the baby and parents and not on overromanticized and dramatic statements about improved marital relationships. Educate both partners about family planning so that future pregnancies can be mutually planned. Refer either partner, or both, to psychological counseling when necessary, especially if antisocial behavior is seen or if there has been fetal loss.

During labor you do necessary physical care, but you may also act as a coach for the mother, or you may support the father as he assists his wife. Flexibility in hospital routines for obstetrical patients is usually possible and contribute to the parents' sense of control. In fact, negative feelings about traditional hospital deliveries have become so widespread that home deliveries are increasing in many cities, often attended by a granny midwife instead of a professional doctor or nurse-midwife.

The physician and nurse or nurse-midwife can work as a team with the expectant couple. In some facilities the nurse-midwife assumes primary responsibility for the family unit. Whenever a mother delivers, she has the right to capable, safe care by qualified caretakers. Home deliveries can be carefully planned and safe. And hospital deliveries can be more homelike. Maternity centers could provide families anticipating a normal childbearing experience with antepartum care that is educational in nature; labor and delivery in a homelike setting (but with adequate equipment) with discharge to home whenever it is safe for mother and baby, probably within 12 hours after delivery; and follow-up care by public health nurses in the home during the postpartum course. The labor-delivery rooms can be designed to accommodate the presence of the father or family during delivery and be less traumatic (cold, with intense lights) for the newborn. Following birth, the infant can remain with the mother; the newborn's physical exam can be done in her presence with the father present as well. Childbirth should be a positive, maturing experience for the couple. Expectant parents have the right and responsibility to be involved in planning their care with the health team and to know what is happening. Cultural beliefs should be recognized, respected, and accommodated whenever possible. A positive childbearing experience contributes to a healthy family unit.

Delivery methods are changing in some centers as doctors and midwives follow the trend set by Dr. Leboyer in France. The delivery room lights are dimmed; people speak softly or whisper; the infant is placed on the mother's abdomen in order to maintain body temperature and the prebirth curved position of the spine; the baby is massaged by mother and doctor; and the cord is not cut immediately. The baby is placed in warm water. Precautions are taken when necessary, but apparently delivery does not have to be so traumatic for the baby (22, 76).

In the early postpartum period assess mother and baby and give the mother physical care and assist her as necessary even if she looks well and able. "Mother" the mother (25, 109, 110). Arrange the environment and hospital routines to enhance bonding between mother and baby. Listen to the mother's concerns; answer her questions; support her maternal behavior. In a nonthreatening way, teach the mother how to handle her baby. Help her begin to unlearn preconceived ideas about the baby and herself and perceive herself and the baby positively. Give her special assistance if she is breast-feeding. After the initial "taking-in" period of having received special care and attention, the mother moves to the "taking hold" stage, where she is able to care for the child (109, 110).

The interaction between the infant and primary caretaker is crucial. The mothering person helps the baby feel secure and loved, fosters a sense of trust, provides stimulation, reinforces certain behavior, acts as a model for language development, and trains the baby in basic learning strategies. In turn, maternal behavior is influenced by baby's cries, coos, smiles, activity, and gazes, as well as by how well baby's behavior meets the mother's expectations.

Your significant contribution to the family unit is to promote attachment between parents and baby, encourage continuing contacts between the family and health professionals so that adequate health and illness care are received, and encourage parents to meet the baby's needs adequately. You can help the parents feel good about themselves and the baby.

You can be instrumental in initiating new trends in care to make the hospital or clinic environment more homelike while providing safe, modern care.

Continued Care in the Fourth Trimester

During the fourth trimester, the 6 or 8 weeks after delivery, the mother needs assistance with child care and an opportunity to regain her former self physically and emotionally. Father also needs support as he becomes involved in child-care responsibilities (104). In the nuclear or single-parent family the parent(s) may struggle alone. Visits by a home health nurse may be useful. Some communities have a crisis line for new parents. You may be able to suggest services or help the parent(s) think of people who could be helpful.

As you assess the mother's functioning, consider her physical and emotional energy, support systems, and current level of parenting activity. If she does not appear to be caring adequately for the child, assess for anemia, pain, bleeding, infections, lack of food or sleep, drug use, or other medical conditions that would interfere with her activity level and feelings of caring. Depression and postpartum blues are difficult to differentiate. In depression the mother is immobilized and forgets basic care, but with postpartum blues she may cry but care for the baby's physical needs.

The new mother usually has enough energy to do only top-priority tasks—eating, sleeping, baby care, and essentials for other family members. A house that is too clean is a danger signal that she is neglecting the baby, herself, or both (18).

The mother's support system is crucial for her energy maintenance, physical as well as emotional. She needs direct support and assistance with daily tasks, plus moral support, a listener, a confidant. Support comes from personal and professional sources—the partner, parents, friends, other relatives, and the nurse, doctor, social worker, or pastor. Negative attitudes from others can drain emotional energy.

Bishop's (18) and Campbell's and Smith's (26) guides to assess parenting feelings and adequate mothering may be helpful. Actual parenting skills can be manifested in various ways. Touching and cuddling are important, but love can also be shown by a tender, soft voice tone and loving gazes. Ability to obtain adequate medical care is typical of the caring parent; lack of use of medical services for the baby indicates a poor mother-child relationship. Other indications of warm parenting feelings include

1. Calling the baby by name.
2. Expressing enjoyment of the baby and indicating that the baby is attractive or has other positive characteristics.
3. Looking at the baby and into the eyes.
4. Talking to the baby in a loving voice.
5. Taking safety precautions for the baby.
6. Responding to the baby's cues for attention or physical care.

If the baby is progressing in normal fashion, focus on the mother's needs and concerns. Help her find nonprofessional support systems that can assist her when the professional is unavailable or that can help with child care. In addition to concern over child care, we must help the mother grow developmentally. Helping her stay in good physical and emotional health ensures better parenting.

Here are some signs of poor parental adaptation to baby on the part of the mother:

1. Sees baby as unattractive.
2. Perceives aspects of care, such as diapering, as revolting.
3. Gets upset when baby's secretions or body fluids touch the self.
4. Lets head dangle without support.
5. Picks up baby without warning touch or speech, or at times to meet her own needs.
6. Plays roughly with baby, including after eating, even if baby vomits.
7. Does not coo or talk to baby.
8. Avoids eye contact.
9. Thinks baby does not love the parent.
10. Expresses fears that infant might die with minor illness.
11. Is convinced baby has a defect or is behaving unnaturally when there is no sign of either.
12. Does not speak positively of self or find in baby any attribute that is valued in self.
13. Gives inappropriate responses to baby's needs, such as over- or underfeeding, over- or underhandling or talking to (18, 26).

Deterrents to adequate mothering include personal immaturity; stress situations, such as loss of loved object; serious disappointments; fear of or rejection from own or partner's parents or other relatives; financial worries; partner punishing her because of his dependency needs; loss of job for partner; having received depersonalized care in hospital; and discharge from hospital soon after delivery without help at home. Assess for these deterrents; your nurturing of the mother and helping her seek additional help may offset the negative impact of these factors.

You may also work with families whose child was born prematurely or with a defect. Prematurity accounts for 50 percent of neonatal mortality and premature infants who survive contribute significantly to the number of physically, intellectually, and emotionally handicapped children in the United States. Complications of prematurity include major and minor physical abnormalities, general motor incoordination, short attention span, distractibility and hyperactivity, difficulty separating from parents, preoccupation with the body, and scholastic underachievement (39).

The last complications may be more related to an early disturbed mother-child relationship than to the prematurity, perinatal complications, or the child's birth defects. Typically the infant is rushed to the nursery after birth, thereby preventing physical or eye contact between mother and baby. The mother is often isolated from other mothers; professionals and family may avoid conversation about the baby. Mother often sees the baby in the premature or intensive care nursery at a distance and only indistinctly; or the baby may have been transported to a children's hospital at some distance so that visiting the baby after her discharge is difficult. The mother may have no opportunity to form any attachment feelings unless nursing staff foster the involvement in child care to the extent possible and keep her informed of baby's condition and progress. The baby who finally comes home to the parents may be a stranger for whom the mother has no maternal response or commitment. Additionally, the mother has developed little confidence in her mothering abilities and no caretaking regimen (39).

Behavior patterns that strongly suggest a disturbed parent–child relationship and future problems in parenting include parents who

1. Are unable to talk about guilt feelings, fears, and their sense of responsibility for the child's early arrival, with each other or others.
2. Demonstrate no visible anxiety about the baby's condition, deny the reality, or displace anxiety onto less threatening matters.
3. Make little effort to secure information about the baby's condition.
4. Consistently misinterpret or exaggerate either positive or negative information about the baby and display no signs of hope as baby's condition improves.
5. Receive no practical support or help from family or friends, and community resources are lacking.
6. Are unable to accept and use help offered (39).

You may be instrumental in promoting certain procedures that can be used by hospital personnel to promote mother–child relationship:

1. Permit the mother to see and touch the baby as soon as possible, preferably in the delivery room. Or transfer the baby to the mother's room in a portable incubator if the baby remains in the same hospital.
2. Permit the mother to become involved in baby's care as soon as possible. Take the mother to the premature care unit, teaching her to use the necessary aseptic technique in order to touch, care for, and visit with the baby.
3. Provide an atmosphere that encourages questions.
4. Encourage parents to talk with each other, family members, and friends—using others for support.

5. Recognize that parents' excessive questions, demands, and criticisms are a reaction to stress and not personal attacks on the professional worker or hospital.
6. Do not offer reassuring cliches or comforting statements too quickly. Encourage parents to cry, to face the reality of the situation.
7. Do not pressure parents to talk about their feelings all at once, but avoid using the excuse of "not wanting to probe" to avoid talking with them.
8. Encourage the mother to express breast milk if she wishes; the breast milk can be taken to a breast-milk bank and used for the infant. When the baby is sucking well, the mother can help bottle-feed the baby until the baby is strong enough to breast-feed.
9. Arrange for father to visit the baby prior to discharge, calling him about baby's progress at intervals when he is unable to visit.
10. Encourage the parents to handle the baby and do baby's care prior to discharge; teach about baby care as necessary while the parents are engaged in care of their baby (55).

Parent Education

To combat the problems associated with the high adolescent birthrate, some junior and senior high schools are establishing creative programs in parenthood education. Some hospitals and health clinics are initiating specialized prenatal and postnatal services for the adolescent mother and her at-risk infant. You can initiate nontraditional programs in your own community.

Cincinnati General Hospital established an innovative program to help adolescent mothers become more effective parents (9).

The adolescent mother who decides to keep her baby needs all the family and outside help she can get. She fears that whatever personal ambitions she has will be thwarted by the baby. Unmarried and unprepared for employment, she finds it almost impossible to make her own way in the world. Anger, frustration, and ignorance hamper her ability to attach to and appropriately care for the baby. Repeated pregnancies, child neglect and abuse, and welfare dependency often occur (9).

Shaw also describes the formation of a mother's group, consisting of women of various ethnic origins in a lower-income bracket, whose purpose was to provide parent education and support and foster talking about feelings (120). Hiemstra gives suggestions on how to educate parents to use community resources (58).

Your work with the mother may prevent maternal deprivation, insufficient interaction between mother and child, conditions under which the deprivation or even abuse develops, as well as negative effects on the child's development.

Work with Adoptive Families

You can help the adoptive parents in their adjustment. Assure them that attachment develops over time. Help them think through how and when to tell the child that he/she is adopted so that the child understands and is not traumatized. Help the parents anticipate how they will help the child cope when the child is taunted by peers about being adopted. Help them realize that the adopted child will probably seek answers to many questions when he/she gets older. Who were the parents? Their cultural, racial, or ethnic background? Their ages, occupations, interests, appearance? Why was he/she relinquished? What are the medical facts surrounding heredity and birth? Help parents realize that these questions do not mean that the child does not love them. Hammon's article supplies information on adoption procedures, stresses encountered, and how to make adoption a success (56). Other references are also helpful (8, 15, 28, 29, 42, 85, 92, 106, 116, 119).

Work with Single-Parent or Reconstituted Families

The guidelines already discussed will be useful to you as you help the single-parent or reconstituted family adjust to its situation. The single-parent family can be referred to a local chapter of Parents Without Partners if the person seeks support from peers. Do not rush in with answers for these families until you have heard their unique problems. Acknowledge their strengths; help them formulate their own solutions. Often a few sessions of crisis therapy will be sufficient.

Family Care Throughout the Life Cycle

You may be called on to assist families as they meet various developmental crises throughout the life cycle: school entry of the child, the adolescent period, children leaving home, divorce, retirement, death of a member. References at the end of Chapters 8, 10, and 11 and at the end of the chapters in *Nursing Assessment and Health Promotion Through the Life Span* (90) can help you adapt care to the family situation.

Your goal is health promotion and primary prevention. Your intervention early in the family life cycle may help establish a positive health trend in place of its negative counterpart. The care you give to young parents lays the foundation for their children's health.

REFERENCES

1. **Ackerman, Nathan,** *Psychodynamics of Family Life*. New York: Basic Books, Inc., 1958.
2. **Adams, Bert,** *The American Family: A Sociological Interpretation*. Chicago: Markham Publishing Company, 1971.
3. _____, and **Thomas Weirath,** eds., *Readings on the Sociology of the Family*. Chicago: Markham Publishing Company, 1971.
4. **Anderson, Ralph,** and **Irl Carter,** *Human Behavior in the Social Environment*. Chicago: Aldine Publishing Company, 1974.
5. **Andolfi, Maurizio,** *Family Therapy: An Interactional Approach*. New York: Plenum Press, 1979.
6. **Andrews, Ernest,** *The Emotionally Disturbed Family*. New York: Jason Aronson, Inc., 1974.
7. **Anthony, E. James,** and **Therese Benedek,** *Parenthood: Its Psychology and Psychopathology*. Boston: Little, Brown & Company, 1970.
8. **Bach-Wiig, Barbara,** "Adoption Insights: A Course for Adoptive Parents," *Children Today*, 4, no. 1 (1975), 22–25.
9. **Badger, E., D. Burns,** and **B. Rhoads,** "Education for Adolescent Mothers in a Hospital Setting," *American Journal of Public Health*, 66, no. 5 (1976), 469–72.
10. **Ball, Judith,** and **Mary Ann Krickus,** "Family at Work: Traditions, Transitions," *Graduate Woman*, 70, no. 2 (1982), 11.
11. **Balswick, Jack,** and **Charles Reek,** "The Inexpressive Male: A Tragedy of American Society," in *Human Life Cycle*, ed. Wm. Sze. New York: Jason Aronson, Inc., 1975, pp. 497–504.
12. **Bell, Norman,** and **Ezra Vogel,** eds., *The Family*. Glencoe: The Free Press of Glencoe, 1960.
13. **Bell, Robert,** *Marriage and Family Interaction*. Homewood, IL: Dorsey Press, 1963.
14. **Benedek, Theresa,** "Parenthood During the Life Cycle," in *Parenthood: Its Psychology and Psychopathology*, eds. E. J. Anthony and T. Benedek. Boston: Little, Brown & Company, 1970, pp. 185–206.
15. **Berman, Claire,** *We Take This Child*. Garden City, NY: Doubleday & Co., Inc., 1974.
16. **Bernard, Jessie,** "Who Provides the Caring?" *Graduate Woman*, 70, no. 2 (1982), 14–16.
17. **Bischof, Ledford,** *Adult Psychology*. New York: Harper & Row, Publishers, Inc., 1969.
18. **Bishop, Barbara,** "A Guide to Assessing Parenting Capabilities," *American Journal of Nursing*, 76, no. 11 (1976), 1784–87.
19. **Blanch, Rubin,** and **Gertrude Blanch,** *Marriage and Personal Development*. New York: Columbia University Press, 1968.
20. **Bossard, James,** and **Eleanor Boll,** *Sociology of Child Development* (4th ed.). New York: Harper & Row Publishers, Inc. 1960.
21. **Brandwein, Ruth, Carol Brown,** and **Elizabeth Fox,** "Women and Children Last: The Racial Situation of Divorced Mothers and Their Families," *Journal of Marriage and the Family*, August 1974, pp. 498–513.

22. **Braun, Jonathan,** "Born with a Smile Instead of a Slap: The Struggle for Acceptance of a New Birth Technique," *Parade*, November 23, 1975, 16 ff.
23. **Brockhaus, Joyce,** and **Robert Brockhaus,** "Adopting an Older Child–The Emotional Process," *American Journal of Nursing*, 82, no. 2 (1982), 288–94.
24. **Bronfenbrenner, Urie,** "Parents, Bring Up Your Children," *Look Magazine*, January 26, 1971, p. 45.
25. **Brown, Marie,** and **Joan Hurlock,** "Mothering the Mother," *American Journal of Nursing*, 77, no. 3 (1977), 439–41.
26. **Campbell, S.,** and **J. Smith,** "Postpartum: Assessment Guide," *American Journal of Nursing*, 77, no. 7 (1977), 1179.
27. **Carmichael, Carrie,** *Nonsexist Childraising*. Boston: Beacon Press, 1977.
28. **Chambers, Donald,** "Willingness to Adopt Atypical Children," *Child Welfare*, 49, no. 5 (1970), 275–79.
29. **Chema, Regina, L. Fanley, F. Oakley,** and **M. O'Brien,** "Adoptive Placement of the Older Child," *Child Welfare*, 89, no. 8 (1970), 450–58.
30. **Chinn, Peggy,** *Child Health Maintenance*. St. Louis: The C. V. Mosby Company, 1974.
31. **Clark, Ann,** "The Beginning Family," *American Journal of Nursing*, 66, no. 4 (1966), 802–5.
32. **Clavan, Sylvia,** "Women's Liberation and the Family," in *Human Life Cycle*, ed. Wm. Sze. New York: Jason Aronson, Inc., 1975, pp. 532–40.
33. **Coleman, Arthur,** and **Libby Coleman,** *Pregnancy: The Psychological Experience*. New York: Herder and Herder, 1972.
34. **Coser, Rose,** ed., *The Family: Its Structure and Function*. New York: St. Martin's Press, Inc., 1966.
35. **Craig, Grace,** *Human Development*. Englewood Cliffs, NJ: Prentice-Hall, Inc., 1976.
36. **David, Miriam,** and **Elaine Doye,** "First Trimester of Pregnancy," *American Journal of Nursing*, 76, no. 12 (1976), 1945–48.
37. **Downs, Florence,** "Technological Advances and the Nurse-Family Relationships," *Nursing Digest*, 3, no 3 (1975), 22–24.
38. **Duberman, Lucille,** *The Reconstituted Family: A Study of Remarried Couples and Their Children*. Chicago: Nelson-Hall Publishers, 1975.
39. **DuBois, Don,** "Indications of an Unhealthy Relationship Between Parents and Premature Infant," *The Journal of Obstetric, Gynecologic, and Neonatal Nursing*, 4, no. 3 (1975), 21–24.
40. **Duvall, Evelyn,** *Family Development* (5th ed.). Philadelphia: J. B. Lippincott Company, 1977.
41. **Edwards, Margot,** "Unattended Home Birth," *American Journal of Nursing*, 73, no. 8 (1973), 1332–35.
42. **Edwards, M. P.,** and **F. E. Boyd,** "Adoption for Adolescents," *Child Welfare*, 54, no. 4 (1975), 298–99.
43. **Erikson, Erik,** *Childhood and Society* (2nd ed.). New York: W. W. Norton & Co., Inc., 1963.
44. **Fogg, Susan,** "New Views on Child Rearing Make Room for Daddy," *Washington Post–Sunday Sun Times*, November 30, 1980, p. 26.
45. **Fondiller, Shirley,** "Childbearing Center–New Approach to Maternal Care," *The American Nurse*, May 15, 1977, 9 ff.

46. **Fox, Tom,** "Tips on Making the Reunited Family Work," *St. Louis Globe-Democrat*, January 31, 1980, reprinted in *LTC Notes*: The Catholic Health Association, 11, no. 2 (1981), 2–3.
47. **Francke, Linda,** et al., "The Children of Divorce," *Newsweek*, February 11, 1980, pp. 58–63.
48. ____, and **Michael Reese,** "After Remarriage," *Newsweek*, February 11, 1980, p. 66.
49. **Friedman, Marilyn,** *Family Nursing: Theory and Assessment*. New York: Appleton-Century-Crofts, 1981.
50. **Gahman, Betsy,** *Twins: Twice the Trouble; Twice the Fun*. Philadelphia: J. B. Lippincott Company, 1965.
51. **Gordon, Thomas,** *Parent Effectiveness Training*. New York: Peter H. Wyden, Inc., 1970.
52. **Greenberg, Martin,** and **Norma Morris,** "Engrossment: The Newborn's Impact Upon the Father," *American Journal of Orthopsychiatry*, 44, no. 4 (1974), 520–31.
53. **Guerin, Philip,** *Family Therapy: Theory and Practice*. New York: Gardner Press, Inc., 1976.
54. **Haley, Jay,** *Problem-Solving Therapy*. San Francisco: Jossey-Bass, Inc., Publishers, 1976.
55. **Hallum, Jean,** "Nursing Implications," *Nursing Digest*, 4, no. 4 (1976), 58–59.
56. **Hammons, Chloe,** "The Adoptive Family," *American Journal of Nursing*, 76, no. 2 (1976), 251–57.
57. **Herman, Sonya,** "Divorce: A Grief Process," *Perspectives of Psychiatric Care*, 12, no. 3 (1974), 108–12.
58. **Hiemstra, Roger,** "Educating Parents in the Use of the Community," *Adult Leadership*, 23, no. 3 (1974), 85–88.
59. **Hoover, Dorothea,** "The Theory of the Interdependence of Family Members and Its Application in an Emotionally Disturbed Family," *ANA Clinical Sessions*. New York: Appleton-Century-Crofts, 1968, pp. 46-52.
60. **Horowitz, J.,** and **B. Perdue,** "Single Parent Families," *Nursing Clinics of North America*, 12, no. 3 (1977), 503–12.
61. **Hott, Jacqueline,** "The Crisis of Expectant Fatherhood," *American Journal of Nursing*, 76, no. 9 (1976), 1436–40.
62. **Hrobsky, Diane,** "Transition to Parenthood: A Balancing of Needs," *Nursing Clinics of North America*, 12, no. 3 (1977), 457–68.
63. **Hughes, Cynthia,** "An Eclectic Approach to Parent Group Education," *Nursing Clinics of North America*, 12, no. 3 (1977), 469–80.
64. **Hurlock, Elizabeth,** *Developmental Psychology* (4th ed.). New York: McGraw-Hill Book Company, 1975.
65. **Iffrig, Sr. Charitas,** "Body Image in Pregnancy: Its Relation to Nursing," *Nursing Clinics of North America*, 7, no. 4 (1974), 631–39.
66. **Irwin, Victoria,** "Family Life Can Be Center of Man's World, Too," *The Christian Science Monitor*, April 4, 1980.
67. **Kantor, David,** and **William Lehr,** *Inside the Family*. San Francisco: Jossey-Bass, Inc., Publishers, 1975.

68. **Kaseman, Charlotte,** "The Single-Parent Family," *Perspectives of Psychiatric Care*, 11, no. 3 (1974), 113–18.
69. **Kierman, Barbara,** and **Mary Scoloveno,** "Fathering," *Nursing Clinics of North America*, 12, no. 3 (1977), 481–90.
70. **Kimmel, Douglas,** *Adulthood and Aging*. New York: John Wiley & Sons, Inc., 1974.
71. **Kitzman, H.,** "The Nature of Well Child Care," *Nursing Clinics of North America*, 75, no. 10 (1975), 1705–8.
72. **Kraines, Judith,** "What Future for Homemaking?" *Graduate Woman*, 69, no. 4 (1981), 20–23.
73. **Kueck, Bruce,** "What's a Step-Parent to Do?" *St. Louis Globe-Democrat*, August 6–7, 1977, Sec. F, p. 1.
74. **LaFrancois, Guy,** *Of Children: An Introduction to Child Development*. Belmont, CA: Wadsworth Publishing Co., Inc., 1973.
75. **Lang, R.,** *The Birth Book*. Ben Lamond, CA: Genesis Press, 1972.
76. "LeBoyer's Babies," *Science News*, January 22, 1977.
77. **LeMasters, E. E.,** "Parenthood as Crisis," in *Crisis Intervention: Selected Readings*, ed. Howard Parad. New York: Family Service Association of America, 1972.
78. **Lidz, Theodore,** *The Person: His and Her Development Throughout the Life Cycle*. New York: Basic Books, Inc., 1976.
79. **Lindberg, George, C. Schrag,** and **O. Larsen,** *Sociology* (3rd ed.). New York: Harper & Row, Publishers, Inc., 1963.
80. **Lubic, Ruth,** "Developing Maternity Services Women Will Trust," *American Journal of Nursing*, 75, no. 10 (1975), 1685–88.
81. **Lynn, David,** *The Father: His Role in Child Development*. Monterey, CA: Brooks/Cole Publishing Company, 1974.
82. **McBride, Angela,** "Can Family Life Survive?" *American Journal of Nursing*, 75, no. 10 (1975), 1648–53.
83. **McEwan, Margaret T.,** "Readaption with a Minimum of Pain," *Social Casework*, 54, no. 6 (1973), 350–53.
84. **McHugh, Mary, Karen Dimitroff,** and **Nancy Davis,** "Family Support Group in a Burn Unit," *American Journal of Nursing*, 79, no. 12 (1979), 2148–50.
85. **McNamara, Joan,** *The Adoption Advisor*. New York: Hawthorn Books, Inc., 1975.
86. **Mead, Margaret,** "Anomalies in American Postdivorce Relationships," in *Divorce and After*, ed. P. Bohanan. New York: Doubleday & Co., Inc., 1970, pp. 97–112.
87. **Messer, Alfred,** *The Individual in His Family: An Adaptational Study*. Springfield, IL: Charles C Thomas, Publisher, 1970.
88. **Midelfort, C. F.,** "Ethnic and Religious Factors in Family Illnesses," *Bulletin of American Association of Social Psychiatry*, 1, no. 3 (1980), 16–21.
89. **Minuchin, Salvador,** *Families and Family Therapy*. Cambridge, MA: Harvard University Press, 1974.
90. **Murray, Ruth,** and **Judith Zentner,** *Nursing Assessment and Health Promotion through the Life Span* (3rd ed.). Englewood Cliffs, NJ: Prentice-Hall, Inc., 1985.
91. **Napier, Augustus,** and **Carl Whitaker,** *The Family Crucible*. New York: Harper & Row, Publishers, Inc., 1978.

92. **Neikson, J.,** "Placing Older Children in Adoptive Homes," *Children Today*, 1 (1972), 7–13.
93. **Nelson, Elof,** *Prime Time*. Owatonna, MN: Journal Chronicle Company, 1972.
94. **Newland, Kathleen,** "Who Is Mopping the Floor?" *Graduate Woman*, 70, no. 2 (1982), 20–22.
95. **Novak, Michael,** "The Family Out of Favor," *Eastern Review*, 1, no. 2 (1976), 42 ff.
96. **Obrzut, Lee,** "Expectant Father's Perceptions of Fathering," *American Journal of Nursing*, 76, no. 9 (1976), 1440–42.
97. **Otto, H. A.,** "Criteria for Assessing Family Strengths," *Canada's Mental Health*, 6 (1966), 257.
98. **Pannor, Reuben,** "The Forgotten Man," *Nursing Outlook*, 18, no. 11 (1970), 36–37.
99. **Parad, Howard,** and **Gerald Caplan,** "A Framework for Studying Families in Crisis," in *Crisis Intervention: Selected Readings*, ed. H. Parad. New York: Family Service Association, 1969.
100. **Payne, Patricia,** "Day Care and Its Impact on Parenting," *Nursing Clinics of North America*, 12, no. 3 (1977), 525–34.
101. **Perdue, B., J. Horowitz,** and **F. Herz,** "Mothering," *Nursing Clinics of North America*, 12, no. 3 (1977), 491–502.
102. **Queen, Stuart,** and **Robert Habenstein,** *The Family in Various Cultures* (4th ed.). Philadelphia: J. B. Lippincott Company, 1974.
103. **Rhodes, Sonya,** and **Joseleen Welson,** *Surviving Family Life*. New York: Putnam, 1981.
104. **Rising, Sharon,** "The Fourth Stage of Labor: Family Reintegration," *American Journal of Nursing*, 74, no. 5 (1974), 870 ff.
105. **Robbins, Margaret,** and **Thomas Schacht,** "Family Hierarchies," *American Journal of Nursing*, 82, no. 2 (1982), 284–86.
106. **Rondell, Florence,** and **Anne-Marie Murray,** *New Dimensions in Adoption*. New York: Crown Publishers, Inc., 1974.
107. **Rossi, Alice,** "Transition to Parenthood," *Journal of Marriage and Family*, 30 (1968), 26–39.
108. ———, "Transition to Parenthood," in *Human Life Cycle*, ed. Wm. Sze. New York: Jason Aronson, Inc., 1975, pp. 515–29.
109. **Rubin, Reva,** "Attainment of the Maternal Role, Part 1: Processes," *Nursing Research*, 16, no. 3 (1967), 237–45.
110. ———, "Attainment of the Maternal Role: Part II—Models and Referrants," *Nursing Research*, 16, no. 4 (1967), 342–46.
111. **Satir, Virginia,** *Conjoint Family Therapy* (2nd ed.). Palo Alto, CA: Science and Behavior Books, 1967.
112. ———, *Peoplemaking*. Palo Alto, CA: Science and Behavior Books, 1972.
113. ———, "Love, Understanding, Communication Are Vital Elements of Family Health," *Parameters*, 4, no. 3 (1979), 8–10.
114. ———, **James Stachowiak,** and **Harvey Taschmen,** *Helping Families to Change*. New York: Jason Aronson, Inc., 1975.
115. **Sawin, Margaret,** "Learning Through Family Clusters," *The Christian Home*, (December–February 1980–81), p. 10.
116. **Scheppler, Vincenette,** *The Adoption Dilemma: A Handbook for Adoptive Parents*. Rochester, NY: Arvin Publications, 1975.

117. **Schulman, Gertrude L.**, "Myths that Intrude on the Adaptation of the Stepfamily," *Social Casework*, 53, no. 3 (1972), 131–39.
118. **Schulz, David**, *The Changing Family*. Englewood Cliffs, NJ: Prentice-Hall, Inc., 1972.
119. **Sharron, Mary Lou**, "Some Helpful Techniques When Placing Older Children for Adoption," *Child Welfare*, 49, no. 8 (1970), 459–63.
120. **Shaw, Nancy**, "Teaching Young Mothers Their Role," *Nursing Outlook*, 22, no. 11 (1974), 695–98.
121. **Siegel, Earl**, and **Naomi Morris**, "Family Planning: Its Health Rationale," *American Journal of Obstetrics and Gynecology*, 118, no. 7 (1974), 995–1004.
122. **Sklar, Kathryn**, "Who Is Minding the Children?" *Graduate Woman*, 70, no. 2 (1982), 12–13.
123. **Skolnick, Arlene**, and **Jerome Skolnick**, *Family in Transition*. Boston: Little, Brown & Company, 1971.
124. **Smoyak, Shirley**, ed., *Psychiatric Nurse as Family Therapist*. New York: John Wiley & Sons, Inc., 1975.
125. **Souder, Fred**, *Individual and Family Therapy: Toward an Integration*. New York: Jason Aronson, Inc., 1979.
126. **Speer, David**, "Family Systems," in *Human Life Cycle*, ed. Wm. Sze. New York: Jason Aronson, Inc., 1975, pp. 437–93.
127. "Stepfamily Faces Many Problems," *Hickory Daily Record*, January 10, 1983, Sec. A, p. 10.
128. **Sussman, Marvin**, "Family Systems in the 1970's: Analysis, Policies, and Programs," in *Family Health Care*, eds. Debra Hymovich and Martha Barnard. New York: McGraw-Hill Book Company, 1973, pp. 18–37.
129. **Thistleton, Kristin**, "The Abusive and Neglectful Parent: Treatment Through Parent Education," *Nursing Clinics of North America*, 12, no. 3 (1977), 513–24.
130. **Toffler, Alvin**, *Future Shock*. New York: Random House, 1970.
131. **Toman, Walter**, "Birth Order Rules All," *Psychology Today*, 4, no. 7 (1974), 45 ff.
132. ———, *Family Constellation* (3rd ed.). New York: Springer Publishing Co., Inc., 1976.
133. **Tyson, Herb**, "Abuse in Family Remains Hidden," *St. Charles Journal*, April 1982.
134. **Vincent, Clark**, *The Family: Trends and Directions in the Seventies*. A speech to the Eleventh Annual Conference on Prevention and Community Mental Health, St. Louis, April 27, 1973.
135. **Visher, Emily**, and **John Visher**, *Step Families: A Guide to Working with Step Parents and Step Children*. New York: Bruner/Mazel, 1979.
136. **Winch, Robert**, "Permanence and Change in the History of the American Family and Some Speculations as to Its Future," *Journal of Marriage and the Family*, 1, no. 2 (1970), 8–16.
137. **Zimmer, Vanessa**, "Family Affair," *The Saturday Herald* (Dubois County, Indiana), April 12, 1980.

Index

A